Management of
Acute Myocardial Infarction

Frontiers in Cardiology

Series Advisors:

MICHEL BERTRAND
JOHN CAMM
DESMOND JULIAN
NORMAN KAPLAN
ULRICH SIGWART

Forthcoming titles:

Local Drug Delivery and Molecular Interventions
Edited by Elazer R. Edelman

Noninvasive Electrocardiology: Clinical Aspects of Holter Monitoring
Edited by Arthur J. Moss and Shlomo Stern

Management of
Acute Myocardial Infarction

Edited by

Desmond G. Julian
Emeritus Professor of Cardiology, University of Newcastle upon Tyne;
Formerly Director of the British Heart Foundation, London, UK

and

Eugene Braunwald
Hersey Professor of the Theory and Practice of Medicine,
Harvard Medical School; Chairman, Department of Medicine,
Brigham and Women's Hospital, Boston, USA

W. B. Saunders Company Ltd
London • Philadelphia • Toronto • Sydney • Tokyo

W. B. Saunders Company Ltd 24–28 Oval Road
London NW1 7DX

The Curtis Center
Independence Square West
Philadelphia, PA 19106-3399, USA

Harcourt Brace & Company
55 Horner Avenue
Toronto, Ontario M8Z 4X6, Canada

Harcourt Brace & Company, Australia
30–52 Smidmore Street
Marrickville, NSW 2204, Australia

Harcourt Brace & Company, Japan
Ichibancho Central Building, 22-1 Ichibancho
Chiyoda-ku, Tokyo 102, Japan

This book is printed on acid free paper

A catalogue for this book is available from the British Library

ISBN 0-7020-1884-8

Typeset by Paston Press Ltd, Loddon, Norfolk
Printed in Great Britain by The University Press, Cambridge

Contents

Contributors

Elliott M. Antman
Associate Professor of Medicine, Harvard Medical School; Director, Samuel A. Levine Cardiac Care Unit, Department of Medicine, Brigham and Women's Hospital, Boston, MA, USA

Eugene Braunwald
Hersey Professor of the Theory and Practice of Medicine, Harvard Medical School; Chairman, Department of Medicine, Brigham and Women's Hospital, Boston, MA, USA

Margarita T. Camacho
The Cleveland Clinic Foundation, Cleveland, OH, USA

Ronald W. F. Campbell
British Heart Foundation Professor of Cardiology, University of Newcastle-upon-Tyne, New Medical School, Newcastle upon Tyne; Honorary Consultant Cardiologist, Freeman Hospital, Newcastle upon Tyne, UK

Douglas A. Chamberlain
Consultant Cardiologist, Department of Cardiology, Royal Sussex County Hospital, Brighton, UK

Melvin D. Cheitlin
Professor of Medicine, University of California, San Francisco; Chief of Cardiology, San Francisco General Hospital, San Francisco, CA, USA

James H. Chesebro
Professor of Medicine and Associate Director of Research, Cardiac Unit, Harvard Medical School and Massachusetts General Hospital, Boston, MA, USA

Anthony C. De Franco
Section of Interventional Cardiology, The Cleveland Clinic Foundation, Cleveland, OH, USA

Michael E. Farkouh
Assistant Professor, Division of Area Medicine, Mayo Clinic, Rochester, MN, USA

Vincent Figueredo
Assistant Professor of Medicine, University of California, San Francisco; Cardiology Division, San Francisco General Hospital, San Francisco, CA, USA

Marcus D. Flather
Senior Research Fellow, Division of Cardiology, McMaster University, Hamilton, Ontario, Canada

Richard Gorlin
Dr George Baehr Professor of Clinical Medicine, Senior Vice President, The Mount Sinai Medical Center, New York, NY, USA

Judith S. Hochman
Associate Professor of Clinical Medicine, College of Physicians and Surgeons, Columbia University, Director, Cardiac Care Unit, St Luke's Roosevelt Hospital Center, New York, NY, USA

Desmond G. Julian
Emeritus Professor of Cardiology, University of Newcastle upon Tyne; Formerly Director, British Heart Foundation, London, UK

J. Ward Kennedy
Robert A. Bruce Professor of Medicine; Director, Division of Cardiology, University of Washington School of Medicine, Seattle, WA, USA

Charles B. Kim
Cardiology Fellow, Stanford University Medical Center, Palo Alto, CA, USA

Henri E. Kulbertus
Chief of Cardiology, Professor of Medicine, University of Liège, Liège, Belgium

Thierry LeJemtel
Professor of Medicine, Albert Einstein College of Medicine, Bronx, NY, USA

Floyd D. Loop
The Cleveland Clinic Foundation, Cleveland, OH, USA

Gary V. Martin
Associate Professor of Medicine, University of Washington, Division of Cardiology, Veterans Affairs Medical Center, Seattle, WA, USA

Beat J. Meyer
Research Fellow in Cardiology, Cardiac Unit, Harvard Medical School and Massachusetts General Hospital, Boston, MA, USA

Derek D. Muehrcke
The Cleveland Clinic Foundation, Cleveland, OH 44195, USA

Luc A. Piérard
Director, Cardiac Care Unit and Cardiac Rehabilitation Unit, Division of Cardiology, University of Liège, Liège, Belgium

Bertram Pitt
Division of Cardiology, Department of Internal Medicine, University of Michigan Medical Center, Ann Arbor, MI, USA

Eric J. Topol
Chairman, Department of Cardiology; Director, The Center for Thrombosis and Vascular Biology; Professor of Medicine, The Ohio State University School of Medicine, Cleveland Clinic Foundation, Cleveland, OH, USA

Richard Vincent
Consultant Cardiologist and Professor of Medical Science, Department of Cardiology, Royal Sussex County Hospital, Brighton, UK

Lars Wilhelmsen
Department of Medicine, Östra Hospital, Göteborg, Sweden

Salim Yusuf
Director, Division of Cardiology, McMaster University, Hamilton, Ontario, Canada

Preface

Acute myocardial infarction may be considered the quintessential illness of the twentieth century. During the first decade of the century, acute coronary occlusion was considered to be immediately and invariably fatal. In the second decade, it became clear that some patients with coronary thrombosis and resultant myocardial infarction lived to reach the hospital and, indeed, to survive the event. For the next 30 years, the recorded incidence of acute myocardial infarction grew by alarming proportions and by mid-century this condition was recognized as the most common cause of in-hospital death in the industrialized world. Moreover, among survivors, the risk to life and well-being remained high, particularly during the first year following the event. Medical therapy, which consisted of analgesia, bed rest and sedation, had little to offer.

Commencing in the 1960s, however, the tide began to turn. The appreciation of the frequency of sudden death as the terminating event, the development of electrocardiographic monitoring techniques, the availability of new, potent antiarrhythmics and of external cardioverter–defibrillators rapidly led to the establishment of coronary care units in almost all acute-care hospitals. This was rewarded by a decisive reduction of in-hospital mortality secondary to electrical instability.

By the late 1960s, a second major complication of infarction, left ventricular failure secondary to necrosis of large quantities of myocardium, became the major cause of in-hospital death. Efforts were made to reduce the extent of ventricular injury by improving the balance between oxygen supply and demand of the jeopardized heart muscle. A major advance in the field occurred in 1980 with the development of coronary thrombolytic therapy, at first with the drugs administered directly into the culprit coronary artery, and then intravenously. Later in the 1980s, attention focused on ancillary therapy, such as anticoagulants and antiplatelet drugs to enhance the effectiveness of thrombolytic agents and of angiotensin-converting enzyme inhibitors to prevent postinfarct remodeling, often a prelude to late heart failure and death.

During the first half of this, the last decade of the century, there has been a veritable explosion of new information that has altered our understanding of the pathophysiology and treatment of myocardial infarction, both during the acute event and subsequently as well. Based on many carefully designed multicenter trials, virtually every aspect of the management of this condition has undergone intense scrutiny and, in many instances, firm numbers have replaced clinical impressions.

Our goal in preparing *Management of Acute Myocardial Infarction* was to capture the considerable body of information that has recently become available, much of it in the last

I

year or two. All important aspects of the management of the patient with acute myocardial infarction are considered – from pre-hospital care, through medical and mechanical therapy, to postinfarction risk stratification and post-hospital care. We have made every effort to include the most recent information, some of it presented at medical meetings but not yet previously published.

We hope that this book will be useful to all physicians – specialists and generalists – responsible for the care of patients with acute myocardial infarction, as well as to clinical investigators and other serious students of this condition.

We wish to express our appreciation to our talented authors, all respected authorities in their fields, who adhered to a very tight production schedule. The rapid production of the book also required the guidance and effective leadership of our editors Gill Robinson and Tracy Breakell of W. B. Saunders Company Ltd.

DESMOND JULIAN, MD
London

EUGENE BRAUNWALD, MD
Boston

1

Pre-hospital Management

R. Vincent

The management of acute myocardial infarction remains centred on the provision of effective care in hospital. But for the majority of patients the most uncomfortable, turbulent, and dangerous phase of their illness occurs *before* hospital admission.

The extreme vulnerability of patients early in their attack has been known for over 20 years; yet implementing optimum strategies for pre-hospital management has been both slow and patchy. A new impetus has arisen from our recent appreciation that, following coronary occlusion, the beneficial effects of thrombolysis diminish rapidly with time. Minimizing delay to treatment has become a renewed goal and with it a fresh emphasis on pre-hospital care.

In this chapter I will review the rationale, principles, practicalities, and achievements to date of schemes to provide in the community all that the patient needs at this early stage to preserve life and to limit myocardial damage.

Rationale

Acute myocardial infarction poses an immediate threat to life and to the functional reserve of the heart. Studies of natural history and pathology attest to the early instability and the high initial risk of the patient with an evolving infarct. More recently, large-scale trials of thrombolytic therapy have emphasized the value of treatment within the first few hours of major symptoms. These three strands – natural history, pathology and the results of early treatment – provide the rationale for schemes of pre-hospital care.

Natural History

Community studies in the USA and in Europe provide a concordant view that over half of patients dying from acute myocardial infarction do so within the first hour of their illness.[1–6] The majority of deaths are attributable to early ventricular fibrillation, though electromechanical dissociation often due to myocardial rupture is also a prominent cause, particularly in the elderly. The high incidence of ventricular fibrillation within this period is confirmed by studies of patients observed within 1 hour of the onset of major symptoms[7] (Figure 1.1).

These observations illustrate graphically the need for resuscitation facilities as an essential component of early care. They led over 20 years ago to the introduction of coronary care ambulances staffed either by a full medical team[5] or by specially trained ambulance paramedics.[8–10] Subsequently, the value of community-based resuscitation

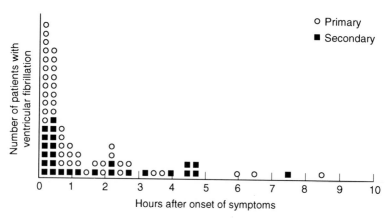

Figure 1.1   Incidence of ventricular fibrillation in 500 patients with myocardial infarction observed within 1 hour of onset of symptoms. (Reproduced with permission from Ref. 8.)

has become well attested, not only for victims of myocardial ischemia, but for a variety of other life-threatening conditions.[11,12]

Pathology

The initiating event for nearly all cases of acute myocardial infarction is the abrupt instability of an atheromatous plaque in an epicardial coronary artery.[13] Fissuring of the overlying fibrous capsule renders the plaque unstable, and a sudden increase in coronary narrowing occurs through several mechanisms: platelet adhesion, fibrin clot formation, enlargement of the atheromatous plaque by intraplaque hemorrhage, abnormal vaso-constriction, and adventitial inflammation (Figure 1.2). The process is dynamic – fluctuation and progression of the occlusion are common.

With the passage of time the composition of the occlusive clot alters. Increasing fibrin deposition and cross-linking extend and stabilize the coronary thrombosis providing

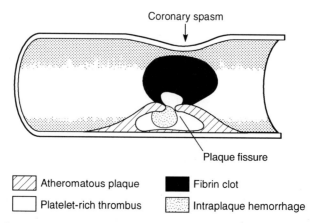

Figure 1.2   Mechanisms causing coronary occlusion that commonly provoke acute myocardial infarction. (Reproduced with permission from Ref. 14.)

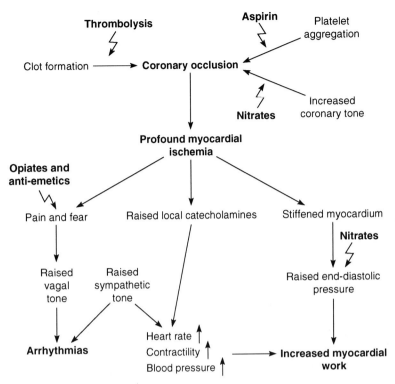

Figure 1.3 Mechanisms in the pathogenesis of acute myocardial infarction illustrating the 'vicious circle' of changes in ventricular muscle and potential sites for therapy.

increasing resistance to the action of thrombolytic drugs and further threatening the myocardium.

In the muscle served by the occluded artery, a rapid adverse change takes place in the metabolic-dependent processes of contraction and relaxation. There is a profound alteration of the extracellular milieu together with cellular swelling, calcium influx and a release of local catecholamines.[15–18] Autonomic imbalance triggered by the ischemic process,[19] and by the pain and distress that results, adds to the instability and progression of the infarction zone. The vicious circle that these changes engender is illustrated in Figure 1.3, together with potential therapeutic interventions likely to halt the downward spiral of myocardial cell death and worsening left ventricular function. Knowledge of these pathogenetic mechanisms gives strong theoretic reasons to suggest that the efficacy of these agents will be enhanced by their use as early as possible after the onset of the attack.

Results of Early Therapy

Thrombolysis

From the outset, experimental models of thrombolytic therapy have predicted maximum benefit from its use as soon as possible after thrombotic coronary occlusion[20] (Figure 1.4). The first major clinical trials to demonstrate the efficacy of thrombolysis for acute myocardial infarction supported these experimental observations. GISSI-1 showed an

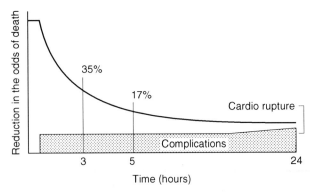

Figure 1.4   Time dependence of benefit and complications of thrombolytic therapy in acute myocardial infarction as shown in an experimental model. (From Ref. 20.)

18% reduction in overall mortality in patients treated with streptokinase compared with placebo;[21] but this figure was increased to 23% for those treated within 3 hours, and to a striking 47% for those receiving streptokinase within the first hour. Benefit was persistent for at least 1 year.

The unique 1-hour data of the GISSI-1 study merits cautious interpretation but other trials have shown a similar if less dramatic trend. The ISIS-2 study showed a more gradual gradient of effect with time: a 53% (13.1 to 6.4%) reduction in mortality from treatment within the first 4 hours compared with a 33% (13.3 to 9.2%) reduction in mortality for therapy given between 4 and 24 hours.[22] Other trials have shown different degrees of time-dependent benefit, but the message remains clear from cumulative data in 58 600 patients that delay to therapy profoundly limits the survival advantage of thrombolysis[23] (Figure 1.5).

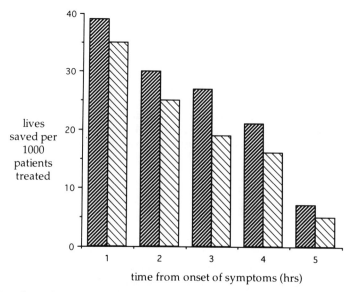

Figure 1.5   Time dependence of the benefit from thrombolytic therapy. ▨, ST elevation or BBB; ▨, all patients. (Data from Ref. 23.)

Finally, early thrombolytic therapy favors not only a decreased early and late mortality, but better arterial patency, enhanced reperfusion and improved left ventricular function.[24–31] Maximum benefit from intravenous thrombolysis appears to be obtained when treatment is given within 2 hours of symptom onset.

Aspirin

Aspirin without thrombolytic therapy is of undoubted benefit in the management of acute myocardial infarction. The ISIS-2 trial recorded a reduction in early mortality of 23% compared with placebo. The mechanism of action of aspirin is unclear, but is likely to be chiefly through the prevention of reocclusion.[32–36]

In contrast to thrombolytic agents, no noticeable time-dependent effect was observed over the 24 hours during which therapy was initiated. However, time dependence of maximum benefit in ISIS-2 was recorded for treatment with a *combination* of streptokinase and aspirin, and data have been reported that aspirin and thrombolytic therapy have a synergistic effect.[37]

Other agents

No data exist to support the concept that benefit from other accepted therapies for acute myocardial infarction diminish with time. Damage limitation seems most likely, however, if their effect can be utilized while the coronary and myocardial pathology are at their most unstable (Figure 1.3).

Time Delays in the Early Management of Acute Myocardial Infarction

Figure 1.6 illustrates a time-line of steps that are the usual experience of patients in the community who sustain a symptomatic myocardial infarction. I will look briefly at each in turn.

Patient Delay

The longest component of pre-hospital delay is determined by the patient. *Median* delays from symptom onset to reaching a decision to call for help have been reported variously as 27, 40, 45, 52, 60, 63, 66, 80, 90, 126 and 300 min,[31,38–44] but the distribution is skewed and there is wide individual variation (15 min to 60 hours).

An early decision to seek help appears to be associated with the severity of the infarction (though not necessarily the severity of pain), a high somatic awareness, and

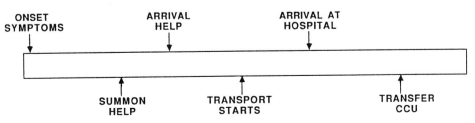

Figure 1.6 Steps on the time-line of care applicable to most patients with a heart attack starting in the community.

developing symptoms away from home. In contrast, female gender and advanced age seem to lengthen delay.[43,45,46] Patients calling their general practitioner take longer to initiate a call than those who summon an ambulance – a median of 70 min versus 40 min in the 1531 patients observed by Birkhead.[39] Patients included in trials of pre-hospital care seem often to have shorter delays to calling for help than those serviced by more conventional systems.[38]

Delay to the Arrival of Medical Help

The time for medical assistance to reach the patient with suspected acute myocardial infarction depends extensively on variations in geography and the local systems available for first response. General practitioners can respond rapidly; a median time of 20 min was noted in an observational study[39] of 886 patients in six UK towns, though this delay is likely to be longer during the period 08.00 to 12.00. Even shorter delays have been reported where there is a special interest in pre-hospital coronary care.[31,47] In a recent study[48] of common UK practice the median time from onset of symptoms to arrival of the general practitioner was 90–100 min. The response time of the general practitioner in this series was calculated to be in the order of 20–30 min.

The response time of ambulances, particularly in urban communities, is likely to be quicker, though this is not inevitable. In the 16 countries participating in the European Myocardial Infarction Project,[42] calls for help in the first 2027 patients resulted in an attendance by the mobile coronary care unit with a median delay of 20 min. In the UK, ambulances attending emergency (999) calls are able to reach patients in densely populated areas in under 10 min. In rural settings delays may be considerably longer, though it is also observed that patients in rural areas are less likely to summon an ambulance than their general practitioner.[39]

Treatment on Site and Overall Delay to Hospital Arrival

Extended treatment on first contact with the patient threatens to increase delay before hospital admission. In trials of pre-hospital thrombolysis (pp. 94–95), median times occupying this phase of treatment have been recorded as 30–50 min. To avoid this delay a 'scoop-and-run' policy may seem preferable; but perceptions of the speed of this time-saving strategy may be over optimistic. In the Cincinnati Heart Project paramedic chiefs servicing 12 acute hospitals perceived the scoop-and-run system to take 28 min from activation of the ambulance system to arrival at hospital. In both retrospective and prospective studies of patients with acute myocardial infarction attended by paramedic crews this figure in practice exceeded 40 min.[49,50] Recording an ECG on site does not appear to significantly extend the pre-hospital period.[51,52]

Cumulative delays to hospital admission therefore reflect the combined effect of the response of both patients and healthcare professionals to the symptoms of a suspected infarct, features of local geography, and the available facilities for pre-hospital care. In the UK, patients who choose to seek help from their general practitioner take a median time to reach hospital of about 90 min whereas those who call an ambulance without being seen first by a doctor arrive more quickly in a median of 41 min.[39]

Delays in Hospital

It is now well recognized that the delay to thrombolytic therapy after arrival in hospital is often substantial.[39,49,53–55] Patients transferred from an emergency department to a cardiac care unit before receiving thrombolytic agents experience greatest delay (a median of 85–120 min); those who receive thrombolysis after direct admission to a cardiac care unit fare better,[56] and those whose thrombolysis is given in the emergency department itself have the shortest recorded delays to treatment (15–30 min).[39,57–60]

In-hospital delays are an important component of the overall time to therapy and deserve further attention (pp. 22–23); but note that comprehensive pre-hospital care (including thrombolysis) will appear to be of greater advantage when in-hospital treatment is *delayed* than when it is prompt.

Strategies for Pre-hospital Care

Minimizing delay to therapy whilst retaining a high level of patient safety is the principal goal of strategies for pre-hospital care. More than 17 schemes involving mobile coronary care units, paramedics, or primary care physicians have been reported in studies that encompass a variety of locations, populations, and protocols for diagnosis and treatment.[31,38,40–42,48,51,61–92] This section will deal with the main principles of such schemes, followed by a review of their practical achievements.

Reducing Patient Delay

Strategies for reducing patient delay have been singularly disappointing. Mass public education has made little impact on the patient's response to ischemic pain, but has increased the number of patients seeking help for pain of a non-cardiac origin. Delay times to calling help for acute myocardial infarction have shown either no improvement or only transient benefit.[93,94] Up to 30% of patients presenting with acute myocardial infarction are already known to have coronary disease. These patients and their relatives might reasonably be targeted for advice on emergency life support and in the correct response to coronary pain at rest. But it is also a group in whom denial of the significance of cardiac symptoms seems stronger than average resulting in longer delays to summon help than in those whose ischemic pain is new.

Schemes for Delivering Pre-hospital Care

Schemes that have been explored for delivering pre-hospital coronary care comprise: (1) physician-manned mobile coronary care units (MCCUs); (2) initial attendance by a physician or general practitioner prior to calling for ambulance assistance; (3) paramedic evaluation with a radio link to the base hospital; (4) paramedic attendance with no immediate link for medical review.

Physician-manned MCCUs

A physician-manned coronary care unit provides comprehensive care combining a high level of medical expertise including ECG interpretation, familiarity with emergency conditions, facilities for advanced life support, and the availability of a wide range of drugs including opioids for pain relief and thrombolytic agents. Transport can be rapid, yet with such a thorough system of care there is usually little need to return to the base hospital with any speed.

The major drawback is cost and availability. MCCUs are predominantly a feature of European patterns of healthcare. They also occur in Canada, but not in the USA. In the UK, MCCUs operate only in Northern Ireland.

Physician evaluation with later ambulance attendance

In this system several advantages of the physician-manned MCCU are retained, but with important caveats. The attending physician will have greater medical expertise than paramedics alone in patient evaluation and may already know the medical and social background of the patient attended. But in practice, for any one family practitioner, attending to a patient with acute myocardial infarction will be a relatively uncommon experience – one to four cases per year in the UK.

The experience of a non-specialist physician in ECG interpretation may be limited; recognition of an unequivocal infarct pattern may be secure, but more subtle hyperacute changes, or patterns of bundle branch block, may be less well recognized. Training and facilities in general practice for defibrillation and other elements of advanced life support are uncommon, though they are being adopted more widely and where used have been highly successful.

The attendance of a physician allows early pain relief by intravenous opiates with antiemetics, as well as refined judgment in the use of aspirin and nitrates where appropriate. The use of these accepted agents in the community management of acute myocardial infarction, however, is still suboptimal;[95] and the routine administration of thrombolytic therapy for pre-hospital treatment by nonspecialist physicians, though not discouraged, has so far proved rare.[96]

Paramedic evaluation with telephone link to the base hospital

Many countries including the USA and (increasingly) mainland UK rely on emergency systems staffed by paramedic ambulance crews. Paramedics are familiar with life-threatening emergencies, including acute cardiac ischemic syndromes, and are skilled and equipped for full advanced emergency life support. Their skills at interpreting cardiac arrhythmias may be high and may be supplemented by single lead telemetry to the base hospital. The advent of reliable cellular ECG transmission has led to improved diagnostic accuracy of myocardial infarction in the field and with the possibility for remote, physician-directed administration of thrombolytic agents.

However, paramedics are limited in the range of therapies available to them for the relief of pain and nausea. Inhaled nitrous oxide appears helpful, but is not in common use. Experience with the nonaddictive opiate agent, nalbuphine, is also limited, but may offer a safe and effective alternative to diamorphine or morphine for use by paramedics.[97]

Paramedic with no hospital link

This group differs from those with access to hospital telemetry only in that no physician support is immediately available to support the diagnosis of myocardial infarction or to direct the administration of thrombolytic or other therapy. Experience with specially trained paramedics supported by on-site interpretative/computerized ECGs has been encouraging and paramedics can undoubtedly develop high levels of expertise in ECG interpretation.

Further to ensure an accurate evaluation of patients for thrombolytic therapy, at least two studies[51,87] have reported the use of check-lists to confirm the presence of adequate indications and the absence of contraindications to the use of thrombolysis in the prehospital phase (Figure 1.7).

Ambulance Thrombolysis Study

	Tick for yes
1. Can you confirm that the patient is not a woman of child-bearing age?	☐
2. Is the patient aged 70 or less?	☐
3. Is the patient conscious and coherent?	☐
4. Has the patient had symptoms characteristic of a coronary heart attack? (i.e. pain in a typical distribution of 20 min duration or more?)	☐
5. Did the continuous symptoms start less then 6 hours ago?	☐
6. Does the electrocardiogram show abnormal ST segment elevation of 2 mm or more (0.08 s after J point) in at least two standard leads or at least two precordial leads? Remember ST elevation can sometimes be normal in V1 and V2.	☐
7. Is the QRS width 0.14 mm or less, and is bundle branch block absent from the tracing?	☐
8. Can you confirm that there is no atrioventricular block greater than first degree?	☐
9. Did the pain build up over seconds and minutes rather than starting totally abruptly?	☐
10. Can you confirm that breathing does not influence the severity of the pain?	☐
11. Can you confirm that the patient has not been treated for a peptic ulcer within the last 12 months?	☐
12. Can you confirm that the patient has not had a stroke of any sort within the last 12 months and no permanent disability from a previous stroke?	☐
13. Can you confirm that the patient has no diagnosed bleeding tendency and has had no recent blood loss?	☐
14. Can you confirm that the patient has not had any surgical operation (including tooth extractions) within the last 6 months?	☐
15. Can you confirm definitely that APSAC/streptokinase has not been given within the last 6 months?	☐
16. Can you confirm that the heart rate is between 50 and 140?	☐
17. Can you confirm that the patient is not on warfarin?	☐
18. Can you confirm that the systolic blood pressure is over 80 mmHg?	☐

Figure 1.7 A check-list used in the Brighton Study of the feasibility of paramedics giving thrombolytic therapy without prior contact with the hospital base.

Studies in Pre-hospital Care

The Prethrombolytic Era

In the prethrombolytic era, studies in the pre-hospital management of acute myocardial infarction focused on the provision of oxygen, pain relief, and facilities for resuscitation. Effective schemes were reported based on mobile coronary care units, paramedic systems, and primary care physicians. Successful resuscitation from ventricular fibrillation was achieved in an important number of cases together with the worthwhile management of other threatening arrhythmias with atropine, lignocaine, and adrenaline.

The introduction in the late 1970s of well-drilled rapid response teams equipped with defibrillators and other measures for advanced life support demonstrated that long-term worthwhile survival from out-of-hospital cardiac arrest could be achieved particularly for patients with primary ventricular fibrillation attended rapidly. The provision of basic life support within 4–5 min and advanced life support (notably defibrillation) within 8–10 min has been shown to result in a rate of survival of over 40% of patients in this category.[98,99] Hospital discharge rates for such patients in centers with a pioneering interest in community resuscitation are maintained at 25–30% although in many other places these rates are substantially lower.[100]

Achieving this degree of continuing success – and a success in patient rescue from other life-threatening conditions – has depended on highly organized response schemes, mostly though not uniquely in urban areas, a level of bystander intervention that can usually be implemented only as a result of widespread public education[101] and the development of agreed resuscitation protocols that encompass the best available knowledge on life support techniques.[102,103] That many localities achieve success rates substantially lower than those quoted is a call to improve facilities and education for implementing each of the steps of the 'chain of survival'[104] particularly for patients at risk of ventricular fibrillation due to profound myocardial ischemia. At least 5% of victims of myocardial infarction develop cardiac arrest in the presence of the attending medical or paramedic staff; and the majority of these patients (80%) will have ventricular tachycardia or ventricular fibrillation.[105]

Resuscitation may have little impact on the overall community mortality from coronary disease, but its value to individual patients and their families is dramatic. The provision of adequate resuscitation facilities in the early management of acute myocardial infarction cannot be overemphasized.

The Thrombolytic Era

With the appreciation of the time-dependent benefit of thrombolysis came a number of investigations of the feasibility, safety, and clinical value of pre-hospital administration using the approaches outlined above. Table 1.1 lists the observations from several of these early trials, many of which were based only on small numbers of patients. In general, confirmation of the feasibility and safety of pre-hospital thrombolysis was obtained, but with a variable experience of additional patient benefit.

More recently, four studies have been published that extend these early observations: the Myocardial Infarction Triage and Intervention Trial, the European Myocardial Infarction Project, the Grampian Region Early Anistreplase Trial, and the UK Royal College of General Practitioners Post-Marketing Surveillance Study.

Myocardial Infarction Triage and Intervention Trial (MITI)

The MITI study[38,51] was based on a paramedic service using cellular transmission of the 12-lead ECG to the base hospital. A total of 19 hospitals participated enrolling 360 patients of the 8863 screened during the 3-year study period. Diagnostic accuracy was high (98%) though this was achieved by additional training of the paramedics, the use of 12-lead interpretative ECG, a screening checklist, and immediate physician review by telephone link of both clinical and electrocardiographic data.

Therapy with aspirin 325 mg and alteplase (rt-PA) 100 mg over 3 hours was administered in an open but randomized manner either in the pre-hospital phase (175 patients) or on arrival at hospital (185 patients). The primary endpoint was a composite score of death/serious bleeding and infarct size.

The median interval between pre-hospital and in-hospital injections – representing the time saved by pre-hospital administration – was 33 min. Ten deaths occurred in the pre-hospital group and 15 in the hospital-treated group giving a mortality reduction ratio of

Table 1.1 Observations from early, small (<200 patients) studies in pre-hospital coronary care

Reference	Thrombolytic agent	System	Observations
Koren et al.[28]	SK	MCCU	Improved LV function (EF 56% vs 47%) for patients with treatment ≤1.5 hours
Fine et al.[62]	SK	MCCU	Improved LV function and QRS score for anterior infarcts when treatment given <2 hours
Mathey et al.[61]	U	MCCU	Smaller anterior infarcts <3.5 hours
Applebaum et al.[63]	SK	MCCU	Delay shortened 30–60 min 'safe and feasible'
Weiss et al.[65]	SK	MCCU	Smaller infarcts and better residual myocardial function
Roth et al.[77]	rt-PA	MCCU	No difference in infarct size, LV function or arterial patency or 60 day mortality
Barbash et al.[78]	rt-PA	MCCU	No difference in arterial patency or LV function between 0–2 hour and 2–4 hour groups but short- and long-term survival significantly improved with earlier therapy
Castaigne et al.[72]	Ani	MCCU	No objective clinical benefit. No increased adverse effects. No additional pre-hospital delay giving thrombolysis
TEAHAT[85]	rt-PA	MCCU	Safety and feasibility of pre-hospital thrombolysis confirmed
Bippus et al.[69]	SK	MCCU	Safety and feasibility of pre-hospital thrombolysis confirmed
Linderer et al.[80]	Ani	MCCU	30% reduction in infarct size when treatment started within 90 min of symptom onset
Purvis et al.[82]	rt-PA	MCCU	90% patency when measured 90 min after thrombolysis
Bossaert et al.[67]	Ani	Ph+MCCU	Safe and feasible, time saved 46–53 min
Castaigne et al.[64]	Ani	Ph+MCCU	Safe and feasible: time saved 60 min
McKendall et al.[81]	Front-loaded rt-PA	Para	Paramedics successfully diagnosed six eligible patients for thrombolysis
Karagounis et al.[52]	–	Para	Pre-hospital ECG speeded in-hospital treatment. (No thrombolytic therapy given.)
Gallagher et al.[89]	U	Para	Paramedic diagnosis of myocardial infarction without telemetry and the use of pre-hospital urokinase was feasible and accurate

Ani, anistreplase; EF, ejection fraction; LV, left ventricle; MCCU, mobile coronary care unit; Para, paramedics; Ph, physician; rt-PA, tissue plasminogen activator; SK, streptokinase; U, urokinase.

0.69 that was nonsignificant. Moreover, the pre-hospital group showed no significant improvement in the composite score, ejection fraction, or infarct size. Secondary analysis, however, did indicate that where treatment was initiated early – within 70 min of symptom onset and whether before or after hospital admission – outcome (composite score, mortality, infarct size) was improved.

European Myocardial Infarction Project (EMIP)

The EMIP study,[41,42] based on physician-manned MCCUs, was conducted at 163 centers in 15 European countries and Canada. It formed a double-blind study in patients seen within 6 hours of the onset of symptoms who had a qualifying 12-lead ECG. Patients were assigned to receive randomly either anistreplase before admission followed by placebo in hospital (the pre-hospital group), or placebo at home followed by anistreplase after hospital arrival. A total of 2750 patients received pre-hospital thrombolytic therapy compared with 2719 patients whose thrombolysis was delayed until admission. The time saved by pre-hospital treatment was a median of 55 min.

The all-cause mortality at 30 days (the primary endpoint of the trial) was reduced in the pre-hospital group by 13% (9.7% vs 11.1%), but this figure failed to reach statistical significance ($P = 0.08$). Deaths from *cardiac* causes, however, were significantly less frequent in the pre-hospital group than those treated after hospital arrival (8.3% vs 5.8%, a 16% reduction; $P = 0.049$).

The majority of patients in this study were entered on the basis of history together with ST segment *elevation* of at least 1 mm in two limb leads, 2 mm in at least two precordial leads, or both (87%). A small proportion were entered on the basis of history together with an ECG that was abnormal but without typical ST segment elevation. In contrast with most other studies no difference in overall 30-day mortality was observed between those with and those without ST segment elevation.

Diagnostic accuracy in the study was high (87.8%), and the complication rate low. The expected adverse effects of thrombolysis were the same in both groups though their *timing* – particularly ventricular fibrillation and symptomatic hypotension – was clearly related to the administration of therapy. These complications were therefore more commonly seen in the pre-hospital phase in those receiving active therapy rather than placebo at home. A similar trend was seen for patients receiving thrombolytic therapy in hospital so that, overall, no difference in the incidence of these complications was recorded between the two groups.

The EMiP trial confirmed the safety and feasibility of administering pre-hospital thrombolysis in an MCCU system, but the mortality benefit was not at all prominent for the group as a whole. A subsequent analysis of deaths according to improvement in pre-hospital delay, though not a predefined endpoint, showed that patients who received anistreplase more than 90 min earlier by pre-hospital use did have a significant mortality reduction (19/261 compared with 29/217; relative risk reduction: 0.58; $P = 0.047$).

Grampian Region Early Anistreplase Trial (GREAT)

This study[31] was conducted amongst general practitioners in Scotland serving 29 rural practices in Grampian Region. The admitting hospital at Aberdeen was on average 36 miles away from the scene of the infarct. Five of the practices had previously taken part in a study of the use of defibrillators in the community.

Three hundred and eleven patients suspected on a history of at least 20 min of chest pain were entered into a randomized double-blind trial of intravenous anistreplase versus placebo given either at home or at hospital. It is noteworthy that although the general practitioners were required to record an ECG, interpretation was unnecessary for trial entry. Another important constraint was that patients were entered only if it were judged possible for them to be seen in hospital within 6 hours of the onset of symptoms, so that all could receive thrombolytic therapy within this 6-hour period. Accepted contraindications for thrombolysis were applied, and as in the EMiP trial, all other concomitant therapies were allowed according to the usual practice of the practitioners involved (253 cases (81%) received opiates and 261 cases (84%) received aspirin as part of their early therapy).

The trial was designed to assess the feasibility, safety, and efficacy of domiciliary thrombolysis; at the outset, no significant mortality reduction was expected because of the small numbers of patients involved.

The final diagnostic accuracy for acute myocardial infarction was 78%, though in only 3/311 cases (1%) did the admitting hospital doctor make an alternative initial diagnosis to the general practitioner.

The outcome of the study is illustrated in Figure 1.8. The time saving of 130 min in the delay to thrombolytic therapy by pre-hospital use was associated with a surprising 49% reduction in mortality at 3 months and an important improvement in left ventricular function. This benefit was sustained to 1 year from trial entry at which time the mortality

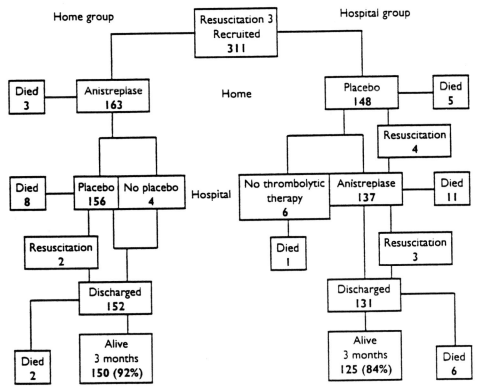

Figure 1.8 The results of the GREAT study.

in the pre-hospital group was 10.4% compared with 21.6% in the hospital group, a 52% relative reduction.[92] Though apparently encouraging these beneficial findings need cautious application to a general population of infarct patients. Patients were preselected as a group that would inevitably receive thrombolysis very early in the course of their illness; the number of patients considered for the trial but rejected because of inappropriate timing is unstated; time saving was substantial because of the rural setting of the study; and close involvement of the trial organizers seemed an essential component of the study to ensure adequate recruitment. Moreover, a mortality analysis, or the timing at which one might be made, was not a predetermined endpoint of the study.

UK Royal College of General Practitioners Post-marketing Surveillance Study (RCGP Study)

This study[48] differed from a conventional clinical trial. It sought to observe rather than influence the practice of doctors in their community management of acute myocardial infarction. In the face of the UK product licence allowing *any* practitioner to use thrombolytic therapy, the Royal College of Physicians was interested to know the manner in which practitioners adopted this new form of therapy. A total of 1339 doctors volunteered to participate in the study and expressed a wish to use anistreplase as an intravenous bolus in the management of their infarct patients. In the event, just 344 of these practitioners became actively involved in the trial. The opportunity was taken also to include a separate group of general practitioners who did not wish to use anistreplase but were prepared to record for comparison their early management of acute infarcts (2237 doctors volunteered of whom 776 became active). Over a 20-month period the two groups attended a total of 888 patients and 2495 patients respectively. Of patients treated in the anistreplase 'user group', only 310 received active therapy.

The interval between onset of symptoms and the doctor's arrival was a median of 90 min for the user group and 100 min for the 'comparison' group. The administration of anistreplase at home increased the interval between the doctor's arrival and transfer to hospital by about 15 min from a median of 30 min for those not receiving thrombolytic therapy. Just over half the patients in each group were seen within 2 hours of the onset of symptoms. Most of the patients seen in the study (93%) were transferred to hospital where in 198 patients (64%) given anistreplase in the community the diagnosis of myocardial infarction was subsequently confirmed by standard criteria. Another 17 patients (5%) were thought to have a probable or possible myocardial infarction. Ultimately, 13 patients (4%) given anistreplase in the community were thought to have non-cardiac conditions.

It was observed that patients in the user group *not* given anistreplase had a poorer 28-day mortality (18.7%) than either those given anistreplase (12.7%) or those in the 'comparison group' (13.9%); but it is important to realize that no control was exerted over patient selection or the criteria for the use of thrombolysis so that any rigorous comparison of these figures is impossible.

Adverse reactions were few, but as observed in other studies, hypotension and bradycardia were reported more frequently in patients given anistreplase than in other groups. Cardiac arrest occurred in 9 patients (2.9%) given domiciliary anistreplase, 12 patients (2.1%) in the user group who did not receive thrombolytic therapy, and 42 patients (1.7%) in the comparison group. User doctors successfully resuscitated 12 of 18 patients (67%) who arrested at home; figures for comparison doctors were 18 of 36 (50%). In many episodes of arrest the general practitioner was assisted by the ambulance staff.

The RCGP Study indicates that while pre-hospital thrombolysis appears feasible and safe, with present agents it is neither easy to arrange in practice nor is it popular.

Pre-hospital Management in Practice

Organization

The profound pathophysiologic instability and high attrition rate that follows acute coronary occlusion warrant a rapid medical response to patients with prolonged chest pain at rest even though many will have an alternative and often benign diagnosis. Reducing patient delay remains a worthwhile goal, but, like advice on the cessation of smoking and the reduction of alcohol intake by drivers, may take many different strategies over many years to achieve. Emphasis on the education of patients known to be at risk (and their relatives) should be encouraged. Written advice together with simple training in the recognition of coronary symptoms and the delivery of basic life support should be adopted as widely as possible.

No one scheme for the early professional review of a patient with chest pain seems optimum, though the most comprehensive care will be provided by the simultaneous attendance of a physician and a paramedic ambulance. In practice this may be achieved by a fully staffed MCCU, but many recognize the high cost of such an option. In the UK, a recent report from the British Heart Foundation recommends that local strategies be developed to ensure wherever possible the joint arrival of the general practitioner and emergency ambulance personnel to attend to a patient with suspected myocardial infarction.

Paramedic systems without physician attendance can attain high levels of skill in the diagnosis and management of patients with chest pain and are often better placed to offer emergency life support including defibrillation. A therapeutic agent providing rapid and powerful analgesia without adverse cardiorespiratory effects or the capacity to cause addiction would give even wider therapeutic potential to the ambulance crew without physician support.

Whatever system is operative in the locality of a receiving hospital, facilities and skills for resuscitation are mandatory. Automated defibrillators are satisfactory when full medical or paramedic skills are not available, and they can also speed the delivery of a shock in highly trained hands. If possible, however, advanced cardiac life support (ACLS) should be available and is likely overall to be more effective in a collapsed patient. For cases of suspected infarction a preadmission ECG and good communication with the base unit will enhance early care.

Efficient systems should be developed for the rapid assessment of and response to calls for help from patients with chest pain whether such calls are directed first to a primary-care physician or to the ambulance service. Those receiving such calls should, ideally, be trained in the evaluation of patients with chest pain syndromes and in telephone-directed emergency life support.

Therapy

The current focus on early thrombolytic therapy should not obscure the value of more established, and perhaps less contentious, treatment in the pre-hospital phase of an acute infarct. Utilization of these drugs (listed below), especially analgesics and aspirin, is still far from optimal.

Oxygen

Oxygen helpfully counters the hypoxemia that even patients with uncomplicated symptoms experience through ventilation/perfusion mismatch.[106,107] Its use becomes mandatory when left ventricular failure is suspected.

Analgesia

Pain relief, beyond bringing comfort, reduces sympathetic tone lessening both myocardial workload and the proarrhythmic effect of catecholamines.[108] Their use should be prompt. Opiates are recommended by slow *intravenous* injection. Diamorphine 5 mg given at 1 mg min^{-1} (or morphine 10 mg at 2 mg min^{-1}) is preferred, using half this dose in the elderly and in patients with important chronic respiratory disease. (It is wise for naloxone always to be at hand in case of an unexpectedly profound effect.) Opiates may be repeated at 10-min intervals until satisfactory pain relief is obtained. In the absence of a doctor in attendance, analgesia may be effected by nitrous oxide or by nalbuphine.[97]

Antiemetics

The combination of high vagal tone and the emetic effect of opiate therapy promotes unwelcome and potentially dangerous nausea and vomiting. An antiemetic should therefore be given with the analgesic agent. Cyclizine 25–50 mg is convenient as it can be used to dissolve the opiate for a single combined injection. Metoclopramide 10–20 mg i.v. is an alternative and should be used when the vasoconstrictor effects of cyclizine must be avoided, i.e. in severe left ventricular failure or cardiogenic shock.[109]

Nitrates

Three vascular territories where nitrates are of potential help in acute myocardial infarction are the coronary arteries themselves (especially at or adjacent to sites of recent plaque disruption), the peripheral arterioles, and the venous capacitance vessels. Oral glyceryl trinitrate spray or tablets should be encouraged as an immediate therapy unless the patient is profoundly hypotensive.

Aspirin

Aspirin now forms part of the early management of all patients with suspected acute myocardial infarction. Its time of administration within the first 24 hours may not be critical, but there seems no good reason to delay therapy once the diagnosis is suspected. The recommended dose is 150–300 mg taken once. A common recommendation is that a chewable aspirin tablet be taken to speed absorption (particularly after opiate therapy), though it seems wise to defer aspirin administration in those who are troubled by nausea or vomiting in the early phase of their illness. Its use is contraindicated in those allergic to salicylates, and it should be used with caution in patients with active peptic ulcer.

Antiarrhythmic agents

While the use of prophylactic antiarrhythmic agents after myocardial infarction is decreasing, the availability of atropine, lidocaine, and adrenaline remains worthwhile for the treatment of important rhythm disorders. Atropine is helpful to counter either a profound bradycardia ($\leq$40 beats min^{-1}) or a less marked bradycardia complicated by poor cardiac output, heart failure, or frequent ventricular premature beats.

Lidocaine is no longer recommended for routine prophylaxis against ventricular arrhythmias, but in a divided dose of 100–200 mg intravenously is appropriate for (1) the first-line treatment of ventricular tachycardia where a pulse is palpable; (2) late in the treatment algorithm for ventricular fibrillation[103]; and (3) to prevent a recurrence of either of these malignant arrhythmias. Epinephrine plays a prominent role in advanced life support following circulatory arrest in ventricular fibrillation, asystole, or electromechanical dissociation.[110] Apart from its effect on cardiac rhythm and contractility, it appears to support the peripheral vascular tree enhancing the effect on the circulation of external chest compression.

Pre-hospital thrombolysis

The value of administering thrombolysis as soon as possible after the onset of major symptoms of myocardial infarction is attested by experimental results and the evidence of most major clinical trials. Though the absolute number of lives saved by thrombolytic therapy is small (at best about seven lives per 100 patients treated) the prospect of improved left ventricular function and the long-term gain of an opened artery have prompted many to find ways of delivering thrombolysis to as many eligible patients as possible with minimum delay.

Pre-hospital administration undoubtedly reduces delay to treatment, but time-gain may vary substantially according to the locality of the patient, the nature of the first response system, and the in-hospital delay at the receiving unit (Table 1.2). A rural setting with a rapid primary-care response and a long journey to hospital coupled with a protracted in-hospital delay will undoubtedly favor community-initiated therapy. An urban setting with rapid ambulance transport and short in-hospital delay is likely to

Table 1.2 Time saved by pre-hospital administration in a selection of studies of pre-hospital thrombolysis

Study	Time saved (min)
Göteborg	40
EMIP	55
MITI	33
GREAT	130
Brighton	40
Belfast	70
Jerusalem	50
Tel Aviv	40

show no more than a modest benefit in the speed with which thrombolytic agents can be administered.

The value of reducing delay to treatment depends not only on the magnitude of time saved, but on *when* in the course of the illness the time-saving is achieved (Figure 1.9). In pre-hospital trials, benefit has been more noticeable when delays have been reduced by an absolute value of 90 min or more, or when delay reduction has allowed patients to receive thrombolytic therapy within the first 2-hours of the onset of major symptoms. It has been argued that reducing delay by as little as 30 min would be worth while if the patient seeks help early in their attack. Patient delay, however, is still an important rate-limiting factor, one that remains challenging to overcome.

In spite of the many trials reported since 1978, pre-hospital thrombolysis has failed to excite an enthusiastic response from cardiologists, or to find widespread implementation in practice. In part this reflects the hospital-directed focus of many who have pioneered, or continue to practice, the current high standards of care for the infarct patient. However, other factors are contributory: concerns that the *diagnosis* will be sufficiently accurate to choose patients who will benefit from thrombolysis without increased risks of adverse effects; that thrombolytic therapy will prove unsafe in pre-hospital use; that the practicalities and/or cost of therapy will substantially limit its availability; and that in practice the number of patients suitable for pre-hospital thrombolysis will be so small compared to those initially considered for its use that healthcare resources might better

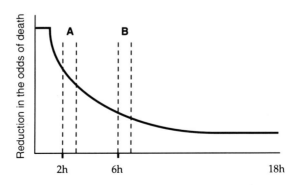

Figure 1.9 Time dependence of the value of shortening delay to thrombolytic therapy. A 1-hour time saving at **A** is likely to produce greater benefit than a similar reduction in delay at **B**.

Table 1.3   Diagnostic accuracy for myocardial infarction in a selection of studies of pre-hospital care

Study	System	Diagnostic accuracy (%)
EMIP		
All patients	MCCU	88
Those with ST elevation	MCCU	91
TEAHAT	MCCU	42
MITI	Paramedic	98
Brighton	Paramedic	96
GREAT	GP	78
RCGP (Thrombolysis Group)	GP	67

GP, general practitioner; MCCU, mobile coronary care unit.

be allocated to hastening hospital admission and reducing in-hospital delay before thrombolytic therapy.

Diagnostic accuracy

Table 1.3 lists the diagnostic accuracy recorded in a number of studies of pre-hospital thrombolysis. The proportion of patients judged to be suffering myocardial infarction in whom this was confirmed at hospital discharge or death varied from 40 to 98%. Greatest accuracy, though still short of 100%, was achieved where the diagnosis was made by a physician-based MCCU with ECG confirmation. Diagnostic accuracy was lowest (40%) in the TEAHAT study where no ECG was recorded. In studies involving UK general practitioners a diagnostic accuracy of 64–78% was achieved. In these studies ECGs were not mandatory for diagnosis, though were recorded in many cases.

Paramedics have achieved similar results, whether through independent operation or supported by transtelephonic links or computerized ECG interpretation. The overall diagnostic accuracy of pre-hospital systems based on clinical assessment and the ECG appears acceptable. Moreover the benefit of thrombolysis appears greatest in patients whose ECGs show the most striking – and hence the most easily recognized – abnormalities of ST segment elevation or left bundle branch block.

Assessment of contraindications and safety

Few data exist directly to show the effectiveness of pre-hospital evaluation in identifying potential contraindications to thrombolysis. The check-lists used by several paramedic-based ambulance schemes appear highly successful.[51,87] General practitioners appear, if anything, to be oversensitive to pre-existing conditions or treatments that could endanger the patient from the adverse effects of thrombolysis.

Most studies attest to the freedom from adverse effects experienced by patients receiving thrombolysis before hospital admission. As might be expected, none occur that have not been observed during thrombolytic therapy in hospital. Bleeding and allergic reactions are rare; bradycardia and symptomatic hypertension are more common, but rarely require treatment. These changes are often self-limiting or respond rapidly to intravenous atropine.

Ventricular fibrillation is known to occur earlier in patients receiving thrombolytic therapy than in controls, but with a lower incidence overall. The EMIP study highlighted the increased propensity to ventricular fibrillation soon after active thrombolytic treatment, whether this was given at home or in hospital. Other studies have produced conflicting results. However, this phenomenon should not be overemphasized. To be unduly concerned that skills and equipment for defibrillation are mandatory only for those wishing to initiate thrombolysis in the community is to miss the vital message of the prethrombolytic era that *all* patients with myocardial infarction require access to defibrillation as soon as possible after the onset of their attack. Early, potentially arrhythmic death remains a fatal plague on which advances in pharmacotherapy have made very little impact.

Concerns that it may be unsafe to administer thrombolysis before hospital admission are understandable, but gain little support from published studies.

Practicality and cost

For pre-hospital use, the administration of thrombolytic therapy by *bolus* rather than by intravenous infusion substantially improves the ease (and therefore the likelihood) of successful treatment. Anistreplase was a compound designed for bolus administration and is therefore the single agent most commonly studied in experimental pre-hospital schemes. It has no current rival for bolus use, but changing views of the initial dosing regimen for rt-PA, and the possibility that urokinase could be given by bolus injection, present alternatives for the future.

In cost-conscious health delivery systems, the responsibility for purchasing thrombolytic agents for pre-hospital use has dampened the enthusiasm of many. And costs extend beyond that of the thrombolytic agent itself. Training, ECG and transmission equipment, or even the provision of specially equipped vehicles, will add to the total cost depending on the scheme adopted.

Poor recruitment

Even when enthusiasm for pre-hospital thrombolysis has been high, the rate of recruitment of patients eligible for thrombolysis has proved surprisingly low. Those who subsequently received active thrombolytic agents have been even fewer.

In the 6 months of the Milwaukee Chest Pain Project,[111] a paramedic emergency system using ECG transmission, 680 patients with chest pain were attended. Of these, 91 (21%) proved to have an acute myocardial infarction and just 12 were selected for pre-hospital thrombolysis. Six patients received active therapy.

Other studies in the USA similarly report rates of eligibility for pre-hospital thrombolysis of 4–5%.

The EMIP study recruited an impressive number of subjects (5469) of which half received thrombolytic therapy in the field. The original intention, however, was to enter 10 000 patients. In order to include at least 5000–6000 patients (to give results judged to be 'worthwhile') participating centers were broadened to include Canada, and the length of the study extended from 24 to 40 months. Moreover, the study failed to report how many patients with either chest pain or acute myocardial infarction considered for inclusion failed to meet the entry criteria.

The GREAT study demonstrated the capacity for rural general practitioners to identify and treat patients with acute myocardial infarction and, with the close encouragement of the chief investigator, to recruit an average of 3.5 patients per general practitioner during the 3 years of the study. It is salutary to note, however, that since the completion of this study several of the general practitioners involved have ceased to administer domiciliary thrombolytic therapy.

Low recruitment rates for pre-hospital thrombolysis were also demonstrated by the RCGP Study.[48] At the outset it proved easier to include general practitioners who did *not* wish to give thrombolytic agents as part of their routine management (776 doctors) than those who did (344 doctors). More patients were treated in the 'comparison group' than

Table 1.4 Reasons why anistreplase was not given by general practitioners in the RCGP Study

	Number of patients	Proportion in user group (%)
Recognized contraindication	249	28.0
Uncertain diagnosis	189	21.3
Patient died before treatment possible	11	1.2
Other reason specified	267	30.1
Anistreplase not available	118	
History of conditions thought to preclude use	28	
Treatment thought to be inappropriate	28	
Other practical reasons	15	
ECG did not confirm myocardial infarction	14	
Adverse clinical state of patient	14	
Prompt admission thought to be preferable	12	
Patient being managed at home	8	
Cardiac arrest before treatment	6	
Other miscellaneous reasons	13	
No reason given	3	

NB More than one reason could be given, so total number of reasons exceeds the 578 patients in the user group not given anistreplase.

in the 'user group' (2495 vs 888 or 3.2% vs 2.6 patients per doctor), though one might have expected a particular interest in infarct management by practitioners using thrombolytic therapy. In the event, during the 20-month study, anistreplase was given in the community to just 310 patients.

Table 1.4 gives an interesting insight into the reasons why thrombolytic therapy was withheld, a mixture of diagnostic uncertainty, perceived contraindications, and the poor availability of the active agent.

The low rate of eligibility of patients for pre-hospital thrombolysis understandably tempers enthusiasm to press for its universal adoption, but should not preclude its use where the infarct is readily apparent by definite ST segment elevation on the ECG, and where delays to hospital treatment are likely – for whatever reason – to be substantial.

Reducing In-hospital Delay

While optimum pre-hospital schemes to enhance the early treatment of patients with acute myocardial infarction are worth while, they should not distract from a pressing need to improve the initial phase of in-hospital care. Minimizing delay to the initial in-hospital treatment is a matter of organization, education, and continuing audit.[57–60]

In facilities accustomed to receiving emergencies of all types and grades of severity, the organization to provide rapid and informed attention to the patient with a suspected infarct requires:

1. A senior, vigorous protagonist of a fast response scheme, who is clearly involved with the running of the emergency services and who is both sympathetic to and knowledgeable concerning the management of patients with chest pain.
2. The 24-hour availability of a member of staff with sufficient experience to provide immediate triage of patients presenting with chest pain.

3. Immediate access to electrocardiography preferably undertaken while preliminary questions are still being addressed to the patient.
4. The ready availability of a resident doctor who is aware of the need to respond rapidly to cases of suspected infarction (if necessary by temporarily leaving lower priority patients).
5. An understanding by attending staff that the identification of acute myocardial infarction in patients most likely to benefit from thrombolytic therapy can be achieved rapidly through a *limited* history, examination, and characteristic ST segment elevation ('fast track' patients); also that important contraindications to thrombolysis in ideal candidates can be identified similarly without protracted consultation.
6. The education of all attending staff of the short- and long-term value to patients with myocardial infarction of immediate pain relief, access to monitoring, resuscitation skills, and early thrombolysis.

The identification of suitable patients for thrombolysis may be helped by publishing flow charts for wall-display or for carrying in the doctor's pocket. On-going education will be required for the encouragement and updating of existing staff, and for the introduction of new staff to the theory of maintaining a rapid response to this clinical emergency. A continuing audit of early care, particularly of the administration of thrombolytic therapy to 'fast-track' cases (the so-called 'door-to-needle' time), is mandatory to provide useful feedback to those involved in the scheme. Finally, the financial costs of the organization, education, and audit that promote optimal in-hospital management are likely to be small when compared with the benefits such schemes provide to patients.

Where a fast-track system in a general emergency facility is not appropriate, direct admission to a coronary care unit is advocated.[54] The golden rule applies throughout, however, that wherever the patient is first admitted, immediate triage to identify candidates for early therapy is the key to gaining the greatest value from therapies already proven to enhance the outcome from acute myocardial infarction.

Cost-effectiveness of Out-of-hospital Therapy

Calculating the cost-effectiveness of out-of-hospital therapy for acute myocardial infarction is a complex task. Costs will be influenced substantially by the nature of the *system* invoked for pre-hospital care and by the range of *treatments* offered, particularly thrombolytic agents (from $320 for streptokinase/aspirin to $2,300 for accelerated t-PA).[30]

System costs will be determined mainly by the type and number of staff employed to service the first response, by the cost of equipment (electrocardiographs, defibrillators, other devices for advanced life support, communications systems), and by training requirements for the personnel involved. Since proportionately few episodes of chest pain in the community result from a demonstrable infarct,[48,91,111] a physician-manned MCCU available only to service patients with chest pain or collapse is likely to be an expensive solution, particularly on a cost-per-infarct basis. Using existing hospital-based staff on a 'call-out' basis, however, may limit the costs of such a scheme and seems a practical option.

Systems designed to service a wider range of medical emergencies but providing comprehensive treatment for infarct patients will reduce the marginal costs of their pre-hospital care. Costs will be low, while retaining adequate protection from early arrhythmic death, if care is given by paramedics working independently. Survival is not inexpensive, however. For paramedic-resuscitated victims of out-of-hospital cardiac arrest, Valenzuela *et al.*[116] have measured the cost per life saved as $8,886. In the UK, the *additional* attendance of an on-call general practitioner is likely to extend the scope of, but

Table 1.5 Suggested attributes of a system for pre-hospital coronary care

Easy accessibility by patients seeking help:
  to give effective early triage of patient's reported condition
Good communication with base hospital:
  but not necessarily requiring ECG transmission
Facilities and skills for advanced life support:
  including defibrillation and the use of cardioactive drugs
Ability to record a 12-lead ECG without undue delay:
  with on-site capability of recognizing important arrhythmias, left bundle branch block and major changes of infarction
Ability to give effective analgesia and antiemetics if necessary:
  a powerful, safe agent for paramedic use would be ideal
The practice of developing and working within agreed local strategies for pre-hospital care:
  for some areas this may include discussion of the use of pre-hospital thrombolysis

add relatively little to, the cost of pre-hospital care. However, GP-initiated defibrillation, based on the experience[117] of using 200 defibrillators supplied by the British Heart Foundation from 1985–1991 seems costly at about £30,000 ($45,000) per survivor.

A cost-effectiveness model for coronary thrombolysis reperfusion therapy developed by Laffel *et al.*[118] showed that, whatever therapeutic scheme was adopted, the highest cost–benefit ratio was obtained when treatment was initiated within 2 hours. Hugenholz[119] concludes that 'although no detailed cost–benefit analyses have been carried out for the MITI, EMIP, GREAT, or REPAIR studies, the low mortality alone as well as the low complication rates indicate, without much complex calculation, a high benefit-to-cost ratio.' The results of a cost-effectiveness project in the Netherlands on pre-hospital care are awaited with interest.

Conclusions

The management of patients with acute myocardial infarction begins as soon as help has been summoned. A pre-hospital phase of care is inevitable, but how best should this be organized?

Table 1.5 indicates suggested attributes of an appropriate system for pre-hospital coronary care. It is worthwhile considering these from the standpoint first of the patient who develops chest pain, potentially indicating an acute myocardial infarction. The system chosen to service these patients will inevitably vary from country to country. Patient idiosyncrasy will determine the first agency summoned to help even in the face of well-publicized recommendations. Whatever system is adopted, the importance cannot be overemphasized of a rapid response to patients with chest pain, effective early triage, good communication between pre-hospital and hospital personnel, and agreed, well-practised local strategies that are sensitive to geography and available facilities but provide well for patients' needs at the most critical phase of their attack.[112–115]

References

1. Bainton, C.R. and Petersen, D.R. (1963) Deaths from coronary heart disease in persons fifty years of age and younger. *N. Eng. J. Med.*, **268**, 569–75.
2. Gordon, T. and Kannel, W.B. (1971) Premature mortality from coronary heart disease. The Framingham Study. *JAMA*, **125**, 1617–25.
3. Armstrong, A., Duncan, B. and Oliver, M.F. (1972) Natural history of acute coronary attacks. A community study. *Br. Heart J.*, **34**, 167–80.

4. Kinlen, L.J. (1973) Incidence and presentation of myocardial infarction in an English Community. *Br. Heart J.*, **35**, 616–22.
5. Pantridge, J.F. and Geddes, J.S. (1967) A mobile intensive care unit in the management of myocardial infarction. *Lancet*, **ii**, 271–3.
6. Tunstall-Pedoe, H. (1991) The Health of the Nation: Responses: coronary heart disease. *BMJ*, **303**, 701–4.
7. O'Doherty, M., Taylor, D.I., Quinn, E. *et al.*, (1983) Five hundred patients with myocardial infarction monitored within one hour of symptoms. *BMJ*, **286**, 1405–8.
8. White, N.M., Parker, W.S., Binning, R.A. *et al.* (1973) Mobile coronary care provided by ambulance personnel. *BMJ*, **iii**, 618–22.
9. Nazel, E.L., Liberthson, R.R., Hirschman, J.C. and Nussenfeld, S.R. (1975) Emergency Care. *Circulation*, **52** (suppl. III), III-216–18.
10. Cobb, L.A., Werner, J.A. and Troughbaugh, B.G. (1980) Sudden cardiac death, 1: a decade's experience with out-of-hospital resuscitation. *Mod. Concepts Cardiovasc.*, **49**, 31–6.
11. Lewis, S.J., Holmberg, S., Quinn, E. *et al.* (1993) Out-of-hospital resuscitation in East Sussex: 1981–1989. *Br. Heart J.*, **70**, 568–73.
12. Vincent, R., Martin, V., Williams, G. *et al.* (1984) A community training scheme in cardiopulmonary resuscitation. *BMJ*, **288**, 617–20.
13. Davies, M.J. and Thomas, A.C. (1985) Plaque fissuring – the cause of acute myocardial infarction, sudden ischaemic death and crescendo angina. *Br. Heart J.*, **53**, 363–73.
14. Skinner, D.V. and Vincent, R. (1993) *Cardiopulmonary Resuscitation*. Oxford: Oxford University Press.
15. Tennant, R. (1935) Factors concerned in the arrest of contraction in an ischaemic myocardia area. *Am. J. Physiol.*, **113**, 677–82.
16. Poole-Wilson, P.A. (1990) The myocardium in ischaemic heart disease. In: Poole-Wilson, P.A. and Sheridan, D.J. *Atherosclerosis in Ischaemic Heart Disease 2: Myocardial Consequences*, pp. 3.1–3.56. London: Science Press.
17. Steenbergen, C., Murphy, E., Levy, L. and London, R.E. (1987) Elevation in cytosolic free calcium concentration early in myocardial ischaemia in perfused rat heart. *Circ. Res.* **60**, 700–7.
18. Webb, S.C., Rickards, A.F. and Poole-Wilson, P.A. (1993) Coronary sinus potassium concentration during coronary angioplasty. *Br. Heart J.*, **50**, 146–8.
19. McCance, A.J., Thompson, P.A. and Forfar, J.C. (1993) Increased cardiac sympathetic nervous activity in patients with unstable coronary heart disease. *Eur. Heart J.*, **14**, 751–7.
20. Reimer, K.A., Lowe, J.E., Rasmussen, M.M. and Jennings, R.B. (1977) The wave front phenomenon of ischaemic cell death. 1. Myocardial infarction size vs duration of coronary occlusion in dogs. *Circulation*, **56**, 786–90.
21. Gruppo Italiano per lo Studio della Streptokinasi nell'Infarto Miocardico (GISSI) (1986) Effectiveness of intravenous thrombolytic treatment in acute myocardial infarction. *N. Engl. J. Med.*, **314**, 1465–71.
22. ISIS-2 (Second International Study of Infarct Survival) Collaborative Group (1988) Randomised trial of intravenous streptokinase, oral aspirin, both, or neither among 17 187 cases of suspected acute myocardial infarction: ISIS-2. *Lancet*, **ii**, 349–60.
23. Fibrinolytic Therapy Trialists (FTT) Collaborative Group (1994) Indications for fibrinolytic therapy in suspected acute myocardial infarction: collaborative overview of early mortality and major morbidity results from all randomised trials of more than 1000 patients. *Lancet*, **343**, 311–22.
24. van de Werf, F. and Arnold, A.E.R. (1988) Intravenous tissue plasminogen activator and size of infarct, left ventricular function, and survival of acute myocardial infarction. *BMJ*, **287**, 1374–9.
25. ISAM Study Group (1986) A prospective trial of intravenous streptokinase in acute myocardial infarction. *N. Engl. J. Med.*, **314**, 1465–71.
26. Vermeer, F., Simoons, M., Bar, F. *et al.* (1986) Which patterns benefit most from early thrombolytic therapy with intracoronary streptokinase? *Circulation*, **74**, 1379–89.
27. Kennedy, J., Martin, G., Davis, K. *et al.* (1988) The Western Washington Intravenous Streptokinase Trial in acute myocardial infarction randomised trial. *Circulation*, **77**, 345–52.
28. Koren, G., Weiss, A.T., Hasin, Y. *et al.* (1985) Prevention of myocardial damage in acute myocardial ischaemia by early treatment with intravenous streptokinase. *N. Engl. J. Med.*, **313**, 1384–9.
29. AIMS Trial Study Group (1988) Effect of intravenous APSAC on mortality after acute myocardial infarction: preliminary report of a placebo-controlled clinical trial. *Lancet*, **i**, 545–9.
30. The GUSTO Investigators (1993) An international randomised trial comprising four thrombolytic strategies for acute myocardial infarction. *N. Engl. J. Med.*, **329**, 673–82.
31. GREAT Group (1992) Feasibility, safety, and efficacy of domiciliary thrombolysis by general practitioners: Grampian region early anistreplase trial. *BMJ*, **305**, 548–53.
32. Ellis, S.G., Topol, E.J., George, B.S. *et al.* (1989) Recurrent ischaemia without warning. Analysis of risk factors for in-hospital ischaemic events after successful thrombolysis with intravenous tissue plasminogen activator. *Circulation*, **80**, 1159–65.
33. Hisa, J., Hamilton, W.P., Kleiman, N. *et al.* (1990) A comparison between heparin and low-dose aspirin as adjunctive therapy with tissue plasminogen activator for acute myocardial infarction. *N. Engl. J. Med.*, **323**, 1433–7.
34. Norris, R.M., White, H.D., Cross, D.B. *et al.* (1993) Aspirin does not improve early arterial patency after streptokinase treatment for acute myocardial infarction. *Br. Heart J.*, **69**, 492–5.
35. Jang, I.-K., Fuster, V. and Gold, H.K. (1992) Antiplatelets. *Coronary Artery Dis.*, **3**, 1030–6.

36. Roux, S., Christeller, S. and Ludin, E. (1992) Effects of aspirin on coronary reocclusion and recurrent ischaemia after thrombolysis: a meta-analysis. *J. Am. Coll. Cardiol.*, **19**, 671–7.
37. Baskinski, A. and Naylor, C.D. (1991) Aspirin and fibrinolysis in acute myocardial infarction: meta-analytic evidence of synergy. *J. Clin. Epidemiol.*, **44**, 1085–96.
38. Weaver, D.W., Cerqueira, M., Halstrom, A.P. *et al.* (1993) Pre-hospital-initiated vs hospital-initiated thrombolytic therapy. The Myocardial Infarction and Triage Intervention Trial. *JAMA*, **270**, 1211–16.
39. Birkehead, J.S. (1992) Time delays in provision of thrombolytic treatment in six district hospitals. *BMJ*, **305**, 445–8.
40. Schofer, J., Buttner, J., Geng Gutschmidt, K. *et al.* (1990) Prehospital thrombolysis in acute myocardial infarction. *Am. J. Cardiol.*, **66**, 1429–33.
41. European Myocardial Infarction Project (EMiP) Subcommittee (1988) Potential time saving with pre-hospital intervention in acute myocardial infarction. *Eur. Heart J.*, **9**, 118–24.
42. European Myocardial Infarction Project Group (1993) Prehospital thrombolytic therapy in patients with suspected acute myocardial infarction. *N. Engl. J. Med.*, **329**, 383–9.
43. Rawles, J.M., Metcalfe, J.M., Shirreffs, C. *et al.* (1990) Association of patient delay with symptoms, cardiac enzymes and outcome in acute myocardial infarction. *Eur. Heart J.*, **11**, 643–8.
44. Ridker, P.M., Manson, J.E., Goldhaber, S.Z. *et al.* (1992) Comparison of delay times to hospital presentation for physicians and non-physicians with acute myocardial infarction. *Am. J. Cardiol.*, **70**, 10–13.
45. Schmidt, S.B. and Borsch, M.A. (1990) The prehospital phase of acute myocardial infarction in the era of thrombolysis. *Am. J. Cardiol.*, **65**, 1411–15.
46. Kenyon, L.W., Ketterer, M.W., Gheorghiade M. and Goldstein (1991). Psychological factors related to prehospital delay during acute myocardial infarction. *Circulation*, **84**, 1969–76.
47. Rawles, J.N. and Haites, N.E. (1988) Patient and general practitioner delays in acute myocardial infarction. *BMJ*, **296**, 882–4.
48. Hannaford, P., Vincent, R., Ferry, S. *et al.* (1994) Can general practitioners use thrombolysis safely? Evidence from the Royal College of General Practitioners Myocardial Infarction Study. *J.R. Coll. Gen. Prac.* (in press).
49. Kereiakis, D.J., Weaver, W.D., Anderson, J.L. *et al.* (1990) Time delays in the diagnosis and treatment of acute myocardial infarction: a tale of eight cities. *Am. Heart J.*, **120**, 773–9.
50. Gibler, W.B., Kereiakes, D.J., Dean E.N. *et al.* (1991) Prehospital diagnosis and treatment of acute myocardial infarction: A North–South perspective. *Am. Heart J.*, **121**, 1–10.
51. Weaver, W.D., Eisenberg, M.S., Martin, J.S. *et al.* (1990) Myocardial triage and intervention project – phase I: patient characteristics and feasibility of prehospital initiation of thrombolytic therapy. *J Am. Coll. Cardiol.*, **15**, 925–30.
52. Karagounis, L., Ipsen, S.K., Jessop, M.R. *et al.* (1990) Impact of field-transmitted electrocardiography on time to in-hospital thrombolytic therapy in acute myocardial infarction. *Am. J. Cardiol.*, **60**, 786–91.
53. Sharkey, S.W., Brunnette, D.D., Ruiz, E. *et al.* (1989) An analysis of time delays preceding thrombolysis for acute myocardial infarction. *JAMA*, **262**, 3171–4.
54. Pell, A.C.H. and Miller, H.C. (1990) Delays in admission of patients with acute myocardial infarction to coronary care: implications of thrombolysis. *Health Bull.*, **48**, 225–31.
55. Ridker, P., Buring, J., Manson, J. *et al.* (1990) Time to presentation for acute MI in the US Physicians Health Study. *J. Am. Coll. Cardiol.*, **15** (suppl. 2), 167A.
56. Burns, J.M.A., Hogg, K.J., Rae, A.P. *et al.* (1989) Impact of a policy of direct admission to a coronary care unit on use of thrombolytic treatment. *Br. Heart J.*, **61**, 332–5.
57. MacCallum, A., Stafford, P., Jones, C. *et al.* (1990) Reduction in hospital time to thrombolytic therapy by audit of policy guidelines. *Eur. Heart J.*, **11**, 48–52.
58. Dalton, H., Chappel, D. and Climie, R. (1989) Thrombolysis for acute myocardial infarction in a district general hospital. *J. R. Soc. Med.*, **82**, 394–5.
59. Moses, H.W., Bartolozzi, J.J., Koester, D.L. *et al.* (1991) Reducing delay in the emergency room in administration of thrombolytic therapy for myocardial infarction associated with ST elevation. *Am. J. Cardiol.*, **68**, 251–3.
60. Pell, A.C.H., Miller, H.C., Robertson, C.E. and Fox, K.A.A. (1992) Effect of 'fast track' admission for acute myocardial infarction on delay to thrombolysis. *BMJ*, **304**, 83–7.
61. Mathey, D.G., Schofer, J., Sheenhan, F.H. *et al.* (1985) Intravenous urokinase in acute myocardial infarction. *Am. J. Cardiol.*, **55**, 872–82.
62. Fine, D.G., Weiss, A.T., Sapoznikov, D. *et al.* (1986) Importance of early initiation of intravenous streptokinase therapy for acute myocardial infarction. *Am. J. Cardiol.*, **58**, 411–17.
63. Applebaum, D., Weiss, A.T., Koren, G. *et al.* (1986) Feasibility of pre-hospital fibrinolytic therapy in acute myocardial infarction. *Am. J. Emerg. Med.*, **4**, 201–4.
64. Castaigne, A.D., Duval, A.M., Dubois-Rande, J.L. *et al.* (1987) Prehospital administration of anisoylated plasmin-ogen streptokinase activator complex in acute myocardial infarction. *Drugs*, **33** (suppl. 3), 231–4.
65. Weiss, A.T., Fine, D.G., Applebaum, D. *et al.* (1987) Prehospital coronary thrombolysis, a new strategy in acute myocardial infarction. *Chest*, **92**, 124–8.
66. Martens, U., Lange-Braun, P., Langer, R. *et al.* (1987) Systemische Fruhlyse des akuten Myokardinfarkts. *Deutsche Med. Wochenschr.*, **112**, 910–14.
67. Bossaert, L.L., Denney, H.E., Colemont, L.J. *et al.* (1988) Prehospital thrombolytic treatment of acute myocardial infarction with anisoylated plasminogen activator complex. *Crit. Care Med.*, **16**, 823–30.
68. Villemant, D., Barriot, P., Bordeman, P. *et al.* (1988) At home thrombolysis and myocardial infarction, a real saving of time (abstract). *Eur. Heart J.*, **103**, 394.

69. Bippus, P., Haux, H. and Schroder, R. (1988) Prehospital intravenous streptokinase in evolving myocardial infarction: a randomised study about feasibility safety in time gain (abstract). *Eur. Heart J.*, **130**, 395.
70. Nicholas, J., Higginson, J.D.S. and McBoyle, D. (1988) Early intervention in myocardial infarction with streptokinase at home and in accident and emergency department (abstract). *Eur. Heart J.*, **212**, P1198.
71. Greenberg, H., Sherrid, M., Lynn, S. *et al.* (1988) Out-of-hospital paramedic administered streptokinase for acute myocardial infarction. *Lancet*, **ii**, 1187–92.
72. Castaigne, A.D., Herve, C., Duval-Moulin, A. *et al.* (1989) Prehospital use of APSAC: results of a placebo-controlled study. *Am. J. Cardiol.*, **64**, 30A–33A.
73. Sauval, P., Artigou, J., Cristofini, P. *et al.* (1989) Fibrinolyse prehospitalière par rt-PA dans l'infactus aigu du myocarde. *Arch. Mal. Coeur*, **82**, 1957–61.
74. Cazaux, P., Leclerq, G., Vahanian, A. *et al.* (1989) Thrombolyse intraneineuse par l'activateur tissulaire du plasminogene (rt-PA) à la phase prehospitaliere dans l'infarctus myocardique aigu. *Arch. Mal. Coeur*, **82**, 1967–71.
75. Burke, E., McAleer, B., McElhinney, K. *et al.* (1989) Comparative one year mortality in patients treated with thrombolytic treatment at home and in the coronary care unit (abstract). *Br. Heart J.*, **61**, 72.
76. Picart, N., Bossaert, L., Renard, M. *et al.* (1989) A Belgian multicentre study of prehospital thrombolysis with eminase (APSAC) in acute myocardial infarction (abstract). *Eur. Heart J.*, **123**, 618.
77. Roth, A., Barbarsh, G.I., Hod, H. *et al.* (1990) Should thrombolysis therapy be administered in the mobile intensive care unit in patients with evolving myocardial infarction? A pilot study. *J. Am. Coll. Cardiol.*, **15**, 932–6.
78. Barbash, G., Roth, A., Hod, H. *et al.* (1990) Improved survival but not left ventricular function with early and prehospital treatment with tissue plasminogen activator with acute myocardial infarction. *Am. J. Cardiol.*, **66**, 261–6.
79. Kokott, N., Rutsch, W., Berghofer, G. *et al.* (1990) Prehospital treatment with IV rt-PA in acute myocardial infarction (abstract). *Eur. Heart J.*, **356**, P1972.
80. Linderer, T., Heineking, M., Guhl, B. *et al.* (1990) Infarct size and left ventricular function at day 10 after thrombolysis at patients home (abstract). *Circulation*, **82**(suppl. III), III-280.
81. McKendall, G.R., Woolard, R., Mcdonald, M.J. and Williams, D.O. (1990) Feasibility of prehospital acute myocardial infarction diagnosis: results of the prehospital administration of t-PA (PATS) study (abstract). *Circulation*, **82** (suppl. III), III-667.
82. Purvis, J.A., Trouton, T.G., Dalzell, G.W. *et al.* (1990) Pre-hospital double bolus alteplase in acute myocardial infarction (abstract). *Circulation*, **82** (suppl. III), III-538.
83. Sherrid, M., Greenberg, H., Marsella, R. *et al.* (1990) A pilot study of paramedic-administered prehospital thrombolysis for acute myocardial infarction. *Clin. Cardiol.*, **13**, 421–4.
84. Bouten, M., Simoons, M. and Hartman, J. (1990) Snellere behandeling van het acute myocardinfarct door behandeling met alteplase (rt-PA) voor opname. *Ned. Tijdschr. Geneesk.*, **50**, 2434–8.
85. The Thrombolysis Early in Acute Heart Attack Trial Study Group (1990) Very early thrombolytic therapy in suspected acute myocardial infarction. *Am. J. Cardiol.*, **65**, 401–7.
86. Risonfors, M., Gustarsson, G., Ekstrom, L. *et al.* (1991) Prehospital thrombolysis in suspected acute myocardial infarction: results from the TEAHAT study. *J. Intern. Med.*, **229** (suppl. I), 401–7.
87. Vincent, R. (1991) Does pre-hospital thrombolysis have a favourable benefit/risk ratio? In: Chamberlain, D.A. and Pitt, B. (eds) *Controversies in Thrombolysis and AML*, pp. 11–14. London: Royal Society of Medicine Services.
88. Bouten, M.J.M. and Simoons, M.L. (1991) Strategies for pre-hospital thrombolysis: an overview. *Eur. Heart J.*, **12** (suppl. G), 39–42.
89. Gallagher, D., O'Rourke, M., Healey, J. *et al.* (1992) Paramedic-initiated pre-hospital thrombolysis using urokinase in acute coronary occlusion (TICO 2). *Coronary Artery Dis.*, **3**, 605–9.
90. Kowalenko, T., Kereiakes, D.J. and Gibler, W.B. (1992) Prehospital diagnosis and treatment of acute myocardial infarction: a critical review. *Am. Heart J.*, **123**, 181–90.
91. Bouten, M.J.M., Simoons, M.L., Hartman, J.A.M. *et al.* (1992) Pre-hospital thrombolysis with alteplase (rt-PA) in acute myocardial infarction. *Eur. Heart J.*, **13**, 925–31.
92. Rawles, J. (for the GREAT Group) (1994) Halving of mortality at 1 year by domiciliary thrombolysis in the Grampian Region Early Anistreplase Trial (GREAT). *J. Am. Coll. Cardiol.*, **23**, 1–5.
93. Rowley, J.M., Hill, J.D., Hampton, J.R. and Mitchell, J.R.A. (1982) Early reporting of myocardial infarction; impact of an experiment in patient education. *BMJ*, **284**, 1741–6.
94. Herlitz, J., Hartford, M., Holberg, S. *et al.* (1989) Effects of a media campaign on delay time and ambulance use in suspected acute myocardial infarction. *Am. J. Cardiol.*, **64**, 90–3.
95. Wyllie, H.R. and Dunn, F.G. (1994) Pre-hospital opiate and aspirin administration in patients with myocardial infarction. *BMJ*, **308**, 760–1.
96. Rawles, J. (1992) General practitioners and emergency treatment for patients with suspected myocardial infarction: last chance for excellence? *Br. J. Gen. Pract.*, **42**, 525–8.
97. Stene, J.K., Stotberg, L., MacDonald, G. *et al.* (1988) Nalbuphine analgesia in the pre-hospital setting. *Am. J. Emerg. Med.*, **6**, 634–9.
98. Eisenberg, M.S., Bergner, L. and Hallstrom, A.P. (1979) Cardiac resuscitation in the community. *JAMA*, **241**, 1905–7.
99. Torp-Pedersen, C., Birk-Madsen, E. and Pedersen, A. (1989) The time factor in resuscitation initiated by ambulance drivers. *Eur. Heart J.*, **10**, 555–7.
100. Gray, W.A. (1993) Pre-hospital resuscitation. The good, the bad, and the futile. *JAMA*, **270**, 1471–2.
101. Weaver, W.D., Cobb, L.A., Hallstrom, A.P. *et al.* (1986) Considerations for improving survival from out of hospital cardiac arrest. *Ann. Emerg. Med.*, **15**, 1181–6.

102. Emergency Cardiac Care Committee and Subcommittees, American Heart Association (1992) Guidelines for cardiopulmonary resuscitation and emergency cardiac care. *JAMA*, **268**, 2171–302.
103. European Resuscitation Council Basic Life Support Working Group (1993) Guidelines for basic life support. *BMJ*, **306**, 1587–9.
104. Cummins, R.O., Ornato, J.P., Thies, W.H. and Pepe, P.E. (1991) Improving survival from sudden cardiac arrest: the 'chain of survival' concept. *Circulation*, **83**, 1832–47.
105. Colquhoun, M.C. and Julian, D.G. (1992) Treatable arrhythmias in cardiac arrests seen outside hospital. *Lancet*, **339**, 1167.
106. Fillmore, S.J., Shapiro, M. and Killip, T. (1970) Arterial oxygen tension in acute myocardial infarction: serial analysis of clinical state and blood-gas exchanges. *Am. Heart J.*, **79**, 620–9.
107. Madias, J.E. and Hood, W.B. (1976) Reduction of precordial ST segment elevation in patients with anterior myocardial infarction by oxygen breathing. *Circulation*, **53** (suppl. I), 198–200.
108. Lester, R. (1995) Achieving pain relief with physiologic management and analgesic agents during acute myocardial infarction. In: Califf, R.M. and Wagner, G.H.S. (eds) *Acute Coronary Care: Principles and Practice*, pp. 299–309. Boston: Martinus Nijhoff.
109. Tan, L.B., Bryant, S. and Murray, R.G. (1988) Detrimental haemodynamic effects of cyclizine in heart failure. *Lancet*, **i**, 560–1.
110. European Resuscitation Council Advanced Life Support Working Party (1992) Guidelines for advanced life support. *Resuscitation*, **24**, 111–21.
111. Aufderheide, T.P., Keelan, M.H., Hendley, G.E. *et al.* (1992) Milwaukee Pre-hospital Chest Pain Project – Phase I: Feasibility and accuracy of pre-hospital thrombolytic candidate selection. *Am. J. Cardiol.*, **69**, 991–6.
112. Verheugt, F.W., Funke Kupper, A.J., Sterkman, L.G. *et al.* (1989) Emergency room infusion of intravenous streptokinase in acute myocardial infarction: feasibility, safety and hemodynamic consequences. *Am. Heart J.*, **117**, 1018–21.
113. Wilcox, R.G. and Rowlege, J.M. (1990) Prehospital management of acute myocardial infarction: patient and general practitioner interactions. In: Chamberlain, D.A., Julian, D.G. and Sleight, P. (eds) *The Management of Acute Myocardial Ischaemia*, pp. 133–8. London: Current Medical Literature Ltd.
114. Fox, K.A.A. (1990) Thrombolysis and the general practitioner. *BMJ*, **300**, 867–8.
115. Weston, C.F.M., Penny, W.J. and Julian, D.G. (1994) Guidelines for the early management of patients with myocardial infarction. *BMJ*, **308**, 767–71.
116. Valenzuela, T.D., Criss, E.A., Spaite, D.W. *et al.* (1990) Cost-effectiveness analysis of paramedic emergency services in the treatment of prehospital cardiopulmonary arrest. *Ann. Emerg. Med.*, **19**, 1407–11.
117. Colquhoun, M.C. and Julian, D.G. (1992) Treatable arrhythmias in cardiac arrests seen outside hospital. *Lancet*, **339**, 1167.
118. Laffel, G.L., Fineberg, H.V. and Braunwald, E. (1987) A cost-effectiveness model for coronary thrombolysis reperfusion therapy. *J. Am. Coll. Cardiol.*, **10**, 79B–90B.
119. Hugenholtz, P.G. (1993) Expanding indications for thrombolytic therapy in acute myocardial infarction. *Am. J. Cardiol.*, **72**, 22G–29G.

2

General Hospital Management

E. M. Antman

Coronary Care Unit

All wards admitting patients with acute myocardial infarction should have a system capable of sounding an alarm at the onset of an important rhythm change and of recording the rhythm automatically on an ECG ... the provision of the appropriate apparatus would not be prohibitively expensive if these patients were admitted to special Intensive-Care Units. Such units should be staffed by suitably experienced people throughout the 24 hours.[1]

With these words in 1961 Desmond Julian introduced to the British Thoracic Society the concept of what later became known as the coronary care unit (CCU).[2,3] Based upon the fundamental principles espoused above, CCUs were designed and constructed in thousands of hospitals throughout the world. Over the past three decades of their existence, CCUs have been a life-saving environment for patients and a rich and rewarding laboratory for the 'field study' of acute myocardial infarction in humans.[4] From such units has emerged a clearer understanding of the hemodynamic and electrical consequences of acute myocardial infarction (Chapters 7 and 11). CCUs have also been the setting for trials of countless therapies for acute infarction.[5] Therapeutic programs tested on patients with an acute infarction have been diverse, ranging from administration of simple inexpensive drugs as well as medicinals derived from unusual and exotic sources to relaxation therapy and even prayer![6–9]

Probably more than any other area of medicine, the CCU has been the arena for a broad array of clinical trials. These have included modest size trials enrolling small numbers of patients subjected to detailed physiologic measurements to some of the largest cooperative, multicenter, acute intervention studies in medicine, enrolling between 40 000 and 60 000 patients.[10,11] Only a handful of the many interventions tested in acute infarction patients have emerged as clinically important and therapeutically relevant to modern day coronary care and the details of such interventions are discussed in other chapters of this book.[5,12]

Finally, CCUs have been subjected from their very inception to continuous scrutiny of the costs of such highly specialized care. The costs have been assessed not only for the patient receiving the care, but also the staff charged with the responsibility of delivering it, and the society bearing the burden of funding it.[4,5,13–25]

While refinements of admission and discharge criteria have been proposed, along with a reassessment of the future role of the CCU, it remains an integral element in the fabric of care of the patient with acute myocardial infarction.[25–27] It is estimated that CCUs save nearly 20 000 lives annually in the USA and were responsible for 10–15% of the decline in mortality from coronary heart disease in the USA between 1968 and 1976.[28] Generations of physicians have and will continue to rotate through a CCU during their period of training. The continued existence of the CCU concept, after three decades of rigorous medical investigation and evaluation, stands as a testimony to the vision and insight of the early pioneers in the field of coronary care medicine.

Landmarks in History of Coronary Care (Figure 2.1)

Following a series of anecdotal reports of successful closed-chest cardiac resuscitation and recognition that ventricular fibrillation was responsible for most avoidable deaths in the early phase of acute myocardial infarction, the notion of an intensive coronary care treatment area was developed and the CCU concept was implemented.[2–4] Widespread use of direct current defibrillators was probably the major driving force behind the reduction of in-hospital mortality from acute myocardial infarction, from 30% in the pre-CCU era to approximately 15% in the early CCU era (Figure 2.2).[4]

The first decade of coronary care was also notable for extensive cataloging and vigorous management of cardiac arrhythmias.[3,29,30] The concept of prophylactic lidocaine was promulgated.[31] Later, rigorous analysis of randomized controlled trials confirmed that lidocaine was effective for preventing primary ventricular fibrillation, but is use was associated with a tendency towards increased mortality, probably from an excess of fatal bradycardiac and asystolic arrests.[32,33] Bradyarrhythmias were often aggressively treated with temporary pacemakers so that at one point some centers were employing pacing in as many as one-third of patients admitted to the CCU.[34] Subsequently, prophylactic lidocaine and aggressive transvenous pacing became used much less frequently following recognition of the sharp decline in the incidence of

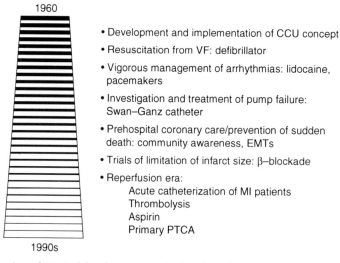

1960

- Development and implementation of CCU concept
- Resuscitation from VF: defibrillator
- Vigorous management of arrhythmias: lidocaine, pacemakers
- Investigation and treatment of pump failure: Swan–Ganz catheter
- Prehospital coronary care/prevention of sudden death: community awareness, EMTs
- Trials of limitation of infarct size: β–blockade
- Reperfusion era:
    Acute catheterization of MI patients
    Thrombolysis
    Aspirin
    Primary PTCA

1990s

Figure 2.1 Prominent historical developments in the last three decades of coronary care medicine. The early CCU era focused on management of cardiac arrhythmias. Clinical attention subsequently broadened to include sophisticated hemodynamic monitoring of infarct patients and efforts to reduce infarct size. The current reperfusion era has further broadened the therapeutic armamentarium available to physicians (depicted schematically by the width of the bar increasing from 1960 to the 1990s).

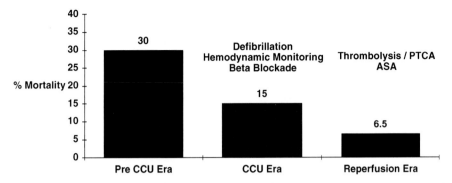

Figure 2.2 The impact of medical therapy for acute myocardial infarction on short-term mortality. In the pre-CCU era the short-term mortality (30 day) from acute myocardial infarction was estimated to be 30%. Implementation of the CCU concept with defibrillation, sophisticated hemodynamic monitoring, and β-blockade reduced the short-term mortality to 15%. A further dramatic reduction in mortality was ushered in by the reperfusion era where combinations of thrombolysis, primary PTCA, and aspirin are now employed.

primary ventricular fibrillation and appreciation of the benign clinical course of sinus bradycardia and atrioventricular (AV) block, particularly associated with inferior myocardial infarction.[35]

Introduction of the pulmonary artery balloon flotation catheter set the stage for bedside hemodynamic monitoring and more precise management of heart failure and cardiogenic shock associated with myocardial infarction.[36] Extension of sophisticated medical care to victims of myocardial infarction prior to hospital arrival (pre-hospital coronary care) was the impetus for development of highly integrated teams of emergency medical technicians and has been the inspiration for numerous community education programs.[26,37]

Beginning in the early 1980s aggressive efforts were made to limit infarct size with a variety of interventions; β-adrenoceptor blockers stand out in numerous analyses as being a consistently beneficial class of drugs of patients across the entire spectrum of acute coronary syndromes.[5,38] It is therefore disappointing to see that inadequate numbers of patients receive β-blockers in acute myocardial infarction.[39]

The groundbreaking studies of DeWood led to the now commonplace practice of acute catheterization of myocardial infarction patients.[40] This initiated the reperfusion era of coronary care marked by the notable introductions of intracoronary and then intravenous thrombolysis, widespread use of aspirin, and development of primary percutaneous transluminal coronary angioplasty (PTCA) for acute myocardial infarction that have all contributed to a further decrement in the short-term mortality of infarction patients (Figure 2.2).

Triage of Patients for Admission to CCU

Despite the extensive numbers of CCUs, the actual availability of a CCU bed for a specific patient in an individual hospital may at times be limited. Selker has reported a gratifying ability of clinicians to adapt to CCU bed shortages without adverse impact on patient outcome.[41]

The decision to admit a patient with suspected acute myocardial infarction to a CCU carries with it important medical consequences for the patient and financial consequences for the healthcare delivery system. It is estimated that annually at least 750 000 to 1 million patients are admitted to CCUs in the USA, and 100 000 in the UK.[26,39] Although precise data are difficult to establish, at least 50% of patients admitted to CCUs in the USA are later proven not to have suffered an acute myocardial infarction, and perhaps as many as 5% of individuals who are seen in an emergency room but are discharged home are later proven to have a myocardial infarction.[28] Physicians evaluating patients in the emergency room for possible admission to the CCU face the difficult task of avoiding unnecessary admissions, but also minimizing the number of patients discharged home inappropriately. Furthermore, with the arrival of the reperfusion era and the desire to minimize 'door-to-needle' time for administration of thrombolytic agents or rapid triage to the catheterization laboratory for primary PTCA in appropriately selected patients, there is a clear need for better methods for prompt identification of patients truly experiencing an acute myocardial infarction as soon as possible.

A variety of triage aids have been evaluated, but the majority have been developed and assessed in the prethrombolytic era.[25] Such tools include identification of high-risk clinical indicators,[42,43] rapid determination of cardiac serum markers,[44,45] two-dimensional echocardiographic screening for regional wall motion abnormalities,[46] myocardial perfusion imaging,[47] and computer-based diagnostic aids.[48,49] Recently a prototype of a clinical and ECG algorithm for predicting the presence of acute myocardial infarction has been incorporated directly into a computerized electrocardiograph along with a statement of the patient's risk of adverse cardiovascular events with and without thrombolysis (Figure 2.3).[50] It is likely that future iterations of such programs will be applied clinically, especially in settings where access to cardiac specialists is limited.

In practice, criteria for admission to the CCU vary among institutions and are often driven more by availability of nursing and medical personnel and concerns about the desired location of a patient should an infrequent but potentially serious complication develop. There is little disagreement that all patients with complicated infarctions (e.g. cardiogenic shock) and/or those requiring sophisticated and labor-intensive treatments (e.g. intraaortic balloon counterpulsation) should be admitted to the CCU. In many hospitals physicians admit low-risk myocardial infarction patients to a coronary observation unit or stepdown unit where automated ECG monitoring and equipment for defibrillation are available although the scope of other medical facilities is reduced in such units (e.g. little if any capability for invasive hemodynamic monitoring and fewer nurses).

General Measures

Previously healthy individuals can be converted into anxious patients experiencing severe pain with an onset of acute myocardial infarction. Concerns about immediate mortality and future functional capacity and productivity can have a devastating impact on the psyche of the patient with acute myocardial infarction. It is mandatory, therefore, that the CCU be designed to provide a sedate professional atmosphere capable of bolstering a patient's confidence. During initial contact with the patient, CCU staff should indicate that the most critical phase of infarction has passed (pre-hospital coronary care) and the purpose of the CCU stay is to provide coordinated surveillance of the recovery process from acute infarction.

Amidst the dazzling array of high-technology equipment in the CCU it is easy to overlook the vitally important physician–patient interaction. Quiet conversation and a confident appearance on the part of the physician coupled with a liberal amount of 'laying on of hands' helps to bolster the patient's optimism and may also contribute to reduction in sympathetic tone and its attendant adverse effects (e.g. tachycardia, hypertension, arrhythmias).

The patient's maintenance medication program should be reviewed and adjusted if necessary to avoid hypoglycemia in diabetics and a drop in systolic blood pressure by

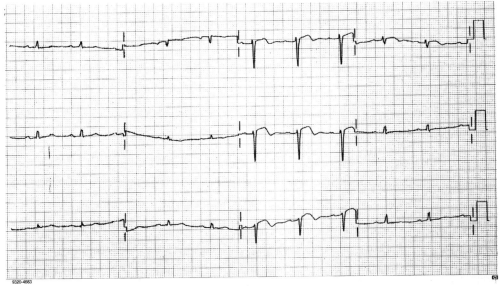

ECG User Input: Gender: **Male** Age: **53** Weight (kg): **100** Hx Diabetes: **no** Hx Hypertension: **no**
Time from symptom onset: **1 hrs 10 min** Blood Pressure: **110 / 60**

ECG Interpretation: HR: **55** Acute MI Location: **Anterior** ST Elevation: **V1, V2, V3, V4**
Abnormal Q waves: **none** QTc: **0.38**

Thrombolytic Predictive Instrument (TPI) Predicted Probabilities of Thrombolysis Outcomes:

if *not* treated with thrombolytic therapy		If treated with thrombolytic therapy	
Acute (30-day) mortality:	**13%**	Acute (30-day) mortality:	**4%**
One year mortality:	**19%**	One-year mortality:	**6%**
Cardiac arrest within 72 hours:	**4%**	Cardiac arrest within 72 hours:	**2%**
		Thrombolysis-related Hemorrhagic Stroke:	**0.2%**
		Thrombolysis-related Major Bleed:	**1.3%**

Figure 2.3 Acute cardiac ischemia time-insensitive predictive instrument (ACI-TIPI). Several investigators have developed mathematically based diagnostic aids to assist emergency department physicians in segregating patients with chest pain into subgroups with different likelihoods of acute myocardial infarction. Selker and coworker have developed a new time-insensitive predictive instrument for prospective real-time clinical use and retrospective medical record review. This triage aid instrument has been incorporated into an electrocardiograph. Under development is a thrombolytic predictive instrument (TPI) to provide clinicians with predicted probabilities of patient outcome with and without thrombolytic therapy. A prototype of the thrombolytic predictive instrument is shown for the case of a 53-year-old male presenting to the emergency department 1 hour and 10 min after the onset of chest pain resulting from an acute anterior myocardial infarct. (Tracing supplied courtesy of Dr Harry Selker, Boston, MA.)

more than 30 mmHg from usual levels. In view of the marked propensity for electrolyte disturbances to precipitate serious ventricular tachyarrhythmias the admission potassium and magnesium levels must be scrutinized.[51] We generally attempt to maintain the serum potassium at or above 4.5 mmol l^{-1} (mEq l^{-1}) and serum magnesium at or above 1.0 mmol l^{-1} (2.0 mEq l^{-1}).

Physical Activity

Experimental models of acute ischemia and infarction have confirmed that physical exercise increases the area of myocardial damage when coronary blood flow is limited.[52] Thus, there is a physiologic basis for placing patients with acute infarction at bedrest

Table 2.1   Activity progression following myocardial infarction

General guidelines
When progressing through the stages noted below specific activities should be stopped for increasing shortness of breath or the patient's perception of fatigue or detection of an increase in the heart rate of >20–30 beats min^{-1}. Vital signs should be monitored before and following progression from one stage to the next and also from one level to the next within each stage. Energy-conserving techniques should be emphasized and the use of prophylactic nitroglycerin should be reviewed with the patient

Stage I (day 1–2)
Use a bedpan/commode. Feed self-prepared tray with arm and back support. Complete assistance with bathing. Passive range of emotion (ROM) to all extremities. Active ankle motion (with footboard if available). Emphasis on relaxation and deep breathing
Partially bathe upper body with back support. Bed to chair transfers for 1–2 hours per day. Active ROM of all extremities 5–10 times (sitting or supine)

Stage II (day 3–4)
Bathe, groom, self-dress sitting on bed or chair. Bed to chair transfers ad lib. Ambulate in room with gradual increase in duration and frequency
May shower or stand at sink to bath. May dress in own clothes. Supervised ambulation outside of room (100–600 feet several times per day) (33–200 meters)
Partially bathe upper body with back support. Bed to chair 20–30 min daily. Active assisted to active ROM, all extremities: 5–10 times (sitting, or supine)

Stage III (day 5–7)
Ambulate 600 feet (200 meters) three times per day. May shampoo hair (e.g. activity with arms over head). Supervised stair walking.
Pre-discharge exercise tolerance test

during the first 6–12 hours. Believing that prolonged rest for a diseased organ was therapeutically beneficial led many clinicians to extend the period of bedrest for infarction patients to as long as 3–6 weeks. In a dramatic departure from this practice, Levine and Lown introduced the concept of early mobilization of the patient to a bedside armchair and reported an uncontrolled clinical experience in 81 patients who experienced a greater sense of well-being and reduction in dyspnea.[53] Several randomized, controlled trials subsequently confirmed the safety of early mobilization and reported a lower incidence of serious complications (recurrent infarction, pulmonary embolism, mortality) in patients mobilized early.[54,55]

Contemporary mobilization schedules are even more accelerated than those introduced just one or two decades ago. During the period of recovery and progressive mobilization it is important that the CCU staff not permit patients with uncomplicated infarction to abdicate responsibilities for self-care during activities of daily life, such as eating, teeth brushing, and shaving. Progression to use of the bedside chair should be encouraged within the first 24 hours and, with appropriate staff supervision, light ambulation about the room should be encouraged within 48 hours. A suggested scheme for activity progression is shown in Table 2.1.

Diet

In view of the clinical instability that may occur during the first 4–12 hours following admission to the CCU, patients should generally either receive nothing by mouth (NPO) or clear liquids only, although appropriate clinical judgment should be exercised on an individual basis. To minimize the risk of precipitation of angina by a heavy meal, the CCU diet should be designed so that the portions are not unusually large or bulky. Liberal quantities of foods containing glucose and electrolytes such as potassium and magnesium are typically recommended, although detailed metabolic balance studies such as those reported for burn patients are lacking in the case of acute infarction.

Table 2.2 Guidelines for diet therapy in the CCU

1. NPO prior to evaluation by physician
2. *Kilocalories and protein:* the diet should initially be planned to provide adequate kilocalories and protein to maintain the patient's initial weight. Caloric restrictions may subsequently be initiated for weight loss if needed
3. *Fats:* the diet should be limited to ≤30% of total calories from fat. Foods high in cholesterol and saturated fats should be avoided. One or two eggs per week may be given if requested and/or to ensure adequate protein intake; egg substitutes should also be available and encouraged
4. *Carbohydrates:* complex carbohydrates should constitute 50–55% of total calories
5. *Fiber:* the diet should contain fiber consistent with a balanced mixed diet, including fresh fruit and vegetable, whole-grain bread, and cereals. Foods that may cause gastrointestinal intolerance should be eliminated on an individual basis
6. *Sodium:* a 'no added salt' (NAS) diet (3–4 g Na$^+$) is recommended, with adjustment as indicated by clinical status. The NAS diet order excludes a salt shaker as well as foods high in sodium (greater than 300 mg per serving).
7. *Potassium:* food high in potassium should be encouraged except for patients with renal insufficiency
8. *Quantity:* small, frequent feedings may be recommended on an individual basis
9. *Fluids:* caffeine intake should be limited to less then 250 mg daily, i.e. use of regular coffee should be moderated. Decaffeinated beverages and weak tea are suggested as substitutes
10. *Education:* the principal goal of patient education and long-term planning is to achieve and maintain ideal body weight and to adhere to dietary adjustments as ordered by the physician

The dietary prescription should provide 30% or less of the total calories from fat by reducing saturated fats in the diet (Table 2.2). Cholesterol should be limited to ≤300 mg per day. Carbohydrates, especially complex carbohydrates, are prescribed for between 50 and 55% of total calories. Patients with documented diabetes or familial triglyceridemia should have simple carbohydrates limited by means of a 'no concentrated sweets' restriction.

The convalescent phase following myocardial infarction is an ideal time to familiarize the patient with the concept of lifestyle and dietary modification. The benefits of a diet low in total cholesterol and saturated fats should be emphasized. Recently the second report of the Expert Panel on Detection, Evaluation, and Treatment of High Blood Cholesterol in Adults (Adult Treatment Panel-II [ATP-II]) was published in the USA and specified that patients with established coronary heart disease and a low-density lipoprotein (LDL) level ≥2.6 mmol l^{-1} (100 mg dl^{-1}) should receive dietary therapy for secondary prevention of coronary events; those patients with an LDL cholesterol ≥3.4 mmol l^{-1} (130 mg dl^{-1}) should receive drug treatment.[56] While these guidelines were not specifically devised for patients with acute myocardial infarction, such individuals are the highest risk group for future events and in most cases there is no compelling reason to delay initiation of hypolipidemic therapy for those patients who qualify for treatment as per the new ATP-II criteria. There are disturbing reports that only a small proportion of patients with documented coronary heart disease and an abnormal lipid profile are actively treated for their disorder, indicating considerable room for improvement in clinical practice.[57]

It should be recalled that there can be a 60% reduction in total plasma cholesterol and LDL cholesterol values within the first few days after a myocardial infarction. However, values obtained within 48 hours of the event are valid measurements for planning long-term treatment needs.[58]

Oxygen

Following acute myocardial infarction, ventilation–perfusion abnormalities are common and are usually secondary to left ventricular dysfunction with an increase in left ventricular end diastolic pressure, ultimately resulting in an increase in lung water. Intrapulmonary shunting of blood may also occur when left ventricular failure develops, further contributing to the hypoxemia that is observed in patients with acute myocardial infarction.

Experimental data and clinical evidence support the concept that increased levels of oxygen in the inspired air protect the ischemic myocardium.[59] Thus, it is a common practice to treat all infarction patients with 100% oxygen, typically delivered via nasal prongs at a rate of $2-4 \, l \, min^{-1}$ for the first 24–48 hours. Preliminary results suggest that hyperbaric oxygen in combination with thrombolysis may reduce infarct size but the additional expense and complexity associated with this therapy necessitates further evaluation in larger clinical trials.[60]

If there is clinical suspicion of significant hypoxemia or if the patient has a history of chronic obstructive lung disease or anemia, arterial blood gases should be obtained and appropriate adjustments in the mode of delivery of supplemental oxygen should be made (e.g. use of a face mask and humidified air) while monitoring the arterial oxygen saturation by noninvasive methods. Patients with severe acute pulmonary edema and hypoxemia should undergo endotracheal intubation and controlled positive pressure ventilation. A variety of mechanical ventilators are available and multiple modes of ventilation are possible. For patients who do not have a depressed sensorium and are capable of initiating spontaneous ventilation, the modes we prefer to use include intermittent mandatory ventilation (SIMV), assist control (AC), or pressure support ventilation (PSV).[61]

Analgesia and Sedation

Patients with acute myocardial infarction typically exhibit overactivity of the sympathetic nervous system. This arises from a combination of chest pain and anxiety. Adverse consequences of sympathetic overactivity include an increase in myocardial oxygen demands via acceleration of the heart rate, elevation of arterial pressure, augmentation of cardiac contractility, and a heightened tendency to ventricular tachyarrhythmias.

Therefore, one of the primary therapeutic strategies during the acute phase of management of myocardial infarction patients is administration of sufficient doses of an analgesic such as diamorphine (utilized commonly in the UK) or morphine sulfate (the drug of choice in the USA). Morphine sulfate can be administered intravenously at a rate of 2–4 mg every 5 min or 4–8 mg every 5–15 min, as dictated by the clinical circumstances.[62,63] It is not uncommon for patients to require as much as 25–35 mg of morphine before adequate pain relief is established. Morphine sulfate should be administered in small increments to avoid paradoxic augmentation of sympathetic nervous system tone, respiratory depression, and hypotension. Respiratory depression related to morphine peaks about 7 min after intravenous administration and is directly related to the total dose administered. Depression of ventilatory efforts results from morphine's effects on the pontine and medullary centers responsible for controlling the rhythm of respiration, and from a morphine-induced reduction in the responsiveness of the brain stem to elevations in P_{CO_2}. Additionally, morphine in small doses can precipitate dramatic depression of ventilatory responses to hypoxia and to hypercapnia, raising the possibility that it may also affect peripheral chemoreceptor function. However, it is important to note that respiratory depression is usually not a significant clinical problem with administration of morphine to patients who have severe chest pain or pulmonary edema. Naloxone 0.4 mg i.v. at up to 3-min intervals to a maximum of three doses may be utilized to relieve any morphine-induced respiratory depression that occurs.

In contrast to the minor and relatively short-lived hemodynamic changes that morphine induces in normal subjects, patients with acute myocardial infarction can develop transient reductions in systemic arterial blood pressure. Peripheral vasodilatation induced by morphine can precipitate dramatic orthostatic hypotension, especially in patients with a decreased effective blood volume due to emesis and diaphoresis, or in the presence of other vasodilating drugs such as intravenous nitroglycerin. The hypotensive effects of morphine sulfate can be treated by having the patient assume the supine position and volume expansion.

Alternative intravenous narcotics that have been utilized in patients with acute infarction include meperidine or pentazocine, but they are generally not recommended because of a high incidence of adverse hemodynamic effects. For example, in a randomized double-blind study comparing morphine and pentazocine, cardiac work was increased by pentazocine due largely to its peripheral vasoconstrictor effects while cardiac work was actually reduced by morphine.[64]

A number of new synthetic and semisynthetic narcotic agents such as fentanyl and sufentanil are used in cardiac anesthesia for open heart surgery, but experience in the acute infarction setting is limited and it is unlikely that they will be shown to offer sufficient advantages over morphine to warrant their greater cost for the patient with routine myocardial infarction.[62,63] While patient-controlled administration of analgesic agents (PCA) such as morphine sulfate is now used commonly for relief of postoperative pain, application of PCA units in the acute infarction setting has not been rigorously evaluated and cannot be endorsed without proper clinical trials. Thoracic epidural anesthesia (TEA) has been shown to have beneficial effects on the ischemic myocardium including reduction in the determinants of myocardial oxygen consumption (blockade of cardiac sympathetic afferent and efferent fibers), attenuation of lactate production, improvement of global and regional left ventricular function, and dilatation of stenotic epicardial coronary segments.[65–67] Application of TEA and other alternative means of pain relief (e.g. intrathecal morphine) in patients with acute infarction remain largely anecdotal at present; these methods may be considered in patients with intractable pain despite more conventional measures and will possibly assume a more prominent role in the CCU management of ischemic pain as additional clinical experience is reported.[62,63,67]

Although used much less frequently in contemporary clinical practice, inhalation of nitrous oxide in a maintenance range of 30–40% blended with oxygen and delivered by face mask has been employed for analgesia in patients with acute myocardial infarction.[68] A 50% mixture of nitrous oxide lowers myocardial oxygen requirements by reducing heart rate and cardiac output.[69] The background sedation also provided by nitrous oxide is an additive benefit, but the side-effects of nausea, vomiting, hyperexcitability, obtundation, and after prolonged administration bone marrow depression, coupled with unfamiliarity of its use on the part of many physicians, has led to a marked decline and near elimination of administration of nitrous oxide in the CCU.[62]

Anxiolytics should be liberally provided to patients with acute infarction. All the benzodiazepines are capable of relieving anxiety and promoting drowsiness, but their proper use is dependent on a thorough understanding of relative potencies and important pharmacokinetic and pharmacodynamic properties.[70] Patients with agitation and delirium (disorientation, impaired memory, disordered sleep) may be seen commonly in the CCU, particularly with complicated myocardial infarctions and protracted stays in an intensive care setting.[70] Many drugs frequently used in the CCU are capable of inducing delirium (Table 2.3). Other causes include low cardiac output, hypoxia, anemia, and central nervous system depression following a cardiac arrest. Patients suffering from delirium that is the result of an adverse reaction to a medication should have the offending agent discontinued. A neuroleptic that can be given safely and effectively even in high doses to cardiac patients is haloperidol.[70] This butyrophenone has a rapid onset of action (11 min) and minimal effects on hemodynamics and respiration. Dosing can begin at 2 mg intravenously for mildly agitated patients and 5–10 mg for progressively

Table 2.3 Common delirium-inducing drugs used in the CCU

Drug group	Agent
Antiarryhythmics	Lidocaine
	Mexiletine
	Procainamide hydrochloride
	Quinidine sulfate
Anticholinergics	Atropine sulfate
Antihistamines	
Nonselective	Diphenhydramine hydrochloride
	Promethazine hydrochloride
H$_2$ blockers	Cimetidine
	Ranitidine hydrochloride
β-Blockers	Propranolol hydrochloride
Narcotic analgesics	Meperidine hydrochloride
	Pentazocine

Reproduced with permission from Ref. 70.

more agitated patients. As emphasized by Stern, intravenous haloperidol is an attractive agent for treatment of agitation in the CCU since the hypotension and endotracheal intubation that may complicate the use of intravenous narcotics and benzodiazepines is rare with intravenous haloperidol.[70]

Monitoring

Noninvasive

Equipment is available in contemporary CCUs for the noninvasive monitoring of the patient's ECG (single and multiple lead) for assessment of cardiac rhythm and ST segment deviation, arterial blood pressure, and arterial oxygen saturation (Figure 2.4).

Although skilled CCU staff can become quite adept at detecting cardiac arrhythmias by continuous visual surveillance of oscilloscopes at the patient's bedside and at central monitoring stations, it has been shown that computer algorithms for detection of arrhythmias is far superior to that of nursing and physician personnel.[71] Technical standards for instrumentation and electrocardiographic monitoring in special care units have been proposed as well as guidelines for integration of the nursing and medical staff with the equipment.[72] Automated ECG monitoring systems perform well in the majority of patients but it should be noted that even sophisticated contemporary units are susceptible to error due to patient movement and artifacts or noise on the signal (Figure 2.5). In addition, there is the possibility, albeit extremely rare, that the low-resistance path formed by the monitoring cables attached to the patient could allow delivery of electrical current from the wall plug with provocation of ventricular fibrillation. This catastrophe can be avoided by periodic preventive maintenance to ensure proper grounding and insulation of all equipment in contact with the patient. Good skin preparation, use of conducting gels, and incorporation of well-designed preamplifiers and buffer amplifiers are important factors that contribute to the integrity of the ECG signal.

Noninvasive monitoring of arterial blood pressure via a sphygmomanometric cuff that undergoes inflation and deflation cycles at programmed intervals can be readily learned and used with a minimum of training and expertise. The atraumatic nature of the monitoring technique and lack of complications (e.g. especially sepsis, which is a serious hazard with indwelling arterial lines) adds to the appeal of this method of blood pressure measurement. Advances in equipment technology and the availability of modules for noninvasive blood pressure (NIBP) measurement that can be transported from one patient's bedside to another have led to the increased popularity of this technique. While NIBP can replace invasive arterial monitoring using an indwelling catheter in many patients and relieve busy nursing staff from the responsibilities of frequent measurements of a patient's blood pressure, there are certain limitations of NIBP that should be recognized. It does not allow direct arterial pressure waveforms to be displayed and the measurements are obtained only on an intermittent basis. Sampling for arterial blood gases and other laboratory tests is not possible with NIBP. The accuracy of NIBP measurements can be adversely affected by mechanical factors such as cuff size, muscle contractions, and serious discrepancies can develop in critically ill patients with peripheral vasoconstriction in whom inaccurate and at times falsely low blood pressure readings may be obtained.

Invasive

While most skilled clinicians can readily distinguish at the bedside those patients with normal hemodynamics and a low risk of mortality from those with peripheral hypoperfusion and pulmonary congestion, it is frequently difficult to plan therapy for the latter group based solely on the physical examination of the patient and review of the chest X-ray and laboratory data. In a classic CCU study, Forrester and colleagues used a pulmonary artery balloon flotation catheter to evaluate the hemodynamics in 200 patients with acute myocardial infarction at the time of hospital admission (Figure 2.6).[73] Since cardiac performance is most appropriately evaluated by assessing the relationship between ventricular filling pressures and cardiac index (or stroke index), these investigators plotted the measured pulmonary capillary wedge pressure and simultaneously calculated cardiac index and correlated these observations with the probability of survival. When cardiac index was $<2.2 \, \mathrm{l \, min^{-1} \, m^{-2}}$ and pulmonary artery wedge pressure $>18 \, \mathrm{mmHg}$ on admission, a higher in-hospital mortality was likely (see the lower right-hand quadrant of Figure 2.6). The hemodynamic subsets proposed by Forrester based on invasive monitoring bear a close relationship but do not overlap completely with the clinically based hemodynamic classification proposed 10 years earlier (1967) by Killip and Kimball (see Table 2.4).[74] The mortality trends listed in Table 2.4 are probably still qualitatively accurate in the current reperfusion era of management of patients with acute myocardial infarction, but the quantitative estimates are grossly inflated compared with what would be observed in contemporary CCU patients who now receive the benefits of two to three decades of advances in coronary care medicine since the original reports by Killip and Kimball and Forrester *et al.*

Undoubtedly, the flow-directed pulmonary artery catheter (Figure 2.7) and invasive arterial line monitoring have revolutionized the practice of critical care medicine by allowing clinicians to perform sophisticated hemodynamic monitoring at the patient's bedside but appropriate selection of patients (Table 2.5) and site of invasive access (Table 2.6) along with operator experience are required to employ these invasive tools safely (Figure 2.8). Interpretation of hemodynamic data and therapeutic management of congestive heart failure, cardiogenic shock, right ventricular infarction, and mechanical complications such as ventricular septal defect and mitral regurgitation are discussed in more detail in Chapter 12. Typical hemodynamic formulae used for hemodynamic monitoring in the CCU are shown in Table 2.7 and profiles of common clinical conditions seen in the CCU are shown in Table 2.8.

(a)

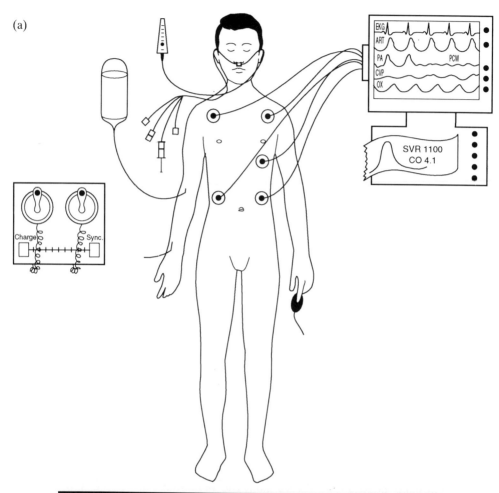

(b)

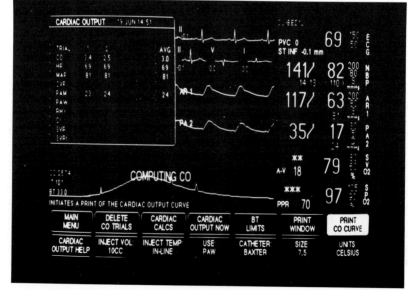

Table 2.4 Hemodynamic classifications of patients with acute myocardial infarction

	A. Based on clinical examination[a]			B. Based on invasive monitoring.[b]	
Class	Definition	Mortality (%)	Subset	Definition	Mortality (%)
I	Rales and S3 absent	8	I	Normal hemodynamics PCWP <18, CI >2.2	2
II	Rales over <50% of lung	30	II	Pulmonary congestion PCWP >18, CI <2.2	10
III	Rales over >50% of lung fields (pulmonary edema)	44	III	Peripheral hypoperfusion PCWP <18, CI >2.2	22
IV	Shock	80–100	IV	Pulmonary congestion and peripheral hypoperfusion PCWP >18, CI < 2.2	56

Reproduced with permission from Rakel, R.A. (1984) *Conn's Current Therapy*. Philadelphia: W.B. Saunders.
[a] Modified from Ref. 74.
[b] Modified from Ref. 73.
PWCP, pulmonary capillary wedge pressure; CI, cardiac index.

Figure 2.4 Invasive and noninvasive monitoring equipment typically used in the CCU. (a) The patient's heart rhythm is monitored via a multilead cable providing a minimum of one ECG lead but ideally programmable so that multiple ECG leads can be monitored simultaneously. In addition, contemporary monitoring devices are capable of on-line assessment of ST segment deviation. The rhythm and ST segment data are displayed at a multichannel bedside oscilloscope, which in turn transmits its information to a central monitoring system capable of displaying electrocardiographic traces from all patients in the intensive care unit in one or more prominent locations in the CCU so that the staff can perform visual surveillance of the electrocardiographic signals. Sophisticated algorithms for automated detection of arrhythmias and ST segment deviation outside of programmable limits trigger alarms locally at the patient's bedside and centrally to alert staff members to potentially significant alterations in the patient's condition. Arterial pressure can be monitored via direct cannulation of the arterial system (typically at the radial artery), but also can be monitored noninvasively with a blood pressure cuff that is programmed to cycle through inflation and deflation sequences at regular intervals (not shown). In addition, through a single multilumen catheter, several pressure waveforms can be displayed simultaneously; typically the CVP (right atrial) pressure and pulmonary arterial (PA) pressure are monitored continuously. Intermittently, as desired by the staff, pulmonary capillary wedge (PCW) pressure can be displayed. Through the same catheter, thermodilution cardiac output (CO) measurements can be obtained. The hemodynamic waveforms and cardiac output curves along with standard calculations (e.g. systemic vascular resistance) can be printed on multichannel strip chart recorders at the bedside. Supplemental oxygen is delivered usually by nasal prongs with a flow rate that is adjusted using a wall-mounted flow meter. Oxygen saturation of the patient's arterial blood can be monitored continuously noninvasively using an oximetric recording method with probes placed on the patient's fingertip or earlobe. Apparatus capable of delivering multiple energy levels of electrical shock for defibrillation or synchronized cardioversion is available either at the bedside or can be rapidly brought to the patient's bedside from a central location in the unit. (b) Example of the use of the multichannel bedside oscilloscope for the management of a patient with acute myocardial infarction. In the top center portion of the figure, ECG lead II is displayed and below that is depicted continuous ST segment monitoring of ECG lead II, a precordial lead (V) and lead I. Two hemodynamic pressures are displayed, systemic arterial pressure (AR1) and pulmonary arterial pressure (PA2). Along the upper right-hand portion of the figure in descending order of appearance are seen the continuous display of heart rate, noninvasive blood pressure (NBP), systemic arterial pressure (AR1), pulmonary arterial pressure (PA2), mixed venous oxygen saturation (SVO2), and oxygen saturation via pulse oximeter (SPO2). A thermodilution cardiac output curve (CO) is displayed along the bottom of the figure. Previous cardiac output curves and associated hemodynamic calculations are provided for reference. The buttons along the bottom provide the user with access to other menu options such as pulmonary capillary wedge measurement, 12-lead ECG acquisition and interpretation, and summary reports of stored data on arrhythmias, hemodynamic measurements, and ST segment deviation. (Courtesy of Marquette Electronics, Milwaukee, WI.)

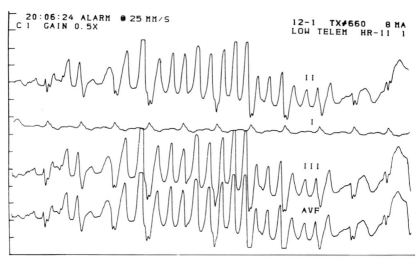

Figure 2.5 'Pseudo-ventricular tachycardia' detected on multiple-lead electrocardiographic monitoring. In this tracing the four ECG leads are recorded simultaneously. One of the monitoring electrodes has lost contact with the patient's skin and skeletal muscle movement from teeth brushing has produced an artifact mimicking ventricular tachycardia. Note, one of the ECG leads continues to record sinus rhythm during the artifact confirming clinical stability of the patient rather than a life-threatening ventricular tachyarrhythmia. This figure reinforces the propensity for even sophisticated ECG monitoring equipment to register artifacts and also illustrates the benefits of simultaneous multiple lead monitoring.

Concern has arisen that the overzealous use of pulmonary artery catheters may be associated with adverse clinical consequences. It is difficult to determine the exact incidence of complications related to use of pulmonary artery catheters. Most large series report an incidence of major complications between 3 and 5%, and, depending upon the definition, minor complications in 20–25% of patients.[75] Gore et al. reported higher case fatality rates in myocardial infarction patients complicated by congestive heart failure or hypotension who underwent invasive hemodynamic monitoring with a pulmonary artery catheter compared to those who were treated without a pulmonary artery catheter.[76] However, inadequacies of medical documentation, changes in medical therapy for myocardial infarction during the period of study, and the possibility of incomplete adjustment for severity of illness suggest a need for caution before declaring a moratorium on the use of pulmonary artery catheters as has been suggested by some authors.[77]

Invasive arterial monitoring is the preferred method for blood pressure measurement in patients with a low-output syndrome and can provide more reliable information for titration of inotropic therapy in patients with severe left ventricular failure. In addition to any local arterial pathology that is present at the site of cannulation, the risks associated with invasive arterial monitoring are directly related to operator experience and the duration of time the catheter remains in the patient's vasculature.

Thrombolytic Therapy: Indications and Selection of Patients
(see Chapter 3)

Randomized controlled trials have demonstrated unequivocally that thrombolytic therapy for acute myocardial infarction with ST segment elevation on the ECG reduces

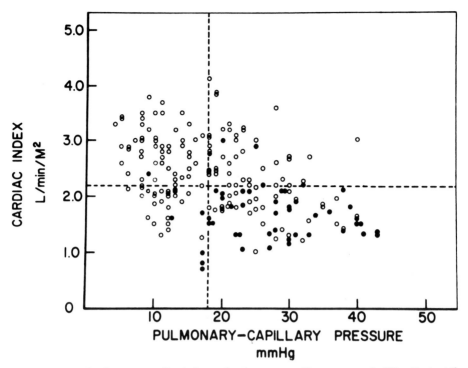

Figure 2.6 Relationship between cardiac index and pulmonary capillary pressure in 200 patients at the time of hospital admission. There is a wide degree of variability in left ventricular performance in patients with acute myocardial infarction. The mortality rate increases as cardiac performance deteriorates. The majority of individuals who are nonsurvivors are those with cardiac indices below $2.21 \text{min}^{-1}\text{m}^{-2}$ and pulmonary capillary wedge pressures above 18 mmHg at admission (see lower right-hand quadrant of figure). ○, Survivors; ●, nonsurvivors. (Reproduced with permission from Ref. 73.)

mortality. Despite the totality of evidence documenting the benefits of thrombolytic therapy and the lack of dispute about the mortality reduction observed in clinical trials, it is disturbing that only approximately 35% of individuals presenting with acute myocardial infarction actually receive thrombolytic therapy in the USA.[78–81] Considerable international variation exists in the proportion of patients with myocardial infarction who receive thrombolytic therapy; about 50% of European patients receive thrombolytics and at least 70% of patients enrolled in the ISIS-4 and GISSI-3 trials were treated with thrombolytics. Paradoxically, those individuals who do not receive lytic therapy are at higher risk for adverse cardiovascular events.[82] Understandably, clinicians carefully weigh the risk–benefit ratio for individual patients. Hesitancy to prescribe thrombolytic therapy arises from uncertainty regarding the eligibility criteria for thrombolysis and uncertainty about contraindications to thrombolytic therapy.[83] Failure to appreciate the magnitude of the benefits of thrombolytic therapy (e.g. streptokinase plus aspirin reduced mortality by 50% in patients treated within 1 hour of the onset of chest discomfort in ISIS-2[84]) coupled with data that patients with acute myocardial infarction who are not treated with thrombolytic therapy because of 'ineligibility' have an unacceptably high mortality rate underscores the continued need for educational programs to disseminate information about this vitally important and life-saving mode of therapy for acute infarction. Funding agencies such as the National Heart, Lung, and Blood Institute in the USA have developed initiatives such as the National Heart Attack Alert Program to close knowledge gaps and shorten the 'door-to-needle' time (Figure 2.9).

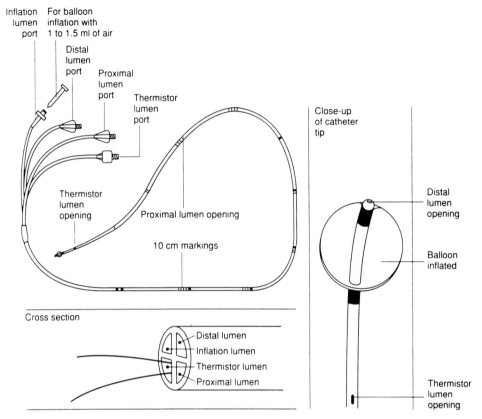

Figure 2.7 Anatomy of the pulmonary artery balloon flotation catheter (Swan–Ganz catheter). This multiple-lumen catheter has distal and proximal ports for hemodynamic monitoring and injection of medications as well as ports for inflation of the balloon and temperature sampling (thermistor lumen). (Reproduced with permission from *Nursing* (1981) **81**, 11[1].)

The fundamental elements that must all be present (although not necessarily exactly at the same time) that serve as standard indications for administration of thrombolytic therapy to patients with acute myocardial infarction are shown in Table 2.9. In view of the risks of bleeding from peptic ulcer disease and aortic dissection, clinicians should be convinced that the patient's chest pain is typical of myocardial ischemia.

ECG Pattern

Since thrombolytic therapy is of benefit in patients with Q-wave myocardial infarction (resulting from thrombotic occlusion of an epicardial coronary artery in 90% of cases) and is of little benefit in patients with unstable angina or non-Q-wave myocardial infarction, current practice dictates that the ECG should be reviewed before administration of thrombolytic therapy. In patients with ischemic-type chest pain, ST segment elevation has a specificity of 91% and sensitivity of 46% for diagnosing acute myocardial infarction.[85] If ST segment elevation or depression is considered, the sensitivity increases to 77% but the specificity falls to 75%.[85] Experience in trials of thrombolytic therapy for unstable angina and non-Q-wave infarction where the presenting electrocardiographic

Table 2.5 Indications for invasive hemodynamic monitoring in acute myocardial infarction

Management of hemodynamically complicated acute myocardial infarction
  Severe left ventricular failure
  Low-output syndrome (cardiogenic shock vs hypovolemic shock)
  Mechanical lesions (severe mitral regurgitation, ventricular septal rupture, subacute cardiac rupture
    with tamponade)
  Right ventricular infarction
  Refractory arrhythmias (e.g. ventricular tachycardia, atrial fibrillation) that may be a result of in-
    adequately treated hemodynamic abnormalities

Evaluating the effects of mechanical ventilation and differentiating pulmonary disease vs left ventricular
failure as the cause of hypoxemia and/or 'rales'

Assessment of the hemodynamic impact of therapeutic maneuvers in selected patients
  Intraaortic balloon counterpulsation
  Atrial versus ventricular pacing
  β-Blockade
  Inotropic therapy
  Afterload reduction for left ventricular failure

Septic shock

abnormality was frequently ST segment depression indicate an increased risk of fatal and nonfatal infarction and reinfarction in the group receiving thrombolysis.[86]
  For the reasons discussed above, and the findings of DeWood and colleagues that the correlation between ST segment depression or T-wave changes on the ECG and intraluminal thrombus is considerably weaker than the correlation with ST segment elevation, thrombolytic agents should only be administered to patients with ST segment elevation ≥ 0.1 mV on the ECG. Data from the ISIS-2 investigators suggest that patients

Table 2.6 Comparison of arterial sites for invasive blood pressure monitoring

Site	Advantages	Disadvantages	Comment
Radial artery	Superficial, easily compressible Good collateral flow Easy to keep sterile	Comparatively small vessel Difficult to cannulate in hypotensive and vasoconstricted patients Necrosis of overlying skin may occur	Most common site for intra-arterial monitoring Use a modified Allen test for adequacy of the collateral circulation Insert cannula as distally as possible
Femoral artery	Large vessel, accessible even with patients in shock or with vasoconstricted states	Difficult to keep sterile and to compress Higher incidence of hematoma and retroperitoneal hemorrhage	Avoid puncturing the artery above the inguinal ligament
Brachial artery	Easily palpable	Less good collateral flow May lead to ischemic loss of hand and forearm Subfascial hematoma may lead to compression syndromes, including median nerve neuropathy and Volkmann ischemic contracture	Avoid routine use Avoid using in patients receiving anticoagulants or with bleeding disorders

Adapted from Amin, D.K., Shah, P.K. and Swan, H.J.C. (1993) The Swan–Ganz catheter: Techniques for avoiding common errors. *J. Critical Illness*, **8**, 1263–71.

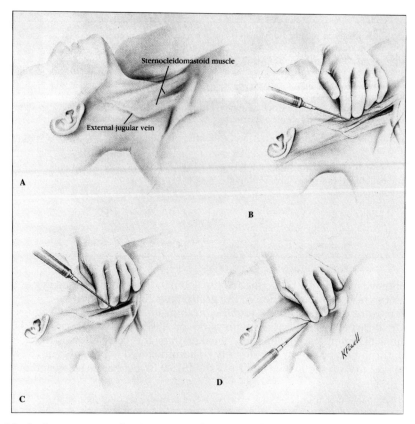

Figure 2.8 Surface anatomy and various approaches to cannulation of the internal jugular vein. Panels A–D illustrate the surface anatomy, anterior approach, central approach, and posterior approach to cannulation of the internal jugular vein. (Reproduced with permission from Rippe, J.M. *et al.* (1985) *Intensive Care Medicine.* Boston: Little, Brown.)

with bundle branch block and a clinical presentation strongly suggesting an evolving acute myocardial infarction should also be considered suitable candidates for thrombolytic therapy.[84]

Timing of Lytic Therapy

Previous recommendations stated that thrombolytic therapy should be initiated within 6 hours of the onset of symptoms. This was derived in part from the experimental pathology studies of Reimer *et al.* illustrating a time-dependent 'wavefront of necrosis' spreading from the subendocardium to subepicardium that is complete in approximately 6 hours in dogs.[87] Since myocardial salvage increases with progressively earlier administration of thrombolytic therapy, five trials have evaluated the relative benefits of prehospital versus hospital administration of thrombolytic agents.[88–92] A variety of lytic agents were studied, and the mean interval from the onset of chest discomfort to administration of thrombolytic therapy between the pre-hospital and hospital groups ranged between 33 and 130 min. Although no individual trial had sufficient power to

Table 2.7 Hemodynamic formulae commonly used in the CCU

Cardiac output (CO) = HR × SV
Cardiac index (CI) = CO/BSA
Stroke volume (SV) = CO/HR
Stroke index (SI) = SV/BSA or CI/HR

$$\text{Left ventricular stroke work index (LVSWI)} = \frac{1.36 \times (\text{MAP} - \text{PCWP}) \times \text{SI}}{100}$$

$$\text{Systemic vascular resistance (SVR)} = \frac{(\text{MAP} - \text{RAP})}{\text{CO}} \times 80$$

$$\text{Pulmonary vascular resistance (PVR)} = \frac{(\text{PAP} - \text{PCWP})}{\text{CO}} \times 80$$

$$\text{Mean arterial pressure (MAP)} = \frac{(2 \times \text{diastolic}) + \text{systolic}}{3}$$

$$\text{Ejection fraction} = \frac{\text{SV}}{\text{end-diastolic volume}} \times 100$$

BSA, body surface area; HR, heart rate; MAP, mean arterial pressure; PAP, mean pulmonary pressure; PCWP, pulmonary capillary wedge pressure; RAP, right atrial pressure; SV, stroke volume.

Table 2.8 Hemodynamic patterns for common clinical conditions

Cardiac condition	Chamber pressures (mmHg)				
	RA	RV	PA	PCW	CI
Normal	0–6	25/0–6	25/0–12	6–12	≥2.5
AMI without LVF	0–6	25/0–6	30/12–18	≤18	≥2.5
AMI with LVF	0–6	30–40/0–6	30–40/18–25	>18	>2.0
Biventricular failure	>6	50–60/>6	50–60/25	18–25	>2.0
RVMI	12–20	30/12–20	30/12	≤12	<2.0
Cardiac tamponade	12–16	25/12–16	25/12–16	12–16	<2.0
Pulmonary embolism	12–20	50–60/12–20	50–60/12	<12	<2.0

Reproduced with permission from Gore, J.M. and Zwerner, P.L. (1990) Hemodynamic monitoring of acute myocardial infarction. In: Francis, G.S. and Alpert, J.S. (eds) *Modern Coronary Care*, pp. 139–64. Boston: Little, Brown and Co.
AMI, acute myocardial infarction; CI, cardiac index; LVF, left ventricular failure; PA, pulmonary artery; PCW, pulmonary capillary wedge; RA, right atrium; RV, right ventricle; RVMI, right ventricular myocardial infarction.

demonstrate a statistically significant effect of the pre-hospital administration of thrombolytic therapy, the pooled results indicate a 17% reduction in the risk of short-term mortality if thrombolytic therapy is administered prior to arrival in the hospital.[92]

A detailed report from one of the studies, the EMIP trial, clearly documented a reduction in cardiovascular mortality in those patients who received thrombolytic therapy (APSAC) prior to hospital arrival but who survived following treatment in the field to have their care continued in the hospital, as compared with those who did not receive thrombolytic therapy until they arrived in the hospital (in-hospital mortality in the pre-hospital group was 7.8% vs in-hospital mortality in the hospital treatment group of 9.6%).[92] Concern was raised about an excess mortality 'in the field' in the pre-hospital treatment group vs the hospital treatment group (1.3% pre-hospital mortality vs 0.9%). Indeed, a small 'early hazard' (excess of deaths early after fibrinolytic therapy on day 0–1)

Speeding Time to Treatment ——————————

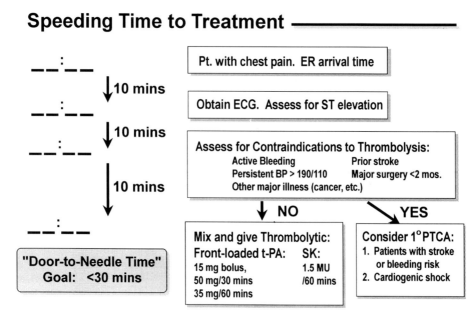

Figure 2.9 Algorithm for rapid triage of patients in the emergency room (ER) to provide thrombolysis with the shortest possible 'door-to-needle' time. (Figure courtesy of Dr Chris Cannon, Brigham and Women's Hospital, Boston, MA.)

in thrombolytic-treated patients has been reported in GISSI-1, ISIS-2, and in a recent collaborative overview of nine large trials by the Fibrinolytic Therapy Trialists (FTT).[84,93,94] The mechanism of the early excessive deaths with fibrinolytic therapy is unclear, but may be due to a combination of reperfusion injury and myocardial rupture. Nevertheless, this small early hazard is far outweighed by the survival advantage experienced in patients who receive thrombolytic therapy, particularly in those cases at higher risk of cardiovascular mortality. Clinicians should strive to quickly identify suitable candidates for thrombolysis (Table 2.9) and expeditiously administer treatment.

Two trials (LATE and EMERAS) evaluated whether the benefits of thrombolytic therapy could be extended beyond a time window of 6 hours from the onset of chest discomfort. These trials evaluated recombinant tissue plasminogen activator (rt-PA) and anisoylated plasminogen streptokinase activator complex (APSAC) respectively in patients treated 6–24 hours after the onset of chest pain.[95,96] A consistent observation between the two trials was that individuals who received thrombolytic therapy between 6 and 12 hours had a significantly lower mortality compared with placebo (albeit a somewhat smaller relative reduction in mortality compared with previously reported results of patients treated within 6 hours). No benefit was seen in patients who were treated with thrombolytic therapy between 12 and 24 hours. In conjunction with subgroup analyses in the ISIS-2 and GISSI-2 studies, these two trials, taken together, now provide the basis for administration of thrombolytic therapy up to 12 hours after the onset of chest pain. On an individual patient basis it may be appropriate to consider administration of thrombolytic therapy even beyond 12 hours (e.g. young individual with continued chest pain, ST segment elevation, and evidence of extensive anterior myocardial infarction on ECG), but insufficient data are available even from overviews of multiple trials to provide firm guidelines about selection of patients for thrombolysis beyond 12 hours from the onset of chest pain.

Table 2.9 Criteria for thrombolysis in acute myocardial infarction

Indications
1. Chest pain consistent with acute myocardial infarction
2. Electrocardiographic changes
   ST-segment elevation >0.1 mv in at least two contiguous leads
   New or presumably new left bundle-branch block
3. Time from onset of symptoms
   <6 hours: most beneficial
   6–12 hours: lesser but still important benefits
   >12 hours: diminishing benefits but still useful

Absolute contraindications
1. Active internal bleeding
2. Suspected aortic dissection
3. Prolonged or traumatic cardiopulmonary resuscitation
4. Recent head trauma or known intracranial neoplasm
5. Diabetic hemorrhagic retinopathy or other hemorrhagic ophthalmic condition
6. Pregnancy
7. Previous allergic reaction to the thrombolytic agent (streptokinase or APSAC)
8. Recorded blood pressure >200/120 mmHg
9. History of cerebrovascular accident known to be hemorrhagic

Relative contraindications[a]
1. Recent trauma or surgery >2 weeks; trauma or surgery more recent than 2 weeks, which could be a source of rebleeding, is an absolute contraindication
2. History of chronic, severe hypertension with or without drug therapy
3. Active peptic ulcer
4. History of cerebrovascular accident
5. Known bleeding diathesis or current use of anticoagulants
6. Significant liver dysfunction
7. Prior exposure to streptokinase or APSAC (this contraindication is particularly important in the initial 6–9-month period after streptokinase or APSAC administration and applies to reuse of any streptokinase-containing agent, but does not apply to rt-PA or urokinase)

Adapted from: AHA Medical/Scientific Statement Special Report (1990) ACC/AHA guidelines for the early management of patients with acute myocardial infarction. *Circulation*, **82**, 664–707; Anderson, H.V. and Willerson, J.T. (1993) Thrombolysis in acute myocardial infarction. *N. Engl. J. Med.*, **329**, 703–9.
[a]These should be considered on a case-by-case analysis or risk vs benefit. In instances where these contraindications (particularly 1 to 5) have paramount importance, such as more recent trauma or surgery or active peptic ulcer with history of bleeding, they become absolute contraindications when weighed against a less than life-threatening, evolving acute myocardial infarction.

Elderly Patients

Large randomized trials of thrombolytic therapy for acute infarction usually excluded patients older than 70–75 years of age because of concerns about an increased risk of bleeding complications. Common barriers to treatment of older patients with acute myocardial infarction in general practice include a greater delay in seeking medical care, a decreased incidence of chest pain, and increased frequency of atypical symptoms and concomitant illnesses, and an increased incidence of nondiagnostic ECGs. Although younger patients achieve a slightly greater relative reduction in mortality compared with older patients, the higher absolute mortality rate in the elderly results in similar absolute mortality reductions (Figure 2.10).[94,97] As expected, advanced age does increase the risk of stroke following acute myocardial infarction. In a recent decision-analytic model to evaluate the cost-effectiveness of thrombolysis in the elderly with acute infarction, Krumholz and colleagues estimated that adminstration of streptokinase to an 80-year-old patient with acute myocardial infarction was associated with a cost of \$21 200 for each year of life saved.[98] The cost-effectiveness ratio did not change significantly for patients a

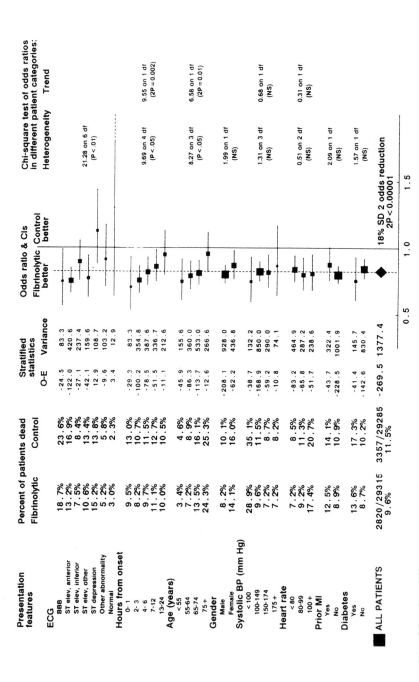

Figure 2.10 Mortality differences during day 0–35 subdivided by presentation features in a collaborative overview of results from nine trials of thrombolytic therapy. The absolute mortality rates are shown for fibrinolytic and control groups in the center portion of the figure for each clinical feature at presentation listed on the left side of the figure. The ratio of the odds of death in the fibrinolytic group to that in the control group is shown for each subdivision (black square) along with its 95% confidence interval (horizontal line). The summary odds ratio at the bottom of the figure corresponds to an 18% proportional reduction in 35-day mortality and is highly statistically significant. This translates to a reduction of 18 deaths per 1000 patients treated with thrombolytic agents. (Reproduced with permission from Ref. 94.)

decade younger ($21 600 per year of life saved for 70-year-old patient) but increased by a factor of 2–2.5 as the risk of stroke and cost of caring for a stroke victim increased about fourfold above the baseline assumptions of an overall rate of stroke of 1.3% and cost of $200 000 to care for a stroke victim.

The excess of deaths on day 0–1 reported earlier from the FTT Collaborative Group Overview was also seen in patients with increasing age, but so too was the reduction in deaths during days 2–35.[94] Thus, neither the increased risk of stroke or 'early hazard' on day 0–1 outweigh the marked reductions in 35-day mortality observed with fibrinolytic therapy in elderly patients and clinicians should therefore not consider advanced age a contraindication to thrombolytic therapy; the elderly have the most to gain in view of their higher absolute mortality risk and therefore should be considered appropriate candidates for life-saving therapies such as thrombolysis.

Location of Infarction

From the data shown in Figure 2.10 it can be seen that patients presenting with anterior ST segment elevation have nearly twice the absolute baseline mortality risk compared with patients presenting with ST segment elevation in the inferior leads. Since the *proportionate* reduction in mortality with thrombolytic therapy is approximately the same for patients with anterior and inferior ST segment elevation, the absolute benefits are larger in patients with anterior ST segment elevation. Probably of at least equal significance to the exact site of infarction is the size of infarction as predicted by the number of ECG leads showing ST segment elevation. Patients with eight to nine leads showing ST segment elevation at presentation have three to four fold higher mortality compared with those with only two to three leads showing ST segment elevation at presentation.[99]

Other Clinical Features

It is possible to integrate numerous clinical variables at presentation and estimate a patient's mortality risk prior to administration of thrombolytic therapy. The TIMI-II investigators classified patients as low risk if they *lacked* any of the following: age ⩾70 years, previous infarction, atrial fibrillation, anterior infarction, rales in more than one-third of the lung fields, hypotension and sinus tachycardia, female gender, and diabetes mellitus.[100] However, scrutiny of Figure 2.10 indicates that clinicians should not *preclude* patients from consideration of thrombolytic therapy based only on gender, presenting systolic blood pressure, heart rate, history of myocardial infarction, or history of diabetes when evaluating potential benefits of thrombolytic therapy.

Based on the short-term (6 week) and long-term (3 year) follow-up of the TIMI-II trial, it is reasonable to conclude that the decision to administer a thrombolytic agent to a patient with an acute myocardial infarction is *not* automatically coupled to an invasive management strategy. The TIMI-II investigators demonstrated that following thrombolysis there was no advantage either in mortality reduction or prevention of reinfarction with an invasive approach compared with a conservative strategy of reserving cardiac catheterization and revascularization for patients with spontaneous or provocable ischemia provided that patients had appropriate access to a catheterization facility in the event of spontaneous or provocable ischemia.[101] Also, the infrequent development of recurrent myocardial infarction during the 2–3 year follow-up of TIMI-II patients suggest that no new advantage for the invasive surgery is likely to be found on longer follow-up.

Risk of Stroke

Treatment with thrombolytic therapy, however, is associated with a slight but significant excess of stroke that occurs early after the start of treatment (predominantly day 0–1).[94] Using a case-control method of data analysis in 150 patients with documented intracranial hemorrhage in five randomized controlled trials, Simoons and colleagues developed a model for the assessment of a patient's risk for the development of intracranial hemorrhage in association with thrombolysis.[102] The following four clinical variables known at hospital admission were shown to predict an increased risk of intracranial hemorrhage: age >65 years (odds ratio and 95% confidence interval for intracranial hemorrhage = 2.2 (1.4–3.5)), weight <70 kg (2.1 (1.3–3.2)), hypertension on presentation (2.0 (1.2–3.2)), and use of rt-PA (1.6 (1.0–2.5)). Based on the number of these risk factors present at the time of evaluation of a patient who is a candidate for thrombolysis, clinicians may estimate the probability of intracranial hemorrhage as illustrated in Figure 2.11.

Following a review of the literature and compilation of clinical experience, consensus recommendations have been published by the American College of Cardiology/ American Heart Association Task Force on Assessment of Diagnostic and Therapeutic Cardiovascular Procedures. Absolute contraindications suggested by this task force, listed in Table 2.9, are designed to exclude patients with an unacceptable risk of bleeding, especially in an incompressible site, and also to exclude patients with a potential for anaphylaxis due to streptokinase-like thrombolytic agents (rt-PA would be an acceptable alternative in such patients).[26] Relative contraindications to thrombolytic therapy are also shown in Table 2.9. Clinicians must weigh carefully the dramatic life-saving potential of thrombolysis vs the potential bleeding risk in an individual patient. Given

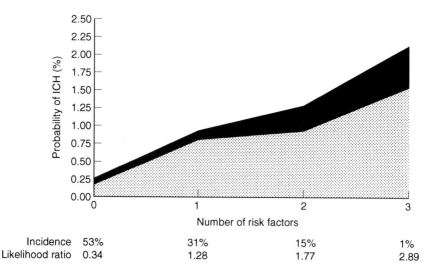

Incidence	53%	31%	15%	1%
Likelihood ratio	0.34	1.28	1.77	2.89

Figure 2.11 Estimation of individual risk for development of intracranial hemorrhage (ICH) during thrombolytic therapy. Along the bottom of the figure is shown the estimated incidence of the frequency of one or more of the following risk factors: age >65 years, weight <70 kg, hypertension on admission, and use of rt-PA in patients with acute myocardial infarction who are potential candidates for thrombolytic therapy. The likelihood ratio describes the probability of finding the risk profile among patients with intracranial bleeding divided by the probability of finding the same risk profile among patients without intracranial bleeding. The curves depict the estimated probability of ICH assuming an overall incidence of 0.5% (□) and 0.75% (■) (bottom and top curves respectively). (Adapted from data in Ref. 102.)

Table 2.10 Dose regimens for intravenous thrombolytic agents for acute myocardial infarction

Streptokinase: 1.5 million units over 1 hour
Tissue plasminogen activator: (front-loaded regimen)
  15-mg bolus, followed by 0.75 mg kg^{-1} (up to 50 mg) over first hour and 0.5 mg kg^{-1} (up to 35 mg) over
  60 min
Anisoylated plasminogen–streptokinase activator complex:
  30 units over 5 min

the overwhelming data on the benefits of thrombolysis, physicians are strongly encouraged to expand their criteria for thrombolysis in acute myocardial infarction with particular emphasis on inclusion of elderly patients and treatment up to 12 hours from the onset of chest pain.

Doses of Lytic Agents and Relative Importance of Selection of Regimen

Recommended doses of the available thrombolytic regimens are shown in Table 2.10. The relative advantages and disadvantages of one treatment regimen versus another are discussed in Chapter 3. It should be remembered, however, that the prognosis of a patient with acute myocardial infarction is a result of a complex interplay of many clinical variables at the time of presentation, virtually all of which weigh more heavily on the probability of surviving the first month after infarction than precisely which thrombolytic agent is used (Figure 2.12).

Other Interventions to be Administered in the CCU

Other beneficial therapeutic interventions that should be routinely prescribed in the CCU are aspirin and β-adrenoceptor blockers (see Chapters 4 and 6). Nitrates and angiotensin-converting enzyme (ACE) inhibitors have only a modest effect on short-term mortality but have been shown to favorably modify ventricular loading conditions and decrease a patient's risk for left ventricular chamber dilatation and remodeling (see Chapters 8 and 9).

Infarct Extension and Expansion

Myocardial infarct extension and expansion are two important complications that must be differentiated both clinically and pathophysiologically (Table 2.11). Myocardial infarct *extension* occurs in approximately 10% of patients with acute infarction during the first 10 days, but in up to 20% of patients who have undergone thrombolytic therapy. Infarct extension following thrombolysis is due to reocclusion of the infarct-related coronary artery. Weisman and Healy have arbitrarily defined myocardial infarct extension as occurring between 24 hours and completion of the in-hospital postinfarction course.[103] Pathologic examination reveals areas of healing myocardial infarction with more recent necrosis usually in the same zone of myocardial tissue perfused by the original infarct-related artery. Myocardial reinfarction is arbitrarily defined as occurring after the in-hospital postinfarction course and may refer to a new infarction occurring within the original infarct zone or infarction in a different zone of myocardium supplied by an artery different from the initial culprit vessel.

It is often clinically difficult to distinguish postinfarction angina from infarct extension. Typically, infarct extension is characterized by more severe and prolonged chest

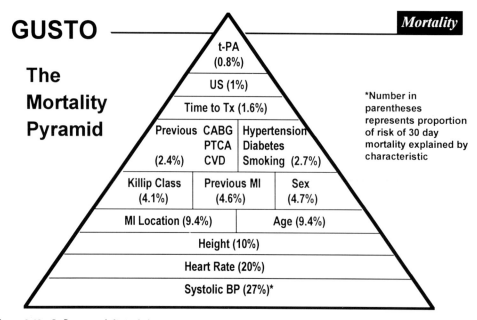

GUSTO

The Mortality Pyramid

Mortality

t-PA (0.8%)

US (1%)

Time to Tx (1.6%)

Previous CABG   Hypertension
PTCA   Diabetes
(2.4%)   CVD   Smoking (2.7%)

Killip Class   Previous MI   Sex
(4.1%)   (4.6%)   (4.7%)

MI Location (9.4%)   Age (9.4%)

Height (10%)

Heart Rate (20%)

Systolic BP (27%)*

*Number in parentheses represents proportion of risk of 30 day mortality explained by characteristic

Figure 2.12   Influence of clinical characteristics on 30-day mortality in thrombolytic-treated patients from the GUSTO trial. Although considerable controversy exists over the absolute differences in mortality observed with different thrombolytic regimens, it is important to emphasize that the exact choice of a thrombolytic agent is far less important than other clinical variables at the time of presentation with infarction. This figure depicts the importance of such clinical variables as calculated from a regression analysis in the GUSTO trial. The numbers in parentheses represent the proportion of risk of 30-day mortality explained by the characteristic. (Adapted from data presented at the 66th Annual Scientific Sessions of the American Heart Association, November 1993.)

discomfort associated with recurrent and persistent electrocardiographic changes including ST–T wave abnormalities and/or QRS abnormalities that may show various stages of evolution. In addition, myocardial infarct extension is associated with reelevation of serum creatine kinase-myocardial bound (CK-MB) after the initial peak from the index infarction (Figure 2.13). Because serum cardiac markers may be difficult to interpret early after thrombolysis, the diagnosis of recurrent infarction within 18 hours after the start of thrombolytic therapy should be based on the presence of recurrent severe ischemic discomfort of at least 30 min duration and recurrent ST segment elevation of at least 0.1 mV in at least two contiguous leads. Eighteen hours after administration of thrombolytic therapy the diagnosis of recurrent infarction can be based on a reelevation of CK-MB to above the upper limit of normal and increased by at least 50% over the previous value. If multiple CK and CK-MB specimens are available prior to the episode of suspected recurrent infarction, the directional trend should be consistent with the diagnosis of recurrent infarction.

Myocardial infarct extension occurs in about 15–20% of fatal infarctions and is seen in the majority of patients who experience cardiogenic shock. Patients who undergo myocardial infarct extension experience a mortality several fold higher than that of patients in whom extension did not occur (Figure 2.14). Clinical risk factors for its development include obesity, female gender, non-Q-wave myocardial infarction, diabetes mellitus, a previous myocardial infarction, and an early peaking CK-MB curve (<15 hours).[104]

Fewer than 50% of patients with infarct extension actually experience recurrent ischemic pain or develop ECG changes, indicating that this complication is likely to be

Table 2.11 Comparison of infarct expansion, extension, and reinfarction

Expansion	Extension	Reinfarction
Incidence		
Up to 70% of all fatal infarctions	About 15–20% of fatal infarctions	About 10–20% in most studies: higher incidence among women
About 35–45% of anterior transmural infarctions	Clinical incidence varies according to diagnostic criteria and patient selection, but probably is between 10% and 20% in the general population	
Lower incidence seen at other sites		
Time course		
Hours to several days after infarction	Arbitrarily defined as occurring between 24 hours and completion of the in-hospital postinfarction course	Arbitrarily defined as occurring after the in-hospital postinfarction course
Pathologic features		
Gross pathology	Gross pathology: healing myocardial infarction with surrounding foci or more recent necrosis usually within the same vascular risk region	Gross and histologic pathology: remote healed myocardial infarction with new infarction in the same or a different vascular risk region
Infarct thinning and dilatation		
Secondary global dilatation (possibly)		
Histology	Histology: contraction band necrosis present in the newer foci of necrosis	
Myocyte slippage		
Consequences		
Congestive heart failure	Actual increase in infarct size	Increase in total infarct mass
Increased mortality	Congestive heart failure	Congestive heart failure
Left ventricular dilatation (regional and global)	Cardiogenic shock	Cardiogenic shock
Mural thrombus	Increased mortality	Increased mortality
Cardiac rupture	Infarct expansion?	
Left ventricular aneurysm		
Infarct extension?		
Postinfarction angina?		

Reproduced with permission from Ref. 103.

underdiagnosed unless frequent sampling of cardiac serum markers is performed (not practical). Patients with a high-risk factor profile for myocardial infarct extension, as discussed above, should be considered candidates for early cardiac catheterization and possible revascularization with angioplasty or coronary artery bypass graft surgery.

Following acute myocardial infarction, a series of events are initiated that ultimately cause remodeling of the left ventricular chamber.[105] Patients who undergo extensive alterations of left ventricular geometry are at great risk for the development of congestive heart failure, left ventricular aneurysms, and a significantly higher mortality rate. The process of remodeling of the left ventricular chamber is a combination of hypertrophy of residual noninfarcted myocardium and changes in left ventricular dimension.[105] The two most important factors impacting on changes in left ventricular dimension are infarct-artery patency and ventricular loading conditions, although size and distensibility of the infarct and activation of tissue hormonal systems play important contributory roles. The metabolic state of the adjacent and remote myocardium helps determine the timing and extent of hypertrophy of the residual noninfarcted myocardium.

The term myocardial infarct *expansion* was introduced to refer to a serious complication that may be seen in nearly three-quarters of fatal infarctions and one-third to one-half of

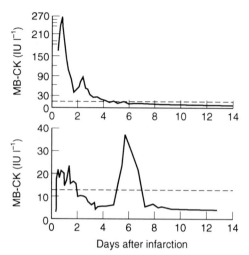

Figure 2.13   MB creatine kinase (MB-CK) time–activity curves for patient in whom myocardial extension developed prior to return of plasma MB-CK to baseline (top panel) and a patient in whom extension occurred after return of MB-CK to baseline (bottom panel). (Reproduced with permission from Muller, J.E. (1988) *Ann. Intern. Med.*, **108**, 1.)

anterior Q-wave myocardial infarctions.[103] It is characterized by disproportionate thinning and dilatation of the necrotic zone prior to development of a well-healed scar. Clinically, myocardial infarct expansion may be seen within several hours of the onset of chest pain or may be delayed for several days. Patients typically experience chest discomfort, although it may be of a slightly different nature than the original pain experienced with infarction. Minor nonspecific ST–T wave abnormalities may be detected on the ECG but there is no reelevation of CK-MB values. Individuals with infarct expansion exhibit signs of hemodynamic compromise including new or louder gallop sounds and new or worsening pulmonary rales.

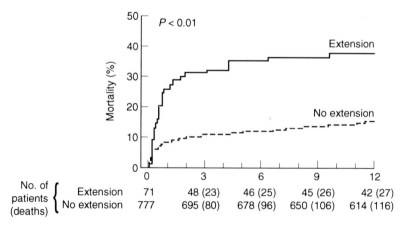

Figure 2.14   Cumulative mortality curves in patients with and without myocardial infarct extension. The early mortality in patients with extension is several-fold higher than that seen in patients without extension. (Reproduced with permission from Muller, J.E. (1988) *Ann. Intern. Med.*, **108**, 1.)

The process of left ventricular chamber dilatation following myocardial infarction commences as infarct expansion but over the long term also involves viable regions. The magnitude of overall left ventricular chamber remodeling has important adverse prognostic consequences.

Therapeutic maneuvers that may favorably impact on the development of remodeling of the left ventricle include reperfusion of the infarct-related artery, even beyond the time when myocardial salvage may occur (see Chapter 5) and administration of nitrates and ACE inhibitors to modify the loading conditions and tissue hormonal responses following myocardial infarction (see Chapters 8, 9 and 15).

Bradycardia and AV Conduction Disturbances

Sinus bradycardia occurs frequently (30–40% of patients) within the first hour of infarction and is seen more commonly with inferior infarction, especially in association with reperfusion of the right coronary artery when it may be accompanied by hypotension (Bezold–Jarisch reflex). Management of sinus bradycardia depends on the timing of the arrhythmia and whether hypotension and/or a low-output syndrome accompanies the slow heart rate. Isolated sinus bradycardia should simply be observed in view of the generally good prognosis and possible protective effects against ventricular arrhythmias. When sinus bradycardia is associated with hemodynamic compromise, atropine should be administered intravenously in increments of 0.3 mg to a total dose of 2.0 mg. Factors known to precipitate episodes of sinus bradycardia include chest pain as well as narcotic analgesics and nitroglycerin typically administered early in the course of treatment in the CCU (Figure 2.15). Junctional escape rhythms represent a normal escape mechanism

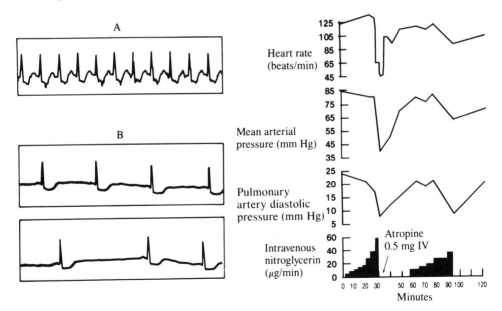

Figure 2.15 Sinus bradycardia and hypotension provoked by intravenous nitroglycerin in a patient with acute myocardial infarction. Intravenous nitroglycerin at a dose of 20–40 μg min^{-1} in a patient with acute anteroseptal myocardial infarction and sinus tachycardia (A) provoked profound sinus bradycardia (B) and hypotension. This was quickly reversed with intravenous atropine 0.5 mg, but recurred after reinstitution of intravenous nitroglycerin. (Reproduced with permission of the American Heart Association Inc. from Come, P.C. and Pitt, B. (1976) *Circulation*, **54**, 624.)

when automaticity of the sinus node drops below that of the AV junction. Treatment is indicated only if the loss of the atrial contribution to ventricular filling causes hemodynamic compromise and consists of acceleration of the sinus rate with atropine or atrial pacing.

Heart block may develop in 6–14% of patients with myocardial infarction.[106–111]. In-hospital mortality is increased in patients who develop heart block in association with myocardial infarction, although for those patients surviving to hospital discharge the long-term survival is equivalent to those who did not develop heart block.[107,108,110] With rare exceptions (e.g. patients who develop profound bradycardia in an unmonitored setting or in whom measures to accelerate the heart rate are delayed), the increased mortality is not a direct result of heart block itself but is a function of the severity of infarction as assessed by peak CK values or the extent of wall-motion abnormalities.[106,110,111] In the TIMI-II trial 13% of patients developed heart block within 24 hours after treatment with rt-PA and the 21-day mortality was 7.1%.[109] Of note, the infarct-related artery was occluded in 28% of patients with heart block, compared to 16% of patients without heart block at catheterization 18–48 hours after thrombolysis.[109]

Several factors modify the general prognosis of high-degree heart block. While heart block occurring more than 24 hours after myocardial infarction is not associated with increased long-term mortality, heart block in the setting of right ventricular infarction is associated with a 41% mortality, compared to 14% for right ventricular infarction without heart block and 11% for heart block without right ventricular infarction.[106,112] Although the incidence of heart block is twice as high with inferior infarction compared with anterior infarction, because a larger mass of infarcted myocardium occurs in the latter, mortality is higher in patients with heart block and anterior rather than inferior infarction.[11]

Patients who develop AV block in the setting of acute myocardial infarction can usually be grouped into two broad categories according to the site of block. Although it is not possible to pinpoint the location of conduction block on the basis of noninvasive tests, certain generalizations are appropriate. First-degree AV block and Mobitz type I second-degree block are generally supra-Hisian and considered proximal blocks. Mobitz type II second-degree, and third-degree AV block are usually infra-Hisian and considered distal blocks. Table 2.12 summarizes important diagnostic and therapeutic features of these two groups.

Digitalis

Digitalis glycosides have been used for treating cardiovascular illness for over two centuries. The two indications for prescription of digitalis in patients with myocardial infarction are control of the ventricular rate in atrial fibrillation and acute management of left ventricular dysfunction in patients with sinus rhythm. There is little debate about the first of these indications for digitalis but most clinicians now turn to other inotropic agents such as dopamine or dobutamine for treatment of left ventricular dysfunction after myocardial infarction in view of the slow onset of action of digitalis, long half-life, and narrow therapeutic range. In addition, in a direct comparison of patients who received captopril or digoxin for prevention of left ventricular remodeling and dysfunction after anterior myocardial infarction, Bonaduce and colleagues found that patients in whom captopril therapy was initiated 7–10 days after onset of infarction had less left ventricular remodeling and more well-preserved global left ventricular function than patients receiving digitalis.[113] Observations such as these plus the favorable effects of ACE inhibitors on short-term mortality reported by the ISIS-4, GISSI-3, and the Chinese investigators make ACE inhibitors a more attractive therapeutic option than digitalis for

Table 2.12 Features of AV conduction disturbances in acute myocardial infarction

	Location of AV conduction disturbance	
	Proximal	Distal
Site of block	Intranodal	Infranodal
Site of infarction	Inferoposterior	Anteroseptal
Compromised arterial supply	RCA (90%), LCX (10%)	Septal perforators of LAD
Pathogenesis	Ischemia, necrosis, hydropic cell swelling, excess parasympathetic activity	Ischemia, necrosis, hydropic cell swelling
Predominant type of AV nodal block	First degree (PR > 200 ms) Mobitz type I second degree	Mobitz type II second degree, Third degree
Common premonitory features of third-degree AV block	(a) First→second-degree AV block (b) Mobitz I pattern	(a) Intraventricular conduction block (b) Mobitz II pattern
Features of escape rhythm following third degree block (a) Location (b) QRS width (c) Rate (d) Stability of escape rhythm	(a) Proximal conduction system (His bundle) (b) $<0.12\,\text{s}^a$ (c) 45–60 min^{-1} but may be as low as 30 min^{-1} (d) Rate usually stable; asystole uncommon	(a) Distal conduction system (bundle branches) (b) $>0.12\,\text{s}^a$ (c) Often $< 30\,\text{min}^{-1}$ (d) Rate often unstable with moderate to high risk of ventricular asystole
Duration of high-grade AV block	Usually transient (2–3 days)	Usually transient but some form of AV conduction disturbance and/or intraventricular defect may persist
Associated mortality rate	Low unless associated with hypotension and/or congestive heart failure	High because of extensive infarction associated with power failure or ventricular arrhythmias
Pacemaker therapy (a) Temporary (b) Permanent	(a) Rarely required; may be considered for bradycardia associated with left ventricular power failure, syncope, or angina (b) Almost never indicated, since conduction defect is usually transient	(a) Should be considered in patients with anteroseptal infarction and acute bifascicular block (b) Indicated for patients with high grade AV block with block in His–Purkinje system and those with transient advanced AV block and associated bundle branch block

Modified from Antman, E.M. and Rutherford, J.D. (1986) *Coronary Care Medicine. A Practical Approach.* Boston: Martinus Nijhoff; Dreifus, L.S. *et al.* (1991) Guidelines for implantation of cardiac pacemakers and antiarrhythmia devices. *J. Am. Coll. Cardiol.*, **18**, 1.
[a] Some studies suggest that a wide QRS escape rhythm (>0.12 s) following high-grade AV block in inferior infarction is associated with a worse prognosis.
RCA   right coronary artery;
LCX   left circumflex coronary artery;
LAD   left anterior descending coronary artery.

treatment of left ventricular dysfunction following myocardial infarction and prevention of development of abnormal left ventricular geometry (see Chapter 9). Long-term therapy with ACE inhibitors in patients with left ventricular dysfunction has also been shown to be associated with marked reductions in mortality, rehospitalization for congestive heart failure, and recurrent myocardial infarction (see Chapter 15).

An additional serious concern about digitalis glycosides has been the observation that chronic administration of digitalis following infarction may be associated with an increased mortality risk. Mølstad recently reviewed the data from 10 trials providing information on possible hazards of chronic administration of digitalis in patients after myocardial infarction.[114] In 1981, Moss and colleagues reported a 30% (18% to 42%) increase in mortality after 4 months of treatment with digitalis in a group of high-risk patients post infarction who experienced congestive heart failure in the CCU and also exhibited ventricular premature beats on a predischarge ambulatory electrocardiographic recording.[115] Ryan and associates reviewed data from the Coronary Artery Surgery Study (CASS) registry and found a nonsignificant trend towards an association between digitalis treatment and an increase in mortality following myocardial infarction.[116] Madsen in 1984 presented equivocal data on an association between digitalis and mortality in a 1-year follow-up of 1599 patients followed after myocardial infarction.[117] Bigger and associates performed a Cox regression analysis of 504 patients followed for 3 years after myocardial infarction and reported a relative risk of 1.58 (95% confidence interval 0.97–2.60) of mortality in patients receiving digitalis.[118]

Because of these alarming reports the databases of two large trials were scrutinized. Analysis of 1921 placebo-treated patients from the Beta Blocker Heart Attack Trial (BHAT) and 903 patients who survived the hospital phase of acute myocardial infarction in the Multicenter Investigation of the Limitation of Infarct Size (MILIS) using logistic regression analyses and Cox proportional models reported no increase in mortality in patients receiving digitalis after adjusting for other baseline variables.[119,120]

In 1987 the Digitalis Subcommittee of the Multicenter Post-Infarction Research Group reported the results of a 24–48 month follow-up in 867 patients who survived an acute myocardial infarction.[121] Of these patients 31% were taking digitalis, and this therapy was associated with a significantly increased mortality risk after adjustment for 22 baseline variables (relative risk 2.3; 95% confidence interval 1.4–3.7, $P < 0.001$).

An additional report from the CASS registry on 1114 patients with a proximal stenosis of the left anterior descending or circumflex artery provided additional information about potential risks of digitalis.[122] This was not strictly a postinfarction study, but 61% of the patients had experienced a prior myocardial infarction. Using a Cox survival analysis model, digitalis emerged as a significant predictor of mortality with advanced age and several angiographic markers of depressed left ventricular function. Two other reports, both from Scandinavia, using Cox survival analyses also found digitalis therapy to be a significant predictor of mortality with relative risks of 1.4 (1.07–1.86) and 1.8 (1.2–2.5) respectively.[123,124]

Despite the strong suggestion of mortality hazard associated with chronic digitalis therapy following myocardial infarction, from a review of these 10 studies the crucial question of whether digitalis is contraindicated for chronic administration following acute myocardial infarction remains unanswered. There was considerable variation in trial design and all of the reports are retrospective analyses of trials originally designed for other purposes rather than studying the long-term mortality risks of digitalis. Attempts to adjust for imbalances in baseline characteristics using either a multiple logistic regression technique or a Cox proportional hazards model cannot be considered definitive since failure to identify key baseline imbalances may have led to underadjustment of the risk of digitalis, while introduction of a large number of variables may have overadjusted for the risks of digitalis.[114] Utilizing a specialized meta-analytic technique on those studies that provided details of their Cox survival analysis, a pooled relative risk of 1.40 (1.23–1.59) for mortality associated with chronic digitalis therapy emerges. However, such meta-analytic analyses are subject to bias since the negative studies cited above could not be included because of insufficient data on the details of their analytic techniques in the original reports.

Some authorities have suggested a large-scale randomized controlled trial is required to determine definitively whether chronic digitalis therapy is associated with an increased risk of mortality following myocardial infarction.[125] Burchell has raised an interesting moral dilemma regarding the call for such a trial.[126] Since few data exist suggesting long-term mortality benefit in patients receiving chronic digitalis therapy, the question at hand is whether there is an excess mortality risk associated with chronic digitalis therapy. Thus, patients in a hypothetical randomized trial of chronic digitalis administration following myocardial infarction would be asked to participate in an experiment to confirm whether a particular therapy created harm rather than reduced mortality.

Perhaps because of conundrums such as this, no formal survival trial of digitalis therapy following myocardial infarction has been reported to date. However, a large-scale survival trial organized by the Digitalis Investigators Group (DIG) is evaluating approximately 7500 patients with congestive heart failure, some of whom will have a history of myocardial infarction, to determine whether digitalis provides a survival advantage. Enrollment was concluded in August 1993, and the results of the trial are expected to be available within 18–24 months.

Based upon the available data to date, it seems reasonable to administer digitalis in the acute setting of infarction for control of the ventricular rate in atrial fibrillation and as a possible short-term adjunct to other treatments for management of left ventricular dysfunction in sinus rhythm. The abundance of data indicating benefit from long-term ACE inhibitor treatment in patients with left ventricular dysfunction after myocardial infarction (based largely on the SAVE trial) has led the Food and Drug Administration to approve new labeling for the ACE inhibitor captopril. It is now indicated for use in patients with left ventricular dysfunction after myocardial infarction to improve long-term survival and reduce the incidence of heart failure and need for hospitalization. Thus, patients with left ventricular dysfunction following myocardial infarction who have no contraindications should receive an ACE inhibitor beginning in the CCU to be continued on a long-term basis.

Pericarditis and Dressler Syndrome

Pericarditis occurs in the setting of acute myocardial infarction as a result of extension of myocardial necrosis through to the epicardium. Pathologic reports indicate that virtually all patients with transmural acute myocardial infarction develop at least a localized fibrinous pericarditis.[127] Typical symptoms associated with pericarditis include anterior chest pain that may be confused with and raise concern about recurrent myocardial ischemia. Important clinical clues to the pericardial origin of discomfort include: (1) a pleuritic component to the discomfort; (2) radiation to the trapezius muscles – a site of radiation of discomfort virtually never seen with myocardial ischemia;[128] (3) a pericardial friction rub; (4) low-grade fever (38.1–38.6 °C); (5) J point elevation, concave-upward ST segment elevation, and PR segment depression on the ECG.

Patients with pericarditis experience a higher incidence of pericardial effusion and may be at increased risk for cardiac tamponade and the rare complication of constrictive pericarditis following myocardial infarction.[129–131] In the acute stage, symptoms are frequently mild so that no therapy is required. Dramatic and reliable relief of more severe symptoms can be provided with corticosteroids and indomethacin, although because of the tendency to scar thinning and myocardial rupture with the former and increase in coronary vascular resistance with the latter, these agents should not be used except in refractory cases.[132] The drug of choice for treatment of pericarditis in the setting of acute infarction is aspirin, an agent that virtually all patients should be receiving by the time they enter the CCU.[133] The regular postinfarction maintenance dose of aspirin is 150–325 mg, but higher doses (650 mg every 4–6 hours) may be required for relief of pericardial discomfort.

The presence of acute pericarditis should cause clinicians to reevaluate the risk–benefit ratio for continuing antithrombotic therapy (e.g. heparin). Clinical signs of cardiac tamponade would be a clear indication for discontinuation of antithrombotic therapy. If the situation is unclear, a bedside ECG can be obtained to search for a pericardial effusion and assess its hemodynamic significance.

A syndrome characterized by fever, pericardial pain, pleuritis, and sometimes pneumonitis, occurring 1–6 weeks after infarction, referred to as Dressler syndrome, previously was a more common clinical problem than in the current coronary care era.[134,135] The syndrome is probably due to an immune antoantibody response against certain pericardial–myocardial antigens exposed to the immune system at the time of infarction. Therapy for Dressler syndrome is similar to that for pericarditis. For reasons that are unclear, the incidence of Dressler syndrome has declined dramatically, causing some authorities to question whether it has actually disappeared.[136] One possible factor contributing to the reduction in the incidence of Dressler syndrome is the widespread use of aspirin.

Shoulder–Hand Syndrome

Another clinical syndrome that was seen much more commonly in the past and has become a rarity in coronary care medicine at present is the shoulder–hand syndrome.[137–138] This is characterized by pain, swelling, and limitation of movement of the upper extremity. Onset of the syndrome can be slow or rapid and it is accompanied by vasomotor changes (such as in the Raynaud phenomenon), muscular atrophy, and eventual stiffness of the wrist and shoulder. The underlying pathophysiologic process is probably a form of reflex sympathetic dystrophy that is most effectively treated by physiotherapy with heat and exercise, combined with analgesia and antiinflammatory agents. The current practice of early mobilization of postinfarction patients has probably relegated this entity to a chapter in the history of coronary care medicine since it is no longer a current clinical problem.

Stepdown Unit

The duration of hospitalization ('length of stay') for patients with acute myocardial infarction has decreased from approximately 3–6 weeks in the pre-CCU era to about 1 week in the current reperfusion era.[139] Some reports have suggested that selected patients who achieve early reperfusion and have a negative predischarge exercise test, as well as individuals sustaining an uncomplicated Q-wave infarction but who do not receive thrombolysis, may be discharged home in 3–5 days with no adverse impact on mortality.[140,141] However, as emphasized by Goldstein, such low-risk individuals comprise only 15–25% of the infarct population and this proportion may decline as greater numbers of elderly patients are admitted to CCUs.[142] Despite the present economic pressures on the healthcare delivery system, it is unclear that such rapid discharge practice is clinically wise and decisions must be individualized based on a patient's ability to grasp advice about rehabilitation and the social support available after discharge.[142]

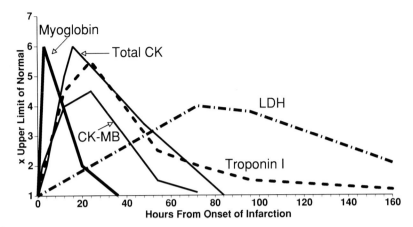

Figure 2.16 Time course of elevations of serum markers after acute myocardial infarction. This figure summarizes the relative timing, rate of rise, peak values, and duration of elevation above the upper limit of normal for multiple serum markers following acute myocardial infarction. While traditionally total CK, CK-MB, and lactic dehydrogenase (LDH (with isoenzymes)) are measured, the relatively slow rate of rise above normal for CK and potential confusion with noncardiac sources of enzyme release for both total CK and LDH has inspired the search for additional serum markers. The smaller molecule myoglobin is released quickly from infarcted myocardium but is not cardiac specific. Therefore, elevations of myoglobin that may be detected quite early after the onset of infarction require confirmation with a more cardiac-specific marker such as CK-MB or troponin I. Troponin I (and troponin T) (not shown) rise more slowly than myoglobin and may be useful for diagnosis of infarction even up to 3–4 days after the event. Assays for troponin I and troponin T are under development using monoclonal antibodies.

The majority of individuals with uncomplicated myocardial infarction typically spend about 2 days in the CCU and then are transferred to a less intensively monitored setting – the intermediate care unit or stepdown unit, sometimes referred to as the telemetry unit because of the frequent application of ECG monitoring via radiofrequency transmitters in ambulatory patients. Radiotelemetry has been shown to be an inexpensive method for detection of serious arrhythmias in patients transferred from the CCU.[143] The ability to continue monitoring the patient in an intermediate care unit allows more rapid turnover of CCU beds, an issue that is becoming increasingly important with the more widespread use of thrombolysis and primary PTCA. The intermediate care area is also an ideal setting for reinforcement of patient education that was initiated in the CCU. Dietary counseling and behavior modification (e.g. cessation of cigarette smoking[144]) are key topics for discussion by the nursing staff with the patient. In addition, hospital staff may continue to monitor the patient's activity progress, checking for the development of undue dyspnea, acceleration of the heart rate beyond 100 beats min^{-1}, or marked hypertension or hypotension with exercise.

Because of the high volume of patients with suspected acute myocardial infarction and the increasing costs of cardiac intensive care, considerable pressure has developed to contain costs. Physicians often play the role of 'gatekeeper' and ration the availability of CCU beds, creating a distinct disadvantage for elderly patients.[22,23] Lee and Goldman have reported that 77% of infarctions were clinically detected in the CCU within 12 hours and 96% were detected within 24 hours.[28] A reasonable strategy therefore, is expeditiously to confirm or exclude the diagnosis of myocardial infarction so that patients who 'rule out' within 12–24 hours can be transferred out of the CCU to the stepdown unit.[145] The availability of new serum markers of myocardial damage (Figure 2.16) has made this strategy a reality in contemporary coronary care medicine.[146]

Table 2.13 The 'low-risk' myocardial infarction patient

The absence of all of the following variables suggests that a patient is at a lower risk of mortality and may be safely discharged from the CCU within 24–36 hours of admission:

1. History of previous myocardial infarction
2. Anterior infarction
3. Rales in more than one-third of the lung fields
4. Hypotension and sinus tachycardia
5. Female gender
6. Diabetes mellitus
7. Persistent ischemic pain
8. Heart block
9. Complex ventricular arrhythmias
10. Atrial fibrillation
11. Age ⩾70 years

Adapted from data in: Gheorghiade, M., Anderson, J., Rosman, H. *et al.* (1988) Risk identification at the time of admission to coronary care unit in patients with suspected myocardial infarction. *Am. Heart J.*, **116**, 1212–17; and Refs 100, 147 and 148.

Even facilitated transfer of patients out of the CCU following exclusion of a myocardial infarction would not unburden the system sufficiently. Additional strategies for risk stratification have been proposed.[147,148] Patients may be classified as low risk and transformed out of the CCU within 24–36 hours after admission if they do not have a history of previous myocardial infarction, persistent ischemic pain, congestive heart failure, hypotension, heart block, or significant ventricular arrhythmias (Table 2.13). Such individuals are unlikely to experience in-hospital deaths or require transfer back to the CCU.

Future Directions

While contemporary CCUs contain the essential elements originally proposed by Julian, Day and Lown, considerable evolution has occurred.[2–4] Rapid implementation of infarct size-reducing therapies such as thrombolysis and primary PTCA is commonplace and is anticipated to increase in the future. Since reocclusion of an initially successful reperfused infarct-related artery is related to inadequate antithrombotic therapy, many CCUs have implemented procedures for bedside monitoring of a patient's coagulation status.[149] There are several ongoing clinical trials with novel direct antithrombins that do not require antithrombin III as a cofactor, and have a more constant antithrombotic effect (TIMI 9, GUSTO-2, TIMI 8). These studies should provide information over the next 2 years indicating whether heparin will be superseded as the antithrombin of choice for acute coronary syndromes by newer agents such as hirudin and Hirulog and whether it really is essential to monitor the activated partial thromboplastin time at the patient's bedside.

The CCU has also evolved into a cardiac intensive care area serving the needs not only of patients with acute myocardial infarction, but those with cardiomyopathy (before and after cardiac transplantation), individuals who have been resuscitated from sudden cardiac death, and patients with complicated forms of organic heart disease such as congenital cardiac lesions and endocarditis. The premium on cardiac intensive care beds makes it imperative that alternatives to the CCU be developed for patients with a low-risk myocardial infarction or an acute coronary syndrome such as unstable angina pectoris (Figure 2.17).

Future developments include enhancements of the stepdown unit with more sophisticated radiotelemetry of ECG signals and the use of wireless Ethernet systems for

Triage of Patients with Acute Myocardial Infarction and Other Coronary Syndromes

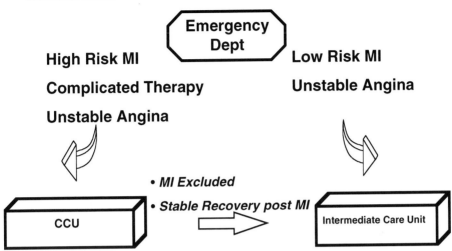

Figure 2.17 Triage flow pattern of patients with acute myocardial infarction and other coronary syndromes. Individuals presenting to the emergency department with acute coronary syndromes should be rapidly evaluated by the staff. Patients with a low-risk myocardial infarction (see Table 2.13) and unstable angina that responds rapidly to initial medical therapy may be admitted to an intermediate care unit. Individuals with high-risk myocardial infarction, those requiring complicated therapeutic interventions (e.g. intraaortic balloon counterpulsation), or those individuals with recurrent bouts of unstable angina despite medical therapy should be admitted to the CCU where a higher nurse–patient ratio is available. As discussed in the text, for individuals in whom a myocardial infarction is excluded and those who have a stable recovery course following a documented myocardial infarction may be transferred from the CCU to the intermediate care unit to free up beds in the CCU for new patients that present to the emergency department.

telemeterized hemodynamic monitoring. Cross-training of nursing personnel between the CCU and stepdown unit and a high level of electronic data integration using advanced computer technology are no longer to be considered theoretical luxuries for some distant time in the future, but must be actively pursued to provide truly cost-effective modern coronary care. It is now possible for physicians and nurses caring for acutely ill cardiac patients to retrieve at bedside computer terminals laboratory data as well as the results of critical tests that the patient may have had including cardiac catheterization, echocardiograms, ECGs, and vascular noninvasive studies.[150] In the very near future it will be possible to actually view selected images of important studies such as PTCA, transesophageal echocardiography, and CAT scans at the same bedside computer terminals. Ideally, ECG and hemodynamic monitoring data acquired on the patient from the time of admission to the CCU can be carried out directly to the stepdown unit and ultimately downloaded into an electronic database that will be accessible, should the patient be readmitted in the future. As diagnostic and treatment algorithms are refined further it should be possible to introduce sophisticated artificial intelligence and expert systems into the CCU environment to help the staff integrate the wealth of data that are now located in disparate areas.[151] Not only will this eliminate some of the present time- and labor-intensive practices in CCU medicine but it will also make the latest technologic advances accessible to hospital settings where specialists are not readily available and primary-care physicians assume greater responsibilities for care of patients with acute myocardial infarction.

References

1. Julian, D. (1961) Treatment of cardiac arrest in acute myocardial ischaemia and infarction. *Lancet*, **ii**, 840–4.
2. Day, H. (1963) An intensive coronary care area. *Dis. Chest*, **44**, 423–7.
3. Lown, B., Fakhro, A.M., Hood, W.B. and Thorn, G.W. (1967) The coronary care unit. New perspectives and directions. *JAMA*, **199**, 188–98.
4. Julian, D.G. (1987) The history of coronary care units. *Br. Heart J.*, **57**, 497–502.
5. Yusuf, S., Sleight, P., Held, P. and McMahon, S. (1990) Routine medical management of acute myocardial infarction. Lessons from overviews of recent randomized controlled trials. *Circulation*, **82**, II-117–II-134.
6. Sodi-Pallares, D., Testelli, M., Fishleder, B. *et al.* (1962) Effects of an intravenous infusion of a potassium–glucose–insulin solution on the electrocardiographic signs of myocardial infarction: A preliminary clinical report. *Am. J. Cardiol.*, **9**, 166.
7. Maroko, P., Hillis, L., Muller, J. *et al.* (1977) Favorable effects of hyaluronidase on electrocardiographic evidence of necrosis in patients with acute myocardial infarction. *N. Engl. J. Med.*, **296**, 898.
8. Guzzetta C.E. (1989) Effects of relaxation and music therapy on patients in a coronary care unit with presumptive acute myocardial infarction. *Heart Lung*, **18**, 609–16.
9. Byrd, R.C. (1988) Positive therapeutic effects of intercessory prayer in a coronary care unit population. *South. Med. J.*, **81**, 826–9.
10. ISIS-3 (Third International Study of Infarct Survival) Collaborative Group (1992) ISIS-3: A randomized trial of streptokinase vs tissue plasminogen activator vs anistreplase and of aspirin plus heparin vs aspirin alone among 41,229 cases of suspected acute myocardial infarction. *Lancet*, **339**, 753–70.
11. The GUSTO Investigators. (1993) An international randomized trial comparing four thrombolytic strategies for acute myocardial infarction. *N. Engl. J. Med.*, **329**, 673–82.
12. Yusuf, S., Wittes, J. and Friedman, L. (1988) Overview of results of randomized clinical trials in heart disease. I. Treatments following myocardial infarction. *JAMA*, **260**, 2088–93.
13. Mather, H., Morgan, D., Pearson, N. *et al.* (1976) Myocardial infarction: a comparison between home and hospital care for patients. *BMJ.*, **i**, 925–9.
14. Walsh, M.J. (1987) The coronary care unit: a reappraisal. *Ir. Med. J.*, **80**, 394–6.
15. Waters, D.D. and Theroux, P. (1987) Whither the coronary care unit? *Can. Med. Assoc. J.*, **136**, 17–19.
16. Reznik, R., Ring, I., Fletcher, P. and Siskind, V. (1987) Differences in mortality from acute myocardial infarction between coronary care unit and medical ward: treatment or bias? *BMJ*, **295**, 1437–40.
17. Hill, J., Hampton, J. and Mitchell, J. (1978) A randomised trial of home versus hospital management for patients with suspected myocardial infarction. *Lancet*, **i**, 837–41.
18. Field, D. (1989) Emotional involvement with the dying in a coronary care unit. *Nurs. Times*, **85**, 46–8.
19. Eagle, K., Mulley, A., Skates, S. *et al.* (1990) Length of stay in the intensive care unit. Effects of practice guidelines and feedback. *JAMA*, **264**, 992–7.
20. Karlson, B.W., Herlitz, J., Wiklund, O. *et al.* (1992) Characteristics and prognosis of patients with acute myocardial infarction in relation to whether they were treated in the coronary care unit or in another ward. *Cardiology*, **81**, 134–44.
21. Holthof, B. and Selker, H.P. (1992) A cost-savings analysis of the use of a predictive instrument for coronary-care-unit admission decisions. *Health Care Manage. Rev.*, **17**, 45–50.
22. Dudley, N.J. and Burns, E. (1992) The influence of age on policies for admission and thrombolysis in coronary care units in the United Kingdom. *Age Ageing*, **21**, 95–8.
23. Fleming, C., D'Agostino, R.B. and Selker, H.P. (1991) Is coronary-care-unit admission restricted for elderly patients? A multicenter study. *Am. J. Public Health*, **81**, 1121–6.
24. Ehrenfeld, M. (1991) Social correlates of satisfaction and stress among Israeli nurses within intensive coronary care units (I.C.C.U.s). *Int. J. Nurs. Stud.*, **28**, 39–45.
25. Davison, G., Suchman, A.L. and Goldstein, B.J. (1990) Reducing unnecessary coronary care unit admissions: a comparison of three decision aids. *J. Gen. Intern. Med.*, **5**, 474–9.
26. Gunnar, R.M., Bourdillon, P.D.V., Dixon, D.W. *et al.* (1990) ACC/AHA Guidelines for the early management of patients with acute myocardial infarction. *Circulation*, **82**, 664–707.
27. Alpert, J. (1991) Myocardial infarction: general considerations. In: Rippe, J.M., Irwin, R.S., Alpert, J.S. and Fink, M.P. (eds) *Intensive Care Medicine*, pp. 364–74. Boston: Little, Brown and Company.
28. Lee, T.H. and Goldman, L. (1988) The coronary care unit turns 25: historical trends and future directions. *Ann. Intern. Med.*, **108**, 887–94.
29. Julian, D., Valentine, P. and Miller, G. (1984) Disturbances of rate, rhythm and conduction in acute myocardial infarction. *Am. J. Med.*, **37**, 915–27.
30. Meltzer, L. and Kitchell, J. (1966) The incidence of arrhythmias associated with myocardial infarction. *Prog. Cardiovasc. Dis.*, **9**, 50–63.

31. Lown, B. and Vassaux, C. (1968) Lidocaine in acute myocardial infarction. *Am. Heart J.*, **76**, 586–7.
32. MacMahon, S., Collins, R., Peto, R. *et al.* (1988) Effects of prophylactic lidocaine in suspected acute myocardial infarction. An overview of results from the randomized, controlled trials. *JAMA*, **260**, 1910–16.
33. Hine, L., Laird, N., Hewitt, P. and Chalmers, T. (1989) Meta-analytic evidence against prophylactic use of lidocaine in acute myocardial infarction. *Arch. Intern. Med.*, **149**, 2694–8.
34. Meltzer, L. and Kitchell, J. (1972) The development and current status of coronary care. In: Meltzer, L.M. and Dunning, A.J. (eds) *Textbook of Coronary Care*, pp. 3–25. Amsterdam: Excerpta Medica.
35. Antman, E.M. and Berlin, J.A. (1992) Declining incidence of ventricular fibrillation in myocardial infarction: implications for the use of lidocaine. *Circulation*, **84**, 764–73.
36. Swan, H., Ganz, W., Forrester, J. *et al.* (1970) Cardiac catheterization with a flow-directed balloon-tipped catheter. *N. Engl. J. Med.*, **283**, 447–51.
37. Geddes, J. (1986) Twenty years of pre-hospital coronary care. *Br. Heart J.*, **56**, 491–5.
38. Maroko, P., Kjekshus, J., Sobel, B. *et al.* (1971) Factors influencing infarct size following experimental coronary artery occlusion. *Circulation*, **43**, 67–83.
39. Collins, R. and Julian, D. (1991) British Heart Foundation surveys (1987 and 1989) of United Kingdom treatment policies for acute myocardial infarction. *Br. Heart J.*, **66**, 250–5.
40. DeWood, M., Sores, J., Notske R. *et al.* (1980) Prevalence of total coronary occlusion during the early hours of transmural myocardial infarction. *N. Engl. J. Med.*, **303**, 897–902.
41. Selker, H.P., Griffith, J.L., Dorey F.J. and D'Agostino, R.B. (1987) How do physicians adapt when the coronary care unit is full? A prospective multicenter study. *JAMA*, **257**, 1181–5.
42. Fuchs, R. and Scheidt, S. (1981) Improved criteria for admission to cardiac care units. *JAMA*, **246**, 2037–41.
43. Nattel, S., Warnica, J. and Ogilvie, R. (1980) Indications for admission to a coronary care unit in patients with unstable angina. *Can. Med. Assoc. J.*, **122**, 180–4.
44. Eisenberg, J., Horowitz, L., Busch, R. *et al.* (1979) Diagnosis of acute myocardial infarction in the ER: a prospective assessment of clinical decision making and the usefulness of immediate cardiac enzyme determination. *J. Community Health*, **4**, 190–8.
45. Seager, S. (1980) Cardiac enzymes in the evaluation of chest pain. *Ann. Emerg. Med.*, **9**, 346–9.
46. Horowitz, R. and Morganroth, J. (1982) Immediate detection of early high-risk patients with an acute myocardial infarction using two-dimensional echocardiographic evaluation of left ventricular regional wall abnormalities. *Am. Heart J.*, **103**, 814–22.
47. Wackers, F., Kie, K., Liem, K. *et al.* (1979) Potential value of thallium-201 scintigraphy as a means of selecting patients for the coronary care unit. *Br. Heart J.*, **41**, 111–17.
48. Pozen, M., D'Agostino, R., Selker, H. *et al.* (1984) A predictive instrument to improve coronary-care-unit admission practices in acute ischemic heart disease. *N. Engl. J. Med.*, **310**, 1273–8.
49. Goldman, L., Cook, E., Brand, D. *et al.* (1988) A computer protocol to predict myocardial infarction in emergency department patients with chest pain. *N. Engl. J. Med.*, **318**, 797–803.
50. Selker, H., Griffith, J. and Beshansky, J. (1994) The acute cardiac ischemia time-insensitive predictive instrument (ACI-TIPI): a decision aid for emergency department triage and a measure of appropriateness of coronary care unit use. In: Califf, R.M., Mark, D.B. and Wagner, G.S. (eds) *Care in the Thrombolytic Era*, 22/e. Mosby-Year Book, Inc. (in press).
51. Nordrehaug, J.E. and Lippe, G.V.D. (1983) Hypokalemia and ventricular fibrillation in acute myocardial infarction. *Br. Heart J.*, **50**, 525–9.
52. Vatner, S., McRitchie, R., Maroko, P. *et al.* (1974) Effects of catecholamines, exercise, and nitroglycerin on the normal and ischemic myocardium in conscious dogs. *J. Clin. Invest.* **54**, 563.
53. Levine, S. and Lown, B. (1952) 'Armchair' treatment of acute coronary thrombosis. *JAMA*, **148**, 1365–9.
54. Bloch, A., Maeder, J., Haissly, J. *et al.* (1974) Early mobilization after myocardial infarction. A controlled study. *Am. J. Cardiol.*, **34**, 152–7.
55. Abraham, A., Sever, Y., Weinstein, M. *et al.* (1975) Value of early ambulation in patients with and without complications after acute myocardial infarction. *N. Engl. J. Med.*, **292**, 719–22.
56. Expert Panel on Detection Evaluation and Treatment of High Blood Cholesterol in Adults (1993) Summary of the Second Report of the National Cholesterol Education Program (NCEP) Expert Panel on Detection, Evaluation, and Treatment of High Blood Cholesterol in Adults (Adult Treatment Panel II). *JAMA*, **269**, 3015–23.
57. Cohen, M., Byrne, M., Levine, B. *et al.* (1991) Low rate of treatment of hypercholesterolemia by cardiologists in patients with suspected and proven coronary artery disease. *Circulation*, **83**, 1294–304.
58. Ryder, R., Hayes, T., Mulligan, I. *et al.* (1984) How soon after myocardial infarction should plasma lipid values be assessed? *BMJ*, **289**, 1651–3.
59. Maroko, P., Radvany, P., Braunwald, E. and Hale, S. (1975) Reduction of infarct size by oxygen inhalation following acute coronary occlusion. *Circulation*, **52**, 360.
60. Ellestad, M., Shandling, A., Hart, G. *et al.* (1992) Hyperbaric oxygen and thrombolysis in myocardial infarction. The 'hot MI' study. *Circulation*, **86**, I-47.
61. Hyzy, R. and Popovich, J. (1993) Mechanical ventilation and weaning. In: Carlson, R.W. and Geheb, M.A. (eds) *Principles and Practice of Medical Intensive Care*, pp. 924–43. Philadelphia: W.B. Saunders.
62. Pasqualucci, V. (1984) Advances in the management of cardiac pain. In: Benedetti, C. *et al.* (eds) *Advances in Pain Research and Therapy*, pp. 501–19. New York: Raven Press.
63. Herlitz, J. (1989) Analgesia in myocardial infarction. *Drugs*, **37**, 939–44.

64. Lee, G., DeMaria, A., Amsterdam, E. *et al.* (1976) Comparative effects of morphine, meperidine, and pentazocine on cardiocirculatory dynamics in patients with acute myocardial infarction. *Am. J. Med.*, **60**, 949–55.
65. Blomberg, S., Emanuelsson, H. and Ricksten, S. (1989) Thoracic epidural anesthesia and central hemodynamics in patients with unstable angina pectoris. *Anesth. Analg.* **69**, 558–62.
66. Blomberg, S., Emanuelsson, H., Kvist, H. *et al.* (1990) Effects of thoracic epidural anesthesia on coronary arteries and arterioles in patients with coronary artery disease. *Anesthesiology*, **73**, 840–7.
67. Kock, M., Blomberg, S., Emanuelsson, H. *et al.* (1990) Thoracic epidural anesthesia improves global and regional left ventricular function during stress-induced myocardial ischemia in patients with coronary artery disease. *Anesth. Analg.*, **71**, 625–30.
68. Thompson, P. and Lown, B. (1976) Nitrous oxide as an analgesic in acute myocardial infarction. *JAMA*, **235**, 924–7.
69. Wynne, J., Mann, T., Alpert, J. *et al.* (1980) Hemodynamic effects of nitrous oxide administered during cardiac catheterization. *JAMA*, **243**, 1440–3.
70. Stern, T.A. (1987) Psychiatric management of acute myocardial infarction in the coronary care unit. *Am. J. Cardiol.*, **60**, 59J–67J.
71. Romhilt, D., Bloomfield, S., Chou, T. *et al.* (1973) Unreliability of conventional electrocardiographic monitoring for arrhythmia detection in coronary care units. *Am. J. Cardiol.*, **31**, 457.
72. Mirvis, D., Berson, A., Goldberger, A. *et al.* (1989) Instrumentation and practice standards for electrocardiographic monitoring in special care units. *Circulation*, **79**, 464–71.
73. Forrester, J., Diamond, G., Chatterjee, K. *et al.* (1976) Medical therapy of acute myocardial infarction by the application of hemodynamic subsets. *N. Engl. J. Med.*, **295**, 1356–62.
74. Killip, T. and Kimball, J. (1967) Treatment of myocardial infarction in a coronary care unit. A two year experience with 250 patients. *Am. J. Cardiol.*, **20**, 457.
75. Paglairello, G. (1993) The pulmonary artery (Swan–Ganz) catheter. *Int.J. Technology Assessment in Health Care*, **9**, 202–9.
76. Gore, J., Goldberg, R., Spodick, D. *et al.* (1987) A community-wide assessment of the use of pulmonary artery catheters in patients with acute myocardial infarction. *Chest*, **92**, 721–7.
77. Robin, E. (1987) Death by pulmonary artery flow-directed catheter. *Chest*, **92**, 727–31.
78. Muller, D.W.M. and Topol, E.J. (1990) Selection of patients with acute myocardial infarction for thrombolytic therapy. *Ann. Intern. Med.*, **113**, 949–60.
79. Lee, T.H., Weisberg, M.C., Brand, D.A. *et al.* (1989) Candidates for thrombolysis among emergency room patients with acute chest pain. Potential true- and false-positive rates. *Ann. Intern. Med.*, **110**, 957–62.
80. Murray, N., Lyons, J., Layton, C. *et al.* (1987) What proportion of patients with myocardial infarction are suitable for thrombolysis? *Br. Heart J.*, **57**, 144–7.
81. Doorey, A.J., Michelson, E.L., Weber, F.J. and Dreifus, L.S. (1987) Thrombolytic therapy of acute myocardial infarction: emerging challenges of implementation. *J. Am. Coll. Cardiol.*, **10**, 1357–60.
82. Pfeffer, M.A., Moyé, L.A., Braunwald, E. *et al.* (1991) Selection bias in the use of thrombolytic therapy in acute myocardial infarction. *JAMA*, **266**, 528–32.
83. Braunwald, E. (1990) Optimizing thrombolytic therapy of acute myocardial infarction. *Circulation*, **82**, 1510–13.
84. ISIS-2 (Second International Study of Infarct Survival) Collaborative Group (1988) Randomised trial of intravenous streptokinase, oral aspirin, both, or neither among 17,187 cases of suspected acute myocardial infarction: ISIS-2. *Lancet*, **ii**, 349–60.
85. Rude, R.E., Poole, W.K., Muller, J.E. *et al.* (1983) Electrocardiographic and clinical criteria for recognition of acute myocardial infarction based on analysis of 3,697 patients. *Am. J. Cardiol.*, **52**, 936–41.
86. The TIMI IIIB Investigators (1994) Effects of tissue plasminogen activator and a comparison of early invasive and conservative strategies in unstable angina and non-Q-wave myocardial infarction. *Circulation*, **89**, 1545–56.
87. Reimer, K., Lowe, J., Rasmussen, M. *et al.* (1977) The wave-front phenomenon of ischemic cell death. I: Myocardial infarct size vs duration of coronary occlusion in dogs. *Circulation*, **56**, 786–94.
88. Castaigne, A., Herve, C., Duval-Moulin, A. *et al.* (1989) Prehospital use of APSAC: results of a placebo-controlled study. *Am. J. Cardiol.*, **64**, 30A–33A.
89. Schofer, J., Buttner, J., Geng, G. *et al.* (1990) Prehospital thrombolysis in acute myocardial infarction. *Am. J. Cardiol.*, **66**, 1429–33.
90. GREAT Group (1992) Feasibility, safety, and efficacy of domiciliary thrombolysis by general practitioners: Grampian region early anistreplase trial. *BMJ*, **305**, 548–53.
91. Weaver, W.D., Cerqueira, M., Hallstrom, A.P. *et al.* (1993) Prehospital-initiated vs hospital-initiated thrombolytic therapy. The Myocardial Infarction Triage and Intervention Trial. *JAMA*, **270**, 1211–16.
92. The European Myocardial Infarction Project Group. (1993) Prehospital thrombolytic therapy in patients with suspected acute myocardial infarction. *N. Engl. J. Med.*, **329**, 383–9.
93. Gruppo Italiano Per Lo Studio Della Streptochinasi Nell'Infarto Miocardico (GISSI) (1986) Effectiveness of intravenous thrombolytic treatment in acute myocardial infarction. *Lancet*, **i**, 397–402.
94. Fibrinolytic Therapy Trialists' (FTT) Collaborative Group (1994) Indications for fibrinolytic therapy in suspected acute myocardial infarction: collaborative overview of mortality and major morbidity results from all randomised trials of more than 1000 patients. *Lancet*, **343**, 311–22.
95. LATE (Late Assessment of Thrombolytic Efficacy) Study Group. (1992) Late assessment of thrombolytic efficacy (LATE) study with alteplase 6–24 hours after onset of acute myocardial infarction. *Lancet*, **342**, 759–66.

96. EMERAS (Estudio Multicentrico Estreptoquinasa Republicas de America del Sur) Collaborative Group. (1993) Randomized trial of late thrombolysis in acute myocardial infarction. *Lancet*, **342**, 767–72.

97. Maggioni, A., Maseri, A., Fresco, C. *et al.* (1993) Age-related increase in mortality among patients with first myocardial infarctions treated with thrombolysis. *N. Engl. J. Med.*, **329**, 1442–8.

98. Krumholz, H.M., Pasternak, R.C., Weinstein, M.C. *et al.* (1992) Cost effectiveness of thrombolytic therapy with streptokinase in elderly patients with suspected acute myocardial infarction. *N. Engl. J. Med.*, **327**, 7–13.

99. Mauri, F., Gasparini, M., Barbonaglia, L. *et al.* (1989) Prognostic significance of the extent of myocardial injury in acute myocardial infarction treated by streptokinase (the GISSI trial). *Am. J. Cardiol.*, **63**, 1291–5.

100. Hillis, L., Forman, S., Braunwald, E. and the Thrombolysis in Myocardial Infarction (TIMI) Phase II Co-Investigators (1990) Risk stratification before thrombolytic therapy in patients with acute MI. *J. Am. Coll. Cardiol.*, **16**, 313–15.

101. Terrin, M., Williams, D., Kleiman, N. *et al.* (1993) Two- and three-year results of the Thrombolysis in Myocardial Infarction (TIMI) Phase II Clinical Trial. *J. Am. Coll. Cardiol.*, **22**, 1763–72.

102. Simoons, M., Maggioni, A., Knatterud, G. *et al.* (1993) Individual risk assessment for intracranial hemorrhage during thrombolytic therapy. *Lancet*, **342**, 1523–8.

103. Weisman, H. and Healy, B. (1987) Myocardial infarct expansion, infarct extension, and reinfarction: pathophysiologic concepts. *Prog. Cardiovasc. Dis.*, **30**, 73–110.

104. Marmor, A., Sobel, B. and Roberts, R. (1981) Factors presaging early recurrent myocardial infarction ('extension') *Am. J. Cardiol.*, **48**, 603–9.

105. Pfeffer, M.A., Braunwald, E. and Jugdutt, B.I. (1990) Ventricular remodelling after myocardial infarction. Experimental observations and clinical implications. *Circulation*, **81**, 1161–72.

106. Sugiura, T., Iwasaka, T., Takahashi, N. *et al.* (1990) Factors associated with late onset of advanced atrioventricular block in acute Q wave inferior infarction. *Am. Heart J.*, **119**, 1008–13.

107. Behar, S., Zissman, E., Zion, M. *et al.* (1993) Complete atrioventricular block complicating inferior acute wall myocardial infarction: short- and long-term prognosis. *Am. Heart J.*, **125**, 1622–7.

108. Clemmensen, P., Bates, E.R., Califf, R.M. *et al.* (1991) Complete atrioventricular block complicating inferior wall acute myocardial infarction treated with reperfusion therapy. TAMI Study Group. *Am. J. Cardiol.*, **67**, 225–30.

109. Berger, P.B., Ruocco, N.A. Jr, Ryan, T.J. *et al.* (1992) Incidence and prognostic implications of heart block complicating inferior myocardial infarction treated with thrombolytic therapy: results from TIMI II. *J. Am. Coll. Cardiol.*, **20**, 533–40.

110. Nicod, P., Gilpin, E., Dittrich, H. *et al.* (1988) Long-term outcome in patients with inferior myocardial infarction and complete atrioventricular block. *J. Am. Coll. Cardiol.*, **12**, 589–94.

111. McDonald, K., O'Sullivan, J.J., Conroy, R.M. *et al.* (1990) Heart block as a predictor of in-hospital death in both acute inferior and acute anterior myocardial infarction. *Q. J. Med.*, **74**, 277–82.

112. Mavric, Z., Zaputovic, L., Matana, A. *et al.* (1990) Prognostic significance of complete atrioventricular block in patients with acute inferior myocardial infarction with and without right ventricular involvement. *Am. Heart J.*, **119**, 823–8.

113. Bonaduce, D., Petretta, M., Arrichiello, P. *et al.* (1992) Effects of captopril treatment on left ventricular remodeling and function after anterior myocardial infarction: comparison with digitalis. *J. Amer. Coll. Cardiol.*, **19**, 858–63.

114. Mølstad, P. (1993) Digitalis in patients after myocardial infarction. *Herz*, **18**, 118–23.

115. Moss, A.J., Davis, H.T., Conard, D.L. *et al.* (1981) Digitalis-associated cardiac mortality after myocardial infarction. *Circulation*, **64**, 1150–6.

116. Ryan, T.J., Bailey, K.R., McCabe, C.H. *et al.* (1983) The effects of digitalis on survival in high-risk patients with coronary artery disease. *Circulation*, **67**, 735–42.

117. Madsen, E.B., Gilpin, E., Henning, H. *et al.* (1984) Prognostic importance of digitalis after myocardial infarction. *J. Am. Coll. Cardiol.*, **3**, 681–9.

118. Bigger, J.T., Fleiss, J.L., Rolnitzky, L.M. *et al.* (1985) Effect of digitalis treatment on survival after acute myocardial infarction. *Am. J. Cardiol.*, **55**, 623–30.

119. Byington, R., Goldstein, S. for the BHAT Research Group (1985) Association of digitalis therapy with mortality in survivors of acute myocardial infarction: observations in the beta-blocker heart attack trial. *J. Am. Coll. Cardiol.*, **6**, 976–82.

120. Muller, J.E., Turi, Z.G., Stone, P.H. *et al.* (1986) Digoxin therapy and mortality after myocardial infarction. *N. Engl. J. Med.*, **314**, 265–71.

121. Digitalis Subcommittee of the Multicenter Post-Infarction Research Group (1987) The mortality risk associated with digitalis treatment after myocardial infarction. *Cardiovasc. Drugs Ther.*, **1**, 125–32.

122. Zack, P.M., Chaitman, B.R., Davis, K.B. *et al.* (1989) Survival pattern in clinical and angiographic subsets of medically treated patients with combined proximal left anterior descending and proximal circumflex artery disease (CASS). *Am. Heart J.*, **118**, 220–7.

123. Mølstad, P. and Abdelnoor, M. (1991) Digitoxin-associated mortality in acute myocardial infarction. *Eur. Heart J.*, **12**, 65–9.

124. Køber, L., Torp-Pedersen, C., Hildebrandt, C. *et al.* (1992) Digoxin is an independent risk factor for long term mortality after acute myocardial infarction. *Eur. Heart J.*, **13**(suppl.), 1897.

125. Yusuf, S., Garg, R., Held, P. and Gorlin, R. (1992) Need for a large randomized trial to evaluate the effects of digitalis on morbidity and mortality in congestive heart failure. *Am. J. Cardiol.*, **69**, 64G–70G.

126. Burchell, H.B. (1990) Digitalis associated mortality in patients after a myocardial infarction: moral responsibilities in recommending clinical trials. *Int. J. Cardiol.*, **29**, 105–7.

127. Erhardt, L. (1974) Clinical and pathological observations in different types of acute myocardial infarction: A study of 84 patients deceased after treatment in a coronary care unit. *Acta Med. Scand. (Suppl.)* **560**, 1.
128. Spodick, D. (1990) Pericardial complications of myocardial infarction. In: Francis, G.S. and Alpert, J.S. (eds) *Modern Coronary Care*, pp. 331–9. Boston: Little, Brown and Co.
129. Gore, J.M., Haffajee, C.I., Love, J.C. and Dalen, J.E. (1984) Isolated right ventricular tamponade after pericarditis from acute myocardial infarction. *Am. J. Cardiol.*, **53**, 372–3.
130. Karim, A.H. and Salomon, J. (1985) Constrictive pericarditis after myocardial infarction. Sequela of anticoagulant-induced hemopericardium. *Am. J. Med.*, **79**, 389–90.
131. Cheung, P.K., Myers, M.L. and Arnold, J.M. (1991) Early constrictive pericarditis and anemia after Dressler's syndrome and inferior wall myocardial infarction. *Br. Heart J.*, **65**, 360–2.
132. Kloner, R., Fishbein, M., Lew, H. *et al.* (1978) Mummification of the infarcted myocardium by high dose corticosteroids. *Circulation*, **57**, 56.
133. Bermen, J., Haffajee, C.I. and Alpert, J.S. (1981) Therapy of symptomatic pericarditis after myocardial infarction: retrospective and prospective studies of aspirin, indomethacin, prednisone, and spontaneous resolution. *Am. Heart J.*, **101**, 750–3.
134. Kossowsky, W., Epstein, P. and Levine, R. (1973) Post-myocardial-infarction syndrome: An early complication of acute myocardial infarction. *Chest*, **63**, 35.
135. Lichstein, E. (1983) The changing spectrum of post-myocardial infarction pericarditis. *Int. J. Cardiol.*, **4**, 234–7.
136. Lichstein, E., Arsura, E., Hollander, G. *et al.* (1982) Current incidence of postmyocardial infarction (Dressler's) syndrome. *Am. J. Cardiol.*, **50**, 1269.
137. Minter, W.T. 3rd (1967) The shoulder–hand syndrome in coronary disease. *J. Med. Assoc. Ga.*, **56**, 45–9.
138. Woodhouse, S.P. (1968) Shoulder–hand syndrome following myocardial infarction. *NZ Med. J.*, **68**, 387–8.
139. McNeer, J., Wagner, G., Ginsburg, P. *et al.* (1978) Hospital discharge one week after acute myocardial infarction. *N. Engl. J. Med.*, **298**, 229–32.
140. Topol, E., Burek, K., O'Neill, W. *et al.* (1988) A randomized controlled trial of early hospital discharge three days after myocardial infarction in the era of reperfusion. *N. Engl. J. Med.*, **318**, 1083–8.
141. Sanz, G., Betriu, A., Oller, G. *et al.* (1993) Feasibility of early discharge after acute Q wave myocardial infarction in patients not receiving thrombolytic treatment. *J. Am. Coll. Cardiol.*, **22**, 1795–801.
142. Goldstein, S. (1993) Early discharge after a myocardial infarction: what's the hurry? *J. Am. Coll. Cardiol.*, **22**, 1802–3.
143. Turkie, W. and Brown, A.K. (1990) The use of radiotelemetry after discharge from the coronary care unit. *J. R. Coll. Physicians Lond.*, **24**, 277–80.
144. Rigotti, N.A., Singer, D.E., Mulley, A.G. Jr and Thibault, G.E. (1991) Smoking cessation following admission to a coronary care unit. *J. Gen. Intern. Med.*, **6**, 305–11.
145. Collinson, P.O., Ramhamadamy, E.M., Stubbs, P.J. *et al.* (1993) Rapid enzyme diagnosis of patients with acute chest pain reduces patient stay in the coronary care unit. *Ann. Clin. Biochem.*, **30**, 17–22.
146. Adams, J. III, Abendschein, D. and Jaffe, A. (1993) Biochemical markers of myocardial injury. Is MB creatine kinase the choice for the 1990s? *Circulation*, **88**, 750–63.
147. Pozen, M., Stechmiller, J. and Voigt, M. (1977) Prognostic efficacy of early clinical categorization of myocardial infarction patients. *Circulation*, **56**, 816–19.
148. Krone, R. (1992) The role of risk stratification in the early management of a myocardial infarction. *Ann. Intern. Med.*, **116**, 223–37.
149. Vacek, J., Hibiya, K., Rosamond, T. *et al.* (1991) Validation of a bedside method of activated partial thromboplastin time measurement with clinical range guidelines. *Am. J. Cardiol.*, **68**, 557–9.
150. Booth, F. (1993) Computers in critical care. In: Carlson, R.W. and Geheb, M.A. (eds) *Principles and Practice of Medical Intensive Care*, pp. 88–95. Philadelphia: W.B. Saunders.
151. Kowalewski, D. and Carlson, R. (1993) Artificial intelligence and expert systems in critical care medicine. In: Carlson, R.W. and Geheb, M.A. (eds) *Principles and Practice of Medical Intensive Care*, pp. 95–108. Philadelphia: W.B. Saunders.

3

Choice of Thrombolytic Agent

G. V. Martin and J. W. Kennedy

Rationale for Reperfusion Therapy in Myocardial Infarction

Myocardial infarction (MI) usually results from complete or near total obstruction of an epicardial coronary artery by a ruptured atherosclerotic plaque with adherent thrombus. High-energy phosphate depletion, glycolytic endproduct accumulation and tissue acidosis quickly follow. The exact mechanism of cell death is uncertain, but animal studies indicate that progression from reversible cell injury to cell death is time dependent and related to the severity of the ischemia. For example, in the dog myocytes begin to die as early as 20 min following abrupt coronary occlusion,[1] while lesser ischemia may be tolerated for much longer periods, and perhaps indefinitely, due to metabolic 'down-regulation'.[2] Little is known about the exact time course of cell death in humans, but there are considerable data supporting the concept that reperfusion within the first several hours (especially in the first hour) limits tissue necrosis.

The fundamental goal of reperfusion therapy for MI is to prevent tissue necrosis by restoring blood flow to ischemic myocardium. The adequacy of blood flow cannot be expressed in absolute terms, but must be sufficient to meet the metabolic needs of the residual viable tissue. Ideally, reperfusion should minimize infarct size and the clinical sequelae of myocardial injury without causing adverse systemic effects. Since the progression from reversible to irreversible myocyte injury is time dependent, the amount of tissue salvage should relate to the rapidity of reperfusion.

This chapter will review pertinent clinical data regarding thrombolysis as a method of reperfusion. The general strengths and limitations of this approach are discussed and the available thrombolytic agents are compared with respect to clinical endpoints, including mortality. Suggestions regarding the use of thrombolytic agents in specific subsets of patients with MI are provided.

Thrombolytic Therapy

Historical Perspective

The modern era of thrombolytic therapy began with the first use of intracoronary streptokinase (SK) therapy by Chazov[3] and Rentrop.[4] During the 4 or 5 years during the early 1980s that intracoronary SK was widely used a great deal of valuable information was accumulated about the clinical and angiographic characteristics of thrombolytic therapy. The principal advantage of intracoronary therapy was the opportunity to observe the process of clot lysis by performing frequent angiograms of the infarct vessel,

71

often every 15 min, during SK infusion. Typically, intravenous SK was delivered at a rate of about 4000 u min^{-1} either as a bolus every minute or as a continuous infusion for a total of 250 000–300 000 u. In one randomized trial using this protocol, the average time from onset of the infusion to vessel opening was 31 min with 67% of those with totally occluded vessels achieving patency.[5] By observing the progress of therapy, it soon became clear that at times vessels opened abruptly and normal flow was established almost immediately, while in other patients the vessel opened and closed during the course of the infusion and flow varied from moment to moment. Occasionally, proximal thrombi were observed to embolize downstream occluding the distal vessel but, usually, the next angiogram demonstrated that the distal occlusion had lysed and flow had been reestablished.

Intracoronary SK therapy proved to be very effective at opening vessels and was associated with a low rate of serious complications. Since the usual dose of SK was about one-sixth the usual dose of intravenous SK, the most dread complication, intracerebral hemorrhage, was rarely encountered. The major problems with the use of intracoronary SK were logistic and related to the difficulty of providing rapid 24-hour access to the cardiac catheterization laboratory. The first major improvement in thrombolytic therapy for acute MI occurred when Schroder *et al.* demonstrated that intravenous SK given in a dose of 1.5 million u over 1 hour resulted in a high early infarct-related patency rate.[6] This finding was rapidly confirmed by a series of small randomized trials comparing intracoronary and intravenous SK therapy.[7–10] Other studies demonstrated there was little overall difference in vessel patency at 24 hours and beyond and no apparent difference in clinical outcome with intravenous as compared to intracoronary therapy. Thus, by 1985 or 1986 most clinical centers in the USA and in Europe had converted from intracoronary to intravenous therapy. The use of immediate coronary angiography in patients with acute MI had another important effect for it demonstrated in many thousands of patients that angiography carried out by experienced cardiologists was a safe procedure even in these often unstable patients. The safe use of acute coronary angiography thereby set the stage for the future use of primary and early secondary percutaneous transluminal coronary angioplasty (PTCA) for the management of patients with acute MI.

Once intravenous SK had been established as an effective therapy, numerous trials were initiated to compare thrombolytic therapy with routine treatment. These trials were of two types: large trials with mortality as the major endpoint such as GISSI[11] and ISIS-2,[12] and many smaller trials which used infarct size, left ventricular function, or vessel patency as endpoints.

During the beginning of the modern era of thrombolytic therapy in the early 1980s many assumed that SK would soon be replaced by newer thrombolytic agents that would be both safer and more effective. The general approach was to develop more potent plasminogen activators that produced less systemic fibrinolysis, and that also would not be antigenic and thus could be used repeatedly in a patient without the possibility of allergic reactions or reduced efficacy due to the presence of neutralizing antibodies, such as occurs with SK. These efforts led to the development and testing of several compounds, most notably tissue plasminogen activator (t-PA), anisoylated plasminogen streptokinase activator complex (APSAC), and single-chain urokinase-type plasminogen activator (scuPA), and subsequently to studies to compare various thrombolytic agents to determine which was most effective and had the best safety profile.

Characteristics of the Thrombolytic Agents

Drugs used for thrombolytic therapy activate plasminogen, the inactive precursor of the fibrinolytic enzyme plasmin. Three have been tested in large clinical trials to assess their

Table 3.1 Comparison of US FDA-approved thrombolytic agents

	SK	APSAC	t-PA
Dose	1.5 million u in 30–60 min	30 mg in 5 min	100 mg in 90 min[a]
Circulating half-life (min)	20	100	6
Antigenic	Yes	Yes	No
Allergic reactions	Yes	Yes	No
Systemic fibrinogen depletion	Severe	Severe	Moderate
Intracerebral hemorrhage	~0.3%	~0.6%	~0.6%
90-min Recanalization rate[b]	~40%	~63%	~79%
Lives saved per 100	~2.5	~2.5	~3.5[c]
Cost per dose (approx. $US)	200	1 700	2 200
Cost per life saved ($US)	8 000	68 000	62 857

[a]'Accelerated' t-PA is given as follows: 15 mg bolus, then 0.75 mg kg^{-1} over 30 min (maximum, 50 mg), then 0.50 mg kg^{-1} over 60 min (maximum, 35 mg).
[b]Based on published data and assuming that 20% of arteries are already open prior to therapy.
[c]Based on the finding from the GUSTO trial[37] that accelerated t-PA saves one more additional life per 100 than does SK.
APSAC, anisoylated plasminogen streptokinase activator complex; SK, streptokinase; t-PA, tissue plasminogen activator.

effects on mortality. They are SK, t-PA and APSAC. Two other drugs, scuPA and urokinase (UK) have been tested less thoroughly and beneficial effects on survival have not been proven. The drugs are of two basic types: those that extensively activate the fibrinolytic system in the blood, resulting in depletion of plasma proteins including fibrinogen and factors V and VIII (SK, UK and APSAC), and the 'fibrin-specific' plasminogen activators which preferentially activate plasminogen at the fibrin surface (t-PA and scuPA), resulting in less fibrinogen depletion. The agents also differ in a number of other respects (Table 3.1). Various other compounds are also under development.[13]

SK, a protein derived from group C streptococci, is the oldest and most studied of these drugs. SK binds to plasminogen forming a complex which activates plasminogen. One disadvantage of SK is that it may cause hypotension requiring specific supportive measures. Rarely it causes febrile reactions, urticaria, angioedema and more severe anaphylactoid reactions. Exposure to SK results in long-lasting antibody formation, although the clinical implications of SK antibodies have not been defined.[14] However, when retreatment is required in a patient who has received SK or APSAC it is advisable to use t-PA. UK is a direct plasminogen activator isolated from human urine. Despite being the second plasminogen activator to be discovered (after SK), it has not been investigated for efficacy in MI to the same extent as newer agents. APSAC is a derivative of SK which becomes active after deacylation in the plasma. The fibrinolytic properties of APSAC are similar to those of SK, the chief distinction being a relatively longer plasma half-life (40 min) and the resultant convenience of single bolus administration. t-PA is a human protein produced by genetic engineering techniques and has been prepared in both the single-chain (alteplase) or double-chain (duteplase) forms; the former is the widely used commercial form. Along with SK, it is the most commonly used thrombolytic agent worldwide. t-PA is able to lyse clots faster than SK possibly because of less 'plasminogen steal' or loss of clot-bound plasminogen.[15] scuPA is also a human protein produced by recombinant technology. In the circulation it is inhibited by a plasma protein but becomes active in the presence of fibrin. Both t-PA and scuPA have greater thrombolytic potency than SK and share with UK the advantage of being nonantigenic.

Clinical Effects of Thrombolytic Therapy

Thrombus Dissolution

The key morphologic components of acute coronary obstruction have been recognized for nearly 30 years.[16] In most cases, the obstructing mass is made up of a lipid-rich atheromatous plaque with a superimposed thrombus adherent to the site of a tear in the fibrous cap of the plaque. The essential rationale for thrombolytic therapy is that thrombus is responsible for a significant portion of the impedance to blood flow and that thrombus dissolution will restore normal antegrade flow. In no less than about 20% of cases, thrombolytic therapy fails to recanalize the infarct artery. The exact reasons for thrombolytic inefficacy are not known. The possibilities include that (1) the obstructing mass contains little or no clot but rather mostly disrupted plaque elements, (2) the lytic agent does not sufficiently perfuse the clot, or (3) some thrombi (or portions of thrombi) are more resistant to plasminogen activators.[17] One cogent hypothesis is that thrombi which cause MI contain a thrombolysis-resistant, platelet-rich portion adjacent to the plaque rupture site, and a more thrombolysis-sensitive portion comprised mostly of erythrocytes and fibrin which forms the 'tail' of the thrombus.[18]

Although angiograms underestimate the extent of luminal clot,[19] careful quantitative studies have aided our understanding of successful coronary recanalization. Brown and associates[20] studied angiograms from 32 patients with recanalized arteries following intracoronary SK. In all but two it was possible to separately identify the margins of the original atherosclerotic plaque and the superimposed thrombus. At the start of SK treatment, the mean diameter of the original plaque was 1.57 mm, it obstructed 56% of the vessel lumen diameter, and did not change with 60–90 min of SK treatment. The mean diameter of the adjacent thrombus decreased from 1.2 mm to 0.58 mm with SK infusion, while the recanalized lumen increased from 0.08 mm to 0.65 mm. The mean final diameter stenosis of the vessel lumen was 77%. In 9 patients with open vessels 5 weeks post SK, an additional improvement in luminal diameter of 0.34 mm (or roughly half the improvement achieved during the SK infusion) was observed, although thrombus was often still present. In the TEAM-2 study,[21] the mean minimum lumen diameter and per cent diameter stenosis following intravenous SK was 0.71 mm and 77.2% respectively. Following intravenous APSAC the measurements were similar, 0.78 mm and 74%.

Several conclusions may be drawn from these and similar studies. Acute coronary thrombosis most often occurs in arteries with only a moderate underlying narrowing (approximately 50% diameter stenosis)[22] and therefore a substantial fraction of the occlusive mass is comprised of thrombus. Thrombolytic therapy dissolves clot in a time-dependent fashion but usually does not result in complete thrombus resolution by 90 min. Most patients are left with a high-grade (about 75% diameter, or 90% area) stenosis with persistent thrombus accounting for much of the residual obstruction to flow. Late resolution of thrombus occurs but this effect cannot be entirely attributed to thrombolytic treatment per se since thrombus resolution occurs even without thrombolytic therapy. About 20% of patients who do not receive thrombolytic therapy will have a patent artery in the first 24 hours of infarction and roughly half by day 10.[23] It is not known whether or not the more potent plasminogen activators such as t-PA, in addition to lysing clots faster, also remove more clot.

There are several potential implications of persistent thrombus and/or high-grade residual stenosis. Perfusion pressure distal to the lesion may be insufficient for normal tissue perfusion and the presence of thrombus or a tight residual stenosis may predispose to rethrombosis.[24] In the APRICOT study,[25] a residual stenosis of greater than 90% was associated with a greater likelihood of reocclusion by 3 months post infarction. Other investigators have failed to find a predictable relationship between the anatomic appearance of the artery and the risk of reocclusion.[26–28] A tight residual stenosis following thrombolysis may also lead to a greater degree of left ventricular dilatation[29] and to impairment of left ventricular function during exercise.[30]

Angiographic Recanalization and Patency

Studies of coronary patency following thrombolytic therapy have varied markedly with respect to the many factors which affect the patency rate. Important among these are the thrombolytic agent used, the dose, route and timing of administration, and the timing of the posttherapy angiogram. While coronary patency is a useful and relatively convenient endpoint for thrombolytic studies, significant limitations are recognized. The administration of intracoronary nitroglycerin and/or the forceful injection of contrast will affect patency in some vessels which are not open initially. Thus, angiographic studies probably overestimate the true effect of thrombolysis alone in achieving coronary patency. Other important limitations are as follows.

In some cases following clot lysis, contrast fills and clears the affected artery more slowly than in surrounding vessels. To distinguish 'slow' filing from the normal pattern, TIMI investigators developed a grading system in which 0 or 1 signified no or minimal contrast movement past the obstruction, 2 indicated complete but slow filling, and 3 referred to normal prompt filling of the vessel.[31] In the TIMI-1 study, about 15% of patent vessels exhibited grade 2 or slow filling, a finding subsequently confirmed in other trials.[21,32–34] Whereas in most studies angiographic patency has been defined broadly as the complete opacification of the culprit vessel (i.e. TIMI grades 2 or 3), the clinical outcomes of patients with TIMI 2 flow patterns are much inferior to those with TIMI 3 flow[35–37] suggesting that total patency is an imprecise measure of thrombolytic efficacy.

Perhaps the most important limitation is that TIMI 3 patency is not synonymous with effective reperfusion of jeopardized myocardial tissue. A vessel may be successfully opened, but too late to salvage tissue. In such cases angiography may demonstrate TIMI 3 flow while nuclear imaging studies indicate a preponderance of nonviable tissue. Conversely, the vessel may open in time, but flow at the myocyte level could be inadequate due to elevated small vessel resistance in the jeopardized tissue. This might occur secondary to mechanical factors such as microvascular plugging by platelet or fibrin emboli or endothelial cell damage, or dynamic factors such as vasospasm. Using intracoronary injections of ^{99m}Tc microalbumin aggregates, before and after treatment, Schofer and colleagues observed no improvement in scintigraphic defect size in 6 of 14 patients in whom the infarct-related artery was opened using intracoronary thrombolytic therapy.[38] Ito and colleagues[39] also reported that one in four patients with angiographically successful reperfusion fail to demonstrate myocardial flow as assessed by contrast echocardiography. Angiograms also provide only a relatively static picture of the dynamic reperfusion process, and it is possible to miss important flow oscillations (either up or down).

Since recanalization can occur spontaneously only those studies which have documented the status of the artery prior to therapy are able to report true 'recanalization' rates (often referred to as 'reperfusion' rates and indicating the opening of initially closed vessels). For all other studies the reported 'patency' rates overestimate true recanalization rates because about 20% of patients will have a patent artery prior to therapy.[31] Low absolute patency rates, such as with SK, substantially overestimate recanalization rates, while high patency rates, such as with accelerated t-PA, only slightly overestimate recanalization rates (Figure 3.1). For example, assuming a pretherapy patency rate of 20%, a reported posttherapy patency rate of 50% would translate to a recanalization rate

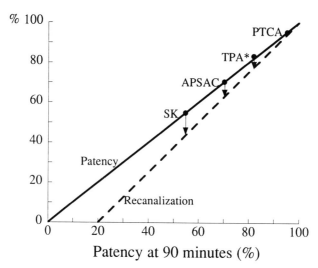

Figure 3.1   The difference between patency rates and recanalization rates for streptokinase (SK), APSAC, accelerated t-PA (t-PA*) and coronary angioplasty (PTCA). The recanalization rates are calculated by assuming that 20% of all treated patients have a patent vessel prior to therapy.

of 38% (or a difference of 12%), while a reported patency rate of 80% would indicate a recanalization rate of 75% (or a smaller absolute difference of 5%).

Table 3.2 summarizes the information from intravenous thrombolytic trials with more than 100 patients and provides both patency rates and estimated recanalization data (assuming a pretherapy patency rate of 20%). Using intracoronary SK, recanalization occurs in about 70% (equivalent to a patency rate of about 76%).[40] With intravenous SK, patency is much less by 90 min following the beginning of treatment (patency = 52.5%, estimated recanalization = 40.2).[31,37,41–43] The efficacy of SK is time dependent, being more effective when administered early after the onset of symptoms.[31] Data from the TEAM-2,[21] PRIMI,[42] and GUSTO[37] trials demonstrate that patency rates continue to increase during the first 24 hours following intravenous SK from 73% at 2–3 hours to about 80% at 24 hours.

With intravenous t-PA (at a dose of about 100 mg given over 180 min) coronary patency is established more rapidly than with SK. At 90 min from the start of therapy, the average patency rate is 72.2% from which a recanalization rate of 65.3% may be estimated.[31,32,44–49] After 2–3 hours, patency is similar to that of SK, about 75%[30,50] and also more than 80% at 24 hours.[45,51] However, as shown in several studies[32,34] including the recent GUSTO trial,[37] even faster patency can be achieved using an 'accelerated' t-PA dosing regimen (100 mg over 90 min, weight adjusted for smaller patients). Patency at 90 min with this regimen is 83.5% corresponding to a recanalization rate of 79.4%. Patency rates at 24 hours are similar to that of SK and t-PA given over 3 hours.[34,37] As shown in Table 3.2, 90-min patency rates for APSAC (70.7%),[34,52] UK (65.8%),[45] and scuPA (71.2%)[42] are superior to those for SK, roughly equal to those for standard t-PA, and less than for accelerated t-PA. Thus, the primary difference between the agents is the *rate* of recanalization as the patency rates with all the drugs are similar at 24 hours. The advantage of accelerated t-PA in this respect is highlighted by data from the RAAMI[32] and TAPS[34] trials which reported *60-min* patency rates of 76% and 73% respectively, which are at least equal to the 90-min patency achieved with standard t-PA and to the 180-min patency with SK. Figure 3.2 shows 60, 90 and 180 min patency data for SK, APSAC, and accelerated t-PA.

Table 3.2 Angiographic patency and estimated reperfusion rates at 90 min following intravenous thrombolytic therapy

Reference	No.	Time to treatment (min)	Patency (%)	Recanalization estimated[a] (%)
SK				
GUSTO[37]	577	165	58.2	47.8
Stack *et al.*[41]	216	180	44.0	30.0
PRIMI[42]	194	140	63.9	54.9
TIMI-1[31]	119	286	42.8	28.5
		Average	52.5	40.2
t-PA				
Topol *et al.*[47]	386	177	74.6	68.3
Topol *et al.*[48]	142	190	71.8	64.8
TIMI-2[44]	131	168	74.8	68.5
TAMI-3[49]	131	165	76.3	70.4
RAAMI[32]	122	162	77.0	71.3
GAUS[45]	121	180	69.4	61.8
TIMI-1[31]	113	286	69.9	62.0
KAMIT[46]	102	180	63.7	54.7
		Average	72.2	65.3
Accelerated t-PA				
GUSTO[37]	291	165	80.8	76.0
TAPS[34]	199	156	84.4	80.5
RAAMI[32]	128	162	85.3	81.6
		Average	83.5	79.4
APSAC				
TAPS[34]	202	150	70.3	62.9
ARMS[52]	156	106	73.0	66.3
		Average	70.7	63.4
UK				
GAUS[45]	117	80	65.8	57.3
scu-PA				
PRIMI[42]	401	140	71.2	64.0

[a]The recanalization rates are calculated assuming that 20% of patients have an open vessel prior to therapy.
APSAC, anisoylated plasminogen streptokinase activator complex; scu-PA, single-chain urokinase-type plasminogen activator; SK, streptokinase; t-PA, tissue plasminogen activator; UK, urokinase.

Reocclusion

Not all vessels that open initially with thrombolysis stay open. Not surprisingly, early reocclusion has been shown to be associated with worsened survival and mechanical function.[53] The reported incidence of reocclusion has varied widely in the range of 5–25% for intravenous SK,[31] intravenous t-PA,[31,54,55] and intravenous APSAC.[56] Platelet activation may play a role in early reocclusion,[57] and experimental studies indicate that antiplatelet therapy may reduce the likelihood of rethrombosis.[58,59] While there are no prospective clinical studies that document the effects of combined antiplatelet and thrombolytic therapy on reocclusion, combined therapy does appear to be safe[60] and a recent meta-analysis[61] of 33 trials suggests that aspirin reduced reocclusion following SK or t-PA from about 25% to 10%.

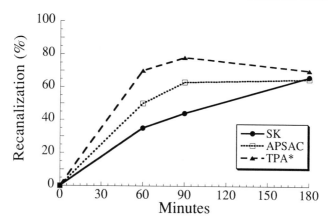

Figure 3.2 Time course of reperfusion for SK, APSAC and accelerated t-PA showing that accelerated t-PA opens about two-thirds of closed vessels by 60 min. APSAC and SK work more slowly, taking about 90 min and 180 min respectively to achieve a 65% recanalization rate.

Thrombolytic therapy also activates the coagulation system *in vivo*.[62–64] Since heparin prevents both the formation and propagation of thrombi it is widely used as an adjunct to thrombolytic therapy. Preliminary studies indicate that full dose intravenous heparin may reduce reocclusion[65] and reinfarction[12] following intravenous SK. In a randomized trial in which patients received either t-PA alone or t-PA and heparin simultaneously, heparin had no effect on 90-min vessel patency.[49] However, heparin given at the start of t-PA infusion does appear to increase overall vessel patency at 1–6 days post MI[66–68] and vessel patency in one study was positively correlated with the level of anticoagulation as assessed by activated partial thromboplastin times.[68] The promising antithrombin agent hirudin was shown to be even more effective than heparin in preventing reocclusion in the TAMI-5 trial.[69] It is likely that new, more effective antithrombotic agents will further reduce the rate of reocclusion following thrombolytic therapy.

As yet there are no definitive answers regarding whether aspirin (or other antiplatelet agents) and heparin (or other antithrombins), used either alone or in combination, decrease coronary reocclusion following successful thrombolysis, and whether such a benefit will apply equally to patients treated with SK, APSAC, and t-PA.[70] However, the experimental data suggest that aspirin and heparin will have a beneficial effect on reocclusion, and the limited clinical data available are supportive to this view. In the recently reported GUSTO trial,[37] in which aspirin and heparin were used routinely, reocclusion between 90 min and 5–7 days was only between 5 and 6% in each of the study arms using intravenous heparin and was 7.7% in patients who received subcutaneous heparin following SK. Several large-scale studies have examined the efficacy of immediate coronary angioplasty following intravenous thrombolytic therapy and provide no evidence of a reduction in angiographic reocclusion rates.[44,71–73]

Summary of the effects of thrombolytic therapy on coronary reperfusion

Thrombolytic therapy recanalizes about two-thirds of occluded infarct-related arteries. Accelerated t-PA works the fastest, taking only 60 min. APSAC is somewhat slower, taking 90 min. SK is much slower, taking about 180 min and is less effective with older clots. However, a conservative interpretation of the available angiographic data suggests that thrombolytic therapy is a successful mode of reperfusion for only a minority of the patients. For 60% of patients receiving thrombolytics, the infarct artery is either already open (20%), never opens (20%), exhibits sluggish (TIMI 2) flow (15%), or reoccludes

(5%). In the remaining 40%, angiographic success is achieved but many of these patients will be reperfused too late or will not have adequate tissue perfusion despite an open vessel. Many who reperfuse will also have significant residual thrombus and a severely narrowed coronary lumen, which may predispose to future ischemic events or precipitate further intervention.

Limitation of Infarct Size

Animal studies have shown that reperfusion following several hours of coronary occlusion results in myocardial salvage, and the same appears to be true for humans. Since most patients who die in the first few days following MI exhibit signs of left ventricular failure, limitation of infarct size is the most cogent explanation for the observed salutary effects of thrombolysis on survival.

A variety of ECG scoring systems, based on the extent and magnitude of ST segment deflection, have been used to assess the effects of thrombolytic therapy. But the correlations of ECG scores with other indices of infarct size have been inconsistent, casting doubt on the reliability of these measurements. Some studies have shown less severe ECG abnormalities following lytic therapy than after conventional therapy[74] and in one trial[75] very early treatment with t-PA resulted in fewer Q-wave infarctions.

In well-controlled animal experiments, measurements of the amount of myocardial enzymes released into the circulation following coronary occlusion is highly correlated with histologic infarct size. Human studies suggest that thrombolytic therapy decreases enzyme release by 20–30%.[76,77] Unfortunately, the kinetics of enzyme washout following reperfused infarcts in humans may be quite different and so the data from animal models may not be applicable to the clinical situation.[78]

The best widely available method for estimating infarct size involves using single photon emission computed tomography (SPECT) imaging following the injection of ^{201}Tl or ^{99m}Tc sestamibi. ^{201}Tl is taken up in the heart in proportion to blood flow,[79] and in experimental preparations infarct size assessed by ^{201}Tl agrees well with histologic measurements.[80] But comparisons of this technique with positron emission tomography (PET) have demonstrated that myocardial viability can be present in the absence of thallium uptake, suggesting that ^{201}Tl may have a tendency to overestimate infarct size.[81] Another general limitation is that this technique does not distinguish old from new infarcts and thus is most useful in patients with first MI.

More recently, ^{99m}Tc sestamibi has been applied to the study of patients with acute MI. Infarct size estimates from SPECT sestamibi studies correlate well with measures of left ventricular function, left ventricular volumes, and myocardial enzymes.[82–90] A potential advantage of this technique is the ability to also obtain estimates of the area at risk and of collateral blood flow, two major independent determinants of infarct size, both prior to and after treatment.[91]

Using ^{201}Tl, it has been estimated that lytic therapy with SK, t-PA, or APSAC reduces infarct size by 20–30%.[92–94] Although no single study has shown a convincing relationship between infarct size and time to treatment, Christian and colleagues studied 89 patients with ^{99m}Tc sestamibi and concluded that the duration of symptoms is an important determinant of infarct size in a multivariate model that incorporates collateral blood flow and myocardium at risk in the analysis.[91]

Figure 3.3 plots thallium infarct size vs the mean time to treatment data from seven thrombolysis trials.[94–100] The data demonstrate a strong linear correlation between the time to treatment and infarct size. Treatment at 60 min from the onset of symptoms reduces infarct size by 75%, salvaging 15% of the left ventricle. Treatment at 3 hours reduces infarct size by 35%, salvaging 7% of the left ventricle. Treatment at 5 hours does not save myocardium. Of course these generalizations will not apply to each individual

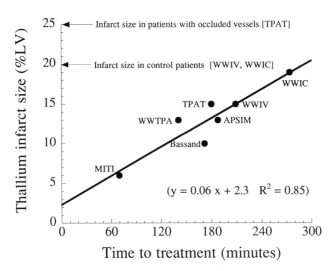

Figure 3.3 Linear relationship between infarct size measured by ^{201}Tl and the time from symptom onset to treatment. Little reduction in infarct size is achieved when treatment is started later than 4 hours from the onset of symptoms. MITI, Myocardial Infarction Triage and Intervention Trial, Ref. 99; Bassand, Ref. 95; WWTPA, Western Washington Myocardial Infarction Registry and Emergency Department Tissue Plasminogen Activator Treatment Trial, Ref. 100; TPAT, Tissue plasminogen activator: Toronto trial, Ref. 98; APSIM, Anisoylated plasminogen streptokinase activator complex (APSAC) in acute myocardial infarction trial, Ref. 94; WWIV, Western Washington Intravenous Streptokinase Trial, Ref. 97; WWIC, Western Washington Intracoronary Streptokinase Trial, Ref. 96. Data from the TPAT trial regarding patients with occluded vessels is given in Ref. 92. Data from the three Western Washington trials and MITI is also summarized in Ref. 93.

patient and they do not take into consideration infarct location. Figure 3.4 shows theoretic relationships between infarct size and time to treatment separately for anterior and inferior MI, assuming linearity and control infarct sizes of 28% of the left ventricle for anterior MI and 14% of the left ventricle for inferior MI.[97] For anterior MI, each 60-min

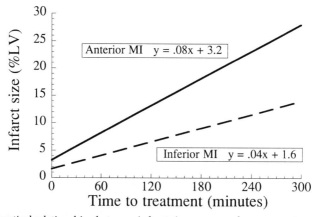

Figure 3.4 Theoretical relationships between infarct size, expressed as a percentage of the left ventricle (LV), and time to treatment separated for anterior and inferior MIs. The plots were constructed assuming a linear relationship as in Fig. 3.3 and by assuming 'contour' infarct size of 28% for anterior MI and 14% for inferior MI.

delay in the initiation of treatment results in the loss of about 5% of the left ventricle, while a similar delay in the treatment of an inferior MI results in the loss of 2.5% of the left ventricle.

Left Ventricular Function

Smaller infarcts result in better contractile function of the myocardium. Accordingly, left ventricular function has been a common endpoint in thrombolysis trials. Left ventricular ejection fraction (EF) and quantitative evaluations of regional wall motion (RWM) are the two measurements most commonly reported. The limitations of these measurements are well recognized. Most importantly, they assess systolic wall motion rather than contractility and thus are load-dependent measures. They are also time dependent. Wall motion may exhibit prolonged postischemic abnormalities due to myocardial stunning,[101] and progressive dilatation may occur up to 6 weeks post MI.[102] Therefore, early measurements may substantially underestimate or overestimate the extent of tissue recovery. EF measurements also do not account for compensatory hyperkinesis of noninfarct zones, which is commonly present in the first weeks following MI. Thus RWM analysis may be a more sensitive and specific indicator of ventricular dysfunction in patients with regional ischemia. The need for validation and limitations of RWM analyses has been reviewed.[103] Despite these limitations, EF and RWM analysis do provide prognostically important information, correlate with other measures of infarct size, and in the context of randomized trials have lent additional support to the concept that thrombolytic therapy preserves myocardium.

Randomized placebo-controlled data on left ventricular function were first obtained in trials of intracoronary SK.[104–107] Results were generally unimpressive, with a statistically significant benefit in favor of SK found only in the trial by Anderson *et al.*[105] In two studies[104,107] EF was measured both before and after treatment and in both trials the late EF was within 3 EF units of the early measurement in both SK and control patients. It is likely that a significant benefit of SK on left ventricular function was not shown in these trials because patients were treated too late. The one intracoronary SK trial that did show an EF difference was the one treating patients the earliest, having randomized only patients presenting within 4 hours of symptom onset.[105]

The EF data for intravenous thrombolysis trials[30,76,94,98,108–114] is summarized in Table 3.3. These studies reported global EF (measured either by contrast or radionuclide ventriculography) at 1–3 weeks post MI. On average, EF for treatment patients was 5 units higher (range −1.0 to 7.0) than for control patients. As with mortality benefits, the salutary effects of thrombolytic therapy on left ventricular function are greater with anterior MI than inferior MI.[76,108–112] Since infarcts in the distribution of the left anterior descending artery are larger than infarcts in the distribution of the right coronary artery, the potential for salvage is greater with anterior infarcts. Collateral vessels are also more frequently observed with occlusion of the right coronary artery[115] and might provide a protective effect in patients failing to reperfuse,[116–119] thus minimizing the relative impact of reperfusion therapy.

The Western Washington[120] and Australian National Heart Foundation[108] trials compared RWM (measured by contrast ventriculography) in treated and control patients at 5–10 days post MI and found no significant differences in wall motion of the infarct zone, although trends in favor of lytic therapy were present in both studies. In the Western Washington trial, wall motion in the infarct zone was expressed in standard deviations from normal wall motion, as assessed in 52 normal subjects. RWM was −2.48 for SK patients and −2.70 for control patients ($P = 0.24$). Benefit was most prominent in patients treated less than 3 hours from symptom onset. In this trial, SK-treated patients did show statistically significant better wall motion in areas remote from the site of infarction. On

Table 3.3 Effects of thrombolysis on global left ventricular function (ejection fraction)

Reference	No.	Drug	Treatment EF (%)	Control EF (%)
ISAM[113]	848	SK	56.8	53.9
Western Washington IV[110]	368	SK	54.3	50.7
White et al.[111]	219	SK	59.0	53.0
Bassand et al.[112]	96	SK	45.0	44.0
		Average	53.8	50.4
Van de Werf and Arnold[76]	721	t-PA	50.7	48.5
National Heart Foundation[108]	144	t-PA	57.7	51.7
Guerci et al.[30]	138	t-PA	53.2	46.4
TICO[108]	126	t-PA	61.0	54.0
TPAT[92]	115	t-PA	53.6	47.8
		Average	55.2	49.6
Meinertz et al.[114] a	256	APSAC	53.0	54.0
APSIM[94]	209	APSAC	53.0	47.0
		Average	53.0	51.0

[a]Data for anterior MI only.
APSAC, anisoylated plasminogen streptokinase activator complex; SK, streptokinase; t-PA, tissue plasminogen activator.

average, SK-treated patients displayed mild hyperkinesis of noninfarct zones while control patients did not.[120] Similar findings for noninfarct regions have been observed by others.[112,121,122]

Studies which compared two or more different agents are shown in Table 3.4.[21,34,37,45,51,95,116,123,124] Most comparative studies have reported no difference between the various thrombolytic agents. Anderson et al.[51] found small but statistically significant EF and RWM differences in favor of t-PA versus APSAC. In GUSTO,[37] a very small but statistically significant difference in favor of accelerated t-PA vs SK was found for RWM but not for EF at both 90 min and 5–7 days.

Table 3.4 Studies comparing the effects of different thrombolytic agents on left ventricular function

Reference	No.	Ejection Fraction (%)	
SK vs t-PA		*SK*	*t-PA*
GUSTO[37]	554	58	59
TIMI-1[116]	290	49	50
White et al.[123]	240	58	58
PAIMS[124]	145	52	56
APSAC vs t-PA		*APSAC*	*t-PA*
TAPS[34]	291	57	57
TEAM-3[51]	277	51	54
Bassand et al.[95]	169	50	52
SK vs APSAC		*SK*	*APSAC*
TEAM-2[21]	370	52	52
UK vs t-PA		*UK*	*t-PA*
GAUS[45]	134	52	53

APSAC, anisoylated plasminogen streptokinase activator complex; SK, streptokinase; t-PA, tissue plasminogen activator; UK, urokinase.

TIMI Phase I[116] data clearly show that left ventricular function benefits occur only when the infarct vessel is open at the time of initial angiography, or with sustained reperfusion. In such cases, there is interval improvement in EF from before therapy to before hospital discharge. When reperfusion does not occur, occurs late, or in the case of reocclusion, EF either decreases or does not change. It is uncertain whether a high-grade residual stenosis has an important bearing on left ventricular function following thrombolysis. Angioplasty after thrombolysis improves the luminal diameter of the infarct vessel, and this is associated with improved exercise but not resting left ventricular function.[30] In GUSTO,[37] a *post-hoc* analysis showed that both EF and RWM were highly correlated with the 90-min TIMI flow grade: EF was 62% in patients with TIMI 3 flow, 56% with TIMI 2 flow, and 54% with TIMI 0 or 1 flow. However the data do not prove a cause-and-effect relationship between left ventricular function and flow status since the baseline left ventricular function, flow, and hemodynamic status in these subgroups is not known.

The most straightforward explanation for improvement of left ventricular function following thrombolysis is that salvage of jeopardized tissue results in a greater mass of tissue capable of systolic contraction. However this hypothesis does not explain benefic-ial effects on noninfarct areas. Compensatory hyperkinesis is associated with better survival among patients with acute MI[121,125] but the mechanism whereby thrombolysis improves the function of noninfarct regions is uncertain. In the Western Washington study, the beneficial effects of SK on hyperkinesis were most prominent in the subset of patients with multivessel disease.[120] Benefit might therefore occur because flow in diseased vessels subserving noninfarct areas no longer is diverted via collaterals to the infarct territory and thereby remains sufficient to support increased myocardial work in the noninfarct area.[126] By mechanisms which are not yet known, reperfusion might also improve left ventricular function by preventing ventricular dilatation even in the absence of myocardial salvage.[127–132] In addition to improved EF, patients treated with thrombolytic agents have smaller end-diastolic and end-systolic volumes.[76,111,122,131–134] Jeremy and colleagues[127] reported that patients with an occluded infarct vessel are more likely to develop ventricular dilatation in the month following myocardial infarction, although Warren *et al.*[135] found no correlation between vessel patency and left ventricular dilatation in patients who reperfused late (greater than 5 hours after the onset of infarction). All else being equal, smaller ventricular volumes are associated with lower wall stress (afterload) and therefore better wall motion in both infarct and noninfarct regions.

It has been difficult to establish an exact relationship between time to treatment and improvement in left ventricular function. In humans, the exact timing of coronary occlusion, which does not necessarily coincide with symptom onset, and of sustained reperfusion are usually unknown. The rate of tissue necrosis may also vary because of collateral blood supply and/or medications, and there may not be a simple relationship between the extent of necrosis and left ventricular dysfunction. None the less, it appears that early treatment results in greater salvage of left ventricular function than does later treatment. Mathey and colleagues[136] measured RWM 2–3 weeks post MI in 69 patients treated with thrombolytic agents (SK or UK). In patients treated within 2 hours of symptom onset, 82% had RWM values in the infarct zone within two standard deviations of normal as compared to only 46% of patients treated 2–5 hours after symptom onset. Other studies[108,113] have also shown EF improvement only for those patients treated within 2–3 hours. Sheehan and colleagues[116] analyzed serial contrast ventriculograms of 45 patients who experienced reperfusion by 90 min following either t-PA or SK (TIMI Phase I) and did not exhibit reocclusion. Treatment within 4 hours resulted in greater improvement in RWM than treatment between 4 and 10 hours. Some patients with collaterals also show improvement in left ventricular function even after relatively late treatment with thrombolytic agents.[116–119]

There is no clear evidence linking preserved left ventricular function following thrombolytic therapy to improved survival.[137] This is not surprising considering the small percentage (3–4%) of treated patients who benefit in terms of survival. Stadius and colleagues reported that left ventricular function measured at a mean of 4.6 hours following thrombolysis was the most powerful predictor of 1-year survival for patients in the Western Washington Intracoronary Streptokinase trial.[138] In GUSTO,[37] the group of patients destined to survive for at least 30 days had better left ventricular function at 90 min than those destined to die. But since it is not possible to separately identify the 3–4% of survivors who would have died in the absence of thrombolysis, the mechanism of their survival remains speculative. Other mechanisms of improved survival are also possible. Although pump failure is the most common cause of death for hospitalized patients with MI, a small percentage of patients also die of lethal arrhythmias.[139]. For example Volpi *et al.*[140] analyzed data from the GISSI trial and concluded that thrombolytic therapy is associated with a 20% decrease in the incidence of in-hospital ventricular fibrillation. A number of small clinical studies have also demonstrated that successful thrombolytic therapy is associated with a decreased incidence of ventricular late potentials[141–151] and inducible ventricular arrhythmias.[152] Whether, given the powerful prognostic value of the EF with respect to survival, the benefits of thrombolytic therapy on left ventricular function convey a longer term survival advantage is also uncertain. However, given the relatively modest overall mean EF differences between patients given thrombolytic therapy and control patients, it is unlikely that any long-term survival benefits would be large.

Summary of the effects of thrombolytic therapy on left ventricular function

Thrombolytic therapy produces beneficial effects that overall are quite modest. Most successfully reperfused patients have severe RWM abnormalities, but only mild global dysfunction. Left ventricular function effects are greatest in those patients with anterior MI, in those treated within 2–4 hours from symptom onset, and in those with sustained TIMI grade 3 flow. Later therapy may also benefit those patients with collaterals to the infarct area. There are no major differences among the various agents with respect to preservation of left ventricular function. Global EF improvements result from beneficial effects on both the infarct zone and remote noninfarct territories. The proposed link between tissue salvage, improved regional myocardial function, and improved survival has not yet been proven.

Reinfarction

Following successful reperfusion with thrombolytic therapy, there is usually residual thrombus and a severe residual stenosis. Somewhat surprisingly, reinfarction is uncommon, occurring with less frequency than angiographic reocclusion. Reinfarction following either SK, t-PA, or APSAC ranges from 1.9 to 4.7% and is about the same as in control patients.[11,12,113,153–156] There are no significant differences in reinfarction rates among the three agents.[157–159] In the GUSTO trial, an additional 19.4% of patients developed recurrent ischemia without infarction.[159]

Hemorrhagic Complications

Thrombolytic therapy causes additional bleeding but by how much is difficult to estimate since aspirin and anticoagulants are usually coadministered. Minor bleeding, usually at venipuncture sites, is relatively common, occurring in nearly one-quarter of patients

Table 3.5 Intravenous thrombolytic therapy: incidence of cerebral hemorrhage (%)

Reference	No.	Control	SK	t-PA	APSAC
ISIS-2[12]	17 187	0.0	0.1	–	–
LATE[155]	5 711	0.0	–	0.4	–
ASSET[153]	5 012	0.1	–	0.3	–
EMERAS[156]	4 534	0.1	0.6	–	–
ISIS-3[158]	46 091	–	0.2	0.7	0.6
GUSTO[159]	41 021	–	0.5	0.7	–
GISSI-2[157]	20 891	–	0.3	0.4	–

APSAC, anisoylated plasminogen streptokinase activator complex; SK, streptokinase; t-PA, tissue plasminogen activator.

treated with SK. However, major bleeding (usually defined as that requiring transfusion or involving the brain or retroperitoneum) is much less common, with an absolute excess rate of occurrence of about 1.0%.[11,12,153–156] While fibrinogen depletion is less with t-PA than for SK and APSAC, the incidence of major bleeding is similar.[157–159] Bleeding following t-PA is more likely in older, female, hypertensive patients and those with lower body weight.[160] Serious bleeding was more common in the elderly in the TIMI trials, in which systemic heparinization and invasive catheterization were routinely employed.[161] However, no significant differences were noted between younger and older patients in either of the GISSI[11] or ISIS-2[12] trials, where urgent invasive procedures were not routinely performed. The use of heparin and/or aspirin increases absolute bleeding rates only slightly.[12]

Cerebral Hemorrhage and Stroke

Cerebral hemorrhage is the most worrisome adverse effect of thrombolytic therapy, and occurs in 0.1–0.7% of patients[12,153,156,159] (Table 3.5). Cerebral hemorrhage is about twice as common following APSAC or t-PA than with SK. Age greater than 65 years, lower body weight (<70 kg), and hypertension have been reported to be risk factors for cerebral hemorrhage.[162–165] The Fibrinolytic Therapy Trialists' Collaborative Group[166] found that among patients with bundle branch block or ST elevation on the ECG, there was a 0.3% absolute excess of strokes due to thrombolytic therapy in the first 35 days following treatment. All of the excess occurred on day 1 and was largely attributed to cerebral hemorrhage. Thereafter, the incidence of stroke was slightly diminished in the patients who received thrombolytic therapy, suggesting that embolic strokes are decreased by thrombolytic therapy. Age was the only presenting clinical feature that significantly increased the early stroke risk in this analysis.

Effects of Thrombolytic Therapy on Mortality

Streptokinase

Great effort has been made in the last 10 or more years to evaluate the effect of thrombolytic therapy on the mortality of patients with acute MI. Few, if any, other medical therapies have been so exhaustively studied. The first studies that reported a benefit on mortality were carried out with the use of intracoronary SK. The first of these was the first Western Washington study carried out in community and teaching hospitals that randomized patients following diagnostic coronary arteriography to either routine coronary care or intracoronary SK.[5] There were 134 patients who received intracoronary SK and 116 randomized to routine care. At 30 days the mortality was 3.7% in the treatment patients and 11.2% for the control patients ($P = 0.02$). The reduction in early mortality was not sustained and by 1 year the mortality difference had narrowed to 8.2% in the intracoronary SK group and 14.7% in the controls ($P = 0.1$). Several of the deaths during follow-up in the treated patients occurred in those who had high-grade residual stenosis following completion of SK therapy. During this early trial, coronary artery angioplasty was not available and if used may have changed the long-term outcome of these patients. The greatest shortcoming of intracoronary SK therapy was the difficulty in providing rapid treatment once the patient arrived at the hospital. This study is an example of this shortcoming with a mean time from the onset of symptoms to treatment of 4.6 hours. This relatively late therapy did not improve left ventricular function in the treatment group as compared to the controls.[96] None the less, patients with open vessels with normal or nearly normal flow (TIMI grade 2 and 3) following completion of the intracoronary SK infusion enjoyed excellent 1-year survival that was significantly greater than those patients with poor or no flow (TIMI grades 0 and 1) in the infarct-related vessel following therapy.[167] This improved survival with late reperfusion, unaccompanied by evidence of improved left ventricular function or reduction in infarction size, helped begin the discussion of the open artery hypothesis that continues to this time.

During the same period of time, four universities in The Netherlands initiated a larger trial of intracoronary SK that later evolved into a trial that utilized both initial intravenous SK as well as coronary artery angioplasty if the vessel was not open at the time of early angiography.[168] Because of this changing protocol it is difficult to compare this study with others, but the early results of the trial from The Netherlands were very similar to those of the Western Washington study. There were 533 patients entered into this trial and the 30-day mortality was 5.2% in the treated patients and 9.8% in the controls ($P = 0.05$). At the end of 5 years, there continues to be a benefit for treated patients with the mortality being 19% for treated patients and 29% for the controls.[169] Thus, both of these initial randomized trials, although small by current standards, provided convincing evidence that thrombolytic therapy, even when applied relatively late by the intracoronary route, markedly reduced early mortality and at 1 year there was a 44% reduction in mortality in both studies. It is interesting to note that few studies since these initial two trials of intravenous SK have demonstrated as much reduction in mortality and none of the large trials of intravenous SK have achieved reductions in mortality in this range. This is probably related to the superior patency rates that are achieved with intracoronary SK, as compared with intravenous SK, and the additional advantage of baseline coronary angiography to guide later therapy that is a requirement of the intracoronary SK approach.

Many randomized placebo-controlled trials designed to evaluate mortality have been performed with intravenous thrombolytic therapy (Table 3.6). The first large trial, ISAM, entered 1741 patients with symptoms of MI of less than 6 hours duration.[113] The patient group as a whole was of low risk judging by the 21-day mortality in the control groups of 7.1%. The treatment group also had a low mortality of 6.3%, but this difference was not significant.

Two other small, randomized trials[110,111] compared intravenous SK with placebo or routine care. The two trials were similar in design with both using a dose of 1.5 million IU of SK, although the New Zealand trial infused the drug over 30 min instead of 1 hour.[111] Neither study used aspirin routinely in either the treatment or the control group. The New Zealand investigators entered 219 patients with symptoms for less than 4 hours. The treated patients had a marked reduction in 30-day mortality of 3.7% as compared

Table 3.6   Effect of intravenous thrombolytic therapy on mortality

| | | | Time | | Mortality (%) | | |
Reference	No.	Drug	(hours)	Follow-up	Treatment	Control	P
GISSI[11]	11 806	SK	<12	Hospital	10.7	13.0	0.002
ISAM[113]	1 741	SK	<6	21 days	6.3	7.1	NS
ISIS-2[12]	17 187	SK	<24	5 weeks	9.3	12.0	0.0001
Western Washington IV[110]	368	SK	<6	14 days	6.3	9.6	0.23
White et al.[111]	219	SK	<4	30 days	3.7	12.5	0.016
AIMS[154]	1 258	APSAC	<6	30 days	6.4	12.1	0.006
German Trial[114]	313	APSAC	<4	28 days	5.6	12.6	0.032
ASSET[153]	5 011	t-PA	<5	30 days	7.2	9.8	0.0011
Van de Werf and Arnold[76]	721	t-PA	<5	14 days	2.8	5.7	0.06
LATE[155]	5 711	t-PA	6–24	35 days	8.9	10.3	NS
LATE[155]	5 711	t-PA	6–12	35 days	8.9	12.0	0.02
EMERAS[156]	4 534	SK	6–24	35 days	11.9	12.4	NS
EMERAS[156]	4 534	SK	7–12	35 days	11.7	13.2	NS

NS, not significant.
APSAC, anisoylated plasminogen streptokinase activator complex; SK, streptokinase; t-PA, tissue plasminogen activator.

with the control mortality of 12.5% ($P = 0.16$). The Western Washington group enrolled 368 patients with symptoms of less than 6 hours. The 14-day mortality in the treatment group was 6.3% as compared with 9.6% in the controls. The 36% reduction in mortality in this small trial was not significant,[110] although of greater magnitude than that reported in many large trials.

Large trials

The first two very large trials of thrombolytic therapy were carried out to evaluate intravenous SK. The first of these was the Gruppo Italiano Per lo Studio della Streptochinasi nell'Infarto Miocardio (GISSI).[11] This remarkable study was carried out during a 17-month period beginning in early 1984 in 176 coronary care units in Italy. These clinical investigators screened more than 30 000 patients and randomized 11 806 to either intravenous SK, in a dose of 1.5 million u infused over 1 hour, or routine cardiac care. Coronary arteriography, PTCA, or revascularization surgery were rarely used in these patients. Aspirin was not routinely prescribed for either study group. Hospital mortality was 10.7% in the intravenous SK group and 13.0% in the controls, a 17.6% reduction in mortality ($P = 0.0002$). Early treatment was more effective than later therapy, with the patients who received intravenous SK within 3 hours of the onset of symptoms having a mortality of 9.2% vs 12.0% for the controls. This important trial was the first to randomize a large number of patients during the first 60 min following the onset of symptoms. Among the more than 1200 patients in this trial treated within 1 hour intravenous SK had a mortality of 8.2% as compared to 15.4% (-47%) in those receiving routine cardiac care.

The 1-year mortality data in the GISSI study demonstrated that the benefits of thrombolytic therapy are sustained without the use of follow-up coronary angiography and the frequent use of coronary artery bypass graft (CABG) surgery or PTCA. In the group overall, the 1-year mortality was 17.2% in the treatment group and 19.0% in the control. Thus, the actual percent difference between the two groups, which had been 2.3% at the time of hospital discharge, was reduced to 1.8% at the time of 1-year follow-up.[170]

The second large trial was the Second International Study of Infarct Survival (ISIS-2). This study evaluated both SK and aspirin using a 2 × 2 factorial design.[12] Patients were entered over 33 months beginning in early 1985. This trial entered 17 187 patients with suspected MI from 417 coronary care units in 16 countries. Patients were randomized to receive oral aspirin, intravenous SK in a dose of 1.5 million u given over 1 hour, both drugs, or placebos. Patients were selected based on their clinical presentation and there were no age limitations or ECG entry criteria. The double-placebo group had a 35-day cumulative vascular mortality of 13.2%, while the mortality was 10.7% (−18.9%) for those receiving aspirin, 10.4% (−21.5%) for those receiving intravenous SK, and 8.0% (−39.4%) for those receiving both drugs, with each group being compared to the patients receiving double placebo. The most striking findings in this large study were the magnitude of benefit for those patients receiving aspirin therapy and the additive benefits of combined aspirin and SK therapy.

Early therapy was more effective then later treatment in ISIS-2 as in other trials, with those receiving both aspirin and SK within the first 4 hours of symptom onset having a mortality of 6.4% as compared with a mortality of 13.1% (−51%) for the corresponding double-placebo group. This was the first large study that suggested that patients with symptoms for more than 12 hours may benefit from thrombolytic therapy. There were a total of 1222 patients that were randomized to either aspirin and SK or double placebo between 12 and 24 hours. The mortality was 7.4% in the SK–aspirin group and 11.5% in the double-placebo group and this difference was significant ($P < 0.05$).

Because ISIS-2 was such a large study there were a number of subgroups of patients to be examined, some of which were large enough to provide definitive information and some that have been useful to develop hypotheses for testing in future trials. Among the most important subgroup observations were that only the patients with ST segment elevation on the ECG, as compared to those with nonspecific ST–T changes or ST depression, had reduced mortality with thrombolytic therapy. Thus, these first two large trials provided a great deal of information on the benefit of SK therapy and the unexpected potency of the combination of SK and aspirin.

Tissue Plasminogen Activator

Soon after t-PA became available two relatively large randomized controlled trials were developed to evaluate the effect of this new thrombolytic agent on mortality. The smaller of the two trials, carried out by the European Cooperative Study Group, randomized 721 patients with symptoms for less than 5 hours to either 100 mg of t-PA given over 3 hours or a placebo infusion.[76] All patients received aspirin and heparin. The 14-day mortality was 2.8% in the treated patients and 5.7% in the controls and this difference was of borderline significance ($P = 0.06$). There was a high cerebral hemorrhage rate in the treated patients of 2.0% as compared to 0.6% in the controls.

The Anglo-Scandinavian Study of Early Thrombolysis (ASSET) began randomizing patients in November 1986. Physicians working in 52 coronary care units evaluated 13 318 patients and entered 5011 of those under the age of 75 years with clinically suspected acute MI into the trial.[153] The treated patients received t-PA 100 mg over 3 hours plus heparin but neither the treatment or the control group received aspirin. There were no ECG criteria for entry into the trial. The 30-day mortality in the treatment group was 7.2% and 9.8% in the controls ($P = 0.0011$). The stroke rate was 1.1% in the treated patients and 1.0% in the controls. Comparing this stroke rate with that observed in the European study suggested that the addition of aspirin to t-PA may have significantly increased the complication of hemorrhagic stroke. The 12-month mortality remained significantly lower in the treatment group as compared to the controls (13.2% vs 15.1%, $P < 0.05$).[171]

APSAC

There have been two relatively large trials that have evaluated the use of APSAC in the management of acute MI and its influence on mortality. The larger of the two trials, the APSAC Intervention Mortality Study (AIMS) enrolled 1258 patients under the age of 71 years with symptoms of acute MI of less than 6 hours duration.[154] Patients were required to have ST elevation on the entry ECG and meet the usual exclusion criteria. They were randomized to receive intravenous APSAC as a 30-mg bolus over 5 min or a placebo. This is one of the few randomized trials of thrombolytic therapy that was terminated prematurely because of a large benefit in reduced mortality for the treated patients. At 30 days the mortality was 6.4% for the treatment group and 12.1% for the control group (-50%, $P = 0.0006$). The remarkable lowering in mortality was achieved without the use of aspirin or other antiplatelet drugs. At 1-year follow-up this reduction in mortality was sustained (11.1% vs 17.7%, $P = 0.0007$).[172]

A much smaller randomized trial of APSAC vs heparin was performed in Germany.[114] This study enrolled 313 patients with symptoms of less then 4 hours duration. The benefit achieved for the treatment group in this trial was similar to AIMS with the 30-day mortality in the treated group being 5.6% vs 12.6% in the heparin group (-55%, $P = 0.032$). Thus, these two trials of APSAC in MI were extremely encouraging and suggested that APSAC may be a superior thrombolytic agent as compared to either SK or t-PA for reducing the mortality of acute MI.

Fibrinolytic Therapy Trialists' (FFT) Collaborative Group

The Fibrinolytic Therapy Trialists' Collaborative Group has gathered all the data available on randomized trials of thrombolytic therapy and has recently provided recommendations for therapy in patients with suspected MI based upon the data from all published trials of more than 1000 patients.[166] The nine trials that comprise this dataset included 58 600 patients of whom 6177 (10.5%) died, 564 (1.0%) had a stroke, and 436 (0.7%) had major noncerebral bleeds. The overall benefit for the 45 000 patients with ST elevation or bundle branch block on the ECG was an absolute mortality reduction of 30 per 1000 for those presenting within 6 hours of the onset of symptoms, 20 per 1000 for those presenting from 7 to 12 hours, and a questionable 10 per 1000 for those presenting between 13 and 18 hours. There were four additional strokes per 1000 in the fibrinolytic group of which two died, one had a moderate or severe disabling neurologic deficit, and one did not. These investigators report that the benefits of thrombolytic therapy were not limited by age, sex, blood pressure, heart rate, or prior history of MI or diabetes.

As might be expected, the reductions in mortality for the pooled result of nine trials are less impressive than the results of the best individual trials. The reduction in 35-day mortality for all patients with and without ST elevation was 18% (9.6% vs 11.5%). There was an excess mortality on day 0 of 5 per 1000 and a minor benefit of 3 per 1000 on day 1 for patients receiving thrombolytic therapy. This excess mortality is thought to be due to intramyocardial hemorrhage and increased rate of ventricular rupture in patients who receive thrombolytic agents later in the course of infarction. Thus, by day 2 there is no benefit achieved with thrombolytic therapy for all treated patients.

Figures 3.5–3.9 summarize the mortality benefits of thrombolytic therapy, expressed as the number of lives saved per 1000 patients treated, in various subsets of patients. The ECG was an important predictor of reduced mortality (Figure 3.5). For patients with bundle branch block or anterior ST segment elevation the number of lives saved per 1000 were 49 and 37 respectively. Patients with inferior ST elevation benefited much less (eight lives saved per 1000) and those with ST depression not at all. Predictably, there was a marked decline in treatment benefit as a function of the time from onset of symptoms to

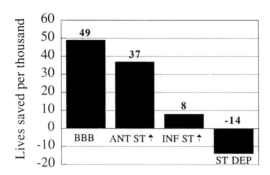

Figure 3.5 The effect of thrombolytic therapy on mortality in various patient subsets classified according to the admission ECG. Patients with bundle branch block (BBB) and anterior ST segment elevation derive the most benefit from thrombolytic therapy. Effects in patients with inferior ST segment elevation are much less, while patients with ST segment depression (ST DEP) do no benefit. (Based on data from Ref. 166.)

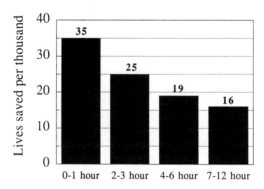

Figure 3.6 The effect of thrombolytic therapy on mortality in various patient subsets classified according to the time from symptom onset to treatment. Patients treated early derive the most benefit. (Based on data from Ref. 166.)

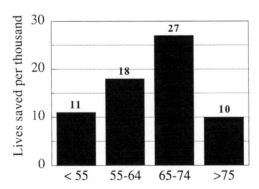

Figure 3.7 The effect of thrombolytic therapy on mortality in various patient subsets classified according to age. Despite a higher overall risk of death patients over the age of 75 years do not derive a greater absolute benefit from thrombolytic therapy than do younger patients. (Based on data from Ref. 166.)

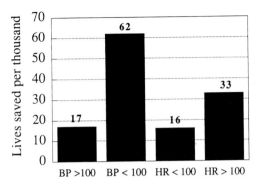

Figure 3.8 The effect of thrombolytic therapy on mortality in various patient subsets classified according to the blood pressure and heart rate. Patients with hypotension or tachycardia benefit the most from thrombolytic therapy, probably because these findings indicate larger infarcts and worse ventricular function. (Based on data from Ref. 166.)

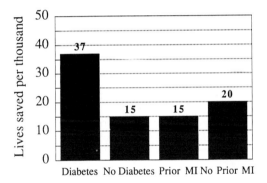

Figure 3.9 The effect of thrombolytic therapy on mortality in various patient subsets classified according to the presence or absence of diabetes or prior infarction. Patients with diabetes are more likely to benefit from thrombolysis than nondiabetic patients. The presence of prior infarction does not predict a greater benefit from thrombolytic therapy. (Based on data from Ref. 166.)

initiation of therapy with twice as many lives saved when treatment is started in the first hour as opposed to 7–12 hours (Figure 3.6). Up to age 75 years there is an increased survival benefit with age, but the very elderly do not achieve an absolute increase in survival with thrombolytic therapy (Figure 3.7). Other subgroups of patients who are most likely to benefit include those with hypotension (blood pressure <100 mmHg), tachycardia (heart rate >100 beats min^{-1}) (Figure 3.8), and those with diabetes (Figure 3.9).

Drug Comparison Trials

Once the safety and efficacy of thrombolytic therapy to reduce the morbidity and mortality of acute MI had been established it remained to be determined which agent or agents were most beneficial. In this evaluation the major endpoint needed to be mortality but rate of reinfarction and the rate of stroke with residual neurologic deficit also had to be established. To compare mortality differences with the use of two or more effective

Table 3.7   Intravenous thrombolytic therapy: comparison of agents and mortality

Trial	No.	Drugs	Time (hours)	Follow-up	Mortality (%)				P
					SK	t-PA[a]	t-PA+SK	APSAC	
GISSI-2/									
Internat. Study[157]	20 891	SK, t-PA	<6	Hospital	8.5	8.9			NS
GUSTO[158]	41 021	SK, t-PA[a], SK + t-PA	<6	30 days	7.3	6.3	7.0		0.001[b]
ISIS-3[159]	46 091	SK, t-PA, APSAC	<24	35 days	10.6	10.3		10.5	NS

[a]t-PA was given in an 'accelerated' dose in the GUSTO study.
[b]Refers to the comparison between SK and accelerated t-PA.
APSAC, anisoylated plasminogen streptokinase activator complex; SK, streptokinase; t-PA, tissue plasminogen activator.

thrombolytic agents requires very large studies, as compared to the much smaller trials that were performed to determine that thrombolytic therapy was superior to placebo. Thus, studies of tens of thousands of patients were initiated to answer these questions. Although there have been several small studies reported that compared one effective thrombolytic agent with another, none of these was large enough to provide definitive information. Three large studies have been reported: GISSI-2,[157] ISIS-3,[158] and GUSTO[159] and each of these will be reviewed in detail. The results of these trials are summarized in Table 3.7.

GISSI-2 International Study

The first of the large drug comparison trials was the Gruppo Italiano Per lo Studio della Streptochinasi nell'Infarto Miocardico (GISSI-2) which compared alteplase (t-PA) with SK and heparin vs no heparin in a factorial design with all patients receiving oral aspirin.[157] The GISSI investigators in Italy entered 12 490 patients while a parallel international study entered an additional 8401 patients for a total of 20 891. Patients with symptoms for less than 6 hours with ST elevation on the ECG were entered into the trial. t-PA was given in a conventional dose of 100 mg over 3 hours, SK was given intravenously 1.5 million u over 1 hour, and heparin was given subcutaneously 12 500 u twice a day with the first dose given 12 hours after thrombolytic therapy. For the combined trial the mortality was 8.5% in the SK group and 8.9% in the t-PA group and this small difference was not significant. The investigators concluded that there was no advantage to be gained with the use of t-PA in place of the less expensive SK.

ISIS-3

The Third International Study of Infarct Survival (ISIS-3) investigators carried out a complex trial in which patients with symptoms of acute MI were entered up to 24 hours from the onset of symptoms.[158] Patients thought to have a clear indication for thrombolytic therapy by their physicians were randomized to one of three thrombolytic agents: SK 1.5 million u over 1 hour, APSAC 30 mg as an intravenous bolus, or t-PA (duteplase) 0.60 Mu kg^{-1} infused over 4 hours. For patients in whom the indication for thrombolytic therapy was not clear, usually because they were seen after 6 hours from the onset of symptoms or did not have ST elevation on the ECG, were randomized equally to one of the three thrombolytic agents or to open control without the use of placebo. In addition, all patients were randomized to receive either aspirin plus subcutaneous calcium heparin given twice daily with the first dose administered 4 hours following the initiation of thrombolytic therapy or aspirin alone. This trial was the largest of the trials up to that time with a total of 41 299 patients enrolled who received thrombolytic therapy. An additional group of patients who were randomized to control were not included in the initial report of ISIS-3. Among the 41 299, 36 381 were considered to have clear indications for therapy. The median time to treatment was 4.0 hours.

The 0–35-day mortality in ISIS-3 was similar for all three treatment groups, with mortality being 10.6% with SK, 10.5% with APSAC, and 10.3% with t-PA. These small differences in mortality were not significant. There were small differences in the 7-day mortality of the patients assigned to heparin plus aspirin vs aspirin alone (7.4% vs 7.9%, $2P = 0.06$) although by 35 days this difference in mortality (10.3% vs 10.6%) was not significant. The definite or probable hemorrhagic stroke rate was significantly higher in the aspirin plus heparin group as compared to those receiving aspirin alone (0.56% vs 0.40%, $2P \leqslant 0.05$) but the rate of total stroke was not different for the two groups (1.28% vs 1.18%).

Because the treatment protocols were similar in ISIS-3 and GISSI-2 it was reasonable to combine the results of the two studies; this was undertaken and published in the initial report of ISIS-3. When the SK and t-PA patients in ISIS-3 are added to the patients taking these drugs in GISSI-2 they total more than 24 000 patients in each treatment group. For these combined SK patients the 35-day mortality was identical to the 10% mortality of the patients who received t-PA. Thus, the overwhelming evidence from these two large trials indicates that there is no difference in mortality of patients with acute MI managed with SK, t-PA or APSAC with or without the use of subcutaneous heparin. Following the publication of the results of these two definitive trials a reasonable physician might conclude that the issue was settled and, with the exception of patients who require retreatment after having previously received SK or APSAC (who should receive t-PA), that standard therapy for nearly all patients would be SK because of the large difference in cost between this and the other two agents. Although many physicians did revert to the use of SK for most patients, many did not because of their belief that t-PA was much more likely to result in early reperfusion than SK and APSAC, and that reduced infarct size and improved long-term survival would result when early reperfusion could be achieved. These physicians also noted that the early (1-day) mortality in ISIS-3 was lower for t-PA (4.7%) than that for SK (5.1%) or for APSAC (5.1%). The mortality for the period 2–7 days was slightly higher for t-PA (3.0%) than for SK (2.6%) and APSAC (2.7%). The difference in mortality between these time intervals might be interpreted as representing better early reperfusion using t-PA, with lower early mortality, and a higher reocclusion rate with a higher mortality during the remainder of the first postinfarction week. This pattern of death might be expected because of the greater perceived need for heparin with the use of t-PA as compared to the other drugs. For these reasons, and probably for additional commercial considerations, an additional large trial (GUSTO) was undertaken, sponsored by the manufacturer of alteplase.

GUSTO

The Global Utilization of Streptokinase and Tissue Plasminogen Activator for Occluded Coronary Arteries (GUSTO) was carried out in 15 countries and 1081 hospitals to determine which of four thrombolytic strategies was superior for the treatment of acute MI.[159] A total of 41 021 patients with symptoms for less than 6 hours and ST segment elevation on the ECG were entered into the trial between December 1990 and February 1993. Patients were randomized to one of four thrombolytic regimens: (1) intravenous SK 1.5 million u over 60 min with subcutaneous heparin 12 500 u every 12 hours with the first dose given 4 hours after the start of thrombolytic therapy; (2) SK as in regimen (1) with intravenous heparin at 1000 u hour^{-1} hour following a 5000-u bolus with recommended adjustments of the dose by body weight and by the partial thromboplastin time during therapy; (3) t-PA (alteplase) given in an accelerated fashion (front-loaded) with a 15-mg bolus followed by 50 mg in the next 30 min and 35 mg given over the next hour for a total of 100 mg over 90 min, with the maximum dose reduced for patients under 67 kg. Heparin was given intravenously in the same way as in regimen (2); or (4) the combination of t-PA at a dose of 1.0 mg kg^{-1} up to a dose of 90 mg given over 1 hour with a 10% bolus combined with SK 1.0 million u over 1 hour given simultaneously through separate catheters along with intravenous heparin as in regimen (2).

The primary endpoint of GUSTO was death from any cause by 30 days with the most important secondary endpoint being death and nonfatal disabling stroke. As expected in such a large trial the baseline characteristics were similar in the four treatment groups. There was no difference in the 30-day mortality between the three SK groups ($P = 0.73$). The 30-day mortality for t-PA (6.3%) was lower than for SK and subcutaneous heparin (7.2%), SK and intravenous heparin (7.4%), and both SK and t-PA plus intravenous heparin (7.0%). The 30-day mortality for accelerated t-PA was significantly lower than the mortality for the combined SK groups with a reduction in risk of 14% ($P = 0.001$). The incidence of hemorrhagic stroke was significantly higher in the t-PA group than in the two SK groups (with intravenous or subcutaneous heparin) with an excess of about 0.2% ($P = 0.03$). The overall stroke rate was 1.55% for the t-PA group and 1.3% for the combined SK groups and this difference was not significant ($P = 0.09$) while the stroke rate was higher in the patients receiving both SK and t-PA plus intravenous heparin (1.64%).

Other complications of acute infarction were generally less frequent with t-PA therapy as compared to the other thrombolytic regimens, with allergic reactions, anaphylaxis, congestive heart failure, cardiogenic shock, sustained hypotension, atrioventricular block, atrial fibrillation or flutter, and sustained ventricular tachycardia all significantly less frequent ($P \leq 0.0001$). In addition, ventricular fibrillation and asystole were also significantly less frequent with t-PA therapy. The decreased frequency of these complications is probably due a higher incidence of early reperfusion with reduction in the duration of myocardial ischemia and, in the case of very early reperfusion a reduction in infarct size as discussed previously.

Pre-hospital Thrombolytic Therapy

In recognition of the marked benefits of very early reperfusion therapy, and of the significant delays which accompany hospital delivery of thrombolytic therapy, several randomized trials of prehospital thrombolytic therapy have been reported.[99,173,174] The Myocardial Infarction, Triage and Intervention Trial (MITI) randomized 360 patients to receive t-PA administered by paramedics in the field or to receive the same therapy after admission to a hospital emergency department.[99] All patients were evaluated in the prehospital setting by paramedics who did a brief history, physical examination and, when clinically eligible for the trial, a 12-lead ECG that was relayed to a monitoring physician by cellular telephone. Only patients with ST segment elevation were entered into the trial. Prehospital therapy resulted in a reduction in the time from symptom onset to treatment from 110 to 77 min. This 33-min reduction in time to treatment did not result in a difference in the composite endpoint of death, or of EF or infarct size at 1 month. A secondary analysis based on time to treatment revealed a marked benefit in this composite endpoint, comparing patients treated within 70 min of the onset of symptoms as compared to those treated between 70 min and 3 hours (composite score, $P = 0.009$; mortality 1.2% vs 8.7%, $P = 0.04$; infarct size 4.9% vs 11.2%, $P < 0.001$; and EF, 53% vs 49%, $P = 0.03$). The GREAT trial was a randomized double-blind trial of APSAC given either at home by general practitioners or in the hospital to 311 patients with suspected acute MI seen at home within 4 hours of symptom onset.[173] Patients treated at home received APSAC 130 min earlier than those treated in the hospital. Adverse events with home treatment were infrequent. There was a strong trend towards a reduction in mortality in patients given thrombolytic therapy at home (6.7% vs 11.5%, $P = 0.1$). The much larger EMIP trial randomized 5469 patients presenting within 6 hours of symptom onset to pre-hospital vs in-hospital APSAC.[174] The average difference in the timing of treatment was 55 min and there was again a strong trend towards reduced 30-day mortality in the pre-hospital group (9.7% vs 11.1%, $P = 0.08$). The EMIP investigators also reported a pooled analysis of all the pre-hospital trials, which showed a 17% reduction in mortality with pre-hospital thrombolytic therapy ($P = 0.03$). These remarkable trials demonstrate the feasibility, safety, and efficacy of pre-hospital thrombolytic therapy in communities where the necessary resources are available.

Late Thrombolytic Therapy

Where there is solid evidence that thrombolytic therapy started within 6 hours of symptom onset improves survival, there is less certainty regarding the possible benefits of later therapy. This issue is important because many patients with MI arrive at the hospital later than 6 hours. Two recently reported trials[155,156] provide compelling evidence that later therapy is also beneficial. The LATE trial[155] randomized 5711 patients with acute MI in a double-blind protocol to intravenous t-PA or placebo between 6 and 24 hours from symptom onset. For patients treated 6–12 hours from symptom onset there was a statistically significant decrease in mortality favoring t-PA (8.9% APSAC vs 12.0% placebo, $P = 0.02$). There was no difference in survival between t-PA and placebo when therapy was given between 12 and 24 hours. The South American trial EMERAS[156] randomized 4534 patients with suspected MI to SK or placebo up to 24 hours from the onset of symptoms. While there was no significant difference in hospital mortality between SK and placebo, a trend towards fewer hospital deaths favoring SK was present in the subset of patients treated between 7 and 12 hours; the mortality was 11.7% in the SK group and 13.2% in the placebo group. Together the data from these trials are consistent with the hypothesis that even relatively late thrombolytic therapy (6–12 hours) in MI is beneficial, reducing mortality by 10–20%. The mechanisms for this benefit remain speculative.

Thrombolytic Therapy in the Elderly

It is well known that the mortality of acute MI is markedly increased with advancing age as well defined by GISSI and ISIS-2. The incidence of stroke also increases with age as do other bleeding complications. The combined effect of this increase in the incidence of serious complications has caused many investigators to limit the enrollment of patients into thrombolytic trials to those under the age of 70 or 75 years of age. Fortunately ISIS-2, ISIS-3, and GISSI-2 did not have age limitations and therefore considerable data are available about the outcome of elderly patients with acute MI with and without thrombolytic therapy. The GISSI-2 investigators have provided an elegant analysis of the effect of age on mortality in 9720 patients having their first MI who were eligible for thrombolytic therapy.[175] All of these patients received either SK or t-PA with or without subcutaneous heparin. The hospital mortality for all patients was 7.9%, was very low in patients under the age of 40 years (1.9%), and increased exponentially by about 6% per year so that patients above the age of 80 years had a hospital mortality of 31.9%. Between hospital discharge and 6-month follow-up the mortality increased an average of 2.7% so that the 6-month mortality for all patients was 10.6% with the risk of death increasing with advancing age in a parallel manner to the increase in hospital mortality by age.

The relative benefit of thrombolytic therapy in elderly patients has been debated with many investigators pointing out that the absolute decrease in mortality achieved with thrombolytic therapy in elderly patients is greater than in younger patients because of the higher absolute mortality in this group. Despite this argument, a very large experience of thrombolytic therapy in the elderly that is now available from the Fibrinolytic Therapy Trialists' Cooperative Group does not demonstrate a significant reduction in mortality in older patients who received thrombolytic therapy.[166] Among the 5035 patients, 75 years and older, who were entered into controlled randomized trials, the 0–30-day mortality was 24.2% for those receiving thrombolytic therapy and 26.0% for the control group (P = NS). Coupling this small benefit with the higher rate of complications and reduced long-term benefit that can be achieved in such old patients makes us cautious in recommending thrombolytic therapy for these patients. In our own practice we restrict thrombolytic therapy in our oldest patients to those who have anterior MI, are hypotensive, or are developing congestive heart failure early in the course of infarction, with the belief that these are the patients most likely to benefit from this therapy. Unfortunately, the elderly are much more likely to have contraindications to thrombolytic therapy than younger patients.[100] In the high-risk elderly patient we often select direct angioplasty as the most effective and least risky method of coronary reperfusion because there is both a higher rate of reperfusion and a lower risk of stroke associated with this form of therapy.[176]

Summary of the Role of Thrombolysis in the Treatment of MI

Thrombolytic therapy is an important advance in the treatment of acute MI. For each 100 patients treated, two to four lives are saved. Beneficial effects on secondary endpoints such as infarct vessel patency, infarct size, and left ventricular wall motion have also been shown, lending credence to the hypothesis that at least one important mechanism for improved mortality is reperfusion leading to myocardial salvage and better contractile function. It is not known whether improvements in vessel patency and contractile function convey additional longer term clinical benefits beyond the short-term (30-day) survival benefit that has been shown. Patients most likely to benefit from this therapy are those who are at greatest risk, most notably those with anterior MI or bundle branch block, and those with unstable hemodynamics (with the possible exception of those in cardiogenic shock for whom a benefit of thrombolysis has not been proven). While patients may receive benefit when treated as late as 12 hours following the onset of symptoms, the greatest benefit is achieved when therapy is initiated in the first hour. Patients with well-developed collaterals to the infarct zone are especially likely to benefit from late treatment. The benefits of thrombolysis can be achieved with relatively small overall risk, but the risk of catastrophic bleeding needs to be carefully considered in the context of the expected benefits in each patient. Survival benefits have been shown for SK, t-PA, and APSAC but the recent GUSTO trial has demonstrated that the use of an 'accelerated' t-PA regimen results in the saving of one additional life per 100 patients as compared to SK, with the benefit most likely due to faster opening of the occluded vessel.

While intravenous thrombolytic therapy has proven to be a very expedient method of reperfusion, important limitations remain with regard to the widespread application of this treatment for acute MI. For each 100 patients with MI, only about 30 are treated with lytic therapy. Of these, only about 10 experience complete (TIMI 3), sustained, myocardial reperfusion. Only a subset of these 10 are likely to get treated in time to limit infarct size, and only one patient will survive who otherwise would have died without therapy. Thus it can be argued that in its present form thrombolytic therapy affords clinically significant benefit to only 1% of the MI population. One way to increase the impact of lytic therapy in MI would be to substantially increase the proportion of MI patients who receive therapy. For example, by considering for treatment patients over the age of 75 years and those who present between 6 and 12 hours from the onset of therapy, close to two-thirds of MI patients could be treated.[177] However, simply treating more patients is not enough. Extending the previous analysis, if treatment were given to 60 of every 100 MI patients, only two lives would be saved. It is also crucial to improve the efficacy of reperfusion therapy, by opening the infarct vessel earlier, and more completely, permanently, and safely than is the case with current thrombolytic regimens. The best therapy (accelerated t-PA) is also quite expensive, about $2200 per dose, leading to real concerns about the cost-effectiveness of this therapy. There is a great need for more cost-effective drugs that dissolve clots more quickly and completely without promoting systemic bleeding, and for improved agents for preventing rethrombosis. There is also a need for improved patient and provider awareness of the necessity for early treatment and the means for delivering this therapy. The role of PTCA in high-risk subgroups also needs to be clarified to maximize the likelihood of early and complete reperfusion at the lowest possible risk.

Specific Treatment Recommendations

Table 3.8 summarizes our specific recommendations for reperfusion therapy in MI. These recommendations apply only to those patients who present within the first 12

Table 3.8 Recommendations for therapy

Patient risk group[a]	Net benefit from thrombolysis[b] (lives saved per 1000)	Additional net benefit with t-PA vs SK[c] (lives saved per 100)	Recommended reperfusion strategy
0–4 hours from symptom onset			
Death high, ICH low	67	14	t-PA
Death high, ICH high	64	10	t-PA
Death low, ICH low	25	6	t-PA
Death low, ICH high	22	2	t-PA or SK
4–12 hours from symptom onset			
Death high, ICH low	37	2	t-PA or SK
Death high, ICH high	34	(−2)	t-PA or SK
Death low, ICH low	13	1	t-PA or SK
Death low, ICH high	10	(−3)	SK or none

[a] High risk of death = any one of anterior MI, bundle branch block, diabetes, Killip 3, heart rate >100 beats min^{-1}, blood pressure <100 mmHg. High risk of intracranial hemorrhage (ICH) = age >65 years.
[b] Net benefit from thrombolysis calculated as number of lives saved − excess ICH. The number of lives saved = baseline death risk × 0.35 for the 0–4 hour patients and baseline death risk × 0.2 for the 4–12 hour patients. The baseline death risk in patients not receiving thrombolytic therapy was assumed to be 20% for the high-risk group (Death high) and 8% for the low-risk patients (Death low). The excess risk of ICH was assumed to be 3 per 1000 for patients at low risk of ICH (ICH low) and 6 per 1000 for patients at high risk of ICH (ICH high).
[c] The additional net benefit from t-PA vs SK was calculated assuming that t-PA is 20% more effective at saving lives when given from 0 to 4 hours and 5% more effective when given from 4 to 12 hours. The excess ICH risk for t-PA was assumed to be equal to SK in the ICH low group but higher in the ICH high group; 8 per 1000 for t-PA vs 4 per 1000 for SK.
SK, streptokinase; t-PA, tissue plasminogen activator.

hours of symptom onset with ST segment elevation or bundle branch block on the ECG. High-risk patients with absolute contraindications to thrombolytic therapy should be treated with primary coronary angioplasty whenever possible, while lower risk patients should be managed conservatively. Patients who present with cardiogenic shock should also be managed with an intraaortic balloon pump support and either PTCA or surgical revascularization when this is feasible. When this is not feasible, initial thrombolytic therapy with transport to a tertiary facility is often the best alternative. Patients with MI who do not have ST segment elevation or bundle branch block should initially receive aggressive medical therapy, excluding thrombolytic therapy, with early coronary angiography for those who remain unstable.

For thrombolysis-eligible patients, we believe that t-PA, delivered in an accelerated dosing regimen, is the most effective fibrinolytic agent. Streptokinase is the second choice, since APSAC has not been proven to be more efficacious than SK and carries a higher risk of cerebral hemorrhage. However, the overall clinical advantages of t-PA over SK (and other modes of therapy) do not apply equally to all patients. In certain patients, t-PA is clearly superior to SK and should be used exclusively. In other groups of patients, the advantages of t-PA over SK are modest, or negligible. It is important to distinguish between these groups of patients since a consideration of cost must enter into every therapeutic decision. We have indicated in Table 3.8 our beliefs regarding the relative merit of t-PA over SK in various subsets of patients. Patients are divided into two main groups: those presenting within 4 hours, and those presenting from 4 to 12 hours. In the 0–4 hour group, reperfusion is likely to limit infarct size and thus the speed of reperfusion is of primary importance; therefore the advantage of t-PA over SK is greatest in these patients. Those presenting from 4 to 12 hours still derive benefit from thrombolytic therapy but infarct size limitation is less likely so that the speed of reperfusion is less important. Patients are further classified by whether they are at high or low risk of death and by whether they are at high or low risk of cerebral hemorrhage. Patients at high risk of death are those with anterior MI, bundle branch block, blood pressure $<100\,mmHg$, heart rate >100 beats min^{-1}, Killip class 3 as well as those with diabetes (see Figures 3.5–3.9). We have not included advanced age in this group since the elderly do not derive an increase in absolute benefit from thrombolysis as compared to younger patients. Patients considered at high risk of cerebral hemorrhage and more susceptible to the greater risk of cerebral hemorrhage with t-PA are those over 65 years old.[37]

In constructing Table 3.8 we have made the following assumptions. Patients treated within 4 hours have an average 35% reduction in mortality, while those treated after 4 hours have an average 20% reduction. High-risk patients have a risk of death in the range of 20% without lytic therapy and low-risk patients have a risk of death in the range of 8%. t-PA is about 20% more effective than SK in saving lives when given in the first 4 hours, but at most only 5% more effective when given from 4 to 12 hours. We have also estimated that the net clinical benefit from thrombolysis is diminished due to an excess of cerebral hemorrhages by, on average three patients per 1000 for patients at low risk of cerebral hemorrhage and by six patients per 1000 for patients at high risk of cerebral hemorrhage. Furthermore, patients at high risk of cerebral hemorrhage have an absolute excess cerebral hemorrhage rate of about four per 1000 (8 vs 4) with t-PA vs SK.

For patients who present early (within 4 hours) from the onset of symptoms, t-PA is the clear choice, except in elderly patients with inferior MI and stable hemodynamics where the advantage of t-PA is minimal. In patients presenting late (4–12 hours), we believe that the drugs are about equal with respect to mortality. In elderly patients with small infarcts who present late, SK may be preferred due to its lower potential for cerebral hemorrhage. Patients in this category derive only a small benefit from thrombolysis overall and in our own practice we often do not treat such patients with thrombolytic therapy.

Based on recent reports and on our own experience it appears that coronary angioplasty is at least as good, and maybe more effective in achieving reperfusion in patients with acute MI than is thrombolysis because of the higher recanalization and lower stroke rate with direct angioplasty (see Chapter 4). Large-scale trials of PTCA are needed before clear recommendations for its use can be made. It is important for the clinician to carefully monitor the course of the patient during thrombolytic therapy. Patients at high risk of death who do not improve during the initial 1–2 hours of therapy should undergo urgent coronary angiography to determine the status of the infarct-related vessel flow. Mechanical revascularization with PTCA or CABG surgery should be considered for those patients who have failed to achieve normal (TIMI 3) flow.

References

1. Jennings, R.B., Sommers, H.M., Smyth, G.A. *et al.* (1960) Myocardial necrosis induced by temporary occlusion of a coronary artery in a dog. *Arch. Pathol.*, **70**, 68–78.
2. Arai, A.E., Pantely, G.A., Anselone, C.G. *et al.* (1991) Active downregulation of myocardial energy requirements during prolonged moderate ischemia in swine. *Circ. Res.*, **69**, 1458–69.
3. Chazov, E.I., Matveeva, L.S., Mazaev, A.V. *et al.* (1976) [Intracoronary administration of fibrinolysin in acute myocardial infarct]. *Ter. Arkh.*, **48**, 8–19.
4. Rentrop, K.P., Blanke, H., Karsch, K.R. *et al.* (1979) Acute myocardial infarction: intracoronary application of nitroglycerin and streptokinase. *Clin. Cardiol.*, **2**, 354–63.
5. Kennedy, J.W., Ritchie, J.L., Davis, K.B. and Fritz, J.K. (1983) Western Washington randomized trial of intracoronary streptokinase in acute myocardial infarction. *N. Engl. J. Med.*, **309**, 1477–82.
6. Schroder, R., Biamino, G., von-Leitner, E.R. *et al.* (1983) Intravenous short-term infusion of streptokinase in acute myocardial infarction. *Circulation*, **67**, 536–48.
7. Valentine, R.P., Pitts, D.E., Brooks-Brunn, J.A. *et al.* (1985) Intravenous versus intracoronary streptokinase in acute myocardial infarction. *Am. J. Cardiol.*, **55**, 309–12.
8. Rogers, W.J., Mantle, J.A., Hood, W.P. Jr *et al.* (1983) Prospective randomized trial of intravenous and intracoronary streptokinase in acute myocardial infarction. *Circulation*, **68**, 1051–61.
9. Alderman, E.L., Jutzy, K.R., Berte, L.E. *et al.* (1984) Randomized comparison of intravenous versus intracoronary streptokinase for myocardial infarction. *Am. J. Cardiol.*, **54**, 14–19.
10. Taylor, G.J., Mikell, F.L., Moses, H.W. *et al.* (1984) Intravenous versus intracoronary streptokinase therapy for acute myocardial infarction in community hospitals. *Am. J. Cardiol.*, **54**, 256–60.
11. Gruppo Italiano per lo Studio della Streptochinasi nell'Infarto Miocardico (GISSI) (1986) Effectiveness of intravenous thrombolytic treatment in acute myocardial infarction. *Lancet*, **i**, 397–402.
12. ISIS-2 (Second International Study of Infarct Survival) Collaborative Group (1988) Randomised trial of intravenous streptokinase, oral aspirin, both, or neither among 17 187 cases of suspected acute myocardial infarction. *Lancet*, **ii**, 349–60.
13. Collen, D. (1993) Towards improved thrombolytic therapy. *Lancet*, **342**, 34–6.
14. Elliott, J.M., Cross, D.B., Cederholm-Williams, S.A. and White, H.D. (1993) Neutralizing antibodies to streptokinase four years after intravenous thrombolytic therapy. *Am. J. Cardiol.*, **71**, 640–5.
15. Torr, S.R., Nachowiak, D.A., Fujii, S. and Sobel, B.E. (1992) 'Plasminogen steal' and clot lysis. *J. Am. Coll. Cardiol.*, **19**, 1085–90.
16. Constantinides, P. (1966) Plaque fissures in human coronary thrombosis. *J. Atheroscler. Res.*, **61**, 1–17.
17. Davies, M.J. (1989) Successful and unsuccessful coronary thrombolysis. *Br. Heart J.*, **61**, 381–4.
18. Jang, I.K., Gold, H.K., Ziskind, A.A. *et al.* (1989) Differential sensitivity of erythrocyte-rich and platelet-rich arterial thrombi to lysis with recombinant tissue-type plasminogen activator. A possible explanation for resistance to coronary thrombolysis. *Circulation*, **79**, 920–8.
19. Sherman, C.T., Litvack, F., Grundfest, W. *et al.* (1986) Coronary angioscopy in patients with unstable angina pectoris. *N. Engl. J. Med.*, **315**, 913–19.
20. Brown, B.G., Gallery, C.A., Badger, R.S. *et al.* (1986) Incomplete lysis of thrombus in the moderate underlying atherosclerotic lesion during intracoronary infusion of streptokinase for acute myocardial infarction: quantitative angiographic observations. *Circulation*, **73**, 653–61.
21. Anderson, J.L., Sorensen, S.G., Moreno, F.L. *et al.* (1991) Multicenter patency trial of intravenous anistreplase compared with streptokinase in acute myocardial infarction. The TEAM-2 Study Investigators. *Circulation*, **83**, 126–40.
22. Ambrose, J.A., Tannenbaum, M.A., Alexopoulos, D. *et al.* (1988) Angiographic progression of coronary artery disease and the development of myocardial infarction. *J. Am. Coll. Cardiol.*, **12**, 56–62.
23. Granger, C.B., Califf, R. M. and Topol, E.J. (1992) Thrombolytic therapy for acute myocardial infarction. A review. *Drugs*, **44**, 293–325.
24. Badger, R.S., Brown, B.G., Kennedy, J.W. *et al.* (1987) Usefulness of recanalization to luminal diameter of 0.6 millimeter or more with intracoronary streptokinase during acute myocardial infarction in predicting 'normal' perfusion status, continued arterial patency and survival at one year. *Am. J. Cardiol.*, **59**, 519–22.

25. Veen, G., Meyer, A., Verheugt, F.W.A. *et al.* (1993) Culprit lesion morphology and stenosis severity in the prediction of reocclusion after coronary thrombolysis: Angiographic results of the APRICOT study. *J. Am. Coll. Cardiol.*, **22**, 1755–62.

26. Gash, A.K., Spann, J.F., Sherry, S. *et al.* (1986) Factors influencing reocclusion after coronary thrombolysis for acute myocardial infarction. *Am. J. Cardiol.*, **57**, 175–7.

27. Wall, T.C., Mark, D.B., Califf, R.M. *et al.* (1989) Prediction of early recurrent myocardial ischemia and coronary reocclusion after successful thrombolysis: a qualitative and quantitative angiographic study. *Am. J. Cardiol.*, **63**, 423–8.

28. Ellis, S.G., Topol, E.J., George, B.S. *et al.* (1989) Recurrent ischemia without warning. Analysis of risk factors for in-hospital ischemic events following successful thrombolysis with intravenous tissue plasminogen activator. *Circulation*, **80**, 1159–65.

29. Leung, W.H. and Lau, C.P. (1992) Effects of severity of the residual stenosis of the infarct-related coronary artery on left ventricular dilation and function after acute myocardial infarction. *J. Am. Coll. Cardiol.*, **20**, 307–13.

30. Guerci, A.D., Gerstenblith, G., Brinker, J.A. *et al.* (1987) A randomized trial of intravenous tissue plasminogen activator for acute myocardial infarction with subsequent randomization to elective coronary angioplasty. *N. Engl. J. Med.*, **317**, 1613–18.

31. Chesebro, J.H., Knatterud, G., Roberts, R. *et al.* (1987) Thrombolysis in Myocardial Infarction (TIMI) Trial, Phase I: A comparison between intravenous tissue plasminogen activator and intravenous streptokinase. Clinical findings through hospital discharge. *Circulation*, **76**, 142–54.

32. Carney, R.J., Murphy, G.A., Brandt, T.R. *et al.* (1992) Randomized angiographic trial of recombinant tissue-type plasminogen activator (alteplase) in myocardial infarction. RAAMI Study Investigators. *J. Am. Coll. Cardiol.*, **20**, 17–23.

33. Neuhaus, K.L., Feuerer, W., Jeep-Tebbe, S. *et al.* (1989) Improved thrombolysis with a modified dose regimen of recombinant tissue-type plasminogen activator. *J. Am. Coll. Cardiol.*, **14**, 1566–9.

34. Neuhaus, K.L., von-Essen, R., Tebbe, U. *et al.* (1992) Improved thrombolysis in acute myocardial infarction with front-loaded administration of alteplase: results of the rt-PA–APSAC patency study (TAPS). *J. Am. Coll. Cardiol.*, **19**, 885–91.

35. Karagounis, L., Sorensen, S.G., Menlove, R.L. *et al.* (1992) Does thrombolysis in myocardial infarction (TIMI) perfusion grade 2 represent a mostly patent artery or a mostly occluded artery? Enzymatic and electrocardiographic evidence from the TEAM-2 study. Second Multicenter Thrombolysis Trial of Eminase in Acute Myocardial Infarction. *J. Am. Coll. Cardiol.*, **19**, 1–10.

36. Vogt, A., von-Essen, R., Tebbe, U. *et al.* (1993) Impact of early perfusion status of the infarct-related artery on short-term mortality after thrombolysis for acute myocardial infarction: retrospective analysis of four German multicenter studies. *J. Am. Coll. Cardiol.*, **21**, 1391–5.

37. The GUSTO Angiographic Investigators (1993) The effects of tissue plasminogen activator, streptokinase, or both on coronary-artery patency, ventricular function, and survival after acute myocardial infarction. *N. Engl. J. Med.*, **329**, 1615–22.

38. Schofer, J., Montz, R. and Mathey, D.G. (1985) Scintigraphic evidence of the 'no reflow' phenomenon in human beings after coronary thrombolysis. *J. Am. Coll. Cardiol.*, **5**, 593–8.

39. Ito, H,. Tommoka, T., Sakai, N. *et al.* (1992) Lack of myocardial perfusion immediately after successful thrombolysis. A predictor of poor recovery of left ventricular function in anterior myocardial infarction. *Circulation*, **85**, 1699–705.

40. Kennedy, J.W., Gensini, G.G., Timmis, G.C. and Maynard, C. (1985) Acute myocardial infarction treated with intracoronary streptokinase: a report of the Society for Cardiac Angiography. *Am. J. Cardiol.*, **55**, 871–7.

41. Stack, R.S., O'Connor, C.M., Mark, D.B. *et al.* (1988) Coronary perfusion during acute myocardial infarction with a combined therapy of coronary angioplasty and high-dose intravenous streptokinase. *Circulation*, **77**, 151–61.

42. PRIMI Trial Study Group (1989) Randomised double-blind trial of recombinant pro-urokinase against streptokinase in acute myocardial infarction. *Lancet*, **i**, 863–8.

43. Hogg, K.J., Gemmill, J.D., Burns, J.M. *et al.* (1990) Angiographic patency study of anistreplase versus streptokinase in acute myocardial infarction. *Lancet*, **335**, 254–8.

44. TIMI II A results. The TIMI Research Group (1988) Immediate vs delayed catheterization and angioplasty following thrombolytic therapy for acute myocardial infarction. *JAMA*, **260**, 2849–58.

45. Neuhaus, K.L., Tebbe, U,. Gottwik, M. *et al.* (1988) Intravenous recombinant tissue plasminogen activator (rt-PA) and urokinase in acute myocardial infarction: results of the German Activator Urokinase Study (GAUS). *J. Am. Coll. Cardiol.*, **12**, 581–7.

46. Grines, C.L., Nissen, S.E., Booth, D.C. *et al.* (1991) A prospective, randomized trial comparing combination half-dose tissue-type plasminogen activator and streptokinase with full-dose tissue-type plasminogen activator. Kentucky Acute Myocardial Infarction Trial (KAMIT) Group. *Circulation*, **84**, 540–9.

47. Topol, E.J., Califf, R.M., George, B.S. *et al.* (1987) A randomized trial of immediate versus delayed elective angioplasty after intravenous tissue plasminogen activator in acute myocardial infarction. *N. Engl. J. Med.*, **317**, 581–8.

48. Topol, E.J., Bates, E.R., Walton, J.A. Jr *et al.* (1987) Community hospital administration of intravenous tissue plasminogen activator in acute myocardial infarction: improved timing, thrombolytic efficacy and ventricular function. *J. Am. Coll. Cardiol.*, **10**, 1173–7.

49. Topol, E.J., George, B.S., Kereiakes, D.J. *et al.* (1989) a randomized controlled trial of intravenous tissue plasminogen activator and early intravenous heparin in acute myocardial infarction. *Circulation*, **79**, 281–6.

50. Topol, E.J., Morris, D.C., Smalling, R.W. *et al.* (1987) A multicenter, randomized, placebo-controlled trial of a new form of intravenous recombinant tissue-type plasminogen activator (activase) in acute myocardial infarction. *J. Am. Coll. Cardiol.*, **9**, 1205–13.

51. Anderson, J.L., Becker, L.C., Sorensen, S.G. *et al.* (1992) Anistreplase versus alteplase in acute myocardial infarction: comparative effects on left ventricular function, morbidity and 1-day coronary artery patency. The TEAM-3 Investigators. *J. Am. Coll. Cardiol.*, **20**, 753–66.

52. Ralik-van-Wely, L., Visser, R.F., van-der-Pol, J.M. *et al.* (1991) Angiographically assessed coronary arterial patency and reocclusion in patients with acute myocardial infarction treated with anistreplase: results of the anistreplase reocclusion multicenter study (ARMS). *Am. J. Cardiol.*, **68**, 296–300.

53. Ohman, E.M,. Califf, R.M., Topol, E.J. *et al.* (1990) Consequences of reocclusion after successful reperfusion therapy in acute myocardial infarction. TAMI Study Group. *Circulation*, **82**, 781–91.

54. Gold, H.K., Leinbach, R.C., Garabedian, H.D. *et al.* (1986) Acute coronary reocclusion after thrombolysis with recombinant human tissue-type plasminogen activator: prevention by a maintenance infusion. *Circulation*, **73**, 347–52.

55. Verstraete, M., Arnold, A.E., Brower, R.W. *et al.* (1987) Acute coronary thrombolysis with recombinant human tissue-type plasminogen activator: initial patency and influence of maintained infusion on reocclusion rate. *Am. J. Cardiol.*, **60**, 231–7.

56. Bonnier, H.J., Visser, R.F., Klomps, H.C. and Hoffmann, H.J. (1988) Comparison of intravenous anisoylated plasminogen streptokinase activator complex and intracoronary streptokinase in acute myocardial infarction. *Am. J. Cardiol.*, **62**, 25–30.

57. Coller, B.S. (1990) Platelets and thrombolytic therapy. *N. Engl. J. Med.*, **322**, 33–42.

58. Mickelson, J.K., Simpson, P.J., Cronin, M. *et al.* (1990) Antiplatelet antibody [7E3 F(ab')2] prevents rethrombosis after recombinant tissue-type plasminogen activator-induced coronary artery thrombolysis in a canine model. *Circulation*, **81**, 617–27.

59. Yasuda, T., Gold, H.K., Fallon, J.T. *et al.* (1988) Monoclonal antibody against the platelet glycoprotein (GP) IIb/IIIa receptor prevents coronary artery reocclusion after reperfusion with recombinant tissue-type plasminogen activator in dogs. *J. Clin. Invest.*, **81**, 1284–91.

60. Kleiman, N.S., Ohman, E.M., Califf, R.M. *et al.* (1993) Profound inhibition of platelet aggregation with monoclonal antibody 7E3 Fab after thrombolytic therapy. Results of the Thrombolysis and Angioplasty in Myocardial Infarction (TAMI) 8 Pilot Study. *J. Am. Coll. Cardiol.*, **22**, 381–9.

61. Roux, S., Christeller, S. and Ludin, E. (1992) Effects of aspirin on coronary reocclusion and recurrent ischemia after thrombolysis: a meta-analysis. *J. Am. Coll. Cardiol.*, **19**, 671–7.

62. Owen, J., Grossman, B., Sobel, J. and Kudryk, B. (1990) Fibrinogen proteolysis and coagulation system activation during thrombolytic therapy. *Adv. Exp. Med. Biol.*, **281**, 401–8.

63. Rapold, H.J., Kuemmerli, H., Weiss, M. *et al.* (1989) Monitoring of fibrin generation during thrombolytic therapy of acute myocardial infarction with recombinant tissue-type plasminogen activator. *Circulation*, **79**, 980–9.

64. Eisenberg, P.R., Sherman, L.A. and Jaffe, A.S. (1987) Paradoxic elevation of fibrinopeptide A after streptokinase: evidence for continued thrombosis despite intense fibrinolysis. *J. Am. Coll. Cardiol.*, **10**, 527–9.

65. Kander, N.H., Holland, K.J., Pitt, B. and Topol, E.J. (1990) A randomized pilot trial of brief versus prolonged heparin after successful reperfusion in acute myocardial infarction. *Am. J. Cardiol.*, **65**, 139–42.

66. Bleich, S.D., Nichols, T.C., Schumacher, R.R. *et al* (1990) Effect of heparin on coronary arterial patency after thrombolysis with tissue plasminogen activator in acute myocardial infarction. *Am. J. Cardiol.*, **66**, 1412–17.

67. Hsia, J., Hamilton, W.P., Kleiman, N. *et al.* (1990) A comparison between heparin and low-dose aspirin as adjunctive therapy with tissue plasminogen activator for acute myocardial infarction. Heparin–Aspirin Reperfusion Trial (HART) Investigators. *N. Engl. J. Med.*, **323**, 1433–7.

68. Arnout, J., Simons, M., de-Bono, D. *et al.* (1992) Correlation between level of heparinization and patency of the infarct-related coronary artery with treatment of acute myocardial infarction with alteplase (rt-PA). *J. Am. Coll. Cardiol.*, **20**, 513–19.

69. Cannon, C.P., McCabe, C.H., Henry, T.D. *et al.* for the TIMI-5 investigators (1993) Hirudin reduces reocclusion compared to heparin following thrombolysis in acute myocardial infarction: Results of the TIMI-5 trial (abstract). *J. Am. Coll. Cardiol.*, **21**(suppl. A), A-136.

70. Sherry, S. and Marder, V.J. (1992) Thrombolytic therapy: reocclusion rates with adjective aspirin and its relation to heparin therapy. *J. Am. Coll. Cardiol.*, **19**, 678–80.

71. Rogers, W.J., Baim, D.S., Gore, J.M. *et al.* (1990) Comparison of immediate invasive, delayed invasive, and conservative strategies after tissue-type plasminogen activator. Results of the Thrombolysis in Myocardial Infarction (TIMI) Phase II-A trial. *Circulation*, **81**, 1457–76.

72. Erbel, R., Pop, T., Diefenbach C. and Meyer, J. (1989) Long-term results of thrombolytic therapy with and without percutaneous transluminal coronary angioplasty. *J. Am. Coll. Cardiol.*, **14**, 276–85.

73. Simoons, M.L., Arnold, A.E., Betriu, A. *et al.* (1988) Thrombolysis with tissue plasminogen activator in acute myocardial infarction: no additional benefit from immediate percutaneous coronary angioplasty. *Lancet*, **i**, 197–203.

74. Clemmensen, P., Grande, P., Saunamaki, K. *et al.* (1990) Effect of intravenous streptokinase on the relation between initial ST-predicted size and final QRS-estimated size of acute myocardial infarcts. *J. Am. Coll. Cardiol.*, **16**, 1252–7.

75. The Thrombolysis Early in Acute Heart Attack Trial Study Group (1990) Very early thrombolytic therapy in suspected acute myocardial infarction. *Am. J. Cardiol.*, **65**, 401–7.

76. Van de Werf, F. and Arnold, A.E. (1988) Intravenous tissue plasminogen activator and size of infarct, left ventricular function and survival in acute myocardial infarction. *BMJ*, **297**, 1374–9.

77. Simoons, M.L., Serruys, P.W., van-den-Brand, M. *et al.* (1986) Early thrombolysis in acute myocardial infarction: limitation of infarct size and improved survival. *J. Am Coll. Cardiol.*, **7**, 717–28.

78. Roberts, R. (1990) Enzymatic estimation of infarct size. Thrombolysis induced its demise: will it now rekindle its renaissance? *Circulation*, **81**, 707–10.

79. Caldwell, J.H., Williams, D.L., Harp, G.D. *et al.* (1984) Quantitation of size of relative myocardial perfusion defect by single-photon emission computed tomography. *Circulation*, **70**, 1048–56.

80. Prigent, F., Maddahi, J., Garcia, E.V. *et al.* (1986) Quantification of myocardial infarct size by thallium-201 single-photon emission computed tomography: experimental validation in the dog. *Circulation*, **74**, 852–61.

81. Tamaki, N., Yonekura, Y., Yamashita, K. *et al.* (1988) Relation of left ventricular perfusion and wall motion with metabolic activity in persistent defects on thallium-201 tomography in healed myocardial infarction. *Am. J. Cardiol.*, **62**, 202–8.

82. Gibbons, R.J., Holmes, D.R., Reeder, G.S. *et al.* (1993) Immediate angioplasty compared with the administration of a thrombolytic agent followed by conservative treatment of myocardial infarction. The Mayo Coronary Care Unit and Catheterization Laboratory Groups. *N. Engl. J. Med.*, **328**, 685–91.

83. Gibbons, R.J. (1991) Perfusion imaging with ^{99m}Tc-sestamibi for the assessment of myocardial area at risk and the efficacy of acute treatment in myocardial infarction. *Circulation*, **84**, 137–42.

84. Christian, T.F., Behrenbeck, T., Gersh, B.J. and Gibbons, R.J. (1991) Relation of left ventricular volume and function over one year after acute myocardial infarction to infarct size determined by technetium-99m sestamibi. *Am. J. Cardiol.*, **68**, 21–6.

85. Christian, T.F., Clements, I.P. and Gibbons, R.J. (1991) Noninvasive identification of myocardium at risk in patients with acute myocardial infarction and nondiagnostic electrocardiograms with technetium-99m-Sestamibi. *Circulation*, **83**, 1615–20.

86. Christian, T.F., Gibbons, R.J. and Gersh, B.J. (1991) Effect of infarct location on myocardial salvage assessed by technetium-99m isonitrile. *J. Am. Coll. Cardiol.*, **17**, 1303–8.

87. Behrenbeck, T., Pellikka, P.A., Huber, K.C. *et al.* (1991) Primary angioplasty in myocardial infarction: assessment of improved myocardial perfusion with technetium-99m isonitrile. *J. Am. Coll. Cardiol.*, **17**, 365–72.

88. Christian, T.F., Behrenbeck, T., Pellikka, P.A. *et al.* (1990) Mismatch of left ventricular function and infarct size demonstrated by technetium-99m isonitrile imaging after reperfusion therapy for acute myocardial infarction: identification of myocardial stunning and hyperkinesia. *J. Am. Coll. Cardiol.*, **16**, 1632–8.

89. Gibbons, R.J., Verani, M.S., Behrenbeck, T. *et al.* (1989) Feasibility of tomographic ^{99m}Tc-hexakis-2-methoxy-2-methylpropyl-isonitrile imaging for the assessment of myocardial area at risk and the effect of treatment in acute myocardial infarction. *Circulation*, **80**, 1277–86.

90. Wackers, F.J., Gibbons, R.J., Verani, M.S. *et al.* (1989) Serial quantitative planar technetium-99m isonitrile imaging in acute myocardial infarction: efficacy for noninvasive assessment of thrombolytic therapy. *J. Am. Coll. Cardiol.*, **14**, 861–73.

91. Christian, T.F., Schwartz, R.S. and Gibbons, R.J. (1992) Determinants of infarct size in reperfusion therapy for acute myocardial infarction. *Circulation*, **86**, 81–90.

92. Morgan, C.D., Roberts, R.S., Haq, A. *et al.* (1991) Coronary patency, infarct size and left ventricular function after thrombolytic therapy for acute myocardial infarction: results from the tissue plasminogen activator: Toronto (TPAT) placebo-controlled trial. TPAT Study Group. *J. Am. Coll. Cardiol.*, **17**, 1451–7.

93. Cerqueira, M.D., Maynard, C. and Ritchie, J.L. (1991) Radionuclide assessment of infarct size and left ventricular function in clinical trials of thrombolysis. *Circulation*, **84**, 1100–8.

94. Bassand, J.P., Machecourt, J., Cassagnes, J. *et al.* (1989) Multicenter trial of intravenous anisoylated plasminogen streptokinase activator complex (APSAC) in acute myocardial infarction: effects on infarct size and left ventricular function. *J. Am. Coll. Cardiol.*, **13**, 988–97.

95. Bassand, J.P., Cassagnes, J., Machecourt, J. *et al.* (1991) Comparative effects of APSAC and rt-PA on infarct size and left ventricular function in acute myocardial infarction. A multicenter randomized study. *Circulation*, **84**, 1107–17.

96. Ritchie, J.L., Davis, K.B., Williams, D.L. *et al.* (1984) Global and regional left ventricular function and tomographic radionuclide perfusion: the Western Washington Intracoronary Streptokinase In Myocardial Infarction Trial. *Circulation*, **70**, 867–75.

97. Ritchie, J.L., Cerqueira, M., Maynard, C. *et al.* (1988) Ventricular function and infarct size: the Western Washington Intravenous Streptokinase in Myocardial Infarction Trial. *J. Am. Coll. Cardiol.*, **11**, 689–97.

98. Armstrong, P.W., Baigrie, R.S., Daly, P.A. *et al.* (1989) Tissue plasminogen activator: Toronto (TPAT) placebo-controlled randomized trial in acute myocardial infarction. *J. Am. Coll. Cardiol.*, **13**, 1469–76.

99. Weaver, W.D., Cerqueira, M., Hallstrom, A.P. *et al.* (1993) Prehospital-initiated vs hospital-initiated thrombolytic therapy. The Myocardial Infarction Triage and Intervention Trial. *JAMA*, **270**, 1211–16.

100. Althouse, R., Maynard, C., Cerqueira, M.D. *et al.* (1990) The Western Washington Myocardial Infarction Registry and Emergency Department Tissue Plasminogen Activator Treatment Trial. *Am. J. Cardiol.*, **66**, 1298–303.

101. Braunwald, E. and Kloner, R.A. (1982) The stunned myocardium: prolonged postischemic ventricular dysfunction. *Circulation*, **66**, 1146–9.

102. Gaudron, P., Eilles, C., Kugler, I. and Ertl, G. (1993) Progressive left ventricular dysfunction and remodeling after myocardial infarction. Potential mechanisms and early predictors. *Circulation*, **87**, 755–63.
103. Sheehan, F.H., Stewart, D.K., Dodge, H.T. *et al.* (1983) Variability in the measurement of regional left ventricular wall motion from contrast angiograms. *Circulation*, **68**, 550–9.
104. Kennedy, J.W., Ritchie, J.L., Davis, K.B. and Fritz, J.K. (1983) Western Washington randomized trial of intracoronary streptokinase in acute myocardial infarction. *N. Engl. J. Med.*, **309**, 1477–82.
105. Anderson, J.L., Marshall, H.W., Bray, B.E. *et al.* (1983) A randomized trial of intracoronary streptokinase in the treatment of acute myocardial infarction. *N. Engl. J. Med.*, **308**, 1312–18.
106. Khaja, F., Walton, J.A. Jr, Brymer, J.F. *et al.* (1983) Intracoronary fibrinolytic therapy in acute myocardial infarction. Report of a prospective randomized trial. *N. Engl. J. Med.*, **308**, 1305–11.
107. Raizner, A.E., Tortoledo, F.A., Verani, M.S. *et al.* (1985) Intracoronary thrombolytic therapy in acute myocardial infarction: a prospective, randomized, controlled trial. *Am. J. Cardiol.*, **55**, 301–8.
108. National Heart Foundation of Australia Coronary Thrombolysis Group (1988) Coronary thrombolysis and myocardial salvage by tissue plasminogen activator given up to 4 hours after onset of myocardial infarction. [Published erratum appears in *Lancet* (1988) ii, 519.] *Lancet*, **i**, 203–8.
109. O'Rourke, M., Baron, D., Keogh, A. *et al.* (1988) Limitation of myocardial infarction by early infusion of recombinant tissue-type plasminogen activator. *Circulation*, **77**, 1311–15.
110. Kennedy, J.W., Martin, G.V., Davis, K.B. *et al.* (1988) The Western Washington Intravenous Streptokinase in Acute Myocardial Infarction Randomized Trial. [Published erratum appears in *Circulation* (1988) 77, 1037.] *Circulation*, **77**, 345–52.
111. White, H.D., Norris, R.M., Brown, M.A. *et al.* (1987) Effect of intravenous streptokinase on left ventricular function and early survival after acute myocardial infarction. *N. Engl. J. Med.*, **317**, 850–5.
112. Bassand, J.P., Faivre, R., Becque, O. *et al.* (1987) Effects of early high-dose streptokinase intravenously on left ventricular function in acute myocardial infarction. *Am. J. Cardiol.*, **60**, 435–9.
113. Schroder, R., Neuhaus, K.L., Leizorovicz, A. *et al.* (1987) A prospective placebo-controlled double-blind multicenter trial of intravenous streptokinase in acute myocardial infarction (ISAM): long-term mortality and morbidity. *J. Am. Coll. Cardiol.*, **9**, 197–203.
114. Meinertz, T., Kasper, W., Schumacher, M. and Just, H. (1988) The German multicenter trial of anisoylated plasminogen streptokinase activator complex versus heparin for acute myocardial infarction. *Am. J. Cardiol.*, **62**, 347–51.
115. Stadius, M.L., Maynard, C., Fritz, J.K. *et al.* (1985) Coronary anatomy and left ventricular function in the first 12 hours of acute myocardial infarction: the Western Washington Randomized Intracoronary Streptokinase Trial. *Circulation*, **72**, 292–301.
116. Sheehan, F.H., Braunwald, E., Canner, P. *et al.* (1987) The effect of intravenous thrombolytic therapy on left ventricular function: a report on tissue-type plasminogen activator and streptokinase from the Thrombolysis in Myocardial Infarction (TIMI Phase I) trial. *Circulation*, **75**, 817–29.
117. Blanke, H., Cohen, M., Karsch, K.R. *et al.* (1985) Prevalence and significance of residual flow to the infarct zone during the acute phase of myocardial infarction. *J. Am. Coll. Cardiol.*, **5**, 827–31.
118. Rentrop, K.P., Feit, F., Sherman, W. *et al.* (1989) Late thrombolytic therapy preserves left ventricular function in patients with collateralized total coronary occlusion: primary end point findings of the Second Mount Sinai–New York University Reperfusion Trial. *J. Am. Coll. Cardiol.*, **14**, 58–64.
119. Habib, G.B., Heibig, J., Forman, S.A. *et al.* (1991) Influence of coronary collateral vessels on myocardial infarct size in humans. Results of phase I thrombolysis in myocardial infarction (TIMI) trial. The TIMI Investigators. *Circulation*, **83**, 739–46.
120. Martin, G.V., Sheehan, F.H., Stadius, M. *et al.* (1988) Intravenous streptokinase for acute myocardial infarction. Effects on global and regional systolic function. *Circulation*, **78**, 258–66.
121. Grines, C.L., Topol, E.J., Califf, R.M. *et al.* (1989) Prognostic implications and predictors of enhanced regional wall motion of the noninfarct zone after thrombolysis and angiography therapy of acute myocardial infarction. The TAMI Study Groups. *Circulation*, **80**, 245–53.
122. Serruys, P.W., Simoons, M.L., Suryapranata, H. *et al.* (1986) Preservation of global and regional left ventricular function after early thrombolysis in acute myocardial infarction. *J. Am. Coll. Cardiol.*, **7**, 729–42.
123. White, H.D., Rivers, J.T., Maslowski, A.H. *et al.* (1989) Effect of intravenous streptokinase as compared with that of tissue plasminogen activator on left ventricular function after first myocardial infarction. *N. Engl. J. Med.*, **320**, 817–21.
124. Magnani, B. (1989) Plasminogen Activator Italian Multicenter Study (PAIMS): comparison of intravenous recombinant single-chain human tissue-type plasminogen activator (rt-PA) with intravenous streptokinase in acute myocardial infarction. *J. Am. Coll. Cardiol.*, **13**, 19–26.
125. Jaarsma, W., Visser, C.A., Eenige-van, M.J. *et al.* (1986) Prognostic implications of regional hyperkinase and remote asynergy of noninfarcted myocardium. *Am. J. Cardiol.*, **58**, 394–8.
126. Homans, D.C., Sublett, E., Elsperger, K.J. *et al.* (1986) Mechanisms of remote myocardial dysfunction during coronary artery occlusion in the presence of multivessel disease. *Circulation*, **74**, 588–96.
127. Jeremy, R.W., Hackworthy, R.A., Bautovich, G. *et al.* (1987) Infarct artery perfusion and changes in left ventricular volume in the month after acute myocardial infarction. *J. Am. Coll. Cardiol.*, **9**, 989–95.
128. Hochman, J.S. and Choo, H. (1987) Limitation of myocardial infarct expansion by reperfusion independent of myocardial salvage. *Circulation*, **75**, 299–306.

129. Force, T., Kemper, A., Leavitt, M. and Parisi, A.F. (1988) Acute reduction in functional infarct expansion with late coronary reperfusion: assessment with quantitative two-dimensional echocardiography. *J. Am. Coll. Cardiol.*, **11**, 192–200.
130. Hale, S.L. and Kloner, R.A. (1988) Left ventricular topographic alterations in the completely healed rat infarct caused by early and late coronary artery reperfusion. *Am. Heart J.*, **116**, 1508–13.
131. Marino, P., Zanolla, L. and Zardini, P. (1989) Effect of streptokinase on left ventricular modeling and function after myocardial infarction: the GISSI (Gruppo Italiano per lo Studio della Streptochinasi nell'Infarto Miocardico) Trial. *J. Am. Coll. Cardiol.*, **14**, 1149–58.
132. Marino, P., Destro, G., Barbieri, E. and Bicego, D. (1992) Reperfusion of the infarct-related coronary artery limits left ventricular expansion beyond myocardial salvage. *Am. Heart J.*, **123**, 1157–65.
133. Bonaduce, D., Petretta, M., Villari, B. *et al.* (1990) Effects of late administration of tissue-type plasminogen activator on left ventricular remodeling and function after myocardial infarction. *J. Am. Coll. Cardiol.*, **16**, 1561–8.
134. Topol, E.J., Califf, R.M., Vandormael, M. *et al.* (1992) A randomized trial of late reperfusion therapy for acute myocardial infarction. Thrombolysis and Angioplasty in Myocardial infarction-6 Study Group. *Circulation*, **85**, 2090–9.
135. Warren, S.E., Royal, H.D., Markis, J.E. *et al.* (1988) Time course of left ventricular dilation after myocardial infarction: influence of infarct-related artery and success of coronary thrombolysis. *J. Am. Coll. Cardiol.*, **11**, 12–19.
136. Mathey, D.G., Sheehan, F.H., Schofer, J. and Dodge, H.T. (1985) Time from onset of symptoms to thrombolytic therapy: a major determinant of myocardial salvage in patients with acute transmural infarction. *J. Am. Coll. Cardiol.*, **6**, 518–25.
137. Van-de-Werf, F. (1989) Discrepancies between the effects of coronary reperfusion on survival and left ventricular function. *Lancet*, **i**, 1367–9.
138. Stadius, M.L., Maynard, C., Fritz, J.K. *et al.* (1985) Coronary anatomy and left ventricular function in the first 12 hours of acute myocardial infarction: the Western Washington Randomized Intracoronary Streptokinase Trial. *Circulation*, **72**, 292–301.
139. Kleiman, N.S., Terrin, M., Mueller, H. *et al.* (1992) Mechanisms of early death despite thrombolytic therapy: experience from the Thrombolysis in Myocardial Infarction Phase II (TIMI II) study. *J. Am. Coll. Cardiol.*, **19**, 1129–35.
140. Volpi, A., Cavalli, A., Santoro, E. and Tognoni, G. (1990) Incidence and prognosis of secondary ventricular fibrillation in acute myocardial infarction. Evidence for a protective effect of thrombolytic therapy. GISSI Investigators. *Circulation*, **82**, 1279–88.
141. Sager, P.T., Perlmutter, R.A., Rosenfeld, L.E. *et al.* (1988) Electrophysiologic effects of thrombolytic therapy in patients with a transmural anterior myocardial infarction complicated by left ventricular aneurysm formation. *J. Am. Coll. Cardiol.*, **12**, 19–24.
142. Malik, M., Kulakowski, P., Odemuyiwa, O. *et al.* (1992) Effect of thrombolytic therapy on the predictive value of signal-averaged electrocardiography after acute myocardial infarction. *Am. J. Cardiol.*, **70**, 21–5.
143. Gang, E.S., Lew, A.S., Hong, M. *et al.* (1989) Decreased incidence of ventricular late potentials after successful thrombolytic therapy for acute myocardial infarction. *N. Engl. J. Med.*, **321**, 712–16.
144. Pedretti, R., Laporta, A., Etro, M.D. *et al* (1992) Influence of thrombolysis on signal-averaged electrocardiogram and late arrhythmic events after acute myocardial infarction. *Am. J. Cardiol.*, **69**, 866–72.
145. Turitto, G., Risa, A.L., Zanchi, E. and Prati, P.L. (1990) The signal-averaged electrocardiogram and ventricular arrhythmias after thrombolysis for acute myocardial infarction. *J. Am. Coll. Cardiol.*, **15**, 1270–6.
146. Chew, E.W., Morton, P., Murtagh, J.G. *et al.* (1990) Intravenous streptokinase for acute myocardial infarction reduces the occurrence of ventricular late potentials. *Br. Heart J.*, **64**, 5–8.
147. Eldar, M., Leor, J., Hod, H. *et al.* (1990) Effect of thrombolysis on the evolution of late potentials within 10 days of infarction. *Br. Heart J.*, **63**, 273–6.
148. Zimmermann, M., Adamec, R. and Ciaroni, S. (1991) Reduction in the frequency of ventricular late potentials after acute myocardial infarction by early thrombolytic therapy. *Am. J. Cardiol.*, **67**, 697–703.
149. Tranchesi, B. Jr, Verstraete, M., Van-de-Werf, F. *et al.* (1990) Usefulness of high-frequency analysis of signal-averaged surface electrocardiograms in acute myocardial infarction before and after coronary thrombolysis for assessing coronary reperfusion. *Am. J. Cardiol.*, **66**, 1196–8.
150. Leor, J., Hod, H., Rotstein, Z. *et al.* (1990) Effects of thrombolysis on the 12-lead signal-averaged ECG in the early postinfarction period. *Am. Heart J.*, **120**, 495–502.
151. Vatterott, P.J., Hammill, S.C., Bailey, K.R. *et al.* (1991) Late potentials on signal-averaged electrocardiograms and patency of the infarct-related artery in survivors of acute myocardial infarction. *J. Am. Coll. Cardiol.*, **17**, 330–7.
152. Kersschot, I.E., Brugada, P., Ramentol, M. *et al.* (1986) Effects of early reperfusion in acute myocardial infarction on arrhythmias induced by programmed stimulation: a prospective, randomized study. *J. Am. Coll. Cardiol.*, **7**, 1234–42.
153. Wilcox, R.G., von-der-Lippe, G., Olsson, C.G. *et al.* (1988) Trial of tissue plasminogen activator for mortality reduction in acute myocardial infarction. Anglo-Scandinavian Study of Early Thrombolysis (ASSET). *Lancet*, **ii**, 525–30.
154. AIMS Trial Study Group (1988) Effect of intravenous APSAC on mortality after acute myocardial infarction: preliminary report of a placebo-controlled clinical trial. *Lancet*, **i**, 545–9.
155. LATE Study Group (1993) Late Assessment of Thrombolytic Efficacy (LATE) study with alteplase 6–24 hours after onset of acute myocardial infarction. *Lancet*, **342**, 759–66.
156. EMERAS (Estudio Multicéntrico Estreptoquinasa Repúblicas de América del Sur) Collaborative Group (1993) Randomised trial of late thrombolysis in patients with suspected acute myocardial infarction. *Lancet*, **342**, 767–72.

157. The International Study Group (1990) In-hospital mortality and clinical course of 20,981 patients with suspected acute myocardial infarction randomized between alteplase and streptokinase with or without heparin. *Lancet*, **336**, 71–5.
158. ISIS-3 (Third International Study of Infarct Survival) Collaborative Group (1992) ISIS-3: a randomised comparison of streptokinase vs tissue plasminogen activator vs anistreplase and of aspirin plus heparin vs aspirin alone among 41,299 cases of suspected acute myocardial infarction. *Lancet*, **339**, 753–70.
159. The GUSTO investigators (1993) An international randomized trial comparing four thrombolytic strategies for acute myocardial infarction. *N. Engl. J. Med.*, **329**, 673–82.
160. Califf, R.M., Topol, E.J., George, B.S. *et al.* (1988) Hemorrhagic complications associated with the use of intravenous tissue plasminogen activator in treatment of acute myocardial infarction. *Am. J. Med.*, **85**, 353–9.
161. Chaitman, B.R., Thompson, B., Wittry, M.D. *et al.* (1989) The use of tissue-type plasminogen activator for acute myocardial infarction in the elderly: results from thrombolysis in myocardial infarction Phase I, open label studies and the Thrombolysis in Myocardial Infarction Phase II pilot study. The TIMI investigators. *J. Am. Coll. Cardiol.*, **14**, 1159–65.
162. Alpert, J.S. (1992) Intracranial hemorrhage after thrombolytic therapy: a therapeutic conflict. *J. Am. Coll. Cardiol.*, **19**, 295–6.
163. De-Jaegere, P.P., Arnold, A.A., Balk, A.H. and Simoons, M.L. (1992) Intracranial hemorrhage in association with thrombolytic therapy: incidence and clinical predictive factors. *J. Am. Coll. Cardiol.*, **19**, 289–94.
164. Anderson, J.L., Karagounis, L., Allen, A. *et al.* (1991) Older age and elevated blood pressure are risk factors for intracerebral hemorrhage after thrombolysis. *Am. J. Cardiol.*, **68**, 166–70.
165. Sloan, M.A. and Gore, J.M. (1992) Ischemic stroke and intracranial hemorrhage following thrombolytic therapy for acute myocardial infarction: a risk–benefit analysis. *Am. J. Cardiol.*, **69**, 21A–38A.
166. Fibrinolytic Therapy Trialists' Group (1994) Indications for fibrinolytic therapy in suspected acute myocardial infarction: Collaborative overview of early mortality and major morbidity results from all randomised trials of more than 1000 patients. *Lancet*, **343**, 311–322.
167. Kennedy, J.W., Ritchie, J.L., Davis, K.B. *et al.* (1985) The Western Washington randomized trial of intracoronary streptokinase in acute myocardial infarction. A 12-month follow-up report. *N. Engl. J. Med.*, **312**, 1073–8.
168. Simoons, M.L., Serruys, P.W., vd-Brand, M. *et al.* (1985) Improved survival after early thrombolysis in acute myocardial infarction. A randomised trial by the Interuniversity Cardiology Institute in The Netherlands. *Lancet*, **ii**, 578–82.
169. Simoons, M.L., Vos, J., Tijssen, J.G. *et al.* (1989) Long-term benefit of early thrombolytic therapy in patients with acute myocardial infarction: 5 year follow-up of a trial conducted by the Interuniversity Cardiology Institute of The Netherlands. *J. Am. Coll. Cardiol.*, **14**, 1609–15.
170. Gruppo Italiano per lo Studio della Streptochi-nasi nell'Infarto Miocardico (GISSI) (1987) Long-term effects of intravenous thrombolysis in acute myocardial infarction: final report of the GISSI study. *Lancet*, **ii**, 871–4.
171. Wilcox, R.G., von-der-Lippe, G., Olsson, C.G. *et al.* (1990) Effects of alteplase in acute myocardial infarction: 6-month results from the ASSET study. Anglo-Scandinavian Study of Early Thrombolysis. *Lancet*, **335**, 1175–8.
172. AIMS Trial Study Group (1990) Long-term effects of intravenous anistreplase in acute myocardial infarction: final report of the AIMS study. *Lancet*, **335**, 427–31.
173. GREAT Group (1992) Feasibility, safety, and efficacy of domiciliary thrombolysis by general practitioners: Grampian region early anistreplase trial. *BMJ*, **305**, 548–53.
174. The European Myocardial Infarction Project Group (1993) Prehospital thrombolytic therapy in patients with suspected acute myocardial infarction. *N. Engl. J. Med.*, **329**, 383–9.
175. Maggioni, A.P., Maseri, A., Fresco, C. *et al.* on behalf of the GISSI-2 investigators (1993) Age-related increase in mortality among patients with first myocardial infarctions treated with thrombolysis. *N. Engl. J. Med.*, **329**, 1442–8.
176. Grines, C.L., Browne, K.F., Marco, J. *et al.* (1993) a comparison of immediate angioplasty with thrombolytic therapy for acute myocardial infarction. The Primary Angioplasty in Myocardial Infarction Study Group. *N. Engl. J. Med.*, **328**, 673–9.
177. Muller, D.W. and Topol, E.J. (1990) Selection of patients with acute myocardial infarction for thrombolytic therapy. *Ann. Intern. Med.*, **113**, 949–60.

4

Angiography and Angioplasty

A. C. De Franco and E. J. Topol

More than 1 million individuals sustain an acute myocardial infarction each year in the USA,[1] and the cumulative mortality at 1 year remains in excess of 11%. Despite the significant mortality reduction demonstrated by the randomized, controlled trials of thrombolytic therapy in the 1980s,[2-6] this cumulative mortality rate must be considered excessive. Two goals for clinical cardiologists in the 1990s are to reduce the mortality and morbidity of myocardial infarction to their lowest possible rates and to do so in a cost-effective manner. Attaining these goals will require the development of the most effective immediate treatments, the most accurate risk stratification methods, and the selective use of revascularization procedures in those patients most likely to benefit. However, the precise role of diagnostic angiography and coronary angioplasty in reaching these goals is controversial. Specifically, clinicians disagree on the appropriate use of diagnostic angiography vs noninvasive methods of risk stratification, as well as the extent to which direct angioplasty should be emphasized over thrombolytic therapy. These controversies have far-reaching implications. The total cost of acute care for myocardial infarction, for risk stratification, and for the revascularization procedures that follow, have staggering implications for health policy.

This chapter evaluates the major indications for diagnostic coronary angiography following myocardial infarction. We review the commonly accepted indications for the procedure during the acute phase, emphasizing the importance of uncoupling the diagnostic angiogram from interventional procedures. The available data on the role of angiography for risk stratification of the uncomplicated postinfarction patient is examined; this analysis supports the use of either routine or selective angiography. We then examine the role of angioplasty in the treatment of acute myocardial infarction, both as a primary therapy for the acute event and its appropriate role following thrombolytic therapy. Although in many areas the available data do not provide conclusive 'proof' of a best approach for *all* patients, currently available data can assist the physician in selecting the appropriate catheterization or angioplasty strategy for an individual patient.

Angiographic Strategies for Myocardial Infarction

Patients with myocardial infarction may undergo one of three general types of cardiac catheterization: emergency, urgent, or elective. These categories are distinguished by their timing and chief purpose.

Emergency Coronary Angiography at Presentation

Emergency coronary angiography is defined as the performance of the procedure as soon as possible after presentation, a priori, regardless of whether thrombolytic therapy has been initiated. The safety of performing coronary angiography in the setting of acute myocardial infarction was clearly established by DeWood and colleagues in 1980,[7] followed by many trials of both thrombolytic therapy and direct angioplasty.[6,8–24] These studies have demonstrated that even in the acute phase of myocardial infarction, diagnostic catheterization carries a risk of mortality (approximately 0.5%) which is only slightly higher than that of elective catheterization.[25] However, there is an increased risk of femoral access site complications, such as local hemorrhage, pseudoaneurysm, and arteriovenous fistulae. In various studies, the incidence of these complications has ranged from 5 to 45%; this variability is due to both the antecedent use of thrombolytic therapy, the use of concomitant medications such as heparin, and to differences in diagnostic criteria of these complications.

Indications

There are three general situations in which the clinician should strongly consider emergency coronary angiography. The first is to confirm the diagnosis of acute myocardial infarction when the patient's clinical presentation is ambiguous. For example, some patients with suggestive clinical symptoms have nondiagnostic ECGs due to left ventricular hypertrophy, left bundle branch block, or prior infarction. Elderly patients are more likely to present with atypical symptoms and nondiagnostic ECGs. The investigators of the Myocardial Infarction Triage and Intervention Study (MITI),[26] reported that more than 40% of patients over the age of 75 years in their study did not have *any* chest pain on presentation. In these clinical situations, confirmation of the diagnosis and definition of the extent of coronary disease can be particularly useful. On the other hand, if emergency angiography excludes the diagnosis of acute infarction, the physician avoids prescribing unnecessary, empiric thrombolytic therapy with its concomitant risks. An additional advantage of this approach is that it also identifies the patency status of the infarct vessel, as well as the overall extent and severity of coronary disease. The physician will manage patients with advanced three-vessel or left main disease differently than those patients with a distal obstruction of a single coronary. Other potential advantages of emergency angiography included the actual enhancement of thrombus dissolution and facilitation of coronary patency by the hydrostatic pressure of contrast injection and the early and accurate identification of patients who are candidates for early hospital discharge based on low-risk coronary anatomy.[27]

A second potential indication for emergency angiography is to evaluate the need for emergency recanalization and, if indicated, to direct the patient to the appropriate form of revascularization. Direct angioplasty (also called primary percutaneous transluminal coronary angioplasty (PTCA)), is defined as the immediate transcatheter recanalization (usually balloon dilatation) of an acute thrombotic occlusion without antecedent thrombolytic therapy. If qualified personnel and an angioplasty suite are immediately available, this strategy is an alternative to intravenous thrombolytic therapy.[4,5,28–32] Patients with a contraindication to thrombolytic therapy, such as those with significant hypotension on presentation, recent surgery or stroke, should undergo emergency angiography with referral to the appropriate form of revascularization.

The third potential indication for emergency angiography occurs in patients who have received thrombolytic therapy but who have clinical symptoms or signs of having failed thrombolysis. Clinical and noninvasive electrocardiographic criteria are insufficient to determine whether reperfusion has occurred.[33,34] In this situation, emergency angiography can identify those who are candidates for rescue angioplasty. These last two indications will be discussed in the section on angioplasty.

Table 4.1 Some commonly accepted indications for emergency or urgent coronary angiography in acute myocardial infarction. (From Ref. 35)

1. To confirm the diagnosis prior to thrombolytic therapy
2. To define the coronary anatomy and to assess candidacy for primary PTCA
3. To assess candidacy for rescue PTCA as a treatment for failed thrombolysis
4. Hypotension or hemodynamic collapse (unexplained or due to ischemia)
5. Clinical or radiographic signs of congestive heart failure
6. Clinical or echocardiographic signs of ventricular septal defect or new mitral insufficiency

Urgent Angiography Prompted by a Clinical Event

Urgent cardiac catheterization refers to an unplanned procedure, prompted by a clinical observation or event, performed at any point from the first few hours to the time of hospital discharge. There are several unequivocal indications for urgent coronary angiography in acute myocardial infarction (Table 4.1); their presence mandates immediate transfer to a facility with angioplasty and coronary bypass capabilities. Auscultatory or echocardiographic findings that suggest new *ventricular septal defect or mitral valvular incompetence* mandate urgent angiography. *Sustained hypotension or cardiogenic shock* suggests severe left ventricular dysfunction and denotes either previous myocardial damage, extensive acute myocardial necrosis, ongoing ischemia with infarct extension, or a combination of these events. These patients have a very poor prognosis that can improve substantially with aggressive management and revascularization.

Patients who initially experience reperfusion with thrombolytic therapy but who develop *suspected reocclusion* also have an indication for urgent angiography. It is important to note that currently available thrombolytic regimens are associated with a relatively high incidence of recurrent ischemia and reinfarction (averaging 12–20% of patients). Data combined from 810 patients enrolled in four of the TAMI trials demonstrated that in the 733 in whom thrombolysis was initially successful, 12.4% (91 patients) had infarct-vessel reocclusion during hospitalization. These patients had a substantial increase in hospital mortality (11% vs 4.5%) as well as significantly higher rates of pulmonary edema (18.7% vs 13.6%), sustained hypotension (25.3% vs 16.5%) and second or third degree heart block (25.3% vs 12.8%). Although the GUSTO-1 trial[6] demonstrated a survival advantage with the strategy of accelerated tissue plasminogen activator (t-PA) and intravenous heparin, there were no differences in the incidence of recurrent ischemia or recurrent infarction compared with streptokinase (Table 4.2). Thus, even the most effective currently available thrombolytic regimens require vigilant observation for signs of recurrent ischemia and reocclusion. In centers where urgent catheterization is not available for patients with suspected reocclusion, readministration of a thrombolytic drug is an alternative management strategy while preparations are made for transfer to a tertiary facility. In the future, new conjunctive therapies (such as direct antithrombin inhibitors and antagonists to the glycoprotein IIb/IIIa receptor) may not only increase rate of brisk and complete infarct vessel reflow, but may also promote coronary artery stabilization, and thereby reduce the need for urgent angiography.

In summary, urgent cardiac catheterization following myocardial infarction is an unplanned procedure prompted by a clinical event; it is performed to define the patency status and lesion severity in the culprit vessel. The findings are often invaluable in the patient's referral to urgent surgical correction, whether it be angioplasty, coronary bypass, or surgical repair of the mitral valve or ventricular septum. Although this strategy is 'standard practice' in most centers in the USA, there are relatively few data that have been reported on its overall effectiveness and long-term clinical outcome. Patients who require urgent angiography for persistent or recurrent ischemia are clearly at a higher risk of immediate complications when compared to patients who do not. Long

Table 4.2 Incidence of cardiogenic shock, pulmonary edema, reinfarction, and recurrent ischemia in the GUSTO trial (numbers are expressed as a percentage). Accelerated tissue plasminogen activator (t-PA) resulted in a lower incidence of cardiogenic shock than the other three regimens tested in the trial and may decrease the requirement for emergency angiography for this indication. (Summarized from Ref. 6.) However, despite the overall improvement in 24-hour and 30-day mortality with accelerated t-PA, in the GUSTO trial there were no differences in the need for emergency angiography, emergency percutaneous transluminal coronary angioplasty (PTCA), or emergency coronary artery bypass graft (CABG) (unpublished data)

	SK (s.c.)	SK (i.v.)	t-PA (accelerated regimen)	t-PA + SK	*P* value (accelerated t-PA vs both SK regimens)
Cardiogenic shock	6.9	6.3	5.1	6.1	<0.001
Pulmonary edema	17.5	16.8	15.2	16.8	<0.001
Reinfarction	3.4	4.0	4.0	4.0	0.26
Recurrent ischemia	19.9	19.6	18.8	19.3	0.14
Emergency angiography	10.2	10.2	9.7	9.4	NS
Emergency PTCA	27.0	26.5	26.0	26.1	NS
Emergency CABG	8.5	8.8	9.5	9.5	NS

NS, not significant; SK, streptokinase.

term, patients who require urgent angiography often have lower residual left ventricular function and suboptimal overall clinical outcomes despite the delivery of aggressive care.

Elective Angiography for Risk Stratification

For uncomplicated patients (those who do not develop hemodynamic or mechanical complications that mandate catheterization) there are two approaches to planned, elective angiography for risk stratification following myocardial infarction: *routine* and *selective*. In the routine approach, coronary angiography is a standard component of the postinfarction risk assessment of all (or nearly all) patients. In the selective approach, catheterization is performed for definite recurrent ischemia or an abnormal functional test that suggests inducible ischemia. In the USA, there is considerable controversy about the appropriate role of elective angiography following myocardial infarction. Although our preferred strategy is to recommend routine catheterization early in the hospital course, there are no definitive data to mandate this approach. Rational arguments support both routine and selective postinfarction angiography.

However, the population of 'postinfarction patients' is of course quite diverse; the most efficient use of resources requires a critical analysis of the available data in two broadly defined, rather different patient subsets. First, there are patients who *complete* an infarction. This may occur due to the patient's late presentation, misdiagnosis, or ineligibility for thrombolytic therapy. Other patients may develop this outcome because thrombolytic therapy is unsuccessful or direct angioplasty is unavailable. Second, there are patients who *present* with threatened infarction but who are successfully treated with thrombolytic therapy; these patients may sustain only partial damage to the infarct zone (on the basis of enzyme analysis, the failure to develop Q-waves, or relative preservation of left ventricular function) or, hopefully, they may escape significant necrosis altogether. Annually, there are at least 400 000 patients who are successfully treated with thrombolytic therapy.[1] In the discussion that follows, we will distinguish between these groups of patients whenever possible. Data regarding the first group are primarily from the prethrombolytic era of the 1970s and 1980s; data on the second group are only becoming available now.

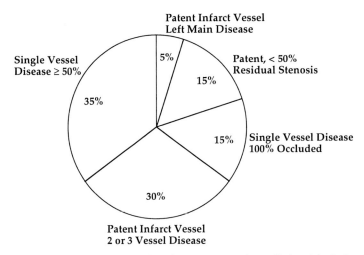

Figure 4.1 Proportion of patients in each of the five anatomic subsets distinguished after thrombolytic therapy. (From Ref. 42; data extrapolated from Refs 16, 18, 38, 74, 103, 104, 160.)

Routine coronary angiography

The rationale for advocating routine coronary angiography is to define the coronary lesion responsible for the infarct, to evaluate the success of thrombolytic therapy, to identify patients with severe coronary artery disease, and to facilitate early hospital discharge and return to work in selected cases. When thrombolytic therapy has been successful on clinical grounds, advocates of routine angiography assume that although the patient has been spared an infarction, he or she remains in the category of patients with an unstable plaque. The early, placebo-controlled trials of thrombolytic therapy support this concept; patients who received this therapy had higher rates of reinfarction than did conventionally managed patients.[2,36,37] Proponents of routine angiography emphasize that it determines the extent of coronary disease most accurately and that therapy can be confidently and efficiently directed on the basis of these findings.

Whether or not a patient has received thrombolytic therapy, precise definition of the anatomic extent of coronary artery disease can be extremely valuable in planning therapeutic strategies to promote long-term survival, free from infarction and angina. On the basis of data from the TIMI, TAMI, and GUSTO trials, patients who undergo routine catheterization after intravenous thrombolysis can be separated into five discrete categories,[15,16,18,38–41] as shown in Figure 4.1. Patients within these categories have different prognoses and require different management strategies.

First, approximately 5% of patients have left main stenosis or its equivalent. It is essential to make this diagnosis in these patients; they deserve consideration for prompt bypass surgery. Although one would hope that noninvasive testing would identify these patients reliably, current noninvasive methods have limitations (discussed below) and they may not accurately identify all members of this critical subset.

Second, roughly 30% of patients have two- or three-vessel coronary artery disease, defined as stenosis of more than 70% in a noninfarct-related vessel; multivessel disease markedly worsens the short-term prognosis.[43] In the TAMI trials, 236 of 855 patients (27.6%) had multivessel disease; their in-hospital mortality was 11.4%, compared with only 4.2% in patients with single-vessel disease.[43] Logistic regression confirmed that the strongest independent predictors of in-hospital mortality were regional wall motion in the noninfarct zone ($P = 0.0057$) and the number of diseased vessels ($P = 0.04$). Of course, although these variables are independent statistically, they are clearly related, since the extent of disease in the noninfarcted arteries will influence wall motion of these territories. The authors conclude that coronary angiography is the procedure of choice for identifying these high-risk patients. Lee and colleagues[44] combined data from several of the TAMI trials[15-17] and used a regression model to predict mortality based on angiographic findings. They concluded that each diseased coronary vessel (in addition to the infarct artery) increases mortality to the same extent as a 16-year increase in age or a 13-point reduction in ejection fraction. In summary, the angiographic documentation of multivessel disease can accurately stratify the patient's risk. Although documenting multivessel disease does not by itself improve prognosis, it can lead to closer surveillance and to a lower threshold for recommending revascularization. Whether angioplasty or bypass surgery is the preferred form of revascularization for these patients is the subject of several ongoing randomized trials.[45]

The third group of patients are the approximately 15% of patients who have an occluded infarct artery at elective angiography; these patients may benefit from delayed angioplasty, if ongoing studies prove that late reperfusion is clinically important. Patients with an occluded artery but without ischemia must be distinguished from those with an occluded vessel and ongoing ischemia, because in the latter setting, rescue angioplasty is clearly beneficial.[46] The fourth group are those patients who have single-vessel disease with a residual stenosis of more than 50%; these patients comprise approximately 35% of patients at angiography. The status of angiography and intervention in both of these subgroups is discussed more fully in the section of this chapter devoted to angioplasty.

The fifth category of patients includes those who have a minimal residual stenosis of the infarct-related vessel; these patients also have an excellent prognosis. In the TAMI trials, this group accounted for approximately 15% of patients;[47] a similar proportion (13%) was identified in the TIMI-2 trial.[37] These patients are often young, more often female, and are more likely to have single-vessel disease; ventricular function is usually good.[47] This 'minimal lesion syndrome' may be due to a relatively small coronary artery plaque (in comparison to older patients with acute myocardial infarction); in addition, a predisposition to more marked vasospasm and/or thrombosis may be present (such as the use of tobacco or oral contraceptives or the presence of an underlying prothrombotic disorder). This group also includes those patients whose infarct-vessel stenosis 'improves' at the time of repeat angiography. In the TAMI-1 trial,[15] in the subgroup of patients randomized to immediate angiography but delayed, elective angioplasty, 14% had spontaneous improvement in their culprit lesion between the time of first catheterization and the second 7 days later. In any case, routine angiography allows the physician to reassure these patients and to recommend intensive risk factor modification, because it provides precise definition of the coronary anatomy and because this diagnosis carries a better 1-year prognosis than that of the typical patient with a high-grade residual stenosis.[47]

Although the percentages of patients in these subsets provide the clinician with a useful framework, it is critically important to note that these data *underestimate* the severity of underlying coronary disease in the entire group of patients with acute myocardial infarction. It is noteworthy that the patients enrolled in the TIMI-2 trial were a select group and had a considerably lower incidence of multivessel disease compared with patients in studies done in the prethrombolytic era. The study design excluded patients with prior bypass surgery, severe hypertension, and prior cerebrovascular disease; these are precisely the groups that would be expected to have a higher prevalence of multivessel disease. Thus, the conclusions from the TIMI-2 trial cannot be applied readily to all patient subsets. Furthermore, the physician who recommends a selective approach should remember that in TIMI-2, the most important trial to evaluate the combination of catheterization and angioplasty, 33% of patients in the 'conservative' strategy required catheterization during the initial hospitalization and a total of 60% ultimately had catheterization within the year following the index infarction.

In summary, coronary angiography can accurately identify the nearly 50% of patients who warrant consideration for revascularization (i.e. those with left main, significant two or three vessel disease, and those with an occluded vessel but viable myocardium beyond the obstruction); when coupled to functional testing, it can reassure both the physician and patient. As we will discuss, it can also potentiate an earlier discharge and return to work. In addition, data from both the prethrombolytic era and from more recent trials identify clinical variables of patients at particularly high risk after myocardial infarction. Ross and colleagues[48] used data from over 1800 patients to derive a decision scheme for coronary angiography after myocardial infarction in order to identify patients at increased risk of death within the first year. According to this analysis, patients under the age of 75 years with a history of a prior myocardial infarction, resting ischemia, left ventricular failure during the initial hospitalization, exercise-induced ischemia or a poor exercise workload, and an ejection fraction of less than 44% are all at significantly increased risk of death in the first year (average mortality 16%). In these patients, the physician should strongly consider catheterization. However, this scheme still predicts that approximately 55–60% of patients will require coronary angiography to complete their risk stratification, and does not take into account the economic impact of the additional tests (such as radionuclide ventriculography) required in many patients, as will be discussed.

Selective coronary angiography

Advocates of this approach offer two broad arguments in support of this strategy. First, they maintain that a selective strategy is practical (i.e. catheterization is expensive and unavailable in many hospitals). In the USA, only 20–25% of the 6000 acute care hospital facilities have a cardiac catheterization laboratory.[49] Therefore, limited use of this procedure would allow continuity of care in local community hospitals and would avoid the need to transfer patients to other hospitals solely for predischarge angiography. Thus, a strategy of selective angiography would theoretically result in fewer unnecessary procedures, hospital transfers, and balloon angioplasty revascularizations. The physician would recommend elective angiography in those patients with documented ischemia and especially if there is evidence of ischemia in several coronary territories. It is often assumed that this strategy would of necessity be less expensive than a strategy of routine angiography.

Second, advocates of the selective approach argue that in the subgroup of patients who receive thrombolytic therapy, both strategies lead to the same clinical outcome with respect to death, reinfarction, and ejection fraction. For example, Rogers and colleagues[8,40,50] in a retrospective analysis of TIMI-2 data compared selective and routine angiography and found that routine angiography did not result in a reduction in either acute or 1-year adverse clinical outcomes. These investigators compared the TIMI-2A strategy of predischarge catheterization without angioplasty to the conservative strategy of selective catheterization from TIMI-2. Interestingly, patients who had catheterization without angioplasty had a higher in-hospital mortality rate of 8% compared to 4% for patients who were considered for angiography selectively. However, although this difference is statistically significant, it is difficult to explain since there were no definite adverse outcomes associated with the angiography itself.

As further evidence that both strategies result in the same clinical outcome, advocates of the selective approach point out that patients randomized to a 'conservative' strategy of 'watchful waiting' in both the TIMI-2 trial[38,40] and in the Should We Intervene Following Thrombolysis? (SWIFT) trial[51] had identical outcomes as patients randomized to an 'invasive' strategy of empiric catheterization coupled to angioplasty (Figures 4.2 and 4.3). Patients randomized to the conservative TIMI-2 trial strategy had a low risk of major events.[38] However, these trials were not designed to test a strategy of routine angiography; instead, they tested a strategy of angiography coupled to angioplasty. In

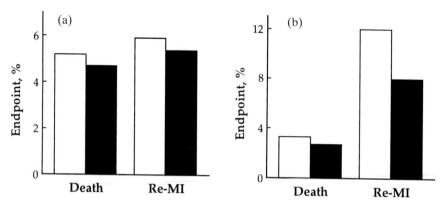

Figure 4.2   Results of randomized trials comparing the prophylactic (□) and selective (■) strategies for cardiac catheterization and coronary angioplasty. (a) Data for death or reinfarction (Re-MI) from 3262 patients in TIMI-2[38] who received tissue plasminogen activator. There was no difference in either endpoint for the two strategies. (b) Data from 8000 patients in the Should We Intervene Following Thrombolysis (SWIFT) trial[51] who received anistreplase show no difference in the death rate but do show a higher rate of reinfarction among patients who had prophylactic angioplasty. (From Ref. 42.)

fact these trials established that angioplasty soon after t-PA resulted in higher rates of acute vessel closure and reinfarction. For example, in the SWIFT trial,[51] stable patients treated with prophylactic angioplasty in the absence of documented ischemia actually had a significantly higher rate of reinfarction than patients treated with a conservative approach (Figure 4.2). In an asymptomatic patient after thrombolysis, for any documented residual stenosis in the infarct-related vessel that is associated with intact regional wall motion, the long-term outcome is usually favorable. When a lesion that is low-risk based on clinical data is dilated solely because of its angiographic appearance, it is probable that angiography was unnecessary.

Whether or not a particular patient has received thrombolytic therapy, many advocates of the selective approach will nevertheless recommend angiography in certain high-risk patients (Figure 4.4). For example, patients who have had a prior myocardial infarction have a higher mortality rate during long-term follow-up. Complex or frequent ventricular arrhythmias may be an indicator of residual ischemia and may correlate with an increased risk of late cardiac morbidity and mortality.[48,52–55] Patients with an ejection fraction less than 45% and those spared from potentially large infarcts (such as a threatened anterior infarct successfully treated with thrombolytics) are also often recommended for 'selective' angiography. In all of these subgroups, the prognosis may improve with early catheterization, as well as with aggressive management of arrhythmias and left ventricular dysfunction.

Which strategy: routine or selective or angiography?

It is critical to note that a 'selective' approach will still require urgent angiography in a substantial proportion of patients who have been successfully reperfused with thrombolytic therapy. In the TIMI-2 trial,[38,40] patients randomized to a 'conservative' strategy of 'watchful waiting' after thrombolysis, with surveillance for clinical indicators of recurrent ischemia, had a 33% rate of angiography before hospital discharge.[38] Similar rates of urgent angiography in patients randomized to a conservative strategy have been observed in other trials. In the TAMI-5 trial,[56] of the 288 patients randomly assigned to delayed catheterization, 26% (75 patients) crossed over to an urgent procedure within 5 days of admission for one or more of the following reasons: chest pain (82%), new ST-segment elevation (60%), or hypotension (35%). Patients who crossed over to urgent

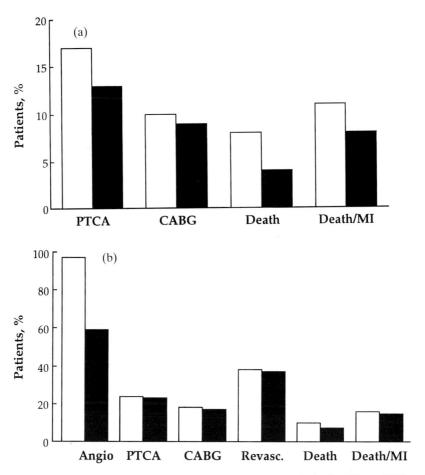

Figure 4.3 A nonrandomized comparison of the routine (□; $n = 197$) and selective (■; $n = 1461$) cardiac catheterization strategies from the TIMI-II trials.[38] (a) Summary of in-hospital procedures and outcomes. The P values for each are as follows: coronary angioplasty (PTCA), $P = 0.15$; coronary artery bypass surgery (CABG), $P > 0.2$; death, $P = 0.013$; and death or reinfarction (MI), $P > 0.2$. (b) Cumulative 1-year follow-up procedure utilization and outcomes. The only significant difference was for angiography (Angio) (97% compared with 59%, $P > 0.001$). Revasc, revascularization. (Modified from Ref. 42.)

angiography had a poorer clinical outcome than patients who did not require this approach; the former group had a higher incidence of pulmonary edema (24% compared with 14%), lower predischarge ejection fractions (51.9% ± 11.3% compared with 54.2% ± 10.8%), and higher in-hospital mortality (7% compared with 3%). These results occurred despite an aggressive approach to myocardial revascularization with either emergency PTCA (49%) or coronary artery bypass graft (CABG) (15%).

Unfortunately, clinical and hemodynamic variables on admission are poor predictors of which patients will require urgent angiography. Furthermore, one cannot assume that the absence of ischemia after thrombolytic therapy is due to significant myocardial salvage and the absence of a significant residual stenosis. Sutton and Topol demonstrated that a high-grade stenosis *without* a perfusion abnormality is often due to more extensive myocardial necrosis (as correlated with peak creatine phosphokinase (CPK) release) despite thrombolytic therapy.[57] The higher the patient's CPK release, the more likely was a negative thallium study.

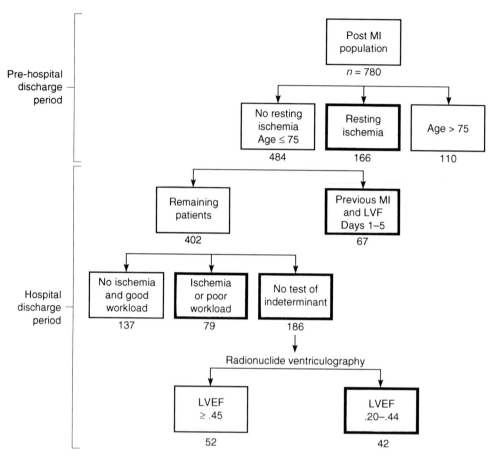

Figure 4.4 Critical analysis of a scheme for selecting patients for coronary angiography as proposed by Ross *et al.*[48] According to this scheme, stratification during the early period is for patients surviving the first 5 days and eliminates patients 75 years of age or older while identifying patients with resting ischemic pain. Stratification at later times is for patients surviving to hospital discharge. Coronary angiography is recommended for selected groups (heavy boxes). Numbers under the boxes show the distribution of patients in a test population on whom the scheme was applied. Although this strategy, if chosen, would reduce the number of angiograms performed following myocardial infarction, it is important to note that angiography would still be recommended for approximately 55% of patients. The sum of those recommended for catheterization (under the heavy boxes) is $186 + 67 + 79 + 42 = 374$; dividing this by 780 (the initial population) yields 55%. This scheme does not include patients with an ejection fraction of less then 20% or patients who had neither an exercise test nor left ventricular ejection fraction determination. LVEF, left ventricular ejection fraction; LVF, left ventricular failure; MI, myocardial infarction. (Modified from Ref. 48.)

Limitations of Noninvasive Testing as a Screening Test

In order to identify patients with residual ischemia, left ventricular dysfunction, or ventricular arrhythmias, the alternative method of risk stratification is noninvasive testing; angiography is then performed on the basis of these results. Proponents of both routine and selective angiography agree that whether or not exercise testing serves as the primary method of risk stratification, it provides essential data on the physiologic significance of coronary stenoses and on the patient's functional capacity. These data are invaluable for prescribing an exercise program and for reassuring the patient.

Table 4.3   Some potential limitations of exercise testing/noninvasive risk assessment following myocardial infarction. (Modified from Ref. 35)

1. Nearly all reported data are derived from patients who did not have myocardial reperfusion therapy; no study has correlated functional tests and long-term clinical outcome following pharmacologic reperfusion
2. The testing may not allow diagnosis of viable, noninfarcted tissue
3. Simple exercise electrocardiographic markers are often difficult to interpret after thrombolysis due to persistent abnormalities
4. Positive predictive accuracy and sensitivity in detecting multivessel coronary disease are lower than in chronic stable angina
5. Reported series in both the prethrombolytic era and more recent studies exclude certain subgroups (the elderly, patients unable to exercise, etc.) that have a high long-term risk of recurrent ischemic events and mortality
6. Follow-up duration is short in most reported studies; when follow-up is adequate, predictive value falls dramatically
7. Submaximal testing may not attain sufficient workload to exclude myocardial ischemia reliably

Although the role of noninvasive testing following myocardial infarction is thoroughly reviewed in Chapter 16, several issues are important to this discussion. In our opinion, there are two distinct difficulties with the use of noninvasive testing as the primary method of risk stratification following myocardial infarction. These limitations of noninvasive testing are summarized in Table 4.3.

First, functional tests in the reperfusion era have not been adequately validated. Although stress testing as a primary means of risk stratification was well-validated in the prethrombolytic era,[58–60] it is not at all clear that these data are immediately applicable to patients who have received thrombolytic therapy. Patients who are eligible for and who have received thrombolytic therapy are a group that is fundamentally different from patients in the prethrombolytic era who completed an infarct and who were then entered into studies of noninvasive testing. Patients who have received thrombolytic therapy are diverse, including those who have completely avoided a large infarct but who remain with a critical stenosis and a significant amount of myocardium at risk, those with a certain amount of damage with some potentially salvageable myocardial tissue within the infarct territory, and those who have no potentially salvageable myocardium but who may benefit from late mechanical revascularization. Although all three of these subgroups existed in the prethrombolytic era, it is intuitive that the different proportions of patients within each subgroup would change the sensitivity and specificity of any form of functional testing. Furthermore, it is highly likely that interpretations of functional tests after intravenous thrombolytic therapy, especially when it is successful, will be extremely difficult. For example, a study of regional or global wall motion may give the false impression that function does not worsen during exercise because of the presence of viable but reversibly injured myocardium. Similarly, after successful thrombolysis, perfusion imaging with thallium may not allow reliable diagnosis of viable, noninfarcted tissue; studies to date have shown a poor sensitivity and specificity for noninfarct vessel anatomy.[61]

Studies of functional tests after intravenous thrombolysis are summarized in Table 4.4;[61–65] each of these studies has raised concerns about the validity of functional testing after reperfusion therapy. These data are especially troublesome when compared to the relatively high predictive accuracy of such testing in the prethrombolytic era.[58–60] Chaitman and colleagues[63] showed that abnormal results on a bicycle ergometry test done before discharge and at 6 weeks after discharge were not predictive of death or reinfarction at 6-month follow-up. Burns and colleagues[61] correlated the findings of quantitative single-photon tomographic thallium scanning and coronary angiography after intravenous thrombolysis; the sensitivity of scintigraphy for diagnosing multivessel disease was only 35%, and specificity for infarct-related vessel disease (>50% stenosis)

Table 4.4 Studies of functional testing after intravenous thrombolysis (Modified from Ref. 42)

Reference	No. of patients	Study design	Test	Major finding
Simoons et al.[62]	533	Streptokinase compared with conventional therapy	Predischarge treadmill exercise	Functional test not predictive of reinfarction or death during 5-year follow-up
Chaitman et al.[63]	1958	t-PA, t-PA compared with catheterization and angioplasty (if suitable)	Predischarge and 6-week postdischarge supine bicycle ergometry and ECG	Functional test not predictive of reinfarction or death during 6-month follow-up
Burns et al.[61]	47	t-PA compared with placebo	Exercise SPECT; thallium on day 8	Sensitivity of detecting substantial stenosis in the infarct-related vessel, 95%; specificity, 14%. For stenosis of a noninfarct-related vessel; sensitivity, 35%; specificity, 79%
Touchstone et al.[64]	21	Streptokinase	Exercise thallium on day 10	Only 25% of patients with preserved regional wall motion have provocable ischemia
Weiss et al.[45]	37	Streptokinase	Exercise-gated blood pool scintigraphy at 7 weeks	46% of patients with early therapy and a significant residual stenosis had a negative test, correlated with reduced evidence of salvage

SPECT, single-photon emission computerized tomography; t-PA, tissue plasminogen activator.

was 14%. Such levels of sensitivity are unacceptable when used for patient screening. Even if a test had a positive predictive accuracy of 95% for cardiac death within 5 years, such a level may be considered inadequate for an otherwise healthy 45-year-old patient.

Simoons and colleagues[62] performed the study with the most extensive follow-up. In 533 patients, event rates during the 5 years after reperfusion therapy were not predicted by a positive functional study. These investigators used a regression model to determine prognostic indices. Five factors were key independent predictors of late prognosis; patient age, previous infarction, ejection fraction, the number of diseased coronary vessels, and the severity of residual stenosis in the infarct-related artery. Unlike the first three variables, the last two predictors can *only* be derived from cardiac catheterization. Furthermore, as mentioned above, Sutton and Topol[57] found that a negative postthrombolytic exercise stress test correlates with greater myocardial necrosis rather than with exercise time or hemodynamics, the time delay to reperfusion, or the severity of the infarct-vessel stenosis. Paradoxically, inadequate myocardial salvage, rather than optimal therapy with no residual ischemia, may be the most likely explanation for this test result. In aggregate, these data suggest that we cannot readily apply data collected during the prethrombolytic era to the group of patients who are excluded from thrombolytic therapy, due to significant differences in these populations.

The second major difficulty with the use of exercise testing as the primary method of risk stratification is that many patients cannot perform the test. In various studies, the percentage of patients unable to do an exercise test has ranged from 20 to 45%.[58–60] The inability to perform an exercise test is a powerful marker of a poor prognosis, with mortality approaching 10–15% within 2 years of the index infarction.[48,66–69] In addition, the elderly have been excluded from many studies of functional testing. As a group, the elderly have a substantially increased risk following infarction. Although newer pharmacologic stress testing with adenosine, dobutamine or dipyridamole may eventually prove adequate for patients who cannot exercise, the predictive values of these tests require further validation. Other important concerns regarding exercise testing as the primary method of risk stratification are listed in Table 4.3.

In summary, it is our opinion that prospective studies with long-term follow-up are warranted in order to determine the accuracy of noninvasive testing in the thrombolytic era. Proponents of stress testing conclude that this method of predischarge risk stratification (in combination with an assessment of left ventricular function and clinical evaluation) has been empirically validated, based on the observation of an excellent 1-year outcome of 'low-risk' patients (those under age 75 years without a history of prior infarction, etc.) in the conservative group of the TIMI-2 trial. On the other hand, proponents of routine catheterization maintain that exercise testing is indeed invaluable: it is most useful when coupled with angiography, to determine the physiologic significance of the coronary lesions present. In the absence of definitive data, this controversy will not be easily resolved.

Economic Considerations in Risk Stratification

One of the major concerns about routine catheterization is cost and effective resource utilization. One analysis suggested that avoiding 50% of catheterizations and related unnecessary coronary revascularization procedures in the USA could provide potential savings of more than $US700 million per year.[41] One of the assumptions following the TIMI-2 study was that a conservative strategy of 'watchful waiting' would be less expensive than an invasive strategy of angiography and angioplasty. However, this is not necessarily true. In a study that illustrates the importance of actual cost analysis, Charles and colleagues[50] reported economic data from the TIMI-2 trial in 310 patients. Although total hospital *charges* were higher for the invasive strategy compared with the conservative strategy ($US15 918 compared to $US12 588, respectively), the difference in actual hospital *costs* was considerably less ($US10 496 compared to $US8826, respectively). Furthermore, follow-up data indicated 'a higher frequency of readmissions for angina pectoris during the first year after myocardial infarction, and during these hospitalizations, more than twice as many patients in the selective group underwent coronary arteriography as did patients in the routine catheterization group during the same time interval'.[40] An adequate cost comparison of the two strategies would obviously have to include the cost of subsequent hospitalizations and, ideally, time lost from work.

Provocative data regarding the importance of examining total cost were recently released from the GUSTO study group.[70] In the GUSTO trial, with the exception of patients enrolled in the angiographic substudy, the patient's attending physician decided whether to recommend postinfarction angiography. There were differences in utilization and differences in outcome. In the USA, angiography was performed in 83% of patients, whereas in Canada it was performed in only 48% (Table 4.5). Importantly, patients who were not sent for angiography had significantly more angina, higher rates

Table 4.5 Comparison of resource utilization in the USA and Canada for patients enrolled in the GUSTO-1 trial. Baseline clinical characteristics were similar in the two groups. Note that angiography was performed far more frequently in the USA; however the total number of physician visits was less in these patients. (From Ref. 70)

	USA	Canada	
No. of patients	2600	400	
Length of stay	8 days	9 days	$P = 0.002$
Angiogram	83%	48%	$P < 0.001$
PTCA	38%	18%	$P < 0.001$
CABG	21%	11%	$P < 0.001$
MD visits	8	12	
Cardiologists	4	3	
FP/internist	2	8	

CABG, coronary artery bypass graft; PTCA, percutaneous transluminal coronary angioplasty.

of hospitalization, and higher rates of costs incurred during the first year following the index infarction.

Despite the cost of the procedure itself, a strategy of routine catheterization does not necessarily result in increased total cost; findings during angiography can result in a shortening of the hospital stay and thus in decreased cost. For example, patients with the minimal lesion syndrome or only single-vessel disease are excellent candidates for an early return to work. This pattern was noted in the early discharge trial.[15] In a randomized trial comparing early (day 4) and conventional (day 7–10) hospital discharge, angiography combined with a functional test permitted 20% of patients with myocardial infarction to be eligible for discharge at day 4.[27] The abbreviated stay was safe and resulted in a 30% reduction in hospital and professional charges ($US5000 saved per patient). Translating these charges to costs and assuming a conservative estimate of 15% of patients eligible, the savings would be nearly $US300 million per year.

Other economic considerations include the small differences in actual cost as opposed to charge data between the invasive (incorporating prophylactic angioplasty) and conservative strategies in TIMI-2,[39,40] the fixed as opposed to variable costs of operating a cardiac catheterization laboratory, the costs of functional tests, and the costs of readmissions. Because of the difficulty in interpreting the ECG in the early days or weeks after myocardial infarction, thallium scintigraphy is frequently used; in most centers the charge is in excess of $US1000. If routine catheterization limits the need for thallium scintigraphy before discharge, at 6 weeks after discharge, or at both times, this may be a trade-off for savings in cost. Finally, the cost of readmission for subsequent catheterization, particularly in facilities where the procedure is not done on an outpatient basis, is an important factor. In fact, 59% of patients in TIMI-2 who were managed using the conservative strategy ultimately underwent cardiac catheterization by 1-year follow-up.[50]

Although the total costs to society are unquestionably part of our responsibility as physicians, so too is the quality of life of our patients. In our analysis of the GUSTO trial cited above, patients who underwent elective angiography scored significantly higher on indices of quality of life.[70] These patients may be more likely to have an earlier return to work; employers and payers view this as a desirable endpoint of treatment. Therefore, a complete functional and anatomic assessment, if performed expeditiously and in a cost-effective manner, can lead to lower hospital costs,[50] earlier discharge[15] and lower total costs to society.

Resolving the Dilemma: A Middle Ground

No definitive data currently exist to recommend selective or routine cardiac catheterization. The guidelines published by the American College of Cardiology and American Heart Association[71] for managing patients with acute myocardial infarction after thrombolytic therapy do not specifically address this issue. It is essential to separate diagnostic angiography, which can be done safely, quickly, and relatively economically, from a therapeutic procedure such as coronary angioplasty. As we have discussed, the trials that have peripherally addressed this issue[38,51] compared a 'package' of angiography and angioplasty with 'no procedure' and analyzed the data using an intention-to-treat principle. Perhaps the best approach would be to use either selective or routine angiography if specific fundamental information can be gained that cannot be determined from noninvasive tests and that may be of value for particular patient subsets. However, despite the data on quality of life noted above, studies have not shown that routine predischarge coronary angiography leads to improved survival or lower reinfarction rates when compared with the selective strategy. Ideally, firm recommendations would be based on a randomized trial comparing 'angiography with angioplasty prophylactic revascularization' with 'no angiography'; unfortunately, such a trial is unlikely to be done.

In our opinion it would be premature for practice guidelines issued by governmental agencies or managed care networks to proscribe routine angiography following myocardial infarction. Unfortunately, Medicare has already refused reimbursement for routine angiography in asymptomatic patients in at least two states (Utah and Nevada). This decision is premature because the data are equivocal. Furthermore, we must emphasize the absolute proscription of revascularization procedures in patients who undergo angiography but who do not have angina or inducible ischemia. As discussed below, there are no data to support aggressive mechanical revascularization in these patients. Within the USA, there is significant variability in the use of angiography after myocardial infarction on a regional basis.[72] This wide variability suggests that there is no single 'standard of clinical practice'. Importantly, the availability of facilities may be related to the increased use of the procedure whereas patients hospitalized in facilities without angiography may be less likely to undergo the procedure. It is critical that additional studies with long-term follow-up be performed comparing both clinical outcome, total cost, and quality of life in order to assess the relative merits of the routine and selective angiography strategies.

Coronary Angioplasty Strategies in Acute Myocardial Infarction

There are four broadly defined strategies of coronary angioplasty following acute myocardial infarction: direct, rescue, empiric, and elective. As with catheterization strategies, different angioplasty strategies are distinguished according to their timing and principal purpose (Table 4.6).

Direct angioplasty

Direct angioplasty (also called primary angioplasty) refers to immediate percutaneous mechanical revascularization of the infarct artery as soon as possible after the patient's initial presentation as an alternative to thrombolytic therapy or conservative management. Before discussing potential merits of this approach, it is useful to distinguish between direct angioplasty as a procedure and direct angioplasty as a therapeutic strategy. As a procedure, direct PTCA refers to the actual transcatheter recanalization of

Table 4.6 Coronary angioplasty strategies for acute myocardial infarction. (Modified from Ref. 35)

Strategy	Prior thrombolytic therapy	Goal	Timing
Direct (primary)	No	Recanalization	As soon as possible
Rescue	Yes	Recanalization when thrombolysis fails	As soon as possible
Empiric	Varies	Prophylactic for recurrent ischemia	Immediate: 12–72 hours after presentation Delayed: 3 days to 2 weeks
Elective	Varies	Treatment of angina or documented ischemia	>2 weeks

the infarct vessel. However, advocates of direct PTCA as a therapeutic strategy emphasize that a substantial percentage of patients do not actually undergo angioplasty; they may require some other form of therapy. Therefore, the strategy might best be described as 'immediate angiography with appropriate triage to the most appropriate form of revascularization'. For example, some cardiologists favor primary angioplasty because the procedure simultaneously determines the extent of disease in other coronary vessels. In approximately 5–8% of patients, the hydrostatic pressure of intracoronary injection of contrast immediately facilitates clot dissolution.[1,15,17,73,74] The initial angiogram will detect significant left main disease in approximately 5% of patients; these patients are often referred for immediate bypass surgery.[21] On the other hand, approximately 5% of patients will not have a severe underlying stenosis in the infarct vessel; these patients can be managed without angioplasty or thrombolytic therapy.[21]

Rationale

If a patient presents to a facility capable of providing direct angioplasty skillfully and rapidly, there are two reasons for the clinician to favor this approach over thrombolytic therapy. First, direct angioplasty is especially useful in patients who have a contraindication to thrombolysis, such as recent surgery, trauma, or stroke.[75] Mechanical reperfusion has a lower risk of hemorrhage complications than thrombolytic therapy. For example, even though a large proportion of the elderly are candidates for thrombolytic therapy, in a significant number these drugs are truly contraindicated. Ineligibility for thrombolytic therapy has dire consequences. Cragg and his colleagues[76] reported on 1471 acute infarction patients treated at a large community hospital; 78% (1144 patients) were treated conventionally without any form of reperfusion therapy. Patients excluded from thrombolytic therapy were older and more likely to have had a prior infarction. Of note, this group had a nearly fivefold increase in mortality (19% vs 4%) when compared to the group that received thrombolytic therapy. These data suggest that patients excluded from thrombolytic therapy have multiple risk factors for a poor outcome; therefore, they may benefit most from an aggressive approach to reperfusion. Although the study was not designed to test this hypothesis, patients treated with primary angioplasty had the same favorable clinical outcome as did patients who were eligible for thrombolytic therapy.

Second, several randomized trials[21–24,77] have shown superior reperfusion rates (>90%) with direct angioplasty. With even the most effective thrombolytic regimen in GUSTO,[6] 46% of patients did not achieve complete reperfusion (i.e. TIMI grade 3). Clinicians have recently appreciated that the traditional method of assessing infarct vessel 'patency' (by considering as equivalent patients with either TIMI grade 2 or grade 3 infarct vessel flow) overestimates the efficacy of thrombolysis. Analyses of this

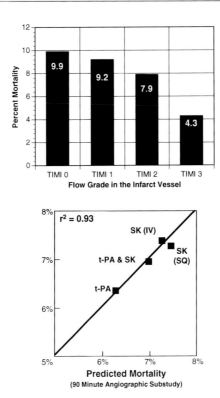

Figure 4.5 *Top:* Mortality in the GUSTO trial according to TIMI flow grade at 90-minute angiography. Combining data from all treatment regimens, TIMI flow grade at 90-min angiography is an excellent predictor of 30 day mortality. *Bottom:* The mortality rate of a particular therapeutic regimen is directly related to its ability to produce TIMI grade 3 flow in the infarct vessel. Overall, these data illustrate that the degree of patency of the infarct vessel at early catheterization are proportionate to mortality. If this relationship is also true for primary angioplasty, then this more invasive approach may prove more effective than *any* thrombolytic regimen, because trials of primary angioplasty have consistently demonstrated TIMI grade 3 flow rates of more than 90%. (Top: modified from Refs 77 and 6; Bottom: from Ref. 78.)

phenomenon[78,79] suggest that contributory factors include insufficiently rapid or incomplete recanalization, incomplete patency with only TIMI grade 2 flow or critical residual coronary stenoses, the absence of tissue perfusion despite patency of the infarct vessel, intermittent coronary occlusion, reocclusion, and reperfusion injury. Therefore, with thrombolytic therapy, truly adequate tissue-level reperfusion may be the exception rather than the rule. In GUSTO-I, only 54% of patients had TIMI grade 3 patency with the most effective therapy at 90 min.[6] On the other hand, direct angioplasty is more likely to achieve complete infarct vessel patency (TIMI grade 3) and to sustain this level of flow. This has been demonstrated recently in several randomized trials.[21–24,77] In the GUSTO angiographic substudy, Simes *et al.* demonstrated that TIMI flow grade in the infarct vessel at 90 min accurately predicts 30-day survival (Fig. 4.5).[80] If TIMI flow grade 90 min after the initiation of therapy is indeed such a powerful predictor of survival, primary angioplasty may be conclusively proven better than any safe, contemporary thrombolytic regimen.

In a recent meta-analysis of direct PTCA observational studies, Eckman *et al.*[81] confirmed that, on average, direct PTCA is associated with a consistently high vessel patency rate of approximately 91%. This analysis included 10 studies with a total of 2073 patients. Overall, the in-hospital mortality rate was 8.3%.

Table 4.7 Randomized trials of primary coronary angioplasty (PTCA) vs intravenous thrombolytic therapy for the treatment of acute myocardial infarction. (From Ref. 82)

Reference	Thrombolytic regimen	No. of patients	Endpoints	Main finding
DeWood[77]	t-PA	43	Patency	No difference
Ribiero et al.[23]	SK	100	Patency Ejection fraction	Favors SK
Zijlstra et al.[24]	SK	56	Patency Ejection fraction	Favors PTCA
Gibbons et al.[22]	t-PA	95	Infarct size (^{99m}Tc sestamibi)	No difference
Grines et al.[12]	t-PA	450	Mortality Reinfarction Recurrent ischemia	Favors PTCA

PTCA, percutaneous transluminal coronary angioplasty; SK, streptokinase; t-PA, tissue plasminogen activator.

Randomized trials

To date, there have been five randomized trials of direct angioplasty (Table 4.7). Gibbons *et al.*[22] performed a trial of 108 patients in whom direct angioplasty was compared with a conventional (i.e. non-front-loaded) t-PA regimen. This study did not demonstrate a difference with respect to myocardial salvage or infarct size, as assessed by acute and predischarge perfusion scans with technetium-99m-sestamibi. However, patients randomized to direct PTCA had a significant reduction in recurrent ischemia, a shorter length of hospital stay, and a trend toward reduced hospital costs. At 6-month follow-up, the PTCA group had fewer readmissions (4% vs 18%, $P = 0.04$) and lower total costs. Zijlstra *et al.*[24] randomized 142 patients to either direct angioplasty or intravenous streptokinase. PTCA achieved acute patency in 98% of patients; this group had lower rates of recurrent ischemia (9% vs 38%, $P = 0.001$) and reinfarction (0% vs 13%, $P = 0.003$). Although this trial demonstrated a higher mean ejection fraction for patients randomized to direct PTCA ($51 \pm 11\%$ vs $45 \pm 12\%$, $P = 0.004$), the thrombolytic regimen used in this study has since been demonstrated to be suboptimal. At late follow-up, angiography confirmed vessel patency in 91% of angioplasty patients compared to only 68% of patients randomized with thrombolytic therapy. Two other small trials of direct angioplasty are summarized in Table 4.7.

The largest trial to date, the Primary Angioplasty and Myocardial Infarction Trial[21] was a multicenter study of 395 patients between the ages of 18 and 75 years randomized to either direct PTCA or intravenous t-PA. Primary PTCA was actually performed in 175 of the 195 patients initially randomized to this strategy; 10 of the remaining patients did not have a hemodynamically significant lesion at the time of the study and another 10 patients went directly to emergency coronary bypass surgery. The success rate of primary angioplasty in those in whom it was actually performed was 97%; no patient in this group required emergency coronary bypass. The combined rate of death and nonfatal reinfarction was 5.1% among the 195 patients randomized to PTCA and 12% among those randomized to t-PA ($P < 0.02$). Among high-risk patients, such as those older than 70 years or patients with anterior infarction, mortality was 2% in the PTCA group compared to 10% in the t-PA group. There was a trend toward a lower reinfarction rate with PTCA (2.6% vs 6.5%, $P < 0.06$). The rate of stroke was 3.5% among t-PA patients (with slightly more than half of these hemorrhagic); there were no strokes in the PTCA group. The higher rate of infarct-vessel patency was also associated with a higher rate of periprocedural hemorrhage from the vascular access site requiring surgical repair (2% vs

0%); this is presumably due to the larger sheath size required for intervention and the longer time period during which the sheath remained in place. In addition, there was a higher rate of periprocedural ventricular fibrillation (6% vs 2%); this is presumably due to more sudden reperfusion of partially infarcted myocardium. The investigators concluded from these results that 'when the necessary facilities and personnel are available, immediate angioplasty is an attractive alternative to intravenous thrombolysis and may even be preferable for high risk patients.'[21]

Although direct angioplasty may be preferable to thrombolytic therapy for the 'right patient, in the right place, at the right time', there are serious deficiencies of the PAMI trial that prevent us from reaching the conclusion that this strategy should be expanded beyond those hospitals currently performing it. First, this trial may have significantly underestimated the potential benefit of thrombolytic therapy. The average time after admission to the hospital until the administration of lytic therapy was 90 min; prompt treatment (within 45–60 min) is attainable and would increase survival in this group.[6] Although the conventional regimen of t-PA used in the trial was the best available at the time the study was begun, more effective regimens have since been documented.[6] The conjunctive therapies used in PAMI have also been criticized; for example, calcium blockers were prescribed more often than β-blockers. Second, the trial has several significant methodologic deficiencies. The combined endpoint of 'death and nonfatal infarction' was selected in a *post-hoc* analysis; there was no statistical difference in the prespecified primary endpoint of left ventricular systolic function. By design, the sample size was too small to allow a direct comparison with respect to mortality. The study did not employ an independent angiographic laboratory to assess the results nor was there a clinical events committee blinded to therapy to adjudicate clinical events such as recurrent ischemia or reinfarction. Third, as Sleight has suggested, the patients randomized to thrombolytic therapy were an 'unlucky lot'. Using the results of the GUSTO trial as a comparison,[6] the stroke rate of the thrombolytic group in PAMI is far higher (3.5% vs 1.4%), as is the rate of catheterization for recurrent ischemia (23.5% vs 5.1%). Whereas the results of lytic therapy are less favorable than expected, the results of angioplasty may be overly favorable. Although the procedural success rate of 93% may be realistic in specialized centers committed to this strategy, it remains unproved in community hospitals that may lack the staff and experience in taking these critically ill patients to the laboratory on a 24-hour basis. Therefore, while we agree with the authors of the PAMI study that primary angioplasty is 'an attractive alternative', the above-mentioned issues prevent the conclusion that primary angioplasty is the new 'standard of care' for acute myocardial infarction.

Other potential advantages of direct angioplasty

Although these deficiencies in study design are important to note, in aggregate these five trials strongly suggest that to date we have underestimated the potential benefits of direct angioplasty. In addition to the potential immediate advantages, a potential long-term advantage is an increase in the long-term vessel patency rate. Until the last few years, many investigators considered that the first few days following thrombolytic therapy was the highest risk period for reocclusion. However, two recent trials of thrombolytic therapy have studied patients both acutely and at late follow-up. In the TAMI-6 trial,[83] angiography was performed acutely and at 6 months after infarction (Figure 4.6). Patients randomized to t-PA (with or without PTCA) had a 6-month patency rate of only 59%, the same as that of the placebo group. In the APRICOT study (Antithrombotics in the Prevention of Reocclusion in Coronary Thrombolysis),[84,85] 300 patients who had a patent infarct vessel 48 hours after streptokinase were treated with either aspirin, coumadin (with continuous heparin until the prothrombin time was therapeutic), or neither. At 3-month follow-up angiography, all three groups had

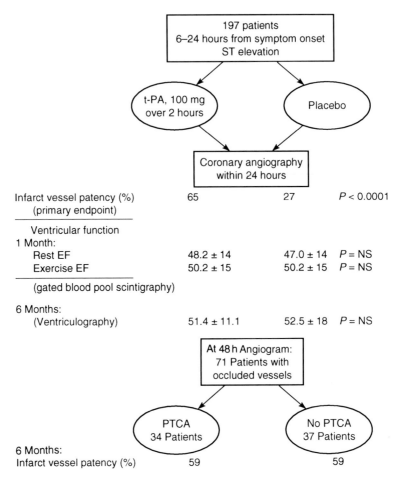

Figure 4.6 Schematic diagram of the TAMI-6 trial.[83] Patients who presented later than 6 but less then 24 hours after symptom onset were randomized to either t-PA or placebo. Coronary angiography within 24 hours of initial presentation established the patency of the infarct vessel; patients with occluded vessels were then randomized to PTCA or no PTCA. The primary endpoint was infarct vessel patency at the time of angiography 6–24 hours after t-PA or placebo administration. Patients who received t-PA had a significantly higher infarct-vessel patency rate; in-hospital mortality was similar as was 6-month mortality. Note that the patients assigned to placebo had an increase in their median end-diastolic volume at a 6-month follow-up, whereas patients randomized to late t-PA therapy did not have an increase in cavity size over the same time period. The second tier of the study examined the role of angioplasty for those patients whose infarct vessels remained occluded at 24–48 hours after initial randomization. At 4–6 weeks, patients randomized to angioplasty had higher rest and exercise ejection fractions although this improvement was not sustained at 6 months. There were no significant differences in clinical events. EF, ejection fraction. (Modified from Ref. 83.)

relatively high patency rates (average, 71%). In contrast, the available data on late patency after direct angioplasty suggest that it is higher (range, 87–91%).[20,24] However, further studies of anticoagulant and antithrombotic regimens after infarction (such as those under investigation in the Coumadin and Aspirin Reinfarction Study) may improve the long-term patency rates of patients treated with either strategy.

Finally, direct angioplasty may reduce costs. In the study by Gibbons *et al.*, patients assigned to direct angioplasty had, on average, shorter hospital stays and a trend toward lower costs. In the PAMI trial, the sum of hospital charges and physician fees were similar in the two groups; this suggests that the 'invasive' approach is at least no more expensive than a 'conservative' one. However, critics of these analyses point out that this similarity in cost between the two regimens is due in part to the high cost of the conservative arm; specifically, the high cost of t-PA as well as the high rate (and cost) of elective angiography. Ultimately, this issue will require further study to determine which strategy is more cost effective. If long-term patency rate is indeed superior with angioplasty, analysis of long-term costs might favor this strategy.

Current status of direct angioplasty

On balance, the currently available data on direct angioplasty demonstrate that in skilled hands PTCA is probably superior to currently available thrombolytic regimens with respect to the time required to reestablish TIMI grade 3 flow, the proportion of vessels which sustain this flow grade, and the proportion of vessels left with a critical residual stenosis at hospital discharge. The GUSTO-II substudy of primary PTCA vs accelerated t-PA will enroll a sufficient number of patients to compare the strategies with respect to the 'hard' endpoints of death and reinfarction. The PAMI-2 trial will also enroll a larger number of patients than its predecessor. Until these results are available (in 1995), we can conclude that direct angioplasty is at least comparable to thrombolytic therapy with respect to mortality reduction, reinfarction, and improvement of left ventricular function. Of particular importance, in patients with a high risk of hemorrhage or other contraindications to lytic therapy, direct PTCA almost certainly reduces the risk of achieving reperfusion. In patients with cardiogenic shock, pulmonary edema or other very high-risk features, direct angioplasty, if available in experienced centers, is clearly the treatment of choice. However, the number of patients studied in prospective, randomized studies of primary angioplasty (approximately 1000 in total) is small in comparison to the number so studied with thrombolytic therapy (approximately 200 000). This disparity prevents one from the conclusion that large portions of health-care delivery systems should shift their resources to this promising but as yet incompletely proven strategy. In addition, for many patients direct PTCA is not a practical option, because it requires immediate transport from the emergency ward to a suitable interventional cardiac catheterization laboratory. These patients can achieve more rapid reperfusion, particularly with newer, accelerated regimens of intravenous t-PA.[6,86,87]

Accessibility issues notwithstanding, for the 'right patient' at the 'right time and place', direct angioplasty is preferable to thrombolytic therapy. The remarkably high procedural success rates of direct angioplasty have led some advocates of this strategy to conclude that the procedure should be expanded even to hospitals without on-site surgical backup. The rationale behind this notion is that the overall mortality rate from direct angioplasty will still be considerably lower than the mortality rate of the same patients treated with thrombolytic therapy. Opponents of this liberal approach point out that only a single study supports allowing centers without cardiac surgery to perform emergency PTCA,[85] and in that study, the same, experienced physicians who routinely perform emergency angioplasty in hospitals *with* surgical back-up (and who are presumably more experienced) are the physicians who performed the procedure in the hospitals *without* backup. The implication is that it would be premature to sanction emergency angioplasty in centers without surgical back-up, since the operators in many of these centers may not have the experience of the operators in this single study. Therefore, the official recommendation of the American College of Cardiology[89] is to sanction primary angioplasty in hospitals without on-site surgical backup *only* as a last resort (for example, in patients with an absolute contraindication to thrombolysis or in patients with cardiogenic shock), and only if transfer to a tertiary site with on-site surgical backup is impractical or impossible.

Rescue Angioplasty

Rescue angioplasty is defined as the performance of the procedure as soon as possible when intravenous thrombolytic therapy has failed to reperfuse the infarct vessel. The rationale for this strategy is that even the most effective currently available thrombolytic regimen (as judged by vessel patency at 90 min) leaves at least 15% of patients with a totally occluded infarct vessel[6,86,87] These patients have an especially poor prognosis.[90] Although some of these thrombolytic failures will recanalize within 48 hours without PCTA,[83] the speed of reperfusion is fundamental to salvage of myocardium. The potential benefits of late vessel patency (beyond the period when actual myocardial salvage is possible) are important enough to warrant a separate chapter in this book (see Chapter 5). In brief, studies suggest that patients who achieve late reperfusion have a higher long-term survival rate when compared to patients with incomplete or no reperfusion.[83] Some studies have documented improvement in various indices of ventricular function[83,91–94] and electrical stability.[83,95–101] In aggregate, these studies suggest that even relatively late reperfusion may improve healing and remodeling of the infarct zone and provide benefits independent of myocardial salvage. A patent epicardial vessel that serves a primarily scarred myocardial region may later serve as a collateral to a distant myocardial region.

Initial studies

A meta-analysis of nonrandomized series and small nonrandomized trials by Ellis *et al*.[102] drew several conclusions about this strategy (Table 4.8). Overall, the procedural success rate was high (71–100%), but was lower than in trials of direct PTCA.[21–24,77,102] This difference is probably because patients who fail intravenous thrombolytic therapy are a more difficult group in whom to perform PTCA, perhaps due to mechanical factors (such as the extent of plaque rupture, clot burden, or low runoff in the distal vessel). Prior to rescue angioplasty, these infarct vessels proved resistant to thrombolytic regimens effective in the majority of patients; as could be expected, the mortality even with rescue PTCA was in the range of 10–20%. Furthermore, in early studies, patients with a successful rescue procedure had a far better survival (ranging from twofold to fourfold) than did those who had an unsuccessful procedure.[10,106,113–115] Therefore, it was unclear whether the potential benefit from successful rescue PTCA outweighed the potential harm from attempted but unsuccessful procedure. In these series, there was little effect on the recovery of systolic function by the time of hospital discharge. In the only randomized trial in this meta-analysis, Belenkie *et al*.[116] randomized 28 patients who presented 3–6 hours after symptom onset. Angioplasty was successful in reestablishing vessel patency in 13 of 16 patients. Rescue PTCA resulted in a trend toward a lower in-hospital mortality rate when compared with patients not randomized to rescue PTCA (7% vs 33%, $P = 0.13$). At follow-up, however, there was no difference in mean left ventricular systolic performance. On average, the hospital mortality was 10.6%.

Although these studies demonstrate that rescue angioplasty improves the patency rate of thrombolytic failures, they do not prove that the *overall* mortality rate is lower. First, there is a discrepancy in reocclusion and mortality rates among different antecedent thrombolytic regimens; patients who receive t-PA have a higher rate of reocclusion and subsequent mortality thereafter (see below). Second, in several series patients who failed to achieve patency with rescue PTCA had an extremely high mortality rate, implying that a failed attempt at rescue angioplasty may be harmful. In balance, the potential effect of failed rescue could outweigh any potential benefit from successes. Prospective, random-ized trials were necessary to settle this dilemma.

Table 4.8 Meta-analysis of series of rescue PTCA prior to the TAMI-5 and RESCUE trials. (From Ref. 102)

Reference	Number of patients	Thrombolytic regimen	Success (%)	Reocclusion (%)	Change in EF	Mortality (%)
Topol et al.[103]	86	rt-PA	73	29	−1	10.4
Califf et al.[104]	15	rt-PA	87	15	+1	NR
	25	UK	84	12	+1	NR
	12	rt-PA + UK	92	0	+2	NR
Belenkie et al.[105]	16	SK	81	NR	+2	6.7
Fung et al.[106]	13	SK	92	16	+10	7.6
Topol et al.[103]	22	rt-PA + UK	86	3	+5	0
Grines et al.[107]	12	rt-PA + SK	100	8	NR	NR
Holmes et al.[108]	34	SK	71	NR	−11	11
Grines et al.[109]	10	rt-PA + SK	90	12	+5	10
O'Connor et al.[110]	90	SK	89	14	−1	17
Baim et al.[111]	37	rt-PA	92	26	NR	5.4
Whitlow[112]	26	rt-PA	81	29	−2	NR
	18	UK	89	25	+1	NR
Ellis[102]	109	rt-PA	79	20	+1	10.1
	5	rt-PA + UK	80	20	+2	20
	59	SK	76	18	+4	10.2
Pooled SK, UK or combination	308		260/308 (84%)	31/223 (14%)	−1	11.2
Pooled rt-PA only	252		191/252 (76%)	38/157 (24%)	−1	9.5
Total	560		451/560 (80%)	69/380 (18%)	−1	10.6

Change in EF, the change in left ventricular ejection fraction from baseline to the measurement before hospital discharge; NR, not reported; rt-PA, recombinant tissue-type plasminogen activator; SK, streptokinase; UK, urokinase.

Large randomized trials

Although the TAMI-5 trial was not specifically a study of rescue angioplasty, it did test the strategy.[104] This trial (Figure 4.7) was a 3 × 2 factorial design in which 575 patients were first randomized to either t-PA, urokinase, or a two-drug combination; thereafter, patients were again randomized to one of two catheterization strategies. Within each lytic arm, one-half of the patients were assigned to an emergency angiogram and rescue PTCA if the infarct vessel was occluded (TIMI flow grade 0 or 1) or to a strategy of delayed coronary angiography 5–7 days later. Rescue PTCA resulted in a high immediate patency rate of 96% and a high predischarge patency rate of 94%. The deferred angiography group had a discharge patency rate of only 90% ($P = 0.065$). In addition, the aggressively treated group had fewer episodes of recurrent ischemia (35% vs 25%, respectively, $P < 0.005$) and thus needed less emergency intervention. Wall motion indices within the infarct zone also improved. Of note, one group of patients who received particular benefit from an aggressive strategy of early angiography and rescue PTCA when indicted were those with a prior myocardial infarction.

The most important study of rescue angioplasty to date has been the RESCUE trial[46] (Figure 4.8). The trial included 151 patients who were within 8 hours of chest pain onset and who had angiographically documented persistent anterior descending occlusion despite intravenous thrombolysis. These patients were randomly assigned to either a 'conservative arm' of vasodilators, aspirin, and heparin, or to a PTCA arm that included these therapies plus angioplasty and additional thrombolytic therapy, as indicated. Exclusion criteria were cardiogenic shock prior to randomization, prior myocardial

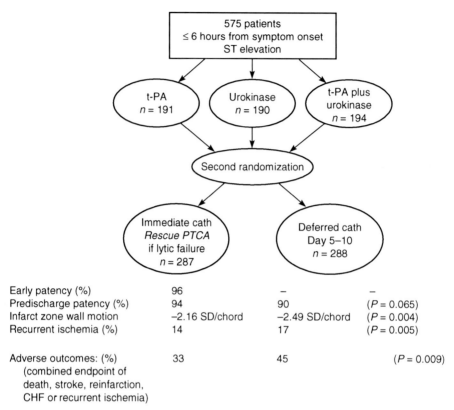

Early patency (%)	96	–	–
Predischarge patency (%)	94	90	(P = 0.065)
Infarct zone wall motion	−2.16 SD/chord	−2.49 SD/chord	(P = 0.004)
Recurrent ischemia (%)	14	17	(P = 0.005)
Adverse outcomes: (%)	33	45	(P = 0.009)
(combined endpoint of death, stroke, reinfarction, CHF or recurrent ischemia)			

Figure 4.7 Schematic diagram of the TAMI-5 trial.[104] This study was a 3 × 2 factorial design in which patients were randomized to one of the lytic regimens shown. Patients in each arm were then randomized again to a strategy of either an emergency angiogram and rescue PTCA if the infarct artery was occluded (TIMI flow grade 0 or 1) or to a strategy of delayed coronary angiography 5–7 days later. Rescue PTCA resulted in a higher immediate patency rate and a higher predischarge patency rate. Note that the aggressively treated group had fewer episodes of recurrent ischemia and a lesser need for acute intervention. Wall motion within the infarct zone was also improved. (Data from Ref. 104.)

infarction, and left main stenosis ≥50%. The technical success rate of 92% compared very favorably with several previous small nonrandomized series. Of note, rescue angioplasty led to a significant reduction in the incidence of the combined endpoint of death and severe (Killip class III or IV) heart failure (1% in the PTCA group vs 7% in the conservatively treated group). In addition, exercise ejection fraction at 30 days was improved in the PTCA group (43% vs 38%, P <0.04). However, there was no difference in the prespecified primary endpoint of resting ejection fraction. This study supports the use of rescue angioplasty in patients with a first myocardial infarction in the distribution of the left anterior descending coronary artery who are treated with thrombolytic therapy but who are suspected not to have achieved early reperfusion within 6–8 hours of the onset of symptoms. This strategy may result in an improvement in 30-day survival and functional status, albeit independent of resting left ventricular ejection fraction.

Current status of rescue angioplasty

A major limitation of identifying patients who could potentially benefit from rescue angioplasty has been the inaccuracy of clinical criteria in determining the patency status of the infarct vessel. Furthermore, the cost of such an expensive 'screening test' to

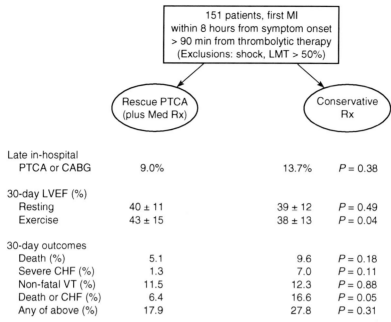

	Rescue PTCA (plus Med Rx)	Conservative Rx	
Late in-hospital			
PTCA or CABG	9.0%	13.7%	$P = 0.38$
30-day LVEF (%)			
Resting	40 ± 11	39 ± 12	$P = 0.49$
Exercise	43 ± 15	38 ± 13	$P = 0.04$
30-day outcomes			
Death (%)	5.1	9.6	$P = 0.18$
Severe CHF (%)	1.3	7.0	$P = 0.11$
Non-fatal VT (%)	11.5	12.3	$P = 0.88$
Death or CHF (%)	6.4	16.6	$P = 0.05$
Any of above (%)	17.9	27.8	$P = 0.31$

Figure 4.8 Schematic diagram of the RESCUE trial.[46] Rescue angioplasty significantly reduced the incidence of the combined endpoint of death and severe heart failure. In addition, the PTCA group had a higher mean exercise ejection fraction at 30 days. CHF, congestive heart failure; LVEF, left ventricular ejection fraction. (Data from Ref. 46.)

identify candidates for rescue angioplasty is considerable. There is no set of clinical criteria that can allow the accurate, noninvasive diagnosis of a patent infarct artery after thrombolytic therapy. The relief of chest discomfort, resolution of electrocardiographic ST-segment elevation, and the presence or absence of ventricular arrhythmias are unreliable guides.[33,34] Data from the TAMI-1 study illustrate this critical point. When chest pain improved following thrombolytic therapy, the probability of a patent infarct artery was 71%; this probability increased to 84% when pain completely resolved. Unfortunately, these indices have limited clinical utility, because they occurred in only 51% and 29% of patients, respectively, who had angiographically confirmed reperfusion. Reduction of initial ST-segment elevation is also an imperfect guide; although ST-segment improvement was associated with an 84% probability of a patent infarct vessel, it occurred in only 38% of patients with angiographically confirmed reperfusion. Complete normalization of the ST segments was associated with a patent infarct artery in 96% of cases, but this improvement occurred in only 6% of patients with an open artery at acute catheterization.[73,117] Overall, electrocardiographic indices have been disappointing; analyses of reperfusion arrhythmias[34] and the signal-averaged ECG[95,118] have not approached the predictive values of ST-segment analysis. Other techniques, such as analysis of creatine kinase isoforms,[119,120] and new radionuclide agents[121–123] are still under investigation. Until the reliability of one or more of these techniques is established, urgent angiography will have to be considered the 'gold standard' by which to triage patients to rescue angioplasty.

Empiric Angioplasty

Empiric angioplasty can be defined broadly as the routine use of the procedure as prophylaxis against recurrent ischemia, in the absence of actual ischemia documented by clinical criteria or functional testing. Empiric angioplasty can be either *immediate*, in which it is performed as soon as possible after the acute infarction or successful thrombolysis, or *deferred*, in which it is performed from 18 hours to 1 week after the event (without provocative testing). Several large clinical trials[18,20,38,73] have investigated immediate empiric angioplasty. Although these trials have limitations the results have been consistent: in the absence of hemodynamic compromise or ischemia, empiric angioplasty does not improve global left ventricular function, nor does it reduce morbidity or mortality when compared to the selective use of PTCA for spontaneous or provokable ischemia. In addition, this use of angioplasty may result in an increased risk of abrupt closure or reocclusion, presumably because the infarct vessel has an unstable, freshly ruptured plaque. Further mechanical damage by an angioplasty device shortly after thrombolytic therapy presumably stimulates platelet aggregation and release of clot-bound thrombin, and stimulates thrombus propagation.

Immediate angioplasty

In the early 1980s, several large randomized trials investigated the strategy of intra-venous thrombolysis followed by immediate angioplasty of the infarct vessel[38,51,83,124-128] (Table 4.9). The presumption behind this strategy was that the occlusive lesion in the infarct vessel consisted of both underlying atherosclerotic plaque and overlying throm-bus. Compared with treating only the overlying thrombus, compressing the plaque with an angioplasty balloon presumably would lead to less recurrent ischemia and an improvement in the patient's functional status. The designs of these trials are summar-ized in Table 4.9.

Although these trials differed somewhat in design and patient population, their results are concordant: for those patients with a significant but not critical stenosis (minimum luminal diameter 50–90% of normal), but without evidence of ischemia, angioplasty is both unnecessary and dangerous. This group of patients comprised approximately 35% of patients who entered the TAMI trials; if they have single-vessel disease, they are at low-risk without an intervention. In an asymptomatic patient after thrombolysis, for any documented residual stenosis in the infarct-related vessel that is associated with intact regional wall motion, the long-term outcome is likely to be favorable.[38,131-134] Long-term follow-up of patients managed with the conservative TIMI-2 strategy showed that such patients are at low risk for major events.[38] In the SWIFT trial[51] prophylactic angioplasty in patients free of hemodynamic instability or documented ischemia actually led to a significantly higher rate of reinfarction when compared to a conservative approach (Figure 4.2). Ellis and associates[135] have shown that the extent of residual stenosis after intravenous thrombolysis does not correlate with likelihood of recurrent ischemic events in the short term. A study by Little and colleagues[136] extends this observation to a longer follow-up period.

In the TAMI 1 trial,[15] 386 patients were treated with intravenous t-PA and underwent emergency angiography at 90 min. Of the total number of patients, 93 (25%) had contraindications to angioplasty, such as extensive multivessel disease or left main trunk obstruction. Ninety-six additional patients (25%) were totally occluded at 90-min angiography. Of the remaining patients, 99 were assigned to immediate PTCA and 98 to a strategy of deferred PTCA. With respect to these last two groups, there was no difference in predischarge left ventricular function. Despite the relatively small numbers of patients in this study, it is important because randomization took place at the time that the coronary anatomy was known, rather than prior to angiography. In the ECSG trial[129] patients were randomized to immediate angioplasty vs no angioplasty following intra-venous t-PA. The protocol of the TIMI 2A[130] trial randomized patients between immedi-ate PTCA and a deferred approach of cardiac catheterization with PTCA if the culprit lesion was suitable for angioplasty (which took place at 18–48 hours from initial presentation).

Table 4.9 Summary of randomized trials of intravenous thrombolysis followed by empiric, immediate angioplasty. (Modified from Ref. 82)

Type of trial	Reference	Randomized no. of patients		Thrombolytic strategy	Control group	Major finding
		PTCA	Control			
Immediate For open or all infarct vessels	TAMI-I[15]	99	98	t-PA	Lysis + delayed PTCA	No advantage of immediate PTCA
	ECSG[129]	183	184	t-PA	No PTCA	No advantage of immediate PTCA
	TIMI-2A[130]	195	194	t-PA	No PTCA	No advantage of immediate PTCA
	O'Neill et al.[20]	63	58	SK	Lysis + PTCA	Direct PTCA superior, less complicated, less expensive
Closed vessels	TAMI-5[104]	287	288	t-PA, UK or t-PA + UK	Lysis + delayed catheterization (5–7 days)	Aggressive strategy had less recurrent ischemia, improved regional vessel motion and patency

EF, ejection fraction; PTCA, percutaneous transluminal coronary angioplasty; SK, streptokinase; t-PA, tissue plasminogen activator; for study acronyms, refer to references.

Angioplasty is often unnecessary in the periinfarction period because many vessels with a significant stenosis in patients without evidence of ischemia will remodel favorably over time, precluding dilatation even on anatomic grounds.[137] In the TIMI and TAMI trials, 15% of patients were found to have a stenosis of less than 50–60% in an infarct-related vessel, and thus did not require intervention.[38,138] This relatively low grade of narrowing presumably relates to continued resolution of thrombus and healing of the plaque rupture or fissure event. The prognosis of these patients is excellent regardless of therapy.

The role of immediate angioplasty in the subset of patients with asymptomatic total occlusion of the infarct vessel is also probably not indicated. This conclusion is less certain because in the TIMI-2 and SWIFT trials[38,51] patients with total occlusions were categorically excluded from angioplasty. Nevertheless, approximately 15% of patients will have an occluded infarct artery. In the TAMI-6 trial[83] patients presenting between 6 and 24 hours after pain onset were randomized to receive an intravenous thrombolytic or placebo. All patients underwent angiography within the next 24 hours; at that time, patients with a closed infarct vessel were again eligible for randomization to either late PTCA (34 patients) or no PTCA (37 patients). Late reperfusion with thrombolytic therapy resulted in a higher infarct-vessel patency than did placebo (65% vs 27%), as well as the avoidance of cavity expansion as reflected in the left ventricular end-diastolic volume (127 ml vs 159 ml). However, patients randomized to late PTCA derived no specific benefit from the procedure. This was probably due to a relatively high rate of reocclusion after successful PTCA and relatively high rate of spontaneous recanalization in the control ('no PTCA') group.

It is noteworthy that the TIMI-2 trial specifically excluded patients with totally occluded infarct vessels from undergoing angioplasty; therefore, the results of this study cannot be applied to this subset of patients. For example, in the Johns Hopkins study[126] comparing t-PA with direct angioplasty, the subset of patients with total occlusion 72 hours after initial presentation who underwent angioplasty had an improvement in their exercise ejection fraction.

Delayed angioplasty

Delayed empiric angioplasty (>48 hours) for a patent vessel is also not indicated following thrombolytic therapy unless the patient has well-documented spontaneous or stress-induced ischemia. The Treatment of Post-Thrombolytic Stenoses trial (TOPS)[128] supports this conclusion. Eighty-seven patients (mean age, 57 years) who had been treated within 6 hours of the onset of chest pain with thrombolytic therapy and who subsequently had a negative functional test were randomized to either medical therapy alone or medical therapy plus PTCA. In the angioplasty group, the procedure was performed between days 4 and 14 since the TIMI[38] and SWIFT[51] trials had shown that the rate of cardiac and peripheral complications was especially high during the first 72 hours. Mean vessel stenosis was 70% prior to randomization; 84% of the patients were male and 7% had multivessel disease. At 6 weeks, there was no difference in left ventricular ejection fraction (the primary endpoint) either at rest or after exercise, as measured by gated blood pool scanning. Although PTCA was successful in 88% randomized to this strategy (38 of the 42 patients), in three of the remaining patients acute vessel closure resulted in a non-Q myocardial infarction. During 12 months of follow-up, there were no cardiac deaths, infarction, or significant differences in angina severity, heart failure, or other clinical characteristics between the two groups. The results of several trials that incorporated the strategy of delayed, empiric angioplasty are summarized in Table 4.10.

Table 4.10 Summary of randomized trials of intravenous thrombolysis followed by empiric, delayed angioplasty. (Modified from Ref. 82)

Reference	Type of trial	Randomized no. of patients		Thrombolytic strategy	Timing of PTCA	Control group	Major finding
		PTCA	Control				
TIMI-2B[38]		1636	1626	t-PA	18–48 hours	i.v. lysis	No difference
SWIFT[51]		397	403	APSAC	<48 hours	No cath./PTCA	No difference in mortality, reinfarction
Van den Brand et al.[24]		113	105	t-PA	2–5 days	i.v. lysis	Less angina at 3 months, otherwise no difference except more cost
SIAM[125]		158	166	SK	14–48 hours	i.v. lysis	No difference
Johns Hopkins[126]		42	43	t-PA	Day 3	No PTCA	Improved exercise ejection fraction with PTCA
Barbash et al.[127]		90	104	t-PA	5 ± 2 days	i.v. lysis	More deaths with invasive strategy
TOPS[128]	Negative exercise test	42	45	Lytic not specified	4–7 days	No PTCA	No advantage for PTCA in patients with negative functional test
TAMI-6[83]	Late Entry patients	34	37	t-PA or placebo	48 hours	No PTCA	Improved 6 weeks rest and exercise, ejection fraction for PTCA, but not persistent at 6 months

APSAC, anisoylated plasminogen streptokinase activator complex; EF, ejection fraction; PTCA, percutaneous transluminal coronary angioplasty; SK, streptokinase; t-PA, tissue plasminogen activator. For study acronyms, refer to references.

Current status of empiric angioplasty

In summary, there is overwhelming evidence to indicate that routine immediate angioplasty after either t-PA or streptokinase is deleterious. Following thrombolytic therapy, patients without ischemia or left ventricular dysfunction have an excellent 1-year prognosis with medical therapy alone. Routine immediate angioplasty does not improve cardiac function, and it increases the risk of acute vessel closure, reinfarction, and short-term mortality. The probable mechanism of these deleterious effects is that the atherosclerotic plaque at the target lesion had preexisting factors favoring thrombosis at the time of its initial rupture; further disruption with an angioplasty balloon exposes more of these elements to the circulation. Particularly in the setting of a nonfibrin-specific agent, these factors combine to aggregate platelets further and promote recurrent thrombosis.

Nevertheless, critics of this analysis argue that this conclusion is flawed on two counts. First, all of these trials assess their primary endpoint (usually left ventricular systolic function) on days 7–16 after initial presentation. Critics have argued that longer follow-up is necessary to prove that the strategy of immediate angioplasty is indeed deleterious. However, data pooled from the TAMI trials with long-term follow-up of up to 6 months has failed to demonstrate a difference in global ejection fraction. Second, critics argue that the addition of platelet glycoprotein IIb/IIIa inhibitors and direct thrombin inhibitors to the immediate angioplasty procedure may result in a lower reocclusion rate and therefore improve the overall effectiveness of the strategy. Although this hypothesis may in fact be true, it remains to be tested in either observational studies or prospective trials.

Despite the overwhelming evidence of these data, it is disturbing to note that functional testing following myocardial infarction and prior to angioplasty is the exception rather than the rule in the USA. An analysis of an insurance claims database of over 2100 angioplasty procedures,[139] only 9% of patients had an exercise test prior to their elective postinfarction angioplasty.

There are no data available to determine whether empiric angioplasty is equally harmful in patients who did not receive thrombolytic therapy, sustained a myocardial infarction, and do not have evidence of spontaneous or stress-induced ischemia thereafter. In the latter patient, in the absence of data to support intervention, empiric PTCA would seem contraindicated. This is especially important in the elderly patient, in whom the risks of the procedure are higher.

Elective Angioplasty

Elective angioplasty following myocardial infarction refers to the performance of the procedure to treat spontaneous postinfarction ischemia or ischemia provoked by functional testing. A complete review of the indications for elective angioplasty vs medical therapy or surgical revascularization is beyond the scope of this review.

Angiography and Angioplasty Strategies in Special Patient Subsets

Patients with Prior Bypass Surgery

Although patients with prior CABG and a new, evolving myocardial infarction are an increasingly common clinical problem, few data are available on the optimal treatment of these patients. In a review of 40 postbypass patients, Kavanaugh and Topol[140] cited several features of these patients that make their diagnosis more difficult and their

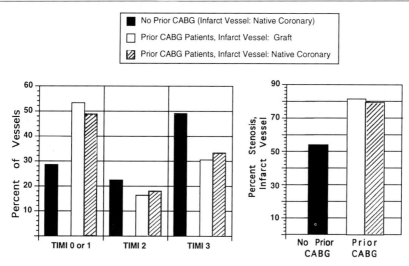

Figure 4.9 Characteristics of patients with previous bypass surgery enrolled in the GUSTO trial. Left: the relationship between TIMI flow grade and the severity of the stenosis in the infarct vessel. Nearly 50% of all infarct vessels in patients with prior bypass had TIMI grade 0 or 1 flow, compared to only 27% of patients without prior bypass. Only 30% of patients with prior bypass had TIMI grade 3 flow, compared to nearly 50% of patients without prior bypass. Right: note that the severity of infarct-vessel stenoses, on average, is greater in patients with prior bypass surgery, regardless of whether the infarct vessel is a native coronary or graft. Overall, these data indicate that patients with prior bypass surgery have more severe infarct-vessel stenoses, and have a much higher likelihood of having an occluded or nearly occluded vessel at the time of angiography. These data argue for routine angiography in this subset of patients. (From Ref. 141.)

treatment less likely to be successful. First, on presentation, the ECG was diagnostic in only 74% of patients. Overall, the ECG changes were less apparent than in patients without prior bypass, with nearly one-half lacking ⩾2 mm ST elevation. These less dramatic changes may be due in part to the more complex, interdependent collateral flow commonly seen in these patients. In these cases, emergency angiography may be required to confirm the diagnosis of acute infarction. In the subset of patients with prior bypass who were enrolled in the GUSTO trial, the mortality rate of patients with prior bypass was significantly higher than that of patients without such a history (10.6% vs 6.4%);[141] by 1 year, mortality in this group increases further (15.8% vs 8.0%). Patients with previous bypass surgery have a higher incidence of other risk factors associated with a poor prognosis[141] (Figure 4.9). Furthermore, regardless of whether the infarct vessel is a native coronary or a vein graft, preliminary data from the GUSTO investigators indicate that patients with prior bypass are more likely to have an occluded or nearly occluded infarct vessel at the time of elective angiography.[141] These data have important implications for the management of patients with previous bypass surgery and an acute infarction. First, the higher likelihood of an occluded or nearly occluded infarct vessel would argue in favor of routine angiography in this patient subset. Second, there are insufficient data to determine whether thrombolytic therapy or transcatheter techniques are superior in these complex patients. Some investigators have suggested that acute mechanical revascularization with PTCA[28] or with newer devices that remove the occlusive thrombus (such as the transluminal extraction catheter) may ultimately prove most effective. Until trials of these approaches are performed, with aggressive thrombolytic regimens and conjunctive therapies as controls, there are no data to mandate a particular strategy in hemodynamically stable postbypass patients.

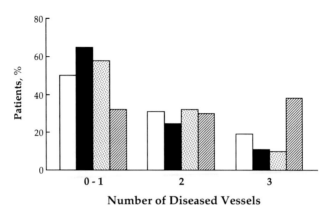

Figure 4.10   Comparison of angiographic findings in recent reperfusion trials with those in studies done in the era before myocardial reperfusion. □, Mayo Clinic data, Ref. 42; ■, TIMI trial data, Ref. 133; ▨, TAMI trial data, Refs 16, 73, 103; and ▨, pooled data from Refs 142–144 before the era of thrombolysis. The data suggest that when compared with historical controls, patients included in thrombolytic trials have less extensive multivessel coronary disease. (Modified from Ref. 42.)

Patients Excluded from Thrombolysis

Patients undergoing angiography in the prethrombolytic era had a higher incidence of severe coronary disease than patients treated with thrombolytics. In these early angiographic studies,[142-144] the incidence of two- or three-vessel disease ranged from 59% to 74% (Figure 4.10). In contrast, the frequency of two- or three-vessel disease in the TAMI and TIMI trials ranged from 27% to 49%. This difference may be due to patient variability with respect to such factors as non-Q-wave infarction among patients in studies antedating thrombolysis, the greater likelihood of multivessel coronary disease in patients with severe hypotension, more advanced age, any previous cerebrovascular disease (which would have excluded patients from the thrombolytic trials), or the performance of angiography earlier during the natural history of coronary artery disease among patients receiving thrombolytic therapy. Given the higher incidence of multivessel coronary disease in patients ineligible for thrombolysis therapy, the physician should consider early angiography in the appropriate clinical context.

Cardiogenic Shock

Although the treatment of patients with cardiogenic shock is briefly mentioned in the section on urgent catheterization, it is worthwhile to mention here in the context of angioplasty. It is also discussed in Chapter 11. Patients with cardiogenic shock are among those who benefit the most from immediate mechanical revascularization, whether it be angioplasty or immediate bypass surgery. Table 4.11 summarizes the published studies to date on the result of angioplasty in the treatment of myocardial infarction and cardiogenic shock. Overall, the expected mortality rate of myocardial infarction and cardiogenic shock is in excess of 80%.[155] The mortality rate with angioplasty in the series ranges from 32 to 55%; on average, the mortality rate is 45%. This rate is consistently lower than that reported in observational series which predate the angioplasty era or in which angioplasty was unavailable. Of particular note is the relative ineffectiveness of thrombolytic therapy in this setting. Presumably, the low systemic pressure leads to less efficient delivery of the peripherally administered drug to the intracoronary thrombus; in addition, the low cardiac output may also predispose to additional thrombus formation.

Table 4.11 Published series on angioplasty in the treatment of myocardial infarction complicated by cardiogenic shock. (From Ref. 82)

Reference	Survival: total no. patients (%)
O'Neill et al.[136]	19/27 (70%)
Lee et al.[146]	12/24 (50%)
Shani et al.[147]	6/9 (66%)
Heuser et al.[148]	7/10 (70%)
Brown et al.[149]	12/28 (43%)
Hibbard et al.[150]	25/45 (56%)
Seydoux et al.[151]	12/21 (57%)
Bengston et al.[152]	25/46 (54%)
Gacioch et al.[153]	22/48 (45%)
Kahn et al.[154]	8/16 (50%)
O'Keefe et al.[28]	23/39 (59%)
Pooled	171/313 (55%)

Thrombolytic therapy should be given only to those patients in shock in whom immediate angiography and appropriate revascularization will clearly be associated with delays (greater than 60–90 min). Thrombolytic therapy in this setting also increases the complication rate from other assist devices that are frequently required, such as the Hemopump, left ventricular assist device, or emergency bypass surgery. These adjunct procedures can be particularly beneficial. For example, Ohman and colleagues[156] have recently shown that in patients with acute myocardial infarction, (even without cardiogenic shock) the use of an intraaortic balloon pump results in less recurrent ischemia and lower rates of reocclusion and reinfarction.

Conclusion

Individualized therapy

With respect to the use of coronary angiography following myocardial infarction, differences between the 'selective' and 'routine' approaches to coronary angiography may be more a matter of degree than of kind. In the final analysis, physicians often make such decisions based on the characteristics and preferences of the specific patient under their care. Those physicians who advocate a 'selective' approach still recommend angiography in a relatively large percentage of cases; even the most ardent supporter of 'routine' angiography does not recommend the procedure in patients with concomitant disease that would preclude mechanical revascularization. Of greater importance than the debate itself is the recognition of two paramount facts. First, the patients at highest risk of mortality often benefit the most from the 'aggressive' or the most invasive therapies. For example, in the treatment of the elderly with thrombolytic therapy, the overall reduction in mortality far outweighs the increased risk of stroke, and the greater is the absolute benefit. Second, as with all medical care, the triage of patients with acute myocardial infarction must be determined in the context of the patient's *overall* clinical status, with careful attention to the patient's values and preferences. 'Conventional' medical treatment without thrombolytic therapy may be appropriate for a particular 65-year-old patient with comorbidity that profoundly decreases life expectancy. On the other hand, thrombolytic therapy, early catheterization and, if necessary, mechanical revascularization may be appropriate for an otherwise healthy 75-year-old patient.

Although these aspects of medical care are fundamental to the daily practice of medicine, they are (or soon will be) the subject of intense debate in the USA. Simplistic algorithms, restrictive practice guidelines or government directives that use specific criteria to apply or to restrict invasive strategies may be arbitrary at best. Similarly, 'scorecard' approaches to evaluating physician competence may paradoxically lower the quality of care, if these practices have the unintended result of discouraging physicians from risking their outcome data by treating high-risk patients. These are precisely the patients who stand to gain the greatest benefit from 'risky' procedures. For example, although the increased mortality of the elderly patient with myocardial infarction is undoubtedly due to age and concomitant illnesses, the lower rate of invasive procedures in this group may also contribute. When comparing patients over 75 years to those under 55 years in the MITI trial, elderly patients were less likely than their younger counterparts to receive mechanical interventions such as PTCA (7% vs 29%, respectively) and bypass surgery (5% vs 11%), despite the higher prevalence of multivessel disease. Unfortunately, there are no data as yet to determine whether this lower utilization rate is due to concomitant illnesses in patients denied these procedures (and might, therefore, be appropriate) or whether some patients are denied treatment simply on the basis of age.

Challenges for the Second Half of the 1990s

The primary reason to advocate a strategy of routine angiography following myocardial infarction is to define the coronary anatomy precisely and to increase the certainty of clinicians' prognosis. If a functional test proved to be highly predictive of cardiac events, routine angiography would be unnecessary. Unfortunately, developing a noninvasive test with this high a predictive accuracy may be difficult or impossible. Reinfarction and recurrent ischemia after thrombolysis are morphologic events due to plaque fissuring or superimposed thrombosis; these events may not be predictable by a physiologic or other noninvasive assessment. Functional testing can only evaluate the degree to which a coronary lesion impairs myocardial blood flow. The issue actually involves the inherent stability of the diseased arterial segment. In the future, an even more direct coronary artery examination with intravascular ultrasonography[157,158] and angioscopy,[159] rather than a noninvasive test, may help select the patients at highest risk. If newer agents (such as antithrombin agents or platelet fibrinogen receptor blockade) prove effective according to the angiographic or ultrasonic characteristics of the culprit lesion, the role of routine cardiac catheterization may change dramatically.

In the next decade we are confronted with several challenges in the care of acute myocardial infarction, including refining the application of invasive diagnostic and therapeutic strategies in various patient groups, developing the most effective thrombolytic regimens and conjunctive therapies for the remaining patients, as well as refining the role of invasive and noninvasive methods of postinfarction risk stratification. Prospective clinical trials will undoubtedly continue to refine the application of both coronary angiography and angioplasty in the management of myocardial infarction.

References

1. American Heart Association (1990) *Heart Facts*. Dallas: American Heart Association.
2. Gruppo Italiano per lo Studio della Streptochinasi nell'Infarto Miocardico (1986) Effectiveness of intravenous thrombolytic treatment in acute myocardial infarction. *Lancet*, i, 871–4.
3. ISIS-2 (Second International Study of the Infarct Survival) Collaborative Study Group (1988) Randomized trial of intravenous streptokinase, oral aspirin, both, or neither among 17,187 cases of suspected acute myocardial infarction: ISIS-2. *Lancet*, ii, 349–60.
4. The AIMS Trial Study Group (1988) Effect of intravenous APSAC on mortality after acute myocardial infarction: Preliminary report of a placebo-controlled clinical trial. *Lancet*, i, 545–9.

5. Wilcox, R.G., Olsson, C.G., Skene, A.M. *et al.* (1988) Trial of tissue plasminogen activator for mortality reduction in acute myocardial infarction. Anglo-Scandinavian study of early thrombolysis (ASSET). *Lancet*, **ii**, 525–30.
6. The GUSTO Investigators (1993) An international randomized trial computing four thrombolytic strategies for acute myocardial infarction. *N. Engl. J. Med.*, **329**, 673–82.
7. DeWood, M., Spores, J., Notske, R. *et al.* (1980) Prevalence of total coronary occlusion during the early hours of transmural myocardial infarction. *N. Engl. J. Med.*, **303**, 897–902.
8. Rentrop, K., Blanke, H., Karsch, K. *et al.* (1979) Initial experience with transluminal recanalization of the recently occluded infarct-related coronary artery in acute myocardial infarction – comparison with conventionally treated patients. *Clin. Cardiol.*, **2**, 92–105.
9. Meyer, J., Merx, W., Schmitz, H. *et al.* (1982) Percutaneous transluminal coronary angioplasty immediately after intracoronary streptolysis of transmural myocardial infarction. *Circulation*, **66**, 905–13.
10. Hartzler, G.O., Rutherford, B.D., McConahay, D.R. *et al.* (1983) Percutaneous transluminal coronary angioplasty with and without thrombolytic therapy for treatment of acute myocardial infarction. *Am. Heart J.*, **106**, 965–73.
11. Simoons, M., Van den Brand, M., de Zwaan, C. *et al.* (1985) Improved survival after early thrombolysis in acute myocardial infarction. *Lancet*, **ii**, 578–82.
12. Kennedy, J., Ritchie, J., Davis, K. *et al.* (1983) Western Washington randomized trial of intracoronary streptokinase in acute myocardial infarction. *N. Engl. J. Med.*, **309**, 1477–82.
13. Rentrop, K., Feit, F., Blanke, H. *et al.* (1984) Effects of intracoronary streptokinase and intracoronary nitroglycerin infusion on coronary angiographic patterns and mortality in patients with acute myocardial infarction. *N. Engl. J. Med.*, **311**, 1458–63.
14. Verstraete, M., Arnold, A., Brower, R. *et al.* (1987) Acute coronary thrombolysis with recombinant human tissue-type plasminogen activator: Initial patency and influence of maintained infusion on reocclusion rate. *Am. J. Cardiol.*, **60**, 231–7.
15. Topol, E.J., Califf, R.M., George, B.S. *et al.* (1987) A randomized trial of immediate versus delayed elective angioplasty after intravenous tissue plasminogen activator in acute myocardial infarction. *N. Engl. J. Med.*, **317**, 581–8.
16. Topol, E.J., Califf, R.M., George, B.S. *et al.* (1988) Coronary arterial thrombolysis with combined infusion of recombinant tissue-type plasminogen activator and urokinase in patients with acute myocardial infarction. *Circulation*, **77**, 1100–7.
17. Topol, E.J., George, B.S., Kereiakes, D.J. *et al.* (1989) A randomized controlled trial of intravenous tissue plasminogen activator and early intravenous heparin in acute myocardial infarction. *Circulation*, **79**, 281–6.
18. Simoons, M.L., Betriu, A., Col, J. *et al.* (1988) Thrombolysis with tissue plasminogen activator in acute myocardial infarction: No additional benefit from immediate percutaneous coronary angioplasty. *Lancet*, **i**, 197–203.
19. DeWood, M.A. (1990) Direct PTCA vs tPA in acute myocardial infarction: Results from a prospective randomized trial. *Thrombolysis and Interventional Therapy in Acute Myocardial Infarction, 5th George Washington University pre-AHA symposium*, pp. 28–29.
20. O'Neill, W.W., Weintraub, R., Grines, C.L. *et al.* (1992) A prospective, placebo-controlled, randomized trial of intravenous streptokinase and angioplasty versus lone angioplasty therapy of acute myocardial infarction. *Circulation*, **86**, 1710–17.
21. Grines, C.L., Browne, K.F., Marco, J. *et al.* (1993) A comparison of immediate angioplasty with thrombolytic therapy for acute myocardial infarction. The Primary Angioplasty in Myocardial Infarction Study Group. *N. Engl. J. Med.*, **328**, 673–9.
22. Gibbons, R.J., Holmes, D.R., Reeder, G.S. *et al.* (1993) Immediate angioplasty compared with the administration of a thrombolytic agent followed by conservative treatment for myocardial infarction. The Mayo Coronary Care Unit and Catheterization Laboratory Groups [see comments]. *N. Engl. J. Med.*, **328**, 685–91.
23. Ribeiro, E.E., Silva, L.A., Carneiro, R. *et al.* (1993) Randomized trial of direct coronary angioplasty versus intravenous streptokinase in acute myocardial infarction. *J. Am. Coll. Cardiol.*, **22**, 376–80.
24. Zijlstra, F., de Boer, M.J., Hoorntje, J.C. *et al.* (1993) A comparison of immediate coronary angioplasty with intravenous streptokinase in acute myocardial infarction. *N. Engl. J. Med.*, **328**, 680–4.
25. Noto, T. Jr., Johnson, L.W., Krone, R. *et al.* (1991) Cardiac catheterization 1990: a report of the Registry of the Society for Cardiac Angiography and Interventions (SCA&I). *Cathet. Cardiovasc. Diagn.*, **24**, 75–83.
26. Weaver, W.D., Litwin, P.E., Martin, J.S. *et al.* (1991) Effects of age on use of thrombolytic therapy and mortality in acute myocardial infarction. The MITI Project Group. *J. Am. Coll. Cardiol.*, **18**, 657–62.
27. Topol, E., Burek, K., O'Neill, W. *et al.* (1988) A randomized controlled trial of hospital discharge three days after myocardial infarction in the era of reperfusion. *N. Engl J. Med.*, **318**, 1083–8.
28. O'Keefe, J.H., Rutherford, B.D., McConahay, D.R. *et al.* (1989) Early and late results of coronary angioplasty without antecedent thrombolytic therapy for acute myocardial infarction. *Am. J. Cardiol.*, **64**, 1221–30.
29. Rothbaum, D.A., Linnemeier, T.J., Landin, R.J. *et al.* (1987) Emergency percutaneous transluminal coronary angioplasty in acute myocardial infarction: A 3 year experience. *J. Am. Coll. Cardiol.*, **10**, 264–72.
30. Ellis, S.G., O'Neill, W.W., Bates, E.R. *et al.* (1989) Coronary angioplasty as primary therapy for acute myocardial infarction 6 to 48 hours after symptom onset: Report of an initial experience. *J. Am. Coll. Cardiol.*, **13**, 1122–6.
31. Prida, X., Holland, J., Feldman, R. *et al.* (1986) Percutaneous transluminal coronary angioplasty in evolving acute myocardial infarction. *Am. J. Cardiol.*, **57**, 1069–74.
32. Miller, P., Brodie, B., Weintraub, R. *et al.* (1987) Emergency coronary angioplasty for acute myocardial infarction. Results from a community hospital. *Arch. Intern. Med.*, **147**, 1565–70.
33. Kircher, R., Topol, E., O'Neill, W. *et al.* (1987) Prediction of infarct coronary artery recanalization after intravenous thrombolytic therapy. *Am. J. Cardiol.*, **59**, 513–15.

34. Califf, R.M., O'Neill, W., Stacks, R.S. *et al.* (1988) Failure of simple clinical measurements to predict perfusion status after intravenous thrombolysis. *Ann. Intern. Med.*, **108**, 658–62.
35. De Franco, A. and Topol, E. (1992) Invasive strategies in acute myocardial infarction in the elderly. *Cardiology in the Elderly*, **2**, 274–89.
36. ISAM (1986) A prospective trial of intravenous streptokinase in acute myocardial infarction (I.S.A.M.). *N. Engl. J. Med.*, **314**, 1465–71.
37. Gruppo Italiano per lo Studio della Streptochinasi nell'Infarto Miocardico (1987) Long-term effects of intravenous thrombolysis in acute myocardial infarction: Final report of the GISSI study. *Lancet*, **ii**, 871–4.
38. TIMI Study Group (1989) Comparison of invasive and conservative strategies after treatment with intravenous tissue plasminogen activator in acute myocardial infarction. Results of the thrombolysis in myocardial infarction (TIMI) phase II trial. *N. Engl. J. Med.*, **320**, 618–27.
39. Rogers, W., Babb, J., Baim, D. *et al.* (1990) Is pre-discharge coronary arteriography beneficial in patients with myocardial infarction treated with thrombolytic therapy? (abstract) *J. Am. Coll. Cardiol.*, **15**, 64A.
40. Rogers, W. Babb, J., Baim, D. *et al.* for the TIMI-II investigators (1991) Selective versus routine predischarge coronary arteriography after therapy with tissue-type plasminogen activator, heparin and aspirin for acute myocardial infarction. *J. Am. Coll. Cardiol.*, **17**, 1007–16.
41. Topol, E. (1994) Thrombolytic intervention. In: Topol, E. (ed.) *Textbook of Interventional Cardiology*, 2nd edn. New York: W.B. Saunders.
42. Topol, E., Holmes, D. and Rogers, W. (1991) Coronary angiography after thrombolytic therapy for acute myocardial infarction. *Ann. Intern. Med.*, **114**, 877–85.
43. Muller, D., Topol, E., Ellis, S. *et al.* and the Thrombolysis and Angioplasty in Myocardial Infarction (TAMI) Study Group (1991) Multivessel coronary artery disease: A key predictor of short-term prognosis after reperfusion therapy for acute myocardial infarction. *Am. Heart J.*, **121**, 1042–9.
44. Lee, K., Sigmon, K., George, B. *et al.* (1988) Early and complete reperfusion – A key predictor of survival after thrombolytic therapy (abstract). *Circulation*, **78**, II-500.
45. Gersh, B. and Robertson, T. (1989) The efficacy of percutaneous transluminal coronary angioplasty (PTCA) in coronary artery disease – Why we need randomized trials. In: Topol, E. (ed.) *Textbook of Interventional Cardiology*, pp. 240–53. Philadelphia: W.B. Saunders.
46. Ellis, S.G., Ribeiro da Silva, E., Heyndrickx, G. *et al.* for the RESCUE Investigators (1993) Final results of the randomized RESCUE evaluating PTCA after failed thrombolysis for patients with anterior infarction (abstract). *Circulation*, **88**, I-106.
47. Kereiakes, D.J., Topol, E.J., George, B.S. *et al.* (1991) Myocardial infarction with minimal coronary atherosclerosis in the era of thrombolytic reperfusion. *J. Am. Coll. Cardiol.*, **17**, 304–12.
48. Ross, J., Gilpin, E., Madsen, E. *et al.* (1989) A decision scheme for coronary angiography after acute myocardial infarction. *J. Am. Coll. Cardiol.*, **79**, 292–303.
49. Topol, E.J., Bates, E.R., Walton, J.J. *et al.* (1987) Community hospital administration of intravenous tissue plasminogen activator in acute myocardial infarction: Improved timing, thrombolytic efficacy and ventricular function. *J. Am. Coll. Cardiol.*, **10**, 1173–7.
50. Charles, E., Rogers, W., Reeder, G. *et al.* (1989) Economic advantages of a conservative strategy for acute myocardial infarction management: rt-PA without obligatory PTCA (abstract). *J. Am. Coll. Cardiol.*, **13**, 152A.
51. The SWIFT (Should We Intervene Following Thrombolysis) Trial Study Group (1991) The SWIFT trial of delayed elective intervention versus conservative treatment after thrombolysis with anistreplase in acute myocardial infarction. *BMJ*, **302**, 555–60.
52. Dwyer, E., McMaster, P., Greenberg, H. *et al.* and the Multicenter Post-Infarction Research Group (1984) Nonfatal cardiac events and recurrent infarction in the year after acute myocardial infarction. *J. Am. Coll. Cardiol.*, **4**, 695–702.
53. Moss, A., DeCamilla, J., Davis, H. *et al.* (1977) Clinical significance of ventricular ectopic beats in the early post-hospital phase of myocardial infarction. *Am. J. Cardiol.*, **39**, 635–40.
54. Bigger, J., Fleiss, J., Kleiger, R. *et al.* and the Multicenter Post-Infarction Research Group (1984) The relationships among ventricular arrhythmias, left ventricular dysfunction, and mortality in the two years after myocardial infarction. *Circulation*, **69**, 250–8.
55. The Multicenter Post-Infarction Research Group (1983) Risk stratification and survival after myocardial infarction. *N. Engl. J. Med.*, **309**, 331–6.
56. Muller, D., Topol, E., Ellis, S. *et al.* (1991) Determinants of the need for early acute intervention in patients treated conservatively after thrombolytic therapy for acute myocardial infarction. *J. Am. Coll. Cardiol.*, **18**, 1594–601.
57. Sutton, J. and Topol, E. (1991) The significance of a paradoxical negative exercise tomographic thallium test in the presence of a critical residual stenosis after thrombolysis for evolving myocardial infarction. *Circulation*, **83**, 1278–86.
58. American College of Physicians (1989) Evaluation of patients after recent acute myocardial infarction. *Ann. Intern. Med.*, **110**, 485–8.
59. Theroux, P., Waters, D., Halphen, C. *et al.* (1979) Prognostic value of exercise testing soon after myocardial infarction. *N. Engl. J. Med.*, **301**, 341–5.
60. Hamm L., Crow, R., Stull, G. *et al.* (1989) Safety and characteristics of exercise testing early after acute myocardial infarction. *Am. J. Cardiol.*, **63**, 1193–7.
61. Burns, R., Freeman, M., Liu, P. *et al.* (1989) Limitations of exercise thallium single photon tomography early after myocardial infarction (abstract). *J. Am. Coll. Cardiol.*, **13**, 125A.

62. Simoons, M.L., Vos, J., Tijssen, J.G. *et al.* (1989) Long-term benefit of early thrombolytic therapy in patients with acute myocardial infarction: 5 year follow-up of a trial conducted by the Interuniversity Cardiology Institute of The Netherlands. *J. Am. Coll. Cardiol.*, **14**, 1609–15.

63. Chaitman, B.R., McMahon, R.P., Terrin, M. *et al.* (1993) Exercise ECG test results in the TIMI II Trial. *Am. J. Cardiol.*, **71**, 131–138.

64. Touchstone, D.A., Beller, G.A., Nygaard, T.W. *et al.* (1988) Functional significance of predischarge exercise thallium-201 findings following intravenous streptokinase therapy during acute myocardial infarction. *Am. Heart J.*, **116**, 1500–7.

65. Weiss, A.T., Maddahi, J., Shah, P.K. *et al.* (1989) Exercise-induced ischemia in the streptokinase-reperfused myocardium: Relationship to extent of salvaged myocardium and degree of residual coronary stenosis. *Am. Heart J.*, **118**, 9–16.

66. Deckers, J., Fioretti, P., Brower, R. *et al.* (1987) Prediction of one year outcome after complicated and uncomplicated myocardial infarction: Bayesian analysis of predischarge exercise test results in 300 patients. *Am. Heart J.*, **113**, 90–5.

67. Krone, R., Gillespie, J., Weld, F. *et al.* and the Multicenter Post-Infarction Research Group (1985) Low-level exercise testing after myocardial infarction: Usefulness in enhancing clinical risk stratification. *Circulation*, **71**, 80–9.

68. Gibson, R., Beller, G, Gheorghiade, M. *et al.* (1986) The prevalence and clinical significance of residual myocardial ischemia two weeks after uncomplicated non-Q wave infarction: A prospective natural history study. *Circulation*, **73**, 1186–98.

69. Krone, R.., Dwyer, E., Greenberg, H. *et al.* and the Multicenter Post-Infarction Research Group (1989) Risk stratification in patients with first non-Q wave myocardial infarction: Limited value of the early low level exercise test after uncomplicated infarcts. *J. Am. Coll. Cardiol.*, **14**, 31–7.

70. Mark, D., Naylor, D., Hlatky, M. *et al.* (1994) Medical resource use and quality of life outcomes following acute myocardial infarction in Canada versus the United States: The Canadian–U.S. Substudy. *N. Engl. J. Med.* (in press).

71. American College of Cardiology/American Heart Association (1990) Guidelines for the early management of patients with acute myocardial infarction. A report of the American College of Cardiology/American Heart Association Task Force on Assessment of Diagnostic and Therapeutic Cardiovascular Procedures (Subcommittee to Develop Guidelines for the Early Management of Patients with Acute Myocardial Infarction). *J. Am. Coll. Cardiol.*, **16**, 249–92.

72. Chassin, M., Brook, R., Park, R. *et al.* (1986) Variations in the use of medical and surgical services by the medicare population. *N. Engl. J. Med.*, **314**, 285–90.

73. Topol, E., Califf, R., Kereiakes, D. *et al.* (1987) The thrombolysis and angioplasty in myocardial infarction (TAMI) trial. *J. Am. Coll. Cardiol.*, **10**, 65B–74B.

74. Topol, E., Califf, R., George, B. *et al.* (1989) Insights derived from the thrombolysis and angioplasty in myocardial infarction (TAMI) trials. *J. Am. Coll. Cardiol.*, **12**, 24A–31A.

75. Topol, E. (1988) Coronary angioplasty for acute myocardial infarction. *Ann. Intern. Med.*, **109**, 970–80.

76. Cragg, D.R., Friedman, H.Z., Bonema, J.D. *et al.* (1991) Outcome of patients with acute myocardial infarction who are ineligible for thrombolytic therapy. *Ann. Intern. Med.*, **115**, 173–7.

77. DeWood, M.A. (1990) Direct PTCA vs intravenous t-PA in acute myocardial infarction: Results from a prospective randomized trial. In: *Thrombolysis and Interventional Therapy in Acute Myocardial Infarction*, pp. 28–9. VI George Washington University Pre-AHA Symposium.

78. Lincoff, A.M. and Topol, E.J. (1993) Trickle down thrombolysis. *J. Am. Coll. Cardiol.*, **21**, 1396–8.

79. Lincoff, A.M. and Topol, E. (1993) The illusion of reperfusion. Does anyone achieve optimal myocardial reperfusion. *Circulation*, **87**, 1792–805. [Erratum (1993) **88**, 1361–75.]

80. Simes, R., Ross, A., Simoons, M. *et al.* for the GUSTO Investigators (1993) Mortality reduction with accelerated tissue plasminogen activator is explained by early coronary patency. *Circulation*, **88**, 291.

81. Eckman, M.H., Wong, J.B., Salem, D.N. *et al.* (1992) Direct angioplasty for acute myocardial infarction. A review of outcomes in clinal subsets. *Ann. Intern. Med.*, **117**, 667–76.

82. Topol, E. (1993) Mechanical interventions for acute myocardial infarction. In: Topol, E. (ed.) *Textbook of Interventional Cardiology*, Vol. I, pp. 292–317. Philadelphia: W.B. Saunders.

83. Topol, E.J., Califf, R.M., Vandormael, M. *et al.* for the TAMI-6 Study Group (1992) A randomized trial of late reperfusion therapy for acute myocardial infarction. *Circulation*, **85**, 2090–9.

84. Meijer, A., Verheugt, F.W., Werter, C.J. *et al.* (1993) Aspirin versus coumadin in the prevention of reocclusion and recurrent ischemia after successful thrombolysis: a prospective placebo-controlled angiographic study. Results of the APRICOT Study [see comments]. *Circulation*, **87**, 1524–30.

85. Veen, G., Meijer, A., Verheugt, F.W. *et al.* (1993) Culprit lesion morphology and stenosis severity in the prediction of reocclusion after coronary thrombolysis: angiographic results of the APRICOT study. Antithrombotics in the Prevention of Reocclusion in Coronary Thrombolysis. *J. Am. Coll. Cardiol.*, **22**, 1755–62.

86. Wall, T., Califf, R., George, B. *et al.* for the TAMI-7 Study Group (1992) Accelerated plasminogen activator dose regimens for coronary thrombolysis. *J. Am. Coll. Cardiol.*, **19**, 482–9.

87. Neuhaus, K., Feuerer, W., Jeep-Teebe, S. *et al.* (1989) Improved thrombolysis with a modified dose regimen of recombinant tissue-type plasminogen activator. *J. Am. Coll. Cardiol.*, **14**, 1566–9.

88. Weaver, W.D., Litwin, P.E., Martin, J.S., Hallstrom, A.P., for the MITI project investigators (1994) Use of thrombolytic therapy — How much impact have we made? (abstract) *J. Am. Coll. Cardiol.*, **23**, 245 A.

89. Ryan, T.J., Bauman, W.B., Kennedy, J.W. *et al.* (1993) Guidelines for percutaneous transluminal coronary angioplasty: A report of the American College of Cardiology/American Heart Association task force on assessment

of diagnostic and therapeutic cardiovascular procedures (Committee on percutaneous coronary angioplasty). *J. Am. Coll. Cardiol.*, **22**(7), 2033–54.

90. Califf, R., Topol, E., George, B. *et al.* (1987) Characteristics and outcomes of patients in whom reperfusion with intravenous tissue-type plasminogen activator fails: Results of the Thrombolysis and Angioplasty in Myocardial Infarction (TAMI) I trial. *Circulation*, **77**, 1090–9.

91. Jeremy, R., Allman, K., Bautovitch, G. *et al.* (1989) Patterns of left ventricular dilation during the six months after myocardial infarction. *J. Am. Coll. Cardiol.*, **13**, 304–10.

92. Touchstone, D.A., Beller, G.A., Nygaard, T.W. *et al.* (1989) Effects of successful intravenous reperfusion therapy on regional myocardial function and geometry in humans: a tomographic assessment using two-dimensional echocardiography. *J. Am. Coll. Cardiol.*, **13**, 1506–13.

93. LATE Study Group (1993) Late Assessment of Thrombolytic Efficacy (LATE) study with alteplase 6–24 hours after onset of acute myocardial infarction. *Lancet*, **342**, 759–66.

94. EMERAS (1993) Randomised trial of late thrombolysis in patients with suspected acute myocardial infarction. *Lancet*, **342**, 767–72.

95. Vatterott, P., Hammill, S., Bailey, K. *et al.* (1991) Late potentials on signal-averaged electrocardiograms and patency of the infarct-related artery in survivors of acute myocardial infarction. *J. Am. Coll. Cardiol.*, **17**, 330–7.

96. Sager, P.T., Perlmutter, R.A., Rosenfeld, L.E. *et al.* (1988) Electrophysiologic effects of thrombolytic therapy in patients with a transmural anterior myocardial infarction complicated by left ventricular aneurysm formation. *J. Am. Coll. Cardiol.*, **12**, 19–24.

97. Volpi, A., Cavalli, A. Santoro, E. *et al.* and the GISSI Investigators (1990) Incidence and prognosis of secondary ventricular fibrillation in acute myocardial infarction. Evidence for a protective effect of thrombolytic therapy. *Circulation*, **82**, 1279–88.

98. Gang, E., Lew, A., Hong, M. *et al.* (1989) Decreased incidence of ventricular late potentials after successful thrombolytic therapy for acute myocardial infarction. *N. Engl. J. Med.*, **321**, 712–16.

99. Hermosillo, A., Dorado, M., Casanova, J. *et al.* (1993) Influence of infarct-related artery patency on the indexes of parasympathetic activity and prevalance of late potentials in survivors of acute myocardial infarction. *J. Am. Coll. Cardiol.*, **22**, 695–706.

100. Boehrer, J.D., Glamann, D.B., Lange, R.A. *et al.* (1992) Effect of coronary angioplasty on late potentials one to two weeks after acute myocardial infarction. *Am. J. Cardiol.*, **70**, 1515–19.

101. Bourke, J., Richards, D., Ross, D. *et al.* (1991) Routine programmed electrical stimulation in survivors of acute myocardial infarction for prediction of spontaneous ventricular tachyarrhythmias during follow-up: Results, optimal stimulation protocol and cost-effective screening. *J. Am. Coll. Cardiol.*, **18**, 780–8.

102. Ellis, S.G., Van de Werf, F., Ribeiro-daSilva, E. *et al.* (1992) Present status of rescue coronary angioplasty: Current polarization of opinion and randomized trials [editorial]. *J. Am. Coll. Cardiol.*, **19**, 681–6.

103. Topol, E., Califf, R., George, B. *et al.* (1987) A randomized trial of immediate versus delayed elective angioplasty after intravenous tissue plasminogen activator in acute myocardial infarction. *N. Engl. J. Med.*, **317**, 581–8.

104. Califf, R.M., Topol, E.J., Stack, R.S. *et al.* (1991) Evaluation of combination thrombolytic therapy and timing of cardiac catheterization in acute myocardial infarction. Results of thrombolysis and angioplasty in myocardial infarction – phase 5 randomized trial. *Circulation*, **83**, 1543–56.

105. Belenkie, I., Knudtson, M.L., Roth, D.L. *et al.* (1991) Relation between flow grade after thrombolytic therapy and the effect of angioplasty on left ventricular function: a prospective randomized trial. *Am. Heart J.*, **121**, 407–16.

106. Fung, A.Y., Lai, P., Topol, E.J. *et al.* (1986) Value of percutaneous transluminal coronary angioplasty after unsuccessful intravenous streptokinase therapy in acute myocardial infarction. *Am. J. Cardiol.*, **58**, 686–91.

107. Grines, C., Nissen, S. Booth, D. *et al.* (1988) Efficacy, safety and cost effectiveness of a new thrombolytic regimen for acute myocardial infarction using half dose tPA with full dose streptokinase. *Circulation*, **78**, II-304.

108. Holmes, D. Jr, Gersh, B.J., Bailey, K.R. *et al.* (1990) Emergency 'rescue' percutaneous transluminal coronary angioplasty after failed thrombolysis with streptokinase. Early and late results. *Circulation*, **81**(3 suppl.), IV51–6.

109. Grines, C., Nissen, S., Booth, D. *et al.* and the Kentucky Acute Myocardial Infarction Trial (KAMIT) Group (1991) A prospective, randomized trial comparing combination half-dose tissue-type plasminogen activator and strepto-kinase with full-dose tissue-type plasminogen activator. *Circulation*, **84**, 540–9.

110. O'Connor, C.M., Mark, D.B., Hinohara, T. *et al.* (1989) Rescue coronary angioplasty after failure of intravenous streptokinase in acute myocardial infarction: in-hospital and long-term outcomes. *J. Inv. Cardiol.*, **1**, 85–95.

111. Baim, D.S., Diver, D.J. and Knatterud, G.L. (1988) PTCA 'salvage' for thrombolytic failures – implications from TIMI II-A (abstract). *Circulation*, **78**, II-112.

112. Whitlow, P.L. (1990) Catheterization/rescue angioplasty following thrombolysis (CRAFT) study: results of rescue angioplasty (abstract). *Circulation*, **82**, III-308.

113. Papapietro, S.E., MacLean, A.H., Stanley, A.W.H. *et al.* (1985) Percutaneous transluminal coronary angioplasty after intracoronary streptokinase in evolving acute myocardial infarction. *Am. J. Cardiol.*, **55**, 48–53.

114. Ellis, S.G., O'Neill, W.W., Bates, E.R. *et al.* (1989) Implications for patient triage from survival and left ventricular functional recovery analyses in 500 patients treated with coronary angioplasty for acute myocardial infarction. *J. Am. Coll. Cardiol.*, **13**, 1251–9.

115. Abbottsmith, C., Topol, E., George, B. *et al.* (1990) Fate of patients with acute myocardial infarction with patency of the infarct-related vessel achieved with successful thrombolysis versus rescue angioplasty. *J. Am. Coll. Cardiol.*, **16**, 770–8.

116. Belenkie, I., Knudtson, M.L., Hall, C.A. *et al.* (1990) Vessel patency, rescue PTCA and mortality in acute myocardial infarction: Results from a prospective randomized reperfusion trial (abstract). *Clin. Invest. Med.*, **13**, 157.

117. Krucoff, M.W., Croll, M.A., Pope, J.E. *et al.* (1993) Continuously updated 12-lead ST-segment recovery analysis for myocardial infarct artery patency assessment and its correlation with multiple simultaneous early angiographic observations. *Am. J. Cardiol.*, **71**, 145–51.

118. Tranchesi, B., Verstraete, M., Van de Werf, F. *et al.* (1990) Usefulness of high-frequency analysis of signal-averaged surface electrocardiograms in acute myocardial infarction before and after coronary thrombolysis for assessing coronary reperfusion. *Am. J. Cardiol.*, **66**, 1196–8.

119. Seacord, L., Abendschein, D., Nohara, R. *et al.* (1988) Detection of reperfusion within one hour after coronary recanalization by analysis of isoforms of the MM creatine kinase isoenzyme in plasma. *Fibrinolysis*, **2**, 151–6.

120. Schofer, J., Ress-Grigolo, G, Voigt, K. *et al.* (1992) Early detection of coronary artery patency after thrombolysis by determination of the MM creatine kinase isoforms in patients with acute myocardial infarction. *Am. Heart J.*, **123**, 846–53.

121. Christian, T., Clements, I. and Gibbons, R. (1991) Noninvasive identification of myocardium at risk in patients with acute myocardial infarction and nondiagnostic electrocardiograms with technetium-99 Sestamibi. *Circulation*, **83**, 1615–20.

122. Gibbons, R. (1991) Perfusion imaging with ^{99m}Tc-Sestamibi for the assessment of myocardial area at risk and the efficacy of acute treatment in myocardial infarction. *Circulation*, **84**(3 suppl.), I37–I42.

123. Wackers, F. (1990) Thrombolytic therapy for myocardial infarction: Assessment of efficacy by myocardial perfusion imaging with technetium-99m sestamibi. *Am. J. Cardiol.*, **66**, 36E–41E.

124. van den Brand, M., Betrui, A., Bescos, L. *et al.* (1992) Randomized trial of deferred angioplasty after thrombolysis for acute myocardial infarction. *Coronary Artery Disease*, **3**, 393–401.

125. Özbek, C., Dyckmans, J., Sen, S. *et al.* (1990) Comparison of invasive and conservative strategies after treatment with streptokinase in acute myocardial infarction: Results of a randomized trial (SIAM) (abstract). *J. Am. Coll. Cardiol.*, **15**, 63A.

126. Guerci, A., Gerstenblith, G., Brinker, J. *et al.* (1987) A randomized trial of intravenous tissue plasminogen activator for acute myocardial infarction with subsequent randomization to elective coronary angioplasty. *N. Engl. J. Med.*, **317**, 1613–18.

127. Barbash, G.I., Roth, A., Hod, H. *et al.* (1990) Randomized controlled trial of late in-hospital angiography and angioplasty versus conservative management after treatment with recombinant tissue-type plasminogen activator in acute myocardial infarction. *Am. J. Cardiol.*, **66**, 538–45.

128. Ellis, S.G., Mooney, M.R., George, B.S. *et al.* for the Treatment of Post-Thrombolytic Restenosis Study Group (1992) Randomized trial of elective angioplasty versus conservative management for patients with residual stenoses after thrombolytic treatment of myocardial infarction. *Circulation*, **86**, 1400–6.

129. Simoons, M., Arnold, A., Betriu, A. *et al.* (1988) Thrombolysis with t-PA in acute myocardial infarction: No beneficial effects of immediate PTCA. *Lancet*, **i**, 197–203.

130. TIMI Research Group (1988) Immediate vs delayed catheterization and angioplasty following thrombolytic therapy for acute myocardial infarction. *JAMA*, **260**, 2849–58.

131. Baim, D.S., Diver, D.J. and Knatterud, G.L. (1988) PTCA 'salvage' for thrombolytic failures – implications from TIMI II-A (abstract). *Circulation*, **78**, II-112.

132. Cheitlin, M. (1988) The aggressive war on acute myocardial infarction: Is the blitzkrieg strategy changing? *JAMA*, **260**, 2894–6.

133. Rogers, W.J., Baim, D.S., Gore, J.M. *et al.* (1990) Comparison of immediate invasive, delayed invasive, and conservative strategies after tissue-type plasminogen activator. Results of the Thrombolysis in Myocardial Infarction (TIMI) Phase-II-A trial [see comments]. *Circulation*, **81**, 1457–76.

134. Sleight, P. (1990) Do we need to intervene after thrombolysis in acute myocardial infarction? *Circulation*, **81**, 1707–9.

135. Ellis, S.G., Topol, E.J, George, B.S. *et al.* (1989) Recurrent ischemia without warning. Analysis of risk factors for in-hospital ischemic events following successful thrombolysis with intravenous tissue plasminogen activator. *Circulation*, **80**, 1159–65.

136. O'Neill, W.W., Erbel, R., Laufer, N. *et al.* (1985) Coronary angioplasty therapy of cardiogenic shock complicating acute myocardial infarction (abstract). *Circulation*, **72**, III-309.

137. Schmidt, W.G., Uebis, R., von Essen, R. *et al.* (1987) Residual coronary stenosis after thrombolysis with rt-PA or streptokinase: Acute results and 3 weeks follow up. *Eur. Heart J.*, **8**, 1182–8.

138. Holmes, D. Jr and Topol, E. (1989) Reperfusion momentum: Lessons from the randomized trials of immediate coronary angioplasty for myocardial infarction. *J. Am. Coll. Cardiol.*, **14**, 1572–8.

139. Topol, E.J., Ellis, S.G., Cosgrove, D.M. *et al.* (1993) Analysis of coronary angioplasty practice in the United States with an insurance-claims data base [see comments]. *Circulation*, **87**, 1489–97.

140. Kavanaugh, K. and Topol, E. (1991) Acute intervention during myocardial infarction in patients with prior coronary bypass surgery. *Am. J. Cardiol.*, **65**, 924–7.

141. De Franco, A.C., Abramowitz, B., Krichbaum, D. and Topol, E.J. for the GUSTO Investigators (1994) Substantial (three-fold) benefit of accelerated t-PA over standard thrombolytic therapy in patients with prior bypass surgery and acute MI: Results of the GUSTO trial (abstract). *J. Am. Coll. Cardiol.*, **23**, 345A.

142. Schulman, S., Achuff, S., Griffith, L. *et al.* (1988) Prognostic cardiac catheterization variables in survivors of acute myocardial infarction: A five year prospective study. *J. Am. Coll. Cardiol.*, **11**, 1164–72.

143. Turner, J., Rogers, W., Mantle, J. *et al.* (1980) Coronary angiography soon after myocardial infarction. *Chest*, **77**, 58–64.

144. Betriu, A., Castaner, A., Sanz, G. *et al.* (1982) Angiographic findings 1 month after myocardial infarction: A prospective study of 259 survivors. *Circulation*, **65**, 1099–105.

145. Topol, E., Holmes, D. and Rogers, W. (1991) Coronary angiography after thrombolytic therapy for acute myocardial infarction. *Ann. Intern. Med.*, **114**, 877–85.
146. Lee, L., Bates, E., Pitt, B. *et al.* (1988) Percutaneous transluminal coronary angioplasty improves survival in acute myocardial infarction complicated by cardiogenic shock. *Circulation*, **78**, 1345–51.
147. Shani, J., Rivera, M., Greengart, A. *et al.* (1986) Percutaneous transluminal coronary angioplasty in cardiogenic shock (abstract). *J. Am. Coll. Cardiol.*, **7**, 149A.
148. Heuser, R., Maddoux, G., Goss, J. *et al.* (1987) Coronary angioplasty for acute mitral regurgitation due to myocardial infarction. *Ann. Intern. Med.*, **107**, 852–5.
149. Brown, T. Jr, Iannone, L., Gordon, D. *et al.* (1985) Percutaneous myocardial perfusion (PMR) reduces mortality in acute myocardial infarction (MI) complicated by cardiogenic shock (abstract). *Circulation*, **72**, III-309.
150. Hibbard, M., Holmes, D., Bailey, K. *et al.* (1992) Percutaneous transluminal coronary angioplasty in patients with cardiogenic shock. *J. Am. Coll. Cardiol.*, **19**, 639–46.
151. Seydoux, C., Goy, J., Beuret, P. *et al.* (1992) Effectiveness of percutaneous transluminal coronary angioplasty in cardiogenic shock during acute myocardial infarction. *Am. J. Cardiol.*, **69**, 968–9.
152. Bengston, J.R., Kaplan, A.J., Pieper, K.S. *et al.* (1992) Prognosis in cardiogenic shock after acute myocardial infarction in the interventional era. *J. Am. Coll. Cardiol.*, **20**, 1482–9.
153. Gacioch, G.M., Ellis, S.G., Lee, L. *et al.* (1992) Cardiogenic shock complicating acute myocardial infarction: the use of coronary angioplasty and the integration of the new support devices into patient management. *J. Am. Coll. Cardiol.*, **19**, 647–53.
154. Kahn, J.K., Rutherford, B.D., McConahay, D.R. *et al.* (1990) Catheterization laboratory events and hospital outcome with direct angioplasty for acute myocardial infarction. *Circulation*, **82**, 1910–15.
155. Goldberg, R., Gore, J., Alpert, J. *et al.* (1991) Cardiogenic shock after acute myocardial infarction. Incidence and mortality from a community-wide perspective, 1975 to 1988. *N. Engl. J. Med.*, **325**, 1117–22.
156. Ohman, E.M., George, B.S., White, C.J. *et al.* (1994) Use of aortic counterpulsation to improve sustained coronary artery patency during acute myocardial infarction. Results of a randomized trial. *Circulation*, **90**, 792–799.
157. Nissen, S.E. and Gurley, J.C. (1991) Application of intravascular ultrasound for detection and quantitation of coronary atherosclerosis. *Int. J. Card. Imaging*, **6**, 165–77.
158. Waller, B.F., Pinkerton, C.A. and Slack, J.D. (1992) Intravascular ultrasound: a histological study of vessels during life. The new 'gold standard' for vascular imaging. *Circulation*, **85**, 2305–10.
159. Mizuno, K., Satomura, K. and Miyamoto, A. (1992) Angioscopic evaluation of coronary-artery thrombi in acute coronary syndromes. *N. Engl. J. Med.*, **326**, 287–91.
160. Topol, E., Ellis, S., George, B. *et al.* (1989) The pivotal role of multivessel coronary artery disease and the remote zone in the reperfusion era (abstract). *J. Am. Coll. Cardiol.*, **13**, 92A.

5

Late Establishment of Patency of the Infarct-related Artery

E. Braunwald and C. B. Kim

It is well established that the benefits of thrombolytic therapy of acute myocardial infarction (AMI) are related inversely to the time interval between the onset of the clinical event and of treatment[1–5] (Figure 5.1). This is readily understandable when the results of studies in experimental animals are considered. It has been shown in the dog that the severe myocardial ischemia consequent to occlusion of a coronary artery leads to a wavefront of myocardial necrosis, generally proceeding from the endocardium to the epicardium.[6] The shorter the time between coronary occlusion and reperfusion the lower the percentage of the area at risk that becomes necrotic. These experimental and clinical

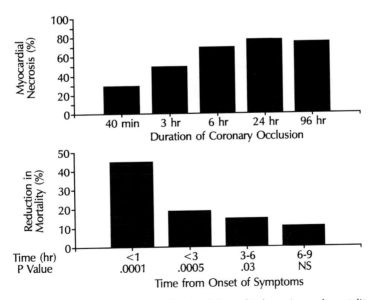

Figure 5.1 Relationship between experimental animal data of infarct size and mortality outcome of GISSI-1 patients as a function of time. The parallelism of these data supports the correlation between salvage of myocardium and the reduction in mortality seen with reperfusion therapy. (From Roberts, R. and Kleiman, N. (1992) The early reperfusion principle. In: *The Open Artery*, p. 5. Hamilton, Ontario: Decker. Modified from Reimer, K.A., Lowe, J.E., Rasmussen, M.M., and Jennings, R.B. (1977) The wavefront phenomenon of ischemic cell death. *Circulation* **56**, 786–94, and Ref. 3.)

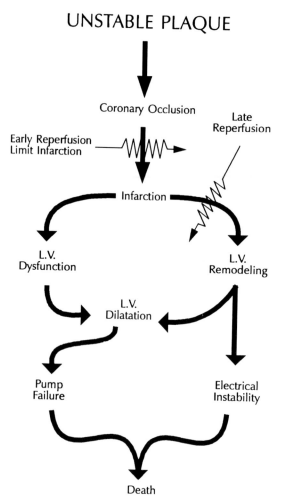

Figure 5.2   Flow chart showing postulated sequence of events from an unstable atherosclerotic plaque to death. The original paradigm is shown at the left; the expanded paradigm is at the right. (From Ref. 10.)

observations have laid the groundwork for the modern management of AMI, which is based on the following straightforward and now widely agreed-upon concept; early reperfusion of an occluded infarct-related artery (IRA) → myocardial salvage → preservation of left ventricular function → improved patient survival (Figure 5.2).

However, there is increasing evidence that relatively late myocardial reperfusion may also exert a favorable influence on clinical outcome, an influence not directly related to myocardial salvage.[7–9] The purpose of this chapter is to summarize this evidence and to consider its implications for the management of AMI. This subject was recently reviewed in detail.[10]

Challenges to the Concept that Restoration of Patency Operates Through Myocardial Salvage

If the benefit of reperfusion therapy resulted entirely from myocardial salvage, it would be anticipated that left ventricular function would be substantially better in patients receiving thrombolytic therapy than those receiving placebo, and that this improvement in function would then be translated into improved survival. However, in several of the early placebo-controlled trials of thrombolytic therapy in which patients were entered relatively late in their course (4–6 hours after the onset of symptoms) left ventricular ejection fraction was not improved by thrombolytic therapy, yet mortality was reduced. [11–15] In contrast, when coronary arterial patency was evaluated angiographically, it was observed that patency of the IRA correlated strongly with survival. For example, in one of the early trials in which all patients received active thrombolytic therapy (the TIMI I trial), patency of the IRA was an important determinant of survival; the 1-year mortality in patients with an open IRA at 90 min was 5.67% compared with 14.8% in patients with a closed IRA, even though the left ventricular ejection fraction (LVEF) in the two groups was similar.[16] In a recent review of all of the TAMI trials, Harrison *et al.* reported that overall thrombolysis did not affect LVEF and produced, on the average, only a slight (14%) improvement in infarct zone regional function.[17] Observations from the aforementioned and other trials, taken together, suggest that even when thrombolytic therapy does not salvage sufficient myocardium to improve LVEF it may improve survival; the latter may be related to the restoration of coronary patency (Figure 5.2).

Evidence that Late Coronary Arterial Patency Improves Left Ventricular Function

While, as indicated above, a dissociation between left ventricular function and survival was demonstrated in some trials, in other studies thrombolytic therapy was found to be associated with improved left ventricular function even when the restoration of patency occurred too late to salvage substantial quantities of myocardium. Two observational studies from the prethrombolytic era demonstrated that spontaneous reperfusion, which usually occurs hours or days after the onset of infarction, is associated with improved left ventricular function. Jeremy *et al.* investigated patients 30 days after a first AMI and reported that left ventricular dilatation, assessed angiographically, occurred uniformly in patients with persistently occluded IRAs and only rarely in patients with patent IRAs.[18] Similarly, Verheugt *et al.* reported that left ventricular function improved more in patients with AMI and patent IRAs than in those with persistent occlusion;[19] during the 2 weeks following AMI, LVEF, measured by radionuclide ventriculography, increased by an average of 15 ejection-fraction units in patients with spontaneous reperfusion and declined by 5 units in those with persistently occluded IRAs.

Similar observations have been made in the thrombolytic era. In the TIMI I trial, in which treatment was begun an average of 4.5 hours after the onset of symptoms, left ventricular end-diastolic and end-systolic volumes rose significantly less between 1 and 6 weeks following AMI in patients with patent vs those with occluded IRAs[20] (Figure 5.3). In the TAMI-6 trial, patients were randomly assigned to treatment with tissue plasminogen activator (t-PA) or placebo 6–24 hours after the onset of symptoms. In the subsequent 6 months, left ventricular end-diastolic volume increased significantly in the placebo-treated patients but remained unchanged in the t-PA treated group.[21] In the same study, angioplasty of occluded IRAs carried out 2 days after the onset of symptoms, too late to salvage substantial quantities of myocardium, resulted in improved left ventricular function. Schroeder *et al.* reported that even when corrections were made for infarct size, patients with a patent IRA 1 month after AMI had significantly better left ventricular function than those with an occluded vessel. This was most marked in patients in whom the IRA was the left anterior descending coronary artery; the LVEF was 52% when the vessel was patent compared with 36% when it was occluded.[22]

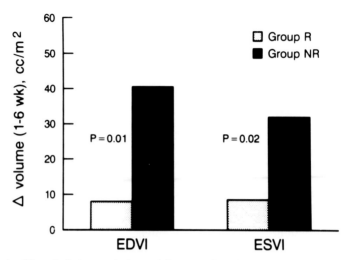

Figure 5.3 Effects of thrombolytic reperfusion on left ventricular volume changes between 1 and 6 weeks following AMI in the TIMI I trial. Differences between patients with successful reperfusion (group R) and those without successful reperfusion (group NR) were significant. EDVI, left ventricular end-diastolic volume index; ESVI, left ventricular end-systolic volume index. (From Ref. 20.)

Leung and Lau studied patients with a first AMI and obstruction limited to the left anterior descending coronary artery. Left ventricular end-systolic and end-diastolic volumes and ejection fractions were similar 7–10 days following infarction in patients with patent and occluded IRAs. However, over the subsequent year, patients with patent IRAs exhibited smaller increases in ventricular volumes and reductions in LVEF than did patients with occluded IRAs[23] (Figure 5.4). Hirayama et al. analyzed patients with AMI

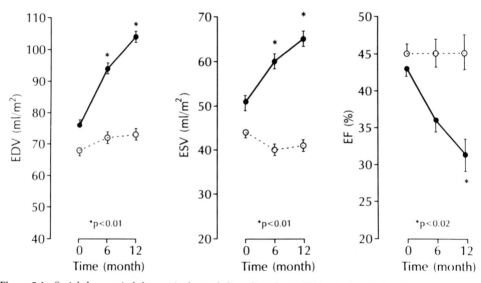

Figure 5.4 Serial changes in left ventricular end-diastolic volume (EDV), end-systolic volume (ESV) and ejection fraction (EF) in patients with occluded versus patent infarct-related arteries at baseline, i.e. 7–10 days after acute myocardial infarction (0), and 6 and 12 months later. Data are expressed as the mean ±SEM. ●——●, total occlusion; ○——○, ≥ 1.5 mm stenosis. (From Refs 3 and 23.)

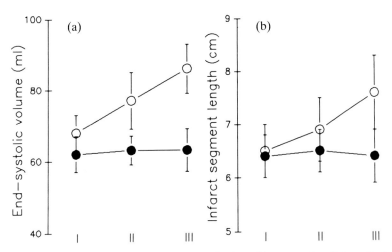

Figure 5.5 End-systolic left ventricular volume (a) and infarct (b) segment length in patients with early reperfused, (≤12 hours), and late reperfused, non-reperfused (>12 hours) CK time to peak during the in-hospital phase of myocardial infarction. There is a progressive increment of ventricular volume and infarct segment length in nonreperfused patients between the first and predischarge echocardiographic examinations, whereas reperfused patients show no change. Error bars are standard error of the mean. CKt, CK time to peak; I, II and III, echocardiographic examinations performed on day 1, 72 hours later, and at discharge, respectively. O——O, CKt >12 hours; ●——●, CKt ≤12 hours. (From Ref. 25.)

according to whether reperfusion was early (<6 hours from the onset of symptoms), late (>6 hours), or did not occur at all. Left ventricular end-systolic and end-diastolic volumes were lower, not only in the early, but importantly also in the late reperfusion group, than in the patients with persistent occlusion.[24] Golia *et al.* compared two groups of patients with AMI, differentiated by the presence or absence of reperfusion, closely matched for clinical characteristics, site of infarction and extent of ventricular asynergy, the latter a variable closely related to infarct size. Patients with patent IRAs exhibited stable end-systolic volumes and infarct segment lengths between admission and discharge, while patients with occluded vessels showed progressive increases in these two echocardiographic measurements (Figure 5.5).[25] Nidorf *et al.* also reported that late opening of the IRA, i.e. after 6 hours, was associated with reduced wall motion abnormalities 3 months later.[26]

Late Coronary Arterial Patency Improves Clinical Outcome

A number of studies have demonstrated the clinical benefit of an open IRA. Cigarroa *et al.* analyzed retrospectively the course of 179 patients with single-vessel coronary artery disease who did not receive thrombolytic therapy. While left ventricular volumes and global ejection fractions were similar in the 64 patients with open and the 115 patients with occluded IRAs at the time of hospital discharge, during 4 years of follow-up no deaths occurred among the former group, compared with 21 deaths among the latter (Figure 5.6). Congestive heart failure also occurred less frequently in patients with patent than in those with occluded IRAs (6% vs 17%).[27]

At least four investigations have shown a patent IRA to be an *independent* predictor of a favorable outcome after AMI. Pfeffer *et al.* demonstrated that among patients experiencing a first anterior MI, persistent occlusion of the left anterior descending coronary artery is an independent predictor for subsequent left ventricular enlargement.[28] In the SAVE

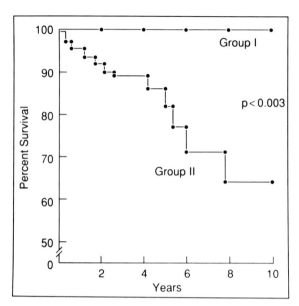

Figure 5.6   Life-table survivorship analysis for groups of patients with myocardial infarction (MI) and single-vessel disease. Left ventricular volume and ejection fractions were similar by 1 month after MI. Group I: open infarct-related artery (IRA), 64 patients; group II: occluded IRA, 115 patients. (From Ref. 27.)

trial, carried out on post-MI patients with impaired ejection fraction, patency of the IRA was identified as an independent predictor of a better clinical outcome. At follow-up averaging 3.5 years after infarction, 36% of the patients with a patent IRA had reached one of the components of the prospectively defined combined endpoint (cardiovascular death, severe heart failure, recurrent infarction, or marked deterioration of LVEF) compared with 51% in those with an occluded IRA.[29] Galvani *et al.* studied 172 patients with single-vessel coronary artery disease who had a first Q-wave MI and, on multiple logistic regression analysis, found patency of the IRA to be an independent predictor of survival.[30] White *et al.* reported on 312 patients with a first AMI who received thrombolytic therapy; cardiac catheterization was carried out at 4 weeks and the patients were then followed for an average of 39 months. Although left ventricular function (reflected in ejection fraction and end-systolic volume) was the most important prognostic factor, on multivariate analysis, patency of the IRA was also an independent predictor of survival.[31]

The importance of patency of the IRA is also supported by the finding that reocclusion is associated with a much poorer prognosis. In an analysis of the TAMI trials of thrombolytic therapy of AMI, Ohman *et al.* noted a distinct gradient in the outcome according to the status of the IRA;[32] failure to achieve IRA patency, the achievement of coronary patency followed by reocclusion, and early and sustained patency were associated with hospital mortality rates of 17%, 11% and 4% respectively. Furthermore, among the patients in whom the IRA opened but became reoccluded following thrombolytic therapy, the failure of rescue angioplasty was associated with twice the mortality observed in patients in whom this procedure was successful.

Benefits of Late Thrombolytic Therapy

Late thrombolytic therapy exerts a favorable, albeit relatively small, beneficial effect on survival. Two trials have examined the value of this approach prospectively. In the LATE trial, 5700 patients were randomized either to t-PA or placebo 6–24 hours following the

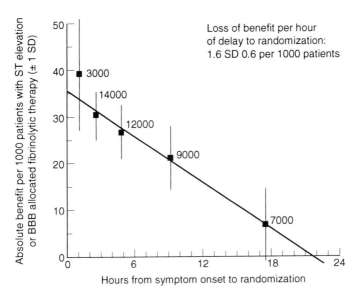

Figure 5.7   Absolute reduction in 35-day mortality vs delay from symptom onset to randomization among 45 000 patients with ST elevation or bundle branch block. (All patients in ASSET and LATE have been included since their tabular information on delay was not subdivided by ECG.) For patients whose delays were recorded as 0–1, 2–3, 4–6, 7–12 and 13–24 hours, the absolute benefit (± 1 SD) is plotted against the mean of their recorded delay times. The area of each block square, and the extent to which it influences the sloping line that is drawn through the five points, is approximately proportional to the number of patients it is based on. (From Ref. 5.)

onset of symptoms. At 6-month follow-up, a 27% reduction in mortality was observed in the patients treated with t-PA 6–12 hours after the onset of symptoms; no survival benefit was seen in patients treated 13–24 hours after the onset of symptoms.[33] In the EMERAS trial, in-hospital mortality showed a nonsignificant trend (14% reduction) in favor of patients treated with streptokinase 6–12 hours after the onset of symptoms.[34] The overview prepared by the fibrinolytic therapy trialists,[5] based on 58 600 patients (which included those enrolled in the LATE and EMERAS trials) demonstrated a straight-line relationship between the time to treatment and the reduction of mortality resulting from thrombolytic therapy (Figure 5.7). The absolute reduction of mortality in patients treated between 7 and 12 hours after the onset of symptoms was about 20 per 1000 patients and might have been even greater were it not for an excess of deaths in the first 2 days in patients receiving a thrombolytic agent.

No angiographic studies on the effectiveness of thrombolytic therapy administered more than 12 hours after the onset of symptoms are available. The lack of any perceptible effect of treatment at this time may be due not to the lack of benefit of late opening of an occluded IRA, but may be related instead to the ineffectiveness of thrombolytics in lysing older thrombi, in which there is firm cross-linking of fibrin and the beginning of collagen deposition.

Potential Mechanisms of Benefit of Late Patency of the IRA

Improved Healing of Infarcted Tissue and Prevention of Ventricular Remodeling

It has been demonstrated in animal experiments[35,36] as well as in patients[37,38] that both infarct expansion and ventricular remodeling contribute to the late deleterious effects of myocardial infarction on left ventricular function. In the hours after AMI, slippage of necrotic fibres occurs, causing thinning and systolic expansion of the infarcted region. However, hyperfunction of the nonischemic, noninfarcted myocardium maintains stroke volume and ejection fraction. The hemodynamic burden on the residual viable myocardium resulting from the combination of loss of contractile tissue and infarct expansion causes remodeling of the left ventricle, which dilates, hypertrophies and becomes more spherical.[39]

Late reperfusion exerts a number of actions which may protect the infarcted ventricle. It causes calcium-induced contraction-band necrosis, intramyocardial hemorrhage, and edema. Even when too late to salvage jeopardized myocardium, these changes may accelerate scar formation, with resultant stiffening of the infarcted tissue,[40] and reduced infarct expansion, ventricular dilatation and remodeling. Late reperfusion also increases the influx of inflammatory cells into the necrotic area, a key early step in the healing process. The importance of this step is reflected in the deleterious effects of the administration of glucocorticoids and nonsteroidal antiinflammatory agents during the first hours of experimentally induced myocardial infarctions.[41] These drugs, which inhibit the inflammatory process, cause greater than normal infarct expansion and thinner scars.

Pevention of Infarct Expansion and Ventricular Remodeling

Late reperfusion, in addition to accelerating myocardial scar formation, provides a blood-filled coronary vascular bed that might serve as a scaffold, diminishing systolic expansion of the necrotic myocardium and limiting infarct expansion, thereby reducing ventricular dilatation.[7,10,42] Experiments in several species support this idea. Lawrence *et al.* have shown in the dog that stiffening of the ischemic myocardium induced by reperfusion enhances global systolic function even without enhancing regional wall motion.[43] Reperfusion 6 hours after coronary occlusion, while too late to salvage myocardium, is associated with an immediate reduction in the diastolic dimensions of the left ventricular cavity[44] and restoration of left ventricular shape. In the rat, reperfusion 2 hours following coronary occlusion, too late to salvage myocardium in this species, diminishes infarct expansion[45] and is associated with a thicker scar[46] (Figure 5.8). Late reperfusion of an occluded IRA in the pig also reduced ventricular dilatation without reducing infarct size.[47]

Similar observations have been made in patients with single vessel coronary artery disease and a first anterior wall MI. Reperfusion has been demonstrated to exert a restraining effect on infarct expansion above and beyond its effect on myocardial salvage.[48] Persistent occlusion of the IRA is associated with greater infarct expansion, left ventricular aneurysm formation, and more severe impairment of left ventricular function.[49,50] On the other hand, AMI patients with a patent IRA rarely develop left ventricular aneurysm, a well-established risk factor for poor outcome following AMI.[49–51] Meizlish *et al.* reported that the 1-year mortality rates were 61% and 9%, respectively, among AMI patients with and without aneurysms.[49] In one series, following a first AMI, aneurysm developed in 7 of 12 patients whose IRA was persistently occluded but in only 1 of 15 patients with successful reperfusion of the IRA.[52]

Coronary arterial patency may have a salutary effect on diastolic as well as on systolic ventricular function. Thus, in the MITI trial, patency of the IRA was associated with a higher early ventricular filling rate.[53]

Perfusion of Hibernating Myocardium

Severely ischemic myocardium, perfused by a markedly stenotic IRA or by collateral vessels, may retain viability without contractile function.[54,55] While such regions of so-

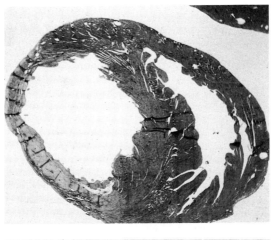

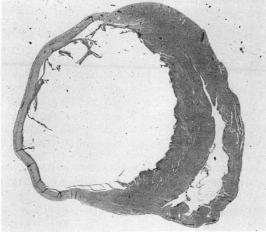

Figure 5.8 Cross-sections of rat hearts with acute myocardial infarction (AMI) obtained 6 weeks after AMI. Top: 2 hours of occlusion followed by reperfusion. Bottom: no reperfusion. Late reperfusion (top) prevented infarct thinning and aneurysm formation. (From Ref. 10. Courtesy of Dr J. Hochman, St Luke's-Roosevelt Hospital, New York.)

called 'hibernating' myocardium bordering an infarct, by definition, do not contribute to left ventricular systolic function, they may nonetheless improve clinical outcome by reducing two of the major complications of large infarctions – left ventricular expansion and electrical instability. Furthermore, it has recently become evident that the contractile performance of hibernating myocardium can be improved even after very late restoration of coronary blood flow. Montalescot *et al.* studied patients with Q-wave MI and patent but markedly stenotic IRAs and reported that angioplasty performed more than 6 weeks post MI improved systolic wall motion in the periinfarct region. This observation indicates that myocardial viability must have been sustained by a patent, though markedly obstructed, IRA for weeks following AMI.[56] Perfusion of the periinfarct region through collateral vessels can also preserve myocardial viability for relatively long periods. Angioplasty of an *occluded* IRA carried out an average of 12 days post MI resulted in an improvement of ventricular function in patients with coronary collaterals.[57] These two investigations provide strong evidence that: (1) even very *low* rates of perfusion of the periinfarct zone are beneficial since they may maintain myocardial viability for long periods following an AMI; and (2) even very *late* increases in flow through an occluded or severly stenotic IRA can restore myocardial function in chronic, severely ischemic, noncontracting, but viable myocardium.

Increased Electrical Stability

Patency of the IRA is associated with greater electrical stability and this may account, in part, for fewer tachyarrhythmias and a more favorable clinical outcome. Dilated hearts display a greater dispersion of refractory periods than do normal hearts,[58] and are more frequently associated with late potentials;[59] left ventricular aneurysm formation is associated with a particularly high incidence of ventricular ectopic activity. Thus prevention of ventricular dilatation by the late restoration of patency of the IRA would be expected to reduce the likelihood of such arrhythmias. Indeed, there is evidence in the dog that myocardial reperfusion is associated with a reduced incidence of late ventricular fibrillation and that this reduction may be independent of myocardial salvage.[60] Similarly, it has been reported that patients who have received thrombolytic therapy and who presumably have a higher incidence of open IRAs have a reduced incidence of late ventricular fibrillation.[61]

Electrophysiologic studies have shown that sustained ventricular tachycardia can be induced much less frequently in patients with AMI who have received thrombolytic therapy. In one series, sustained ventricular arrhythmias could be induced in all 15 patients randomized to treatment with placebo, compared to only 10 of 21 patients randomized to treatment with streptokinase.[62] Saager *et al.* reported in patients with recent anterior wall infarctions that the rate of inducibility was 8% in those who had received thrombolytic therapy compared with 88% in the placebo-treated group[63] (Figure 5.9). By 1 year following implantation of a cardioverter–defibrillator into post-infarct patients with life-threatening arrhythmias, 59% with a closed IRA had experienced automatic firing compared to only 27% with an open IRA.[64] Hii *et al.* reported that a patent IRA was the only independent predictor of response to antiarrhythmic drug therapy during electrophysiologic testing.[65] In a group of survivors of sudden cardiac

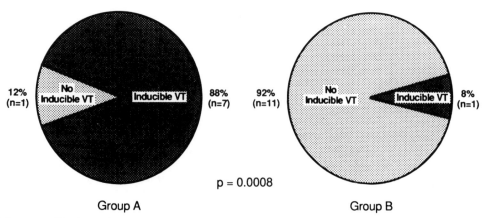

p = 0.0008

Group A   Group B

Figure 5.9 Pie charts showing incidence of ventricular tachycardia (VT) induction by electrophysiologic stimulation in post-AMI patients. Group A, no thrombolytic therapy; group B, thrombolytic therapy. (From Ref. 63.)

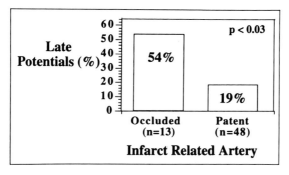

Figure 5.10 The frequency of late potentials was significantly greater in patients with an occluded versus patent infarct-related vessel ($P < 0.03$). (From Ref. 76.)

arrest (likely to include a significant percentage of patients whose arrest was triggered by AMI), late coronary revascularization reduced the incidence of inducible tachyarrhythmias.[66]

Postinfarction patients at increased risk for future arrhythmias may be detected by signal-averaged electrocardiography, which can record late potentials generated by asynchronous conduction through ischemic and/or fibrotic myocardium.[67,68] Approximately one-third of patients with AMI not receiving thrombolytic therapy exhibit late potentials.[69] A closed IRA has been identified as the most powerful independent predictor of late potentials; in one report late potentials were found in 40% and 8% of patients with closed and open IRAs, respectively.[70] Thrombolytic therapy reduces the incidence of late potentials *independently* of LVEF.[71] Among patients receiving thrombolytic therapy the presence of late potentials correlated with persistent occlusion of the IRA[72–76] (Figure 5.10). In one study, multivariate analysis revealed patency of the IRA to be the *only* independent predictor of the absence of late potentials.[77] Steinberg *et al.* found that t-PA treatment 6–12 hours after the onset of symptoms shortened total QRS duration, a powerful predictor of adverse events on signal-averaged electrocardiography.[78] Boehrer *et al.* reported that successful angioplasty of an occluded coronary artery 1–2 weeks after a first MI caused the resolution of signal-averaged electrocardiographic late potentials, while these persisted in conservatively managed patients[79] (Figure 5.11). In patients in whom patency of the IRA was achieved by angioplasty, an average of 12 days after AMI, the *absence* of late potentials was associated with persistently viable myocardium.[80]

The mechanism by which the late achievement of coronary patency reduces late potentials and the propensity for arrhythmias is not clear, but the reduction by an open IRA of ventricular dilatation and ventricular aneurysm, discussed above, may be responsible.

Conclusions

Early restoration of blood flow through the IRA is a major goal in the management of AMI and efforts to shorten the time interval between the onset of clinical manifestations and reperfusion therapy – whether via the administration of a thrombolytic agent or primary angioplasty – should be intensified in order to maximize myocardial salvage. However, as described in this chapter, the late restoration of patency, from 6 hours to several weeks following coronary occlusion, at a time when such restoration is very unlikely to salvage substantial myocardium, may also be beneficial. Thus, the benefits of reperfusion may be twofold (Figure 5.2): (1) time-dependent benefits,[17,81] i.e. myocardial salvage, which

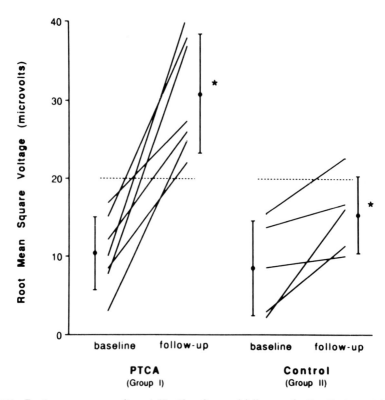

Figure 5.11   Root-mean-square voltage (μV) at baseline and follow-up for 7 patients post AMI who had late angioplasty (group I, left) and 5 not having angioplasty (group II, right). Each line represents data from 1 patient and mean $\pm$ 1 SD is shown on either side of each set of lines. Dotted lines denote lower limit of normal (20 μV). In group I, the root-mean-square voltage increased significantly; at follow-up, it was in the normal range in all 7 patients. In group II, it increased significantly from baseline to follow-up but remained <20 μV in 4 of 5 patients. *$P \leq 0.05$ compared with baseline and the other group at follow-up. PTCA, percutaneous transluminal coronary angioplasty. (From Ref. 79.)

occurs principally in patients in whom reperfusion is achieved during the first 2 or 3 hours following coronary occlusion; and (2) time-independent benefits that result from patency of the IRA. The mechanisms responsible for the latter are not entirely clear but may involve the development of a firmer myocardial scar and a scaffold supplied by the 'erectile force' of a blood-filled coronary vascular bed,[42] both of which limit infarct expansion. Irrespective of the mechanism(s) involved, there is now substantial evidence that the late restoration of blood flow reduces left ventricular dilatation, aneurysm formation, and the proclivity for the development of ventricular tachyarrhythmias. Although there is a growing body of information which suggests that the late restoration of IRA patency is also associated with a better clinical outcome, it must be acknowledged that the evidence for this cannot yet be considered to be definitive.

Myocardial reperfusion is not achieved within the first 6–12 hours in a substantial fraction of patients with AMI. The question of whether or not attempts should be made to achieve late patency in such patients can be resolved only by a prospectively designed randomized trial. Such a trial would require the performance of coronary arteriography sometime after myocardial salvage may be expected to occur, e.g. 6 or 12 hours after the onset of symptoms, followed by randomization of patients with occluded (and perhaps very severely stenotic) IRAs to mechanical revascularization or routine follow-up. Such a trial might be facilitated by the noninvasive detection of failure of reperfusion using serum markers such as creatine kinase isoforms[82] and of reocclusion using sestamibi myocardial perfusion imaging.[83]

Until the results of such a trial are available, late revascularization cannot be recommended on a *routine* basis to post-AMI patients with an occluded IRA. However, given the currently available information it appears appropriate to attempt to identify patients with hibernating myocardium and those in whom ischemia in the territory of the IRA can be induced. If their coronary anatomy is suitable, many such patients with AMI can be expected to benefit from revascularization. It is now agreed that when coronary artery bypass grafting is carried out on patients with chronic ischemic heart disease, the revascularization should be as complete as possible, including the bypass of occluded arteries whenever feasible. Although not without risk and expense, it is likely that a similar approach, i.e. late revascularization of an occluded IRA, even when it occurs after the window for myocardial salvage has closed, will also be found to be beneficial in the treatment of myocardial infarction.

References

1. Cannon, C.P. and Braunwald, E. (1994) GUSTO, TIMI and the case for rapid reperfusion. *Acta Cardiol.*, **49**, 1.
2. Laffel, G.L. and Braunwald, E. (1984) Thrombolytic therapy: A new strategy for the treatment of acute myocardial infarction. *N. Eng. J. Med.*, **311**, 710–17.
3. Gruppo Italiano per lo Studio della Streptochinasi nell'Infarto Miocardico (GISSI) (1986) Effectiveness of intravenous thrombolytic treatment in acute myocardial infarction. *Lancet*, **i**, 397–401.
4. ISIS-2 (Second International Study of Infarct Survival) Collaborative Group (1988) Randomised trial of intravenous streptokinase, oral aspirin, both, or neither among 17 187 cases of suspected acute myocardial infarction: ISIS 2. *Lancet*, **ii**, 349–60.
5. Fibrinolytic Therapy Trialists' (FTT) Collaborative Group (1994) Indications for fibrinolytic therapy in suspected acute myocardial infarction: Collaborative overview of early mortality and major morbidity results from all ransomised trials of more than 1000 patients. *Lancet*, **343**, 311–22.
6. Reimer, K. and Jennings, R.B. (1979) The 'wavefront phenomenon' of myocardial ischemic cell death, II: transmural progression of necrosis within the framework of ischemic bed size (myocardium at risk) and collateral flow. *Lab. Invest.*, **40**, 633–44.
7. Braunwald, E. (1989) Myocardial reperfusion, limitation of infarct size, reduction of left ventricular dysfunction and improved survival: Should the paradigm be expanded? *Circulation*, **79**, 441–4.
8. Van de Werf, F. (1989) Discrepancies between the effects of coronary reperfusion on survival and left ventricular function. *Lancet*, **i**, 1367–9.
9. Califf, R.M., Topol E.J. and Gersh B.J. (1989) From myocardial salvage to patient salvage in acute myocardial infarction: The role of reperfusion therapy. *J. Am. Coll. Cardiol.*, **14**, 1382–8.
10. Kim, C.B. and Braunwald, E. (1993) Potential benefits of late reperfusion of infarcted myocardium: The open artery hypothesis. *Circulation*, **88**, 2426–36.
11. White, H.D., Norris, R.M., Brown, M.A. *et al.* (1987) Effect of intravenous streptokinase on left ventricular function and early survival after acute myocardial infarction. *N. Eng. J. Med.*, **317**, 850–5.
12. Simoons, M.L., Serruys, P.W., Van den brand, M. *et al.* (1986) Early thrombosis in acute myocardial infarction: Limitation of infarct size and improved survival. *J. Am. Coll. Cardiol.*, **7**, 717–28.
13. National Heart Study of Australia, Coronary Thrombolysis Group (1988) Coronary thrombolysis and myocardial salvage by tissue plasminogen activator given up to four hours after onset of myocardial infarction. *Lancet*, **i**, 203–7.
14. Kennedy, J.W., Ritchie, J.L., Davis, K.B. *et al.* (1985) The Western Washington randomized trial of intracoronary streptokinase in acute myocardial infarction; A 12-month follow up report. *N. Eng. J. Med.*, **312**, 1073–8.
15. Meinertz, T., Kasper, W., Schumacher, M., and Just, H. (1988) The German Multicenter Trial of anisoylated plasminogen streptokinase activator complex versus heparin for acute myocardial infarction. *Am. J. Cardiol.*, **62**, 347–51.
16. Dalen, J.E., Gore, J.M., Braunwald, E. *et al.* and the TIMI Investigators (1988) Six- and twelve-month follow of the phase I Thrombolysis in Myocardial Infarction (TIMI) Trial. *Am. J. Cardiol.*, **62**, 179–85.
17. Harrison, J.K., Califf, R.M., Woodlief, L.H. *et al.* and the TAMI Study Group (1993) Systolic left ventricular function after reperfusion therapy for acute myocardial infarction: an analysis of determinants of improvement. *Circulation*, **87**, 1531–41.
18. Jeremy, R.W., Hackworthy, R.A., Bautovich, G. *et al.* (1987) Infarct artery perfusion and changes in left ventricular volume in the month after acute myocardial infarction. *J. Am. Coll. Cardiol.*, **9**, 989–95.
19. Verheugt, F.W.A., Visser, F.C., Van der Wall, E.E. *et al.* (1986) Prediction of spontaneous coronary reperfusion in acute myocardial infarction. *Postgrad. Med. J.*, **62**, 1007–10.

20. Lavie, C.J., O'Keefe, J.H., Chesebro, J.H. *et al.* (1990) Prevention of late ventricular dilatation after acute myocardial infarction by successful thrombolytic reperfusion. *Am. J. Cardiol.*, **66**, 31–46.
21. Topol, E.J., Califf, R.M., Vandormael, M. *et al.* and the Thrombolysis and Angioplasty in Myocardial Infarction-6 Study Group (1992) A randomized trial of late reperfusion for acute myocardial infarction. *Circulation*, **85**, 2090–9.
22. Schroder, R., Neuhaus, K.-L., Linderer, T. *et al.* (1989) Impact of late coronary artery reperfusion on left ventricular function one month after acute myocardial infarction (results from the ISAM Study). *Am. J. Cardiol.*, **64**, 878–84.
23. Leung, W.-H. and Lau, C.-P. (1992) Effects of severity of the residual stenosis of the infarct-related artery coronary artery on left ventricular dilatation and function after acute myocardial infarction. *J. Am. Coll. Cardiol.*, **20**, 307–13.
24. Hirayama, A., Nishidi, K. and Kodama, K. (1992) Prevention of left ventricular dilation without infarct size limitation by late reperfusion in patients with acute myocardial infarction. *Jpn. Circ. J.*, **56** (suppl. 5), 1438–41.
25. Golia, G., Marino, P., Rametta, F. *et al.* (1994) Reperfusion reduces left ventricular dilatation by preventing infarct expansion in the acute and chronic phases of myocardial infarction. *Am. Heart J.*, **127**, 499–509.
26. Nidorf, S.M., Siu, S.C., Galambos, G. *et al.* (1993) Benefit of late coronary reperfusion on ventricular morphology and function after myocardial infarction. *J. Am. Coll. Cardiol.*, **21**, 683–91.
27. Cigarroa, R.G., Lange, R.A. and Hillis, L.D. (1989) Prognosis after acute myocardial infarction in patients with and without residual anterograde coronary blood flow. *Am. J. Cardiol.*, **64**, 155–60.
28. Pfeffer, M.A., Lamas, G.A., Vaughan, D.E. *et al.* (1988) Effects of captopril on progressive ventricular dilatation after anterior myocardial infarction. *N. Eng. J. Med.*, **319**, 80–6.
29. Lamas, G., Flaker, G., Mitchell, G. *et al.* for the SAVE Investigators (1993) Effect of captopril therapy on post MI outcome in patients with and without a patent infarct-related artery (abstract). *J. Am. Coll. Cardiol.*, **21**, 44A.
30. Galvani, M., Ferrini, D., Ottani, D. *et al.* (1992) Prognostic value of infarct artery patency and left ventricular function after Q wave myocardial infarction (abstract). *Circulation*, **86** (suppl. I), I–136.
31. White, H.D., Cross, D.B., Elliott, J.M. *et al.* (1994) Long-term prognostic importance of patency of the infarct-related coronary artery after thrombolytic therapy for acute myocardial infarction. *Circulation*, **89**, 61–7.
32. Ohman, E.M., Califf, R.M., Topol, E.J. *et al.* (1990) Consequences of reocclusion after successful reperfusion therapy in acute myocardial infarction. *Circulation*, **82**, 781–91.
33. LATE Study Group (1993) Late Assessment of Thrombolytic Efficacy (LATE) study with alteplase 6–24 hours after onset of acute myocardial infarction. *Lancet*, **342**, 759–66.
34. EMERAS Collaborative Group (1993) Randomised trial of late thrombolysis in patients with suspected acute myocardial infarction. *Lancet*, **342**, 767–72.
35. Weisman, H.F, Bush, D.E., Mannisi, J.A. *et al.* (1988) Cellular mechanisms of myocardial infarct expansion. *Circulation*, **78**, 186–201.
36. Pfeffer, J.M., Pfeffer, M.A., Fletcher, P.J. and Braunwald, E. (1991) Progressive ventricular remodeling in rat with myocardial infarction. *Am. J. Physiol.*, **260**, H1406–H1414.
37. McKay, R.G., Pfeffer, M.A., Pasternak, R.L. *et al.* (1986) Left ventricular remodeling following myocardial infarction: A corollary to infarct expansion. *Circulation*, **74**, 693–702.
38. Mitchell, G.F., Lamas, G.A., Vaughan, D.E. and Pfeffer, M.A. (1992) Left ventricular remodeling in the year after first anterior myocardial infarction: A quantitative analyis of contractile segment lengths and ventricular shape. *J. Am. Coll. Cardiol.*, **19**, 1136–44.
39. Lamas, G.A., Pfeffer, M.A. and Braunwald, E. (1991) Patency of the infarct-related coronary artery and ventricular geometry. *Am. J. Cardiol.*, **68**, 41D–51D.
40. Pirzada, F.A., Weiner, J.M. and Hood, W.B. Jr. (1978) Experimental myocardial infarction: Accelerated myocardial stiffening related to coronary reperfusion following ischemia. *Chest*, **74**, 190–5.
41. Hammerman, H., Schoen, F.J., Braunwald, E. and Kloner, R.A. (1984) Drug-induced expansion of infarct: Morphologic and functional correlations. *Circulation*, **68**, 446–52.
42. Salisbury, P.F., Cross, C.E. and Rieben, P.A. (1960) Influence of coronary artery pressure upon myocardial elasticity. *Circulation Res.*, **8**, 794–800.
43. Lawrence, W.E., Maughan, W.L. and Kass, D.A. (1992) Mechanism of global functional recovery despite sustained postischemic regional stunning. *Circulation*, **85**, 816–27.
44. Brown, E.J., Swinford, R.D., Gadde, P. and Lillis, O. (1991) Acute effects of delayed reperfusion on infarct shape and left ventricular volume: a potential mechanism of additional benefits from thrombolytic therapy. *J. Am. Coll. Cardiol.*, **17**, 1641–50.
45. Hochman, J.S. and Choo, H. (1987) Limitation of myocardial infarct expansion by reperfusion independent of myocardial salvage. *Circulation*, **75**, 299–306.
46. Hale, S.L. and Kloner, R.A. (1988) Left ventricular topographic alterations in the completely healed rat infarct caused by early and late coronary artery reperfusion. *Am. Heart J.*, **116**, 1508–13.
47. Althaus, U., Gunther, H.P., Baur, H. *et al.* (1977) Consequences of myocardial reperfusion following temporary coronary occlusion in pigs: Effects on morphologic, biochemical and hemodynamic findings. *Eur. J. Clin. Invest.*, **7**, 437–43.
48. Marino, P., Destro, G., Barbieri, E. and Bicego, D. (1992) Reperfusion of the infarct-related coronary artery limits left ventricular expansion beyond myocardial salvage. *Am. Heart J.*, **123**, 1157–65.
49. Meizlish, J.L., Berger, H.J., Plankey, M. *et al.* (1984) Functional left ventricular aneurysm formation after acute anterior transmural myocardial infarction: incidence, natural history and prognostic implication. *N. Eng. J. Med.*, **311**, 1001–6.

50. Forman, M.B., Collins, H.W., Kopelman, H.A. *et al.* (1986) Determinants of left ventricular aneurysm formation after acute myocardial infarction: A clinical and angiographic study. *J. Am. Coll. Cardiol.*, **8**, 1256–62.

51. Visser, C.A., Kan, G., Meltzer, R.S. *et al.* (1986) Incidence, timing and prognostic value of left ventricular aneurysm formation after myocardial infarction: A prospective, serial echocardiographic study of 158 patients. *Am. J. Cardiol.*, **57**, 729–32.

52. Hirai, T., Fujita, M., Nakajima, H. *et al.* (1989) Importance of collateral circulation for prevention of left ventricular aneurysm formation. *Circulation*, **79**, 791–6.

53. Levy, W.C., Cerqueria, M.D., Litwin, P.E. *et al.* and the MITI investigators (1992) A patent infarct related artery improves diastolic filling after thrombolytic therapy: Myocardial Infarction Triage and Intervention (MITI) Trial (abstract). *Circulation*, **86** (suppl. I), I-455.

54. Rahimtoola, S.H. (1989) The hibernating myocardium. *Am. Heart J.*, **117**, 211–21.

55. Braunwald, E. and Rutherford, J.D. (1986) Reversible ischemic left ventricular dysfunction: Evidence for the 'hibernating myocardium'. *J. Am. Coll. Cardiol.*, **8**, 1467–70.

56. Montalescot, G., Faraggi, M., Drobinski, G. *et al.* (1992) Myocardial viability in patients with Q wave myocardial infarction and no residual ischemia. *Circulation*, **86**, 47–55.

57. Sabia, P.J., Powers, E.R., Ragosta, M. *et al.* (1992) An association between collateral blood flow and myocardial viability in patients with recent myocardial infarction. *N. Eng. J. Med.*, **327**, 1825–31.

58. Calkins, H., Maughan, W.L., Weisman, H.F. *et al.* (1989) Effect of acute volume load on refractoriness and arrhythmia development in isolated, chronically infarcted canine hearts. *Circulation*, **79**, 687–97.

59. Zaman, A.G., Morris, J.L., Smylie, J.H. and Cowan, J.C. (1993) Late potentials and ventricular enlargement after myocardial infarction. *Circulation*, **88**, 905–14.

60. Arnold, J.M.O., Antman, E.M., Przyklenk, K. *et al.* (1987) Differential effects of reperfusion on incidence of ventricular arrhythmias and recovery of ventricular function at 4 days following coronary occlusion. *Am. Heart J.*, **113**, 1055–65.

61. Schroder, R. (1988) Ventricular fibrillation complicating myocardial infarction (letter). *N. Engl. J. Med.*, **318**, 381–2.

62. Kersschot, I.E., Brugada, P., Ramentol, M. *et al.* (1986) Effects of early reperfusion in acute myocardial infarction on arrhythmias induced by programmed stimulation: a prospective, randomized study. *J. Am. Coll. Cardiol.*, **7**, 1234–42.

63. Sager, P.T., Perlmutter, R.A., Rosenfeld, L.E. *et al.* (1988) Electrophysiologic effects of thrombolytic therapy in patients with a transmural anterior myocardial infarction complicated by left ventricular aneurysm formation. *J. Am. Coll. Cardiol.*, **12**, 19–24.

64. Horvitz, L.L., Pietrolungo, J.F., Suri, R.S. *et al.* (1992) An open infarct-related artery is associated with a lower risk of lethal ventricular arrhythmias in patients with a left ventricular aneurysm. *Circulation*, **86** (suppl. I), I-315.

65. Hii, J.T.Y., Traboulsi, M., Mitchell, L.B. *et al.* (1993) Infarct artery patency predicts outcome of serial electropharmacological studies in patients with malignant ventricular arrhythmias. *Circulation*, **87**, 764–72.

66. Kelly, P., Ruskin, J.N., Vlahakes, G.J. *et al.* (1990) Surgical coronary revascularization in survivors of prehospital cardiac arrest: Its effect on inducible ventricular arrhythmias and long-term survival. *J. Am. Coll. Cardiol.*, **15**, 267–73.

67. McClements, B.M. and Adgey, A.A.J. (1993) Value of signal-averaged electrocardiography, radionuclide ventriculography, Holter monitoring and clinical variables for prediction of arrhythmic events in survivors of acute myocardial infarction in the thrombolytic era. *J. Am. Coll. Cardiol.*, **21**, 1419–27.

68. Gomes, J.A., Mehra, R., Barreaca, P. *et al.* (1985) Quantitative analysis of the high-frequency components of the signal-averaged QRS complex in patients with acute myocardial infarction: a prospective study. *Circulation*, **72**, 105–11.

69. Kuchar, D.L., Thorburn, C.W. and Sammel, N.L. (1986) Late potentials detected after myocardial infarction: natural history and prognostic significance. *Circulation*, **74**, 1280–9.

70. Lange, R.A., Cigarroa, R.G., Wells, P.J. *et al.* (1990) Influence of anterograde flow in the infarct artery on the incidence of late potentials after acute myocardial infarction. *Am. J. Cardiol.*, **65**, 554–8.

71. Zimmerman, M., Adamec, R. and Ciaroni, S. (1991) Reduction in the frequency of ventricular late potentials after acute myocardial infarction by early thrombolytic therapy. *Am. J. Cardiol.*, **67**, 697–703.

72. Vatterott, P.J., Hammill, S.C., Bailey, K.R. *et al.* (1991) Late potentials on signal-averaged electrocardiograms and patency of the infarct-related artery in survivors of acute myocardial infarction. *J. Am. Coll. Cardiol.*, **17**, 330–7.

73. Gang, E.S., Lew, A.S., Hong, M. *et al.* (1989) Decreased incidence of ventricular late potentials after successful thrombolytic therapy for acute myocardial infarction. *N. Engl. J. Med.*, **321**, 712–16.

74. Eldar, M., Leor, J., Hod, H. *et al.* (1990) Effect of thrombolysis on the evolution of late potentials within 10 days of infarction. *Br. Heart J.*, **63**, 273–6.

75. McClements, B., Trouton, T.G. and Mackenzie, G. (1991) Which factors determine the development of late potentials after first myocardial infarction? A multifactorial analysis. *PACE*, **14**, 1998–2003.

76. Aguirre, F.V., Kern, M.J., Hsia, J. *et al.* (1991) Importance of myocardial infarct artery patency on the prevalence of ventricular arrhythmias and late potentials after thrombolysis in acute myocardial infarction. *Am. J. Cardiol.*, **68**, 1410–16.

77. Pedretti, R., Laporta, A., Etro, M.D. *et al.* (1992) Influence of thrombolysis on signal averaged electrocardiogram and late arrhythmic events after acute myocardial infarction. *Am. J. Cardiol.*, **69**, 866–72.

78. Steinberg, J.S., Hochman, J.S., Morgan, C.D. *et al.* and LATE Ancillary Investigators (1993) The effects of thrombolytic therapy administered 6–24 hours after myocardial infarction on the signal-averaged ECG: Results of a multicenter randomized trial (abstract). *J. Am. Coll. Cardiol.*, **21**, 225A.

79. Boehrer, J.D., Glamman, B., Lange, R.A. *et al.* (1992) Effect of coronary angioplasty on late potentials one to two weeks after acute myocardial infarction. *Am. J. Cardiol.*, **70**, 1515–19.

80. Ragosta, M., Sabia, P.J., Kaul, S. *et al.* (1993) Effects of late (1 to 30 days) reperfusion after acute myocardial infarction on signal-averaged electrocardiogram. *Am. J. Cardiol.*, **71**, 19–23.
81. Lincoff, A.M. and Topol, E.J. (1993) Illusion of reperfusion: Does anyone achieve optimal reperfusion during acute myocardial infarction? *Circulation*, **87**, 1792–805.
82. Devries, S.R., Sobel, B.E. and Abendschein, D.R. (1986) Early detection of myocardial reperfusion assay of plasma MM-creatine kinase isoforms in dogs. *Circulation*, **74**, 567–72.
83. Wackers, F.J., Gibbons, R.J., Verani M.S. *et al.* (1989) Serial quantitative planar technetium-99 m isonitrile imaging in acute myocardial infarction: efficacy for non-invasive assessment of thrombolytic therapy. *J. Am. Coll. Cardiol.*, **14**, 861–73.

6

Aspirin and Anticoagulants

B. J. Meyer and J. H. Chesebro

The aim of thrombolysis is rapid reperfusion of the infarct-related coronary artery, prevention of reocclusion, salvage of ischemic myocardium, improvement of left ventricular function, and reduction of cardiac mortality. The rationale for antithrombotic (including antiplatelet) therapy in acute myocardial infarction will be reviewed with the clinical studies of treatment with or without thrombolysis, and the role of antithrombotic therapy in the prevention of arterial and venous thromboembolism.

Pathogenesis of Acute Coronary Syndromes

It is important to understand the pathogenesis of acute coronary syndromes to design optimal antithrombotic therapy. The major mechanism initiating thrombosis in acute coronary syndromes is disruption of atherosclerotic plaque. Apical left ventricular infarction and dysfunction relates to thromboembolism in peripheral arteries to the lower extremities and the brain even in patients with stable atherosclerotic disease. The population over age 60 years has a higher incidence of thromboembolic events involving the coronary and peripheral arteries which total more that 4% per year (fatal or non-fatal myocardial infarction or stroke).

Disruption of Atherosclerotic Plaques

Disruption of athrosclerotic plaques (deep or type III arterial injury) is the major cause of mural or occlusive thrombosis of coronary arteries leading to the acute coronary syndromes.[1,2] A lesser proportion of myocardial infarctions (approximately one-quarter) involve distal or branch coronary arteries and do not appear to involve plaque disruption but rather are associated with formation of thrombus within a high-grade stenosis associated with endothelial denudation (type II or mild arterial injury).[1–5] Type I injury is endothelial dysfunction which is associated with abnormal vasomotion.[3,4]

Events preceding plaque disruption and development of coronary stenoses involve lipid incorporation into the arterial wall, with the secondary attraction of circulation monocytes that become macrophages, engulf lipid and become foam cells (along with smooth muscle cells). Lesions at risk consist of intracellular and extracellular lipid in a pool which is covered by a fibrous cap. Macrophages within the fibrous cap probably contribute to degradation and thinning of the fibrous cap to a delicate lattice-work of collagen, which is prone to disruption. Immunohistochemical staining of a torn fibrous

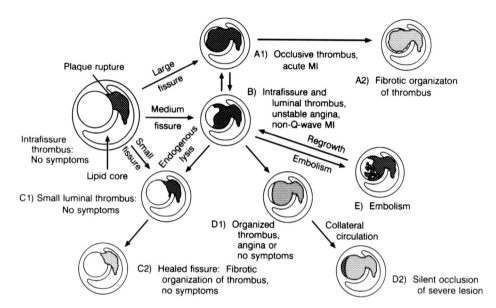

Figure 6.1 Diagram showing major pathogenic modes of progression of coronary disease. Plaque rupture leads to formation of a fissure with flowing blood contacting intraarterial structures and forming an intrafissure thrombus. This may not progress or lead to symptoms (except for possible sudden onset of coronary spasm or vasoconstriction associated with arterial injury). The fissure may be small, medium, or large and may progress immediately to various degrees of luminal obstruction (A1, B, or C1). Sudden progression with a large fissure may be to occlusive thrombus and acute myocardial infarction (MI), A1. Fibrotic organization of the thrombus may occur (A2) or thrombolysis (exogenous or endogenous) may occur and reopen the lumen to partial obstruction (B). A medium-sized fissure may lead to immediate partial obstruction associated with unstable angina or non-Q-wave MI (B); this may progress to total occlusion (A1), partial embolization of thrombus (E), fibrotic organization of thrombus (D1), endogenous lysis to a small thrombus (C1), or no intraluminal thrombus. Residual thrombus may undergo fibrotic or fibromuscular organization (A2, C2 and D1). A severe residual stenosis (D1) may be associated with good collateral circulation and no symptoms. Because of very low antegrade flow and type II injury (endothelial denudation only) but no deep injury, this may silently occlude with a fresh thrombus (D2). A small fissure may lead to a small thrombus without symptoms (C1) and undergo fibrotic organization with progression of disease in the absence of symptoms (C2). (With permission from Ref. 6.)

cap after plaque disruption shows macrophages interspersed within the delicate lattice-work of collagen. Disruption is more often at the margin of attachment of the fibrous cap. This results in fissuring into the plaque with some dissection of blood into the cavity of the lipid pool. Contact of flowing blood with deep arterial structures initiates formation of a platelet-rich thrombus, which is strongly anchored and extends into the arterial lumen. This luminal extension may partially or totally obstruct blood flow.[1-5]

Most plaque disruptions cause minor obstruction to blood flow, result in no symtoms, but appear to contribute to the progression of coronary atherosclerotic disease (Figure 6.1, C). Other mural extensions of thrombus may partially obstruct blood flow and lead to distal ischemia with unstable angina (Figure 6.1, B). Portions of this thrombus may embolize (Figure 6.1, E) and lead to distal microinfarction. Even larger plaque disruptions with formation of larger or longer fissures may lead to larger thrombi which totally occlude the artery causing acute myocardial infarction (Figure 6.1, A1). Mural thrombosis may progress to total occlusion depending upon local and systemic factors and antith-rombotic therapy. Vasoconstriction may also contribute to arterial obstruction and is endothelium dependent (dysfunction or denudation) and platelet dependent.

Local and Systemic Factors in Thrombosis: Role of Thrombin

Local factors for thrombosis include the substrates in the arterial wall and rheologic conditions of blood flow. Deep (type III) arterial injury extends into the tunica media (below the internal elastic lamina) or into the intimal plaque. Substrates in the media and intimal plaque are similar but are often more extensive in plaque (tissue thromboplastin, lipids). Local substrates lead to visible mural thrombus within the arterial lumen. Platelet-rich thrombus covers the entire length of the luminal deep injury. Mild (type II) injury is associated with less thrombogenic substrates and in the absence of a high-grade stenosis leads to only a single layer of platelets or less.[3,4,6]

Injury and arterial wall substrates

Deep injury exposes collagen types I and III which are very thrombogenic.[7,8] By contrast, mild injury exposes collagen types IV and V, which are considerably less thrombogenic and are probably a major reason why only a single layer of platelets forms with mild injury and no stenosis. Lipid in the arterial wall, often in the form of oxidized products, markedly enhances thrombogenicity in part through attraction of macrophages, which produce thromboplastin or stimulate smooth muscle cells to do the same.[8A] In the normal artery, tissue thromboplastin is present in the adventitia but not in the media. Injury to smooth muscle cells and atherosclerotic plaque both stimulate synthesis of tissue thromboplastin in the arterial wall. This tissue thromboplastin stimulates coagulation and thrombin generation.

Normal endothelium protects against thrombosis. Arterial injury destroys the source of this protection. Prostacyclin and endothelium-derived relaxing factor are synthesized by the endothelium and by structures adjacent to the arterial lumen. Local release of both of these substances protects against platelet deposition.[3,4,6]

The matrix of the arterial wall binds α-thrombin, which stimulates platelet and fibrinogen deposition. At least eight to ten times more thrombin appears to be present after deep compared with mild arterial injury as determined by the amount of hirudin (a specific thrombin inhibitor) necessary to totally prevent macroscopic thrombus. In addition, immunohistochemical staining of thrombus adjacent to deep injury is markedly positive for thrombin whereas thrombus adjacent to mild injury stains negative for thrombin.[6] The pivotal role of thrombin after deep arterial injury is documented by the complete inhibition of thrombus by the specific thrombin inhibitor hirudin (which does not inhibit platelet aggregation to thromboxane A$_2$ (TXA$_2$) serotonin, adenosine diphosphate (ADP) or epinephrine).[9,10] Specific receptor inhibitors to TXA$_2$ serotonin, or both do not prevent macroscopic thrombus after deep arterial injury.[6]

Rheology

Rheologic conditions of blood flow also significantly affect platelet and fibrinogen deposition. Shear force is the difference in the cell or fluid velocity at the center of the arterial lumen compared with the periphery and is directly related to flow velocity and inversely to the third power of the lumen diameter. Platelet and fibrinogen deposition increase directly with the shear force. Thus small- and high-flow arteries (e.g. coronary arteries) form more thrombus after deep injury than large arteries with lower shear (carotids, iliac, or aorta). With high shear force, red cells force platelets to the periphery and enhance their deposition. ADP also appears to increase at the cell surface in the presence of high shear forces. After mild injury platelet deposition remains low and reaches a plateau as shear force increases. There may be a transient increase in deposition beyond a single layer, but additional platelets are easily washed away because they are poorly anchored in the presence of mild injury.[3,4,11,12]

After deep injury, platelet deposition increases directly with the severity of stenosis. The greatest platelet deposition is where the luminal diameter of the stenosis is narrowest. Unpublished data from our laboratory shows that the greatest fibrinogen/ fibrin deposition is also associated with greater shear force and stenosis and occurs maximally on the initial layers of thrombus that overly the deep injury, which is consistent with the higher concentration of thrombin observed in thrombus adjacent to deeply injured artery. Distal to a stenosis, relatively more fibrin and red cells compared to platelets are deposited. With angioscopy, a retrograde view distal to a stenosis shows the poststenotic reddish-colored thrombus,[12A] whereas a proximal view looking into the stenosis shows a whitish or platelet-rich thrombus.[11,13] With deep injury and especially in the presence of a stenosis, rapid growth of platelet deposition may suddenly decrease as partial embolization occurs; very rapid regrowth is consistent with accelerated thrombosis due to the high thrombogenicity of residual thrombus and increasing shear force as thrombus formation occurs.[3,4]

Role of thrombin

The pivotal role of thrombin in the formation of platelet-rich arterial thrombus is supported by several studies. Thrombin stimulates platelet aggregation at considerably lower concentrations than those required for conversion of fibrinogen to fibrin.[14] In flowing blood thrombin reaches platelet-stimulating concentrations faster than the TXA_2 analog U-46619.[15] In disseminated intravascular coagulation (a model of thrombosis without significant arterial injury) platelet thrombi are more sensitive to formation by thrombin than fibrin thrombi, since it takes a five times higher plasma level of hirudin (a specific thrombin inhibitor) to inhibit formation of platelet aggregates compared to fibrin thrombi in flowing blood in the pulmonary circulation.[16]

Specific thrombin inhibition with hirudin completely blocks platelet-rich thrombus formation *in vivo* after deep arterial injury.[9,10] Hirudin forms a 1:1 complex with thrombin. Thus the plasma concentration of hirudin required to totally block thrombus formation *in vivo* is proportional to the amount of thrombin generated in each animal model of thrombosis. After deep arterial injury, eight to ten times higher blood levels of hirudin are required compared to other thrombotic stimuli (mild injury, venous thrombosis, AV shunt model). Immunohistochemical staining also documents the increased thrombin associated with deep injury compared with mild injury.[6]

Thrombin generation is accelerated 278 000 times by the formation of an activator complex (prothrombinase complex), which is formed by the assembly of factors X_a and V_a and the Ca^{2+} ion on a lipid membrane (Figure 6.2). The lipid membrane may be the platelet, smooth muscle cell, or other cellular membranes. Thrombin also activates factor V to V_a, which also enhances thrombin generation. In addition to activating platelets, thrombin converts fibrinogen to fibrin, activates factor $XIII–XIII_a$, which cross-links fibrin to stabilize the thrombus, and activates protein C, which in turn inhibits thrombin activation of factor V to V_a and factor VIII to VIII_a. The activation of protein C appears to serve as an auto-feedback control for thrombin generation.

Systemic factors

Arterial thrombosis is also modulated by systemic factors, which usually increase but may decrease thrombus formation. Epinephrine infusion as well as high serum cholesterol levels enhance platelet deposition. High levels of factor VII and fibrinogen are also associated with enhanced thrombotic risk.[17]

Because of the dynamic and simultaneous processes of thrombosis and thrombolysis, factors that decrease fibrinolysis (such as lipoprotein Lp(a)) appear to enhance thrombosis. There is homology of Lp(a) with plasminogen. Thus increased levels of Lp(a) appear to decrease endogenous thrombolysis with a net result of enhancing thrombosis.[18] High

PLATELETS AND COAGULATION

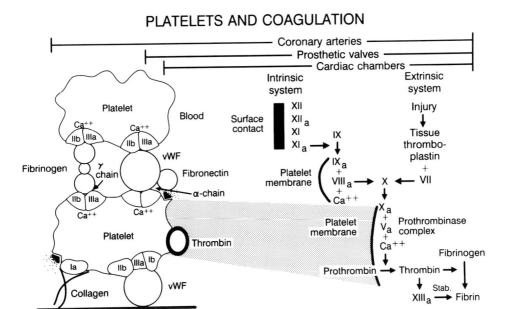

Figure 6.2 Diagram showing biochemical interactions between platelet membrane receptors, vessel wall, and adhesive macromolecules during platelet adhesion and aggregation (left). Also depicted are the intrinsic and extrinsic systems of the coagulation cascade and their interaction with platelet or other cellular membranes, such as the prothrombinase complex, the activator complex for thrombin generation. Coronary thrombosis is associated with coagulation processes that amplify thrombin generation. Thrombin is the primary and major activator of platelets and converts fibrinogen to fibrin. Ca^{2+}, calcium ion; vWF, von Willebrand factor; Ia, glycoprotein Ia; Ib, glycoprotein Ib; IIb/IIIa, glycoprotein IIb/IIIa, Stab., stabilization by cross-linking fibrin. (From Ref. 6 with permission.)

levels of plasminogen activator inhibitor type I (PAI-1) are found in platelets, which serve as the major source of plasma PAI-1. Platelet PAI-1 probably contributes to the resistance of platelet-rich thrombus to thrombolysis compared to a fibrin-rich thrombus.[19] Inhibition of fibrinolysis with aprotinin during aorta–coronary bypass reoperation increased the incidence of thrombosis, myocardial infarction, and death.[20]

Lipoprotein-associated coagulation inhibitor (LACI) is naturally found in animals and humans and interferes with coagulation early in the cascade. LACI inhibits the interaction of tissue factor with factor VII for the activation of factor X to X_a. Thus it is a major systemic factor that may reduce thrombosis. Blood levels of LACI can be measured and are enhanced by heparin. LACI is present in a free and bound state and is highly bound to high-density lipoprotein cholesterol.[21]

Residual Thrombus: the Most Thrombogenic Substrate

Residual thrombus is more thrombogenic than deeply injured arterial wall. In addition, a high-grade stenosis greatly enhances platelet deposition onto residual thrombus. Without a stenosis platelet deposition is doubled on residual thrombus compared to a deeply injured artery. With an 80% stenosis, platelet deposition is increased three to four times on residual thrombus compared to deeply injured artery.[22] Reasons for the enhanced thrombogenicity of residual thrombus are summarized in Figure 6.3.

The high thrombogenicity of residual thrombus and its relative resistance to heparin can be explained by the binding of active thrombin to fibrin and the generation during thrombosis of more thrombin and natural inhibitors to the action of heparin. The binding of fibrin to thrombin masks receptors on thrombin to antithrombin III (AT III) and heparin cofactor II; this markedly diminishes the effectiveness of heparin.[24] In addition, the activation of platelets by thrombin releases platelet factor 4, which is an antiheparin substance. Thrombin converts fibrinogen to fibrin and in the process generates fibrin monomer II, which also interferes with heparin–AT III action against thrombin. Thrombin also may increase its own generation by the activation of factor V to V_a, which is a necessary component of the prothrombinase or activator complex. In addition, binding of factor X_a within the prothrombinase complex to the lipid membrane protects factor X_a from inhibition by heparin–AT III. To further enhance thrombosis, thrombin activates factor XIII–XIII$_a$ which cross-links fibrin and stabilizes the thrombus.[25]

Vasoconstriction after Arterial Injury

Acute arterial injury is associated with acute vasoconstriction.[26,27] This vasoconstriction is both platelet dependent and endothelium dependent and is reduced by nitroglycerin or aspirin.[26–29]

The severity of vasoconstriction is directly related to the log of the number of platelets deposited at the site of arterial injury. Aspirin reduces platelet deposition and vasoconstriction but does not eliminate either one. Thrombin also appears to enhance vasoconstriction because it stimulates release of endothelin, a potent vasoconstrictor.[30] Vasoconstriction is also associated with angioplasty in pigs and humans and can be reduced by the infusion of intravenous nitroglycerin.[27,31] This vasoconstriction associated with angioplasty occurred despite routine use of oral calcium antagonists.[31]

Vasoconstriction is also endothelium dependent. Acute endothelial denudation without severe injury or stretch of the artery causes acetylcholine-induced vasoconstriction

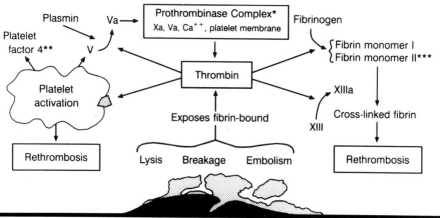

*Protects Xa from heparin-antithrombin III
**Neutralizes heparin
***Inhibits heparin-antithrombin III interaction with thrombin

Figure 6.3 Disturbance of thrombus by lysis (endogenous or exogenous), mechanical breakage (including coronary angioplasty), or spontaneous embolism exposes thrombin bound to fibrin. Thrombin activates platelets, activates factor V to V_a (which leads to generation of more thrombin via the prothrombinase complex), converts fibrinogen to fibrin I and fibrin II, and activates factor XIII to XIII$_a$ (which cross-links fibrin). These processes combine to produce rethrombosis. Heparin may only partially prevent rethrombosis because factor X_a within the prothrombinase complex is protected from heparin–antithrombin III, platelet factor 4 neutralizes heparin, and fibrin monomer II inhibits heparin–antithrombin III. See text for details. (From Ref. 23 with permission.)

only in the region of denudation and not in a distal uninjured region of the same coronary artery.[28] After partial regrowth of endothelium at 4 days in the pig, acetylcholine-induced vasoconstriction persists. Complete endothelial regrowth at 7 days is associated with loss of acetylcholine-induced vasoconstriction.[29] Thus segmental endothelial denudation can lead to segmental vasoconstriction.

Modest elevation of serum cholesterol for 4 months in pigs leads to diffuse acetylcholine-induced vasoconstriction in porcine coronary arteries. This cholesterol feeding is associated with type I injury (endothelial dysfunction without denudation).[32] Four months after stopping cholesterol, there was partial recovery suggesting that a longer term recovery may be necessary. Cholesterol feeding in these pigs is associated with endothelin production in the arterial wall.[33]

Local shear forces may be increased by arterial vasoconstriction and thus may promote platelet deposition and thrombus formation. Vasodilatation with nitroglycerin directly vasodilates and reduces shear force. Nitroglycerin may also indirectly reduce vasoconstriction, because nitroglycerin also directly reduces platelet deposition after deep injury in pigs.[27] Platelet aggregation studies during nitroglycerin infusion in humans suggest that there may be a direct effect against platelet deposition in patients.[34]

Rationale for Antithrombotic Therapy During and After Thrombolysis

Importance of Thorough Lysis

Early administration of thrombolytic agents recanalizes the occluded coronary artery and provides the basis for salvage of ischemic myocardium, reduction of infarct size, preservation of myocardial function, and reduction of early and late mortality in acute myocardial infarction.[35] The hypothesis, that this treatment prompts reperfusion to *normal* flow, preserves myocardium and reduces mortality, has been proven in the angiographic substudy of the GUSTO trial.[36] This study showed that more rapid and complete restoration to *normal* (TIMI grade 3) coronary flow in the infarct-related artery within 90 min of treatment by any lytic strategy (including heparin plus aspirin in all strategies) improved ventricular function and maximally lowered mortality. If at 90 min TIMI grade 3 or normal flow was established, 30-day mortality was 4.4%. For TIMI grade 2 flow, mortality was 7.4%, and for no flow (TIMI grade 0 or 1) mortality was 8.9% (vs 5.7% for any patency, TIMI grade 2 or 3).

Thus the most rational treatment of patients with acute myocardial infarction is thrombolytic therapy with strategies that produce early and sustained coronary artery recanalization with a net clinical benefit over adverse effects. Although the reocclusion rates in this landmark trial were very low (4.9–6.4%), the search for optimal reperfusion strategies (lytic plus antithrombotic agents) continues because major deficiencies remain. Even with the best reperfusion strategy (accelerated recombinant tissue-type plasminogen activator (rt-PA) plus heparin and aspirin) only 54% of patients have TIMI grade 3 (normal) flow of the infarct-related artery at 90 min.

Optimal reperfusion may be limited by insufficiently early or rapid recanalization, incomplete patency (TIMI flow grade 2 or critical residual coronary stenosis[37,38]), inadequate myocardial perfusion despite coronary patency, intermittent coronary patency, and reocclusion. The reported incidences of reocclusion have varied widely due in part to differences in treatment regimens (choice or combination of thrombolytic agents, dose and route of heparin therapy, treatment with aspirin) as well as to inconsistencies in methods of assessment of reperfusion (timing and incidence of angiographic follow-up). In general, treatment with the fibrin-selective agent rt-PA appears to be associated with higher rates of reperfusion at 90 min and reocclusion than the nonselective agents streptokinase, urokinase, or anistreplase.[39–42] Because accelerated administration of rt-PA has been shown to produce the highest infarct-related artery patency at 90 min (of all the thrombolytic strategies), the incidence of reocclusion with this drug regimen is most pertinent to the consideration of optimal reperfusion. In six published studies in which rt-PA was used in conjunction with both aspirin and intravenous heparin[36,39–43] the mean reocclusion rate among more than 2900 patients ranged from 5.7% (GUSTO) to 20%. The occurrence of reocclusion or recurrent ischemic events remains largely unpredictable (from analysis of 174 patients treated with rt-PA) from quantitative or morphologic characteristics of the infarct-related artery assessed during acute coronary angiography.[44] However, reocclusion and recurrent ischemic events are inversely related to adequacy of heparin therapy as measured by the activated partial thromboplastin time (aPTT).[45,46]

Further deterioration of infarct-vessel patency occurs during the period after hospital discharge. Coronary angiography performed at 3–6 months after thrombolytic therapy during the TAMI-6 and the APRICOT (Antithrombotics in the Prevention of Reocclusion in Coronary Thrombolysis) trials demonstrated late reocclusion of 25–40% of previously patent infarct-related arteries.[47,48]

It is likely that thrombotic reocclusion is mediated primarily by the interaction of residual thrombus, blood flow rheology, and hematologic factors, including activated and unactivated platelet aggregates, fibrin-bound and fibrin-split-product-bound thrombin, continued thrombin generation, systemic factors, and unhealed disrupted plaque.[22,49–52]

Evidence for Increased Procoagulant Activity During Thrombolysis

There is now extensive evidence that thrombosis occurs simultaneously with endogenous and exogenous thrombolysis. Even during administration of the fibrinolytic agent, episodes of transient reperfusion followed by reocclusion often precede sustained coronary reperfusion.[53] Thus, the apparent failure to achieve sustained reperfusion may reflect the early or almost immediate recurrence of thrombosis. Active thrombin bound to fibrin and *in situ* fibrin degradation have been demonstrated within pathologic thrombi by immunohistochemical stains.[54] Residual mural thrombus after thrombolysis has a highly active surface, largely due to fibrin-bound thrombin with retained catalytic activity; this surface is even more thrombogenic than deeply injured arterial wall.[22] In addition, plasmin generated during thrombolysis acts on factor V to produce proteolytic fragments with procoagulant activity,[55] and activates factor V to V_a, which contributes to accelerated thrombin generation via the prothrombinase complex as discussed earlier (Figure 6.3). Heparin is effective in inhibiting the procoagulant activity induced by plasmin, but concentrations higher than those typically achieved during intravenous therapy are required.[56]

Platelet activation during thrombolysis with streptokinase or rt-PA leads to the generation of TXA_2, which induces platelet aggregation and vasoconstriction; metabolites of TXA_2 have been detected in plasma and urine in experimental and clinical studies.[57,58] Streptokinase may also induce antibodies that aggregate platelets.[59]

Markers of activated coagulation indicating thrombin activity and generation can be detected in the plasma and include fibrinopeptide A, which is released with the conversion of fibrinogen to fibrin, and thrombin–AT III (TAT). Elevated levels occur with unstable angina and acute myocardial infarction[52] and are increased during both streptokinase and rt-PA infusions. Fibrinopeptide A decreases after the infusion[60,61] or with the coadministration of adequate levels of heparin.[62,63] Levels of thrombin–AT III, a measure of thrombin generation, increased 15 min after infusion of rt-PA or a combination or urokinase and prourokinase.[64] Patients with persistently elevated levels of thrombin–AT III at 120 min were more likely to have angiographic reocclusion 24–36 hours later.[65]

Additonal *in vivo* data show that thrombosis and thrombolysis are simultaneous dynamic processes. Antithrombotic therapy enhances thrombolysis and reduces reocclusion. Effective therapy in animal models includes heparin at high therapeutic concentrations (200–300 u kg^{-1}),[66,67] specific thrombin inhibitors,[68–70] platelet glycoprotein IIb/IIIa receptor inhibitors,[71–75] and TXA$_2$-receptor and serotonin-receptor antagonists (in a mild injury model).[72,76,77] The effectiveness of these agents appears decreased and requires higher doses or combined agents in the presence of deep arterial injury, where platelet deposition and thrombin generation are greater and thrombosis more intense. For example, thrombolytic agents are less effective with platelet-rich thrombi, and platelet glycoprotein IIb/IIIa receptor inhibitors prevent reocclusion in a mild injury model but require adjuvant heparin to prevent reocclusion with deep injury. Only specific thrombin inhibition has been effective alone at preventing mural thrombosis in deep injury.[70] Thrombin inhibition with recombinant-hirudin and other specific thrombin inhibitors accelerates lysis with rt-PA and markedly reduces residual thrombus after thrombolysis compared with conjunctive treatment with heparin or aspirin.[78,78A]

Antithrombotic Therapy During Acute Myocardial Infarction

Aspirin With and Without Thrombolytic Therapy

Thrombolysis produces marked platelet activation.[57,58] Possible mechanisms for this include exposure of thrombin bound to fibrin on the surface of the thrombus, formation of plasmin, or indirect mechanisms through stimulation of other procoagulant systems on the surface of the thrombus. Thrombin binds to receptors on the platelet surface where it activates platelets and stimulates the release of ADP, serotonin, platelet activating factor, and the synthesis and release of TXA$_2$. The platelet agonists, thrombin, ADP and TXA$_2$, bind to their specific receptors on the platelet surface and trigger a series of intracellular biochemical events that culminate in the exposure of a glycoprotein receptor (GP IIb/IIIa) on the platelet surface. Plasma fibrinogen (and von Willebrand factor), a bivalent ligand, binds to GP IIb/IIIa receptor on the surface of adjacent platelets and links them together as platelet aggregates.[79]

Aspirin inhibits platelet aggregation by irreversibly inhibiting the enzyme cyclooxygenase. Cyclooxygenase is responsible for the conversion of arachidonic acid to TXA$_2$ in the platelet, and in vascular wall cells it is responsible for the conversion of arachidonic acid to prostacyclin (PGI$_2$). TXA$_2$ induces platelet aggregation and vasoconstriction while PGI$_2$ inhibits platelet aggregation and induces vasodilatation. Aspirin is effective at potentiating thrombolysis in a canine model of coronary thrombosis but not in a porcine model of deep arterial injury.

Aspirin, if given in oral or intravenous loading doses of at least 2 mg kg^{-1} (i.e. 160 mg in an 80 kg patient) produces a rapid clinical antithrombotic effect due to immediate and near-total inhibition of TXA$_2$ production. Lower doses (e.g. 40–80 mg) take a few days before they develop their full antiplatelet effect.[80,81] Doses less than 80 mg may not be reliably absorbed in all patients. The ISIS-II study,[82] in 17 000 patients with suspected acute myocardial infarction (prolonged chest pain with or without ECG changes), clearly confirms the clinical efficacy of aspirin alone (160 mg daily) or in combination with streptokinase. The major endpoint, 5-week vascular mortality, was reduced 23% by aspirin alone, 25% by streptokinase alone, and 42% by combined streptokinase and aspirin, compared with placebo. The benefit on mortality persisted after a median follow-up of 15 months and for at least 4 years.[83] The in-hospital reinfarction rate was 3.8% in patients who received streptokinase alone compared with 2.9% in those given placebo.

Table 6.1 Reocclusion rate and recurrent ischemia after thrombolysis in patients treated with or without aspirin

| | Reocclusion | | |
	Streptokinase	rt-PA	Ischemia
Aspirin	11% (197)	10% (222)	25% (2977)
No aspirin	24% (334)	26% (179)	41% (721)

Adapted from a meta-analysis in Ref. 84.
Numbers in parentheses indicate total number of patients.
rt-PA, recombinant tissue-type plasminogen activator.

The groups allocated to streptokinase plus aspirin or aspirin alone had reinfarction rates of only 1.8% or 1.9%, respectively, suggesting that aspirin is beneficial for prevention of reocclusion after thrombolysis.

A recent meta-analysis of 32 angiographic studies demonstrated that aspirin (usually combined with heparin) reduced coronary reocclusion and recurrent ischemia after thrombolysis[84] (Table 6.1). The angiographic reocclusion rate in 419 patients treated with aspirin was 11% compared with 25% in 513 patients without aspirin therapy. Recurrent ischemic events were present in 25% of 2977 patients treated with aspirin and 45% of 721 patients treated without aspirin. The effect of aspirin was similar in trials with either streptokinase or rt-PA. The authors speculated that the lower reocclusion rate after thrombolysis seen with aspirin may account for the beneficial effects of aspirin on mortality as demonstrated by ISIS-2.

Bleeding complications and stroke in ISIS-2 are summarized in Table 6.2. Of note, combined streptokinase and aspirin were associated with a reduced overall incidence of stroke (and also of fatal and disabling stroke) during the in-hospital period. Hemorrhagic strokes were slightly more frequent during the first 24 hours in the combined streptokinase plus aspirin group; this was more than offset by a reduced incidence of nonhemorrhagic stroke during the remainder of hospitalization. Not all patients included in the ISIS-2 study had a confirmed myocardial infarction. The liberal entry criteria undoubtedly included patients with noncardiac chest pain or unstable angina (known treatment benefit from aspirin therapy).[85–88] The large size of the study, however, means that this limitation is unlikely to affect the overall conclusions. Aspirin, either alone or in combination with thrombolytic therapy, is of definite benefit in the immediate management of acute myocardial infarction.

Heparin With and Without Thrombolytic Therapy

Heparin has the potential to prevent reocclusion by inactivating free thrombin formed in the vicinity of the lysing thrombus, but its effect is limited by its inability to inhibit clot-bound thrombin.

Table 6.2 Bleeding complications and stroke in ISIS-2

	Total stroke (%)	Major bleeds (%)
Streptokinase+aspirin	0.6	0.6
Streptokinase alone	0.7	0.5
Placebo	1.1	0.3

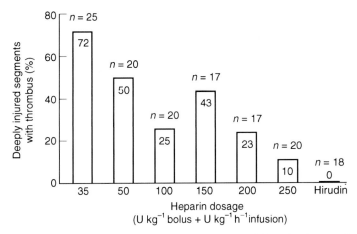

Figure 6.4 Percentage of arterial segments with macroscopic mural thrombus in a porcine carotid model of deep arterial injury produced by balloon dilatation. Heparin produced a dose-dependent reduction in mural thrombus formation, from 72% in the lowest to 10% in the highest heparin dosage group. In comparison, hirudin 1 mg kg^{-1} bolus followed by 1 mg kg^{-1} hour^{-1} (which prolonged the activated partial thromboplastin time to approximately three times the control value) completely abolished mural thrombus formation. (From Ref. 9 with permission.)

Mechanism of action of heparin

Heparin is a mixture of glycosaminoglycans with an average molecular weight of 12 000–15 000. The anticoagulant effect of heparin is mediated largely through its interaction with AT III; this produces a conformational change in AT III and so markedly accelerates its ability to inactivate the coagulation enzymes thrombin, factor X_a and factor IX_a.[89] Heparin also catalyzes the inactivation of thrombin by a second plasma cofactor, heparin cofactor II. This second anticoagulant effect of heparin is specific for thrombin, does not require the unique AT III-binding pentasaccharide, and is achieved only at very high doses of heparin.[90–94]

Thrombin, produced by activation of the coagulation cascade, is the strongest agonist for platelet activation and deposition.[9,95] This suggests that heparin may be a useful adjunct to thrombolysis. Experimentally, heparin produces a dose-dependent reduction in the deposition of platelets and fibrin and in the incidence of macroscopic mural thrombosis at dosages of 30–250 u kg^{-1} administered as a bolus followed by the same dosage per hour, if started prior to deep arterial injury.[9] The higher dosages cannot, however, be safely used in humans, and low dosages are effective against fibrin but not platelets (Figure 6.4).[9] The effect of heparin is also limited by its difficulty in inhibiting thrombin bound to arterial wall matrix and within a thrombus.[51,96] Fibrin binding masks receptors on thrombin to AT III and heparin cofactor II.[24] In addition, platelets release platelet factor 4, which can neutralize heparin,[97] and fibrin monomer II can protect thrombin from inactivation by the heparin–AT III complex. Heparin ≥ 100 u kg^{-1} effectively potentiates lysis when used in combination with a thrombolytic agent.[66,67,98]

Clinical trials of heparin without thrombolytic therapy

An overview of trials from the prethrombolytic era suggests that heparin may be beneficial in acute myocardial infarction.[99–101] Overall, heparin therapy was associated with a 17% reduction in the risk of death, compared with the control group, and a 22% reduction in reinfarction.[102] Most of the studies used heparin dosages of 20 000 u or more daily. The use of heparin in acute myocardial infarction was not only associated with

Table 6.3   Effect of intravenous heparin on infarct-related patency after thrombolytic therapy

Study	n	Treatment group	Control group	Time of angio	Patency
TAMI-3	134	rt-PA[b]+H[c]	rt-PA[b] only	90 min	79% vs 79% NS
Bleich	83	rt-PA+H[d]	rt-PA[a] only	Day 3	71% vs 44% $P < 0.02$
HART	205	rt-PA+H[d]	rt-PA[a]+ASA[e]	18 hours	82% vs 52% $P < 0.001$
ECSG-6	652	rt-PA+H[f]	rt-PA[a]+ASA[g]	48–120 hours	83% vs 75% $P < 0.01$
Australian NHF	241	rt-PA+H[f]	rt-PA[a]+H[f]/24 hours then ASA/D[h]	7–10 days	81% vs 80% NS

ASA, Aspirin; H, Heparin; rt-PA, recombinant tissue-type plasminogen activator; angio, coronary angiography.
[a] rt-PA, 100 mg in 3–4 hours.
[b] rt-PA, 1.5 mg kg^{-1} administered over 4 hours.
[c] H, 10 000-u bolus.
[d] H, aPTT 1.5–2.0.
[e] ASA, 80 mg daily.
[f] H, 5000-u bolus + 1000 u hour^{-1}.
[g] ASA, first day 250 mg i.v. (or 300 mg oral) then 75–125 mg daily.
[h] ASA, 300 mg daily + 300 mg dipyridamole (D).

reduction in mortality and reinfarction but also deep-vein thrombosis, pulmonary embolism, and stroke.[100] These trials do not address whether these beneficial effects will be realized when heparin is given after fibrinolytic therapy and/or aspirin.

Clinical trials of heparin with thrombolytic therapy

Role of heparin in maintaining patency. Several small trials have evaluated the role of heparin in maintaining coronary artery patency after thrombolytic therapy. In TAMI-3 trial, a single intravenous bolus of 10 000 u heparin (given with rt-PA 1.5 mg kg^{-1} over 4 hours) had no appreciable effect on 90-min coronary artery patency (79% in both treatment groups).[103] The authors concluded that early intravenous heparin did not facilitate the fibrinolytic effect of rt-PA at the doses tested (about 143 u kg^{-1} bolus which does not produce a sustained effect and is below the effective dose in animals). It is to be noted that in this study antithrombotic therapy was not continued and coronary patency was assessed only at 90 min. Any effect of heparin on reocclusion could not be ascertained. There was no increased incidence of bleeding complications in patients receiving heparin in addition to rt-PA.

Three randomized angiographic studies have clearly demonstrated that early intravenous heparin with rt-PA improves infarct-artery patency days to weeks after acute myocardial infarction (Table 6.3). This suggests a reduced risk of reocclusion. The beneficial effect of heparin was greater in patients in whom the aPTT was >1.5 times control values.[104,105]

In the first study[106] (Table 6.3), 83 patients with acute myocardial infarction were given rt-PA 100 mg over 3 hours and randomized to heparin (5000-u bolus followed by 1000 u hour^{-1}, titrated to prolong the aPTT to 1.5–2 times control). No aspirin was used in this trial. One patient who received heparin had a major bleeding episode.

The second study[105] employed a similar design (Table 6.3). Two hundred and five patients received rt-PA 100 mg and were randomly allocated to either intravenous heparin (5000-u bolus followed by 1000 u hour^{-1}, titrated to prolong the aPTT 1.5–2 times control) or low-dose aspirin (80 mg orally at the start of rt-PA, then daily). This study indicates a higher patency rate with heparin compared with aspirin. However, aspirin was used in a low dose of 80 mg daily orally; it is therefore possible that after a single oral dose of this size (unlike the 160 mg aspirin chewed in ISIS-2), reduced antiplatelet effect in the first days is observed.

In the third study,[104] a trial of the European Cooperative Study Group, 652 patients with acute myocardial infarction received 100 mg alteplase plus aspirin (250 mg intravenously followed by 75–125 mg on alternate days) and were randomized to adjunctive therapy with heparin (5000 u intravenously followed by 1000 u hourly without dose adjustment) or placebo for heparin (Table 6.3).

In an Australian study,[107] 195 patients received rt-PA followed by heparin for 24 hours (Table 6.3). Patients were randomized to continue heparin therapy or to receive aspirin plus dipyridamole for 7 days. Patency at 7 days was similar in both groups (79.8% vs 82%), suggesting that continuation of heparin beyond 24 hours did not improve results compared with aspirin plus dipyridamole. However today's gold standard is heparin plus aspirin to maximize patency and minimize reocclusion. Angiographic reocclusion was the lowest ever reported for streptokinase or rt-PA in the GUSTO trial (4.9–6.4%).[36]

The value of adjunctive intravenous heparin therapy on coronary patency in patients treated with streptokinase, urokinase, or anisoylated plasminogen streptokinase activator complex (APSAC) has not been established by randomized clinical trials. However, the frequency of recurrent ischemic events after thrombolytic therapy with streptokinase or urokinase is inversely related to the aPTT.[45] Following streptokinase therapy, angiographic reocclusion during administration of aspirin, usually with concomitant heparin, has averaged 11%,[84] and aspirin plus inadequate heparin compared to adequate heparin therapy (all aPTT values >1.5 times control) for 3 weeks resulted in lower patency (46% vs 69% of infarct-related arteries, $P < 0.02$) and more severe residual stenosis (74% vs 57%, $P < 0.02$).[36A]

In addition, there is clinical evidence that streptokinase and urokinase induce marked procoagulant activity, judging from the elevation in plasma concentrations of fibrinopeptide A and thrombin–AT III complexes.[61,65] Heparin appears to attenuate markedly, but not completely prevent, the increased thrombin activity induced by streptokinase.[61]

In conclusion, these studies examining the effect of adjunctive use of intravenous heparin with thrombolytic therapy show that heparin in conventional doses compared with no heparin or aspirin significantly improves early reocclusion rather than enhancing the acute lytic effect. This is consistent with the retrospective analysis of the data derived from the HART and ECSG-6 trials[108] that suggest that the degree of prolongation of aPTT during heparin therapy inversely correlates with the incidence of reocclusion and that inadequate levels or discontinuation of heparin precipitates further myocardial ischemia.[45] Arteries may open and close during initial lysis and may reocclude any time during hospitalization.[39] The benefit of heparin has been demonstrated largely with rt-PA as the thrombolytic agent. Similar benefit of heparin on infarct-artery patency for other thrombolytic agents such as streptokinase and APSAC is strongly suggested but not as firmly established. Finally, the optimal duration of heparinization is not clearly established but probably should be throughout hospitalization to keep reocclusion below 7%.[36A] Additional studies are underway to test the advantage of combined anticoagulation with aspirin after hospitalization (CARS and CHAMPS).

Role of heparin in large clinical trials. Despite sound rationale and favorable experimental results and angiographic evidence of reduced coronary reocclusion when heparin is used adjunctively with thrombolytic therapy at adequate doses, the exact value of heparin in terms of reduced mortality and reinfarction remains very suggestive but uncertain especially when compared with definitive evidence of benefit with the use of aspirin. Uncertainty is in part due to delayed administration, delayed onset of action by the subcutaneous route, and low, inadequate or unmonitored dosing of a drug with a variable dose–activity response due to variable protein binding and natural inhibitors of

Table 6.4 Randomized trials of adjunctive use of subcutaneous heparin with thrombolytic therapy: effect on mortality and bleeding complications

Study	Lytic agent	Adjunctive strategy	n	Mortality (%)	Mortality or disabling stroke (%)	Hemorrhagic stroke (%)	Major bleeds (%)
GISSI-2	SK/t-PA	ASA	10 407	9.4	–	0.4	1.0**
		ASA+H-SC	10 361	9.3	–	0.3	1.0
ISIS-3	SK/t-PA/APSAC	ASA	20 643	10.6	–	0.4*	0.8*
		ASA+H-SC	20 656	10.3	–	0.6	1.0
GUSTO	SK	ASA+H-SC	9 841	7.2	7.7	0.5	0.3
	SK	ASA+H-IV	10 410	7.4	7.9	0.5	0.5
	Acc-t-PA	ASA+H-IV	10 396	6.3	6.9	0.7	0.4
	SK+t-PA	ASA+H-IV	10 374	7.0	7.6	0.9	0.6

*$P < 0.05$, **$P < 0.01$ (all), $P = 0.03$ (SK) and $P < 0.001$ (t-PA no heparin) compared to SC; GUSTO trial did not compare heparin vs no heparin.
APSAC, anisoylated plasminogen streptokinase activator complex; ASA, Aspirin; H-IV, intravenous heparin (aPTT 60–85 s); H-SC, subcutaneous heparin 12 500 u twice daily, started 4 hours (ISIS-3, GUSTO) or 12 hours (GISSI-2) after lytic therapy; SK, Streptokinase; t-PA, tissue-type plasminogen activator.

heparin within thrombi. In addition, beneficial effects of short-term heparin are probably only measurable during its administration because of the long-term healing required after plaque disruption (the thrombotic stimulus) and the now known reactivation of thrombosis with early heparin cessation.

In the two large randomized controlled trials comparing subcutaneous heparin vs no heparin (GISSI-2/ISIS-3), involving over 60 000 patients, there was no benefit or only a short-term benefit on mortality with subcutaneous heparin added to aspirin and thrombolytic therapy. However, heparin dosage was probably too delayed by time and route of administration and as a fixed dose was subtherapeutic in some patients to affect the infarct-related artery.

The GISSI-2 trial and its international extension[109,110] compared the efficacy of two thrombolytic agents plus aspirin (streptokinase and rt-PA) and also tested whether there was an additional net benefit of adding subcutaneous heparin (12 500 u twice daily) initiated 12 hours after the onset of thrombolytic therapy. GISSI-2 found no differences in overall mortality between streptokinase and rt-PA, although streptokinase was associated with slightly fewer strokes. The addition of delayed subcutaneous heparin had no effect on mortality at 35 days (9.3% vs 9.4%) (Table 6.4). However, there was a significant difference in favor of the addition of heparin when in-hospital deaths during the scheduled treatment period were considered (5.4% vs 6.0%, $P < 0.05$) (Table 6.5).

Table 6.5 Thrombolysis in acute myocardial infarction and adjunctive medical therapy: comparison of mortality in patients assigned to subcutaneous heparin plus aspirin (ASA) or aspirin alone

Trial	Antithrombotic comparison Mortality (%)		
	ASA+heparin	ASA alone	P value
ISIS-3	7.4 (1534)	7.9 (1633)	0.06
GISSI-2	5.4 (537)	6.0 (606)	0.05
Combined	6.8 (2071)	7.3 (2239)	0.01

Difference appeared only during treatment period (i.e. in hospital):
ISIS-3, 0–7 days; GISSI-2, 0 to discharge.
Numbers in parentheses indicate total number of patients.

Table 6.6 Effect of heparin therapy 'planned at entry' on 35-day vascular mortality in each of the treatment groups in the ISIS-II study

Heparin	Mortality (%)			
	Streptokinase and aspirin	Streptokinase	Aspirin	Double placebo
Intravenous	6.4 (1024)	8.3 (2054)	8.7 (2048)	13.1 (1023)
Subcutaneous	7.6 (1805)	9.0 (3601)	9.4 (3605)	13.5 (1800)
None	9.6 (1463)	10.1 (2937)	9.8 (2934)	12.9 (1477)

Numbers in parentheses indicate total number of patients.

Similarly, when one analyzes only deaths that occurred after the start of subcutaneous heparin (excluding deaths that occurred when heparin had not yet been started), a significant difference in mortality in favor of heparin emerges.

ISIS-3 compared the efficacy of streptokinase, rt-PA and APSAC plus aspirin and of subcutaneous heparin (12 500 u twice daily, with a 4-hour delay) vs no heparin among 41 299 patients with acute myocardial infarction.[111] ISIS-3 found no differences in overall mortality among the thrombolytic agents tested and the addition of subcutaneous heparin was not associated with a reduction of the reinfarction rate or 35-day mortality (10.3% with heparin vs 10.6% without heparin, Table 6.4). During the scheduled 7 days of heparin use there was a slightly favorable trend toward a lower mortality (7.4% vs 7.9%, $P = 0.06$) and reinfarction rate (3.2% vs 3.5%, $P = 0.09$) with heparin compared with no heparin (Table 6.5).

Pooling the results[111] from GISSI-2 and ISIS-3 shows the 35-day mortality to be 10.0% with, and 10.2% without, heparin. However, during the 7-day treatment period, pooled mortality was lower with heparin (6.8%) than without heparin (7.3%) (Table 6.5).

The SCATI trial[112] enrolled 711 patients with acute myocardial infarction, of whom 433 were admitted within 6 hours of the onset of symptoms and were given streptokinase (1 500 000 u over 1 hour). Those randomly allocated to receive heparin were given an initial bolus of 2000 u intravenously at the time of thrombolysis, followed 9 hours later by 12 500 u subcutaneously every 12 hours to hospital discharge. No aspirin was given. Heparin therapy reduced in-hospital mortality from 8.8% to 4.5% ($P = 0.05$). Patients given heparin without thrombolysis showed a trend toward reduced in-hospital mortality, which was not statistically significant (7.7% with heparin administration and 11.7% in the control group, $P = 0.10$). Recurrent ischemia was reduced from 19.6% to 14.2% ($P = 0.08$) but reinfarction was not. In addition, the rate of left ventricular mural thrombosis was reduced. Bleeding was 4.4% among the heparin-treated patients vs 0.6% among the control group.

Although no anticoagulant therapy was mandated in ISIS-2,[110] some form of heparin was used in more than 60% of patients. There was a trend toward reduced mortality in all treatment groups (streptokinase, aspirin, or both) as the intensity of planned heparin therapy increased. The lowest mortality occurred when streptokinase plus aspirin was used in combination with intravenous heparin (see Table 6.6: intravenous heparin 6.4%, subcutaneous heparin 7.6%, and no heparin 9.6%).

In conclusion, despite experimental and angiographic evidence of reduced coronary reocclusion, the value of therapeutic heparin (aPTT 60–80 s) for reducing mortality and reinfarction needs testing when combined with full-dose aspirin. However, because heparin administration was often 'too little too late' in the large clinical trials, the results of the GISSI-2 and ISIS-3 studies have been criticized.[35,113] The delay (4–12 hours) and mode of administration of heparin in these trials likely led to subtherapeutic aPTT levels during the first 24–48 hours,[114] when reocclusion particularly with rt-PA is most likely to occur.[115] In prespecified subgroups of the same trials (ISIS-2, GISSI-2, ISIS-3) there was a benefit of adjunctive heparin therapy particularly when given intravenously (aPTT >60 s), in spite of major bleeding rates increasing as intensity of heparin therapy increased.

The recent GUSTO trial,[116] although not designed to test the value of heparin, demonstrated no clinical benefit of immediate intravenous heparin (adjusted aPTT between 60 and 85 s for at least 48 hours) compared to subcutaneous heparin (delayed 4 hours, 12 500 u twice daily for 7 days or to hospital discharge) among patients receiving streptokinase and aspirin, but a longer duration of possibly more intense intravenous administration. The lower absolute mortality rates (Table 6.4) and very low reocclusion rates of 4.9–6.4% (angiographic substudy of GUSTO[36]) in all groups suggest a beneficial effect of adjunctive heparin combined with aspirin. However, no large-scale clinical trial has compared aspirin plus intravenous heparin with aspirin and no heparin. In any event, heparin may be an inadequate thrombin inhibitor in the presence of thrombus and during thrombolysis. Newer, more potent and specific thrombin inhibitors such as hirudin may improve the rate and extent of thrombolysis, incidence of reperfusion, and incidence of normal (TIMI grade 3) blood flow with thrombolytic therapy (TIMI-9, GUSTO II). The GUSTO IIa and TIMI 9A trials showed that there is a very narrow therapeutic window for the aPTT (60–85 s) in heparin and hirudin administration so as to avoid intracranial hemorrhage in 2–3% of patients with streptokinase or rt-PA.[116A,116B]

Role of oral anticoagulation in acute myocardial infarction with or without thrombolysis. The appropriate duration of anticoagulant therapy after myocardial infarction is uncertain. Early large trials in the prethrombolytic era suggest that long-term oral anticoagulation after myocardial infarction reduces overall mortality by approximately 20%.[99] Two recent, well-designed clinical trials of long-term anticoagulation after acute myocardial infarction have also shown reduction of mortality, reinfarction, and stroke with acceptable hemorrhagic risk (Sixty Plus Reinfarction Study, International Normalized Ratio (INR) 2.7–4.5; WARIS, INR 2.8–4.8).[117,118] In the WARIS trial patients were enrolled on average 1 month post infarct and followed for the next 37 months. Overall mortality was reduced by 24%, from 20% in the placebo group to 15% in those treated with warfarin; reinfarction was reduced by 34% in the warfarin group. Of particular note, total cerebrovascular accidents (hemorrhagic and nonhemorrhagic) were reduced by 55% with warfarin treatment. Serious bleeding occurred in 0.6% of warfarin-treated patients.

Despite the benefits of long-term warfarin therapy for the reduction of vascular events following myocardial infarction, the use of oral anticoagulants after thrombolysis for secondary prevention needs to be further investigated by directly comparing aspirin to warfarin or both. Heparin followed by short-term oral warfarin therapy for 1 month after intracoronary thrombolysis for acute myocardial infarction may produce further lysis of residual coronary thrombus.[119] This will reduce progression of the original coronary lesion.

Clinical benefits from thrombolysis are significantly compromised by rethrombosis. Reduction of infarct vessel patency occurs during the 3–6 months after hospital discharge when reocclusion of 25–40% of arteries occurs as shown by the TAMI-6 and APRICOT studies.[47,48]

The recently published, placebo-controlled APRICOT study provided important new information on the incidence of late reocclusion (3 months) that correlated with left ventricular dysfunction and the problem of the efficacy of lower-dose antithrombotic therapy in the early phase after thrombolysis. Three hundred patients treated with intravenous thrombolytic therapy (streptokinase 1 500 000 u in 30–60 min [251 patients] or APSAC 30 u in 5 min [33 patients] followed by a fixed low dose of intravenous heparin (20 000 u in 24 hours) were eligible when a patent infarct-related artery was demonstrated at angiography within 48 hours. They were randomized to either 325 mg aspirin daily or placebo with discontinuation of heparin or to coumadin with continuation of heparin until oral anticoagulation was established. (INR 2.8–4.0). After 3 months, in which conservative treatment was intended, vessel patency and ventricular function were reassessed in 248 patients (87% reangiography rate). Reocclusion rates were similar in all groups: 25% with aspirin, 30% with coumadin, and 32% with placebo. However a significant reduction by aspirin over placebo was seen in clinical events including recurrent myocardial infarction (3% vs 8%), need for revascularization (6% vs 16%), and an increase in left ventricular ejection fraction. The effects of coumadin in this study were intermediate between those of aspirin and placebo.

There were two factors in the APRICOT study that may not have been in favor of comparing the coumadin treatment regimen to aspirin. The risk of rethrombosis is highest during the first days after thrombolysis, and immediate antithrombotic protection is needed. Thus, the relatively low dose of intravenous heparin given without a bolus may have contributed to a less favorable outcome in the heparin/coumadin group. Second, the target INR of 2.8–4.0 was not achieved during hospital stay in at least 20% of patients. Because the reocclusion rates are high even with aspirin, the search for better antithrombotic treatment strategies for the prevention of reocclusion should continue.

A new approach of combining aspirin and warfarin is currently being tested in the ongoing Coumadin–Aspirin Reinfarction Study (CARS). This randomized, double-blind study is comparing the efficacy and safety of fixed low doses of coumadin (1 mg or 3 mg) plus aspirin to aspirin alone in the prevention of reinfarction, cardiovascular death, and stroke in 6000 patients after myocardial infarction for up to 4 years. The rationale for the combined use of warfarin and aspirin is a possible synergistic and superior effect of the combination of both agents. Low-dose coumadin may reduce fibrin deposition, but aspirin is probably needed to reduce platelet deposition. The combination of aspirin and warfarin is considered to carry a higher risk of bleeding complication; however lower doses of warfarin and aspirin as used in the ongoing CARS trial (warfarin 3 mg plus aspirin 80 mg, warfarin 1 mg plus aspirin 80 mg, vs 160 mg aspirin alone) are expected to have lower complication rates.

Two recent trials have shown a superior effect of combined warfarin and aspirin. The first was in patients with prosthetic heart valves and a high risk for thromboembolism.[120] The second was in patients with unstable angina or non-Q-wave myocardial infarction where reduced myocardial infarction or death resulted with combined warfarin (INR 2.0–3.0) plus aspirin (162.5 mg per day).[121]

Newer Antithrombotic Therapy

Specific antithrombins

Specific thrombin inhibitors have several potential advantages as antithrombotic agents when compared to heparin. Direct thrombins do not have natural inhibitors and neutralize thrombin directly without the need for a cofactor such as AT III. Heparins are inactivated by the heparin-neutralizing protein platelet factor 4, which is secreted from platelets. Platelet membranes also inhibit the anticoagulant effect of heparin by binding with factor X_a, which protects it from inactivation by the heparin–AT III complex. Thrombin bound to fibrin and extracellular matrix has altered receptors that resist inactivation by heparin–AT III complex and heparin cofactor II but not by direct thrombin inhibitors.[24,51,96] Thrombin-mediated platelet activation is little influenced by heparin, particularly at high shear rate. However, hirudin is an effective inhibitor of thrombin-induced platelet activation[9,10] and is well tolerated in humans and is nonimmunogenic.[122–125] These observations may explain why heparin is less effective in experimental models than hirudin in preventing the formation of arterial thrombosis.

Hirudin is a 65-amino-acid polypeptide isolated from the European leech *Hirudo medicinalis* more than 60 years ago.[126] Hirudin binds thrombin stoichiometrically with extraordinary tightness (K_D 10^{-14} M) and specificity. Recombinant desulfato-hirudin (r-hirudin) is similar (K_D 2.0 × 10^{-13} M). Hirulog is a 20-amino-acid synthetic peptide with hirudin-like tail or exosite and has a lower binding affinity (2.3 × 10^{-9}). Both bind to the catalytic site of thrombin and to the exosite required for thrombin binding to fibrinogen. Hirudin (and probably hirulog) appear to block all of thrombin's *in vivo* actions except the positive feedback activation of factors V and VIII, which increase thrombin generation.[127,128]

New thrombin inhibitors have been shown to be superior to heparin in a number of experimental models of arterial thrombosis and thrombolysis.[126] Data from experimental studies of thrombolysis indicate that hirudin is more effective than heparin in enhancing and sustaining reperfusion with streptokinase[129] or rt-PA[98] at a hirudin dose prolonging the aPTT two or three times the control level. Most importantly, hirudin maximally reduces residual thrombus burden.[98]

Several clinical trials have reported on the safety and preliminary efficacy of the direct antithrombins.[122–126,130,131] The pharmacokinetics of r-hirudin intravenously adminis-tered in patients (mean age 60 years) with chronic coronary artery disease showed a half-life of 2–3 hours compared with 1 hour in younger normal persons.[123] The aPTT values showed little variation, correlated well with plasma levels of r-hirudin, and allowed close titration over a wide range of anticoagulation. The activated clotting time (ACT) and prothrombin time were relatively insensitive for monitoring hirudin administration. No generation of antibodies or increase in bleeding time was observed, and r-hirudin was well tolerated and safe. A study in normal human volunteers showed similar results when r-hirudin was administered subcutaneously.[124]

Hirudin was utilized in two pilot studies in arterial thrombolysis with front-loaded t-PA.[122,125] In the TIMI-V trial[122] 246 patients with acute myocardial infarction were randomized to conjunctive treatment with heparin (aPTT 65–90 s) or r-hirudin in four doses. Hirudin achieved a higher 90-min patency rate than heparin, was more effective in preventing reocclusion and reinfarction, and increased late opening of arteries occluded at 90 min without increasing the rate of spontaneous hemorrhage. Similar results were reported from the HIT trial.[125] r-Hirudin in escalating dosing was given as conjunctive therapy to front-loaded rt-PA in 143 patients with acute myocardial infarction. The effects of hirudin were dose dependent and the highest dose resulted in TIMI grade 3 patency in 76% of 81 patients and reduced reocclusion to 1.2% without excess of spontaneous bleeding.

r-Hirudin was administered for 72–120 hours in a dose-escalating pilot study to patients with unstable angina and coronary angiographic evidence of thrombus at the culprit lesion site. Using the Ciba-Corning 512 monitor (Biotrack, Inc.) for measurement at the bedside (aPTTs may be 10–20 s longer than laboratory measurements), the aPTT appeared to plateau at the 0.2 mg kg^{-1} hour^{-1} infusion dose. A higher proportion of patients treated with hirudin had the maintenance aPTT within a 40-s range (71%) compared to heparin-treated patients (16%). The 116 patients treated with all four doses of hirudin (0.05–0.3 mg kg^{-1} hour^{-1}) tended to show more improvement in the culprit lesion dimensions and TIMI flow grade relative to heparin infusion when considering the average cross-sectional area, minimal cross-sectional area, minimal lumen diameter, and percent diameter stenosis. There were also fewer myocardial infarctions in the hirudin-treated (2.6%) compared to the heparin-treated (8.0%) group. [131] Hirulog administered in a dose-escalating study in patients with unstable angina appeared to have its best effects (aPTT 98 s) in the 14 patients receiving infusions of 1 mg kg^{-1} hour^{-1}.[130]

Thus direct thrombin inhibitors are promising for treatment of acute coronary syn-dromes and large efficacy trials are in progress. The principal objective of the ongoing large-scale Global Use of Strategies to Open Occluded Arteries (GUSTO II) trial is to compare hirudin with heparin in all acute coronary syndromes and/or the reduction of myocardial infarction and death. TIMI-9 is making the same comparisons on patients with acute myocardial infarction with ST elevation undergoing thrombolysis.

Novel antiplatelet agents

The additive effect of aspirin in patients receiving thrombolytic therapy is well established. Since its ability to inhibit thrombin-induced platelet aggregation is limited, other platelet inhibitors including antagonists to receptors in the final common pathway of platelet aggregation (IIb/IIIa integrin, Figure 6.2) have been developed. Study of these receptor antagonists in patients receiving thrombolytic therapy has been limited, owing to concern over serious bleeding complications. Both rt-PA, 7E3, and the monoclonal antibody against GP IIb/IIIa have been used simultaneously in the canine model with acceleration of reperfusion, inhibition of reocclusion, and possible facilitated thrombolysis at reduced rt-PA doses.[74,75] However, if deep arterial injury is present (causing increased thrombin generation) concurrent heparin administration is also required. In patients, 7E3 or other IIb/IIIa receptor antagonists have not yet been administered simultaneously with rt-PA or streptokinase. The only human study was nonrandomized sequential therapy with rt-PA followed by murine Fab (m7E3) at variable times (3, 6 and 15 hours).[132] All 75 patients also received aspirin and heparin. Infarct-vessel patency was assessed 24 hours after therapy. Vessel patency improved in the 7E3 group (92% vs 56%, $P = 0.03$). However, major bleeding events occurred in 25% of patients. The reported 50% increase in bleeding complications in the large EPIC trial, involving 2099 patients with a high-risk percutaneous transluminal coronary angioplasty (PTCA) randomized to 7E3 IIb/IIIa receptor antagonist, also indicates that the increased risk of bleeding associated with this strategy remains a serious concern and is increased with concomitant heparin.[133]

Arterial Thromboembolism

More than 90% of systemic emboli occurring soon after a myocardial infarction originate from a left ventricular apical mural thrombus after an anterior infarction.[134,135] Transmural anterior infarcts especially involve the cardiac apex. The incidence of mural thrombosis is increased if apical wall motion is akinetic or dyskinetic, the ejection fraction is less than 35%,[134,135] or the infarct-related artery is occluded.[136] Other contributing factors to the formation of thrombi include the local inflammatory response,[137] the stasis of the blood in a dyskinetic region of the left ventricle,[134,135] and the generalized hypercoagulable state present during and after an acute infarct.[52] Two-thirds of mural thrombi form within 48 hours[138,139] and 83% develop in the first week after the infarct. Thus immediate and adequate heparin therapy (aPTT $\geq$ 1.5 times control) is mandatory to prevent mural thrombi.

Autopsy studies, despite inherent selection bias, first suggested that anticoagulation may be beneficial. Left ventricular thrombi were found in >50% of patients not treated, compared with 20–25% of those treated with anticoagulants.[140,141] Two-dimensional echocardiography (sensitivity and specificity of 85–90%)[142–144] has become the method of choice for identifying and following changes in thrombus size and morphology, including the effect of anticoagulation.

There are now six prospective, randomized, controlled studies evaluating anticoagulation, started within 12–36 hours of the onset of symptoms, in patients with anterior Q-wave infarcts (Table 6.7).[112,145–149] The two largest studies[112,145] employed a fixed regimen of subcutaneous heparin 12 500 u twice daily; the other smaller studies used heparin (adjusted for the aPTT)[149] or heparin followed by warfarin.[146–148] Data from all six studies combined showed that anticoagulation halved the in-hospital incidence of left ventricular mural thrombus formation from 37% in the control group to 19% in patients who were administered anticoagulants. The delay of as long as 36 hours in initiating anticoagulation with heparin and the delay in reaching therapeutic levels by the subcutaneous route of administration (up to 24–36 hours) probably contribute to the relatively high incidence of ventricular thrombi in those patients administered anticoagulants. Inadequate heparin also increases the incidence of thrombi.

The Canadian study,[145] which used a fixed subcutaneous heparin dosage, found that treatment efficacy correlated with the plasma heparin levels and the prolongation of the aPTT, suggesting that dosage adjusted for the aPTT may have been even more effective in preventing left ventricular mural thrombosis. The control group received low-dose heparin, which was not effective. In addition, an initial heparin bolus (5000 u) to saturate binding sites on endothelium and heparin-binding proteins would generate immediate therapeutic heparin levels.

The other large study, from the SCATI group in Italy,[112] is of particular relevance to current clinical practice because more than half of the patients were also given streptokinase. A substudy of GISSI-2 demonstrated that the incidence of left ventricular thrombi did not differ in patients with acute myocardial infarction treated either with streptokinase or rt-PA.[150] However, a recent meta-analysis suggests[151] that thrombolysis may have a modest benefit in reducing mural thrombus formation particularly in patients with a patent infarct-related artery,[136] perhaps because it improves regional wall motion abnormalities in addition to any direct lytic effect.

Left ventricular mural thrombus formation has been used as a surrogate endpoint for arterial embolism because the embolic event rate is low and no recent study has had sufficient power to detect a reduction in emboli with anticoagulation. The large, randomized studies from the Medical Research Council[152] and Veterans Administration,[141] however, provide strong evidence that anticoagulation with heparin and coumadin is beneficial. Systemic emboli (cerebral plus peripheral) were reduced from 3.4% to 1.3% with anticoagulation in the former, and from 5.4% to 0.8% in the latter.

The more recent studies have focused on patients with anterior Q-wave infarcts, the group at particular risk for left ventricular thrombus formation and embolism. If the in-hospital embolic event rates from the six recent, randomized studies are combined, the incidence of clinically recognized systemic embolism is approximately 4% in the control group and 1% in those patients receiving heparin, in some instances followed by warfarin (Table 6.7). The peak incidence of embolism is during the first 7–10 days post infarct; most of the remaining emboli occur during the next 3 months. Subsequently,

Table 6.7   Randomized studies on the effect of early anticoagulation on left ventricular thrombi in acute anterior myocardial infarction

			No. total patients			
	Entry study (hours)	Treatment	Left ventricular thrombi[a]		Emboli	
Study			Treated	Control	Treated	Control
Nordrehaug et al. [146]	<12	Heparin/warfarin[b]	0/26	7/27	0/26	1/27
Arvan and Boscha [147]	<12	Heparin/warfarin [b]	4/13	6/17	1/13	1/17
Davis and Ireland [148]	<12	Heparin/warfarin [b,c]	14/25	15/27	0/25	1/27
Gueret et al.[149]	<12	Heparin[b]	8/21	13/25	1/21	1/25
Turpie et al.[145]	<36	Heparin [d,e]	10/95	28/88	1/95	4/88
SCATI [112]	<24	Heparin[d]	19/107	34/93	0/107	2/93
Totals			55/287 (19%)	103/277 (37%)	3/287 (1%)	10/277 (4%)
				$P < 0.001$		$P < 0.04$

[a] Echocardiography 7–14 days as at discharge.
[b] Adjusted for aPTT, prothrombin time.
[c] Control group received heparin 5000 u three times daily, 18 of 27 patients also received warfarin.
[d] 12 500 u twice daily.
[e] Control group received heparin 5000 u twice daily.

emboli are generally associated with persistent and severe global left ventricular dysfunction with localized dyskinesis. Anticoagulation is most effective if commenced immediately, because two-thirds of thrombi form within 36–48 hours, emboli may occur before thrombus is visible by echocardiography, and because anticoagulation appears to be more effective at preventing thrombus formation than lysing preexisting thrombi. Furthermore, heparin in combination with thrombolytic therapy prevents the formation of protruding left ventricular thrombi and reduces the risk of embolic events (0.5%) occurring during the hospitalization.[150]

Anticoagulation was still found to be of benefit in two randomized studies of patients with established thrombi.[153,154] Thrombus characteristics associated with an increased likelihood of embolism include large size, protrusion into the luminal cavity, and especially free intracavitary motion of the thrombus.[139,155,156] Echocardiographic thrombus features frequently change spontaneously over time.[138] Although many thrombi disappear during anticoagulation, some recur soon after the anticoagulants are stopped (most often if <3 months duration of therapy).[157] It is not known whether late thrombus recurrence has an associated increased embolic risk. Patients with a left ventricular aneurysm but no diffuse contraction abnormality have a very low incidence of emboli beyond 3 months after infarction of less than 0.5% per year and thus do not appear to require anti-coagulation.[158]

Antiplatelet agents are of no benefit in preventing left ventricular thrombi. Two studies, one using aspirin 100 mg per day,[159] and the other aspirin plus dipyridamole,[160] started within 12–24 hours of a myocardial infarct, found no reduction in the incidence of left ventricular thrombus formation.

Venous Thromboembolism

Much of our current knowledge of the natural history of deep vein thrombosis comes from studies performed in the 1960s and early 1970s, when the management of acute myocardial infarction included prolonged bedrest. Deep leg vein thrombosis begins soon after the infarct (50% develop within 72 hours and 75% within 5–7 days), but usually it takes another 2–3 days to propagate proximally into the popliteal, femoral, or iliac vessels.[161,162] This occurs in approximately one-quarter of calf vein thrombi; conversely, the great majority (90–95%) of proximal thrombi arise from the calf veins.[163,164] Prevention of ileofemoral thrombosis is of major importance because, if untreated, 40–50% will embolize to the lungs. Overall, 10% of deep calf vein thrombi lead to clinical pulmonary embolism, of which one-third prove fatal.

The risk of venous thromboembolism appears similar to that after major surgery, another condition associated with a temporary hypercoagulable state.[165] Factors associated with an increased risk of deep vein thrombosis include heart failure (particularly cardiogenic shock), prolonged immobilization, age over 70 years, previous deep vein thrombosis, obesity, and varicose veins.[166,167]

Early mobilization reduces the incidence of calf vein thrombosis and, more importantly, proximal extension and embolism. This was confirmed in one study using[125] I-labeled fibrinogen to detect venous thrombosis. Leg vein thrombi occurred in 9% of patients mobilized within 1–3 days of their infarct, compared with 63% of those randomly allocated to bedrest for 5 days.[166] This study also documented the importance of heart failure as a major additional risk factor; 22% of those mobilized early and 80% of those mobilized late who had heart failure also had deep vein thrombosis.

The large Medical Research Council[152] and Veterans Administration[141] studies of anticoagulation after acute myocardial infarction reported an incidence of clinically detected pulmonary embolism of 5% in untreated compared to 2% in patients treated with anticoagulation (of moderate intensity). Anticoagulation also reduced deaths from pulmonary embolism and the incidence of pulmonary embolism or infarction detected at autopsy; however, these studies were performed in the era of prolonged immobilization and have limited relevance to current practice.

An alternative prevention of deep venous thrombosis evaluated extensively in surgical patients is subcutaneous heparin 5000 u, two or three times daily. The main effect of low-dose heparin is to increase the rate of AT III-mediated inactivation of activated factor X_a, thereby reducing subsequent amplification of the intrinsic coagulation cascade. This regimen is not effective after thrombus has formed and during brisk thrombin generation via the activator complex (Figures 6.2 and 6.3), and so must be given early to prevent thrombus formation. Since low-dose heparin produces no prolongation of the aPTT, it does not require monitoring, and the risk of bleeding, even in patients undergoing surgery, is not increased. Low-dose heparin, started within 12–18 hours of myocardial infarction and continued for 10 days, reduces the incidence of venous thrombosis from 23% in control to 4% in treated patients.[168–170] This benefit was also evident in higher risk subgroups for thrombosis, such as patients with heart failure. Heparin treatment in higher doses for arterial or left ventricular thrombus will, of course, also prevent venous thrombosis.

Recently, low molecular weight heparins (LMWH) were reported to be as effective as heparin and to produce less bleeding in the prevention and treatment of deep vein thrombosis.[171,172] However, LMWH appear to have little potential for treatment of arterial thrombosis[173] since they have the same disadvantages as unfractionated heparin (Figure 6.3), require higher dosing to measurable aPTTs, and are more expensive.

Practical Implications and Recommendations

In acute myocardial infarction there is immediate activation of the coagulation cascade with thrombin generation, platelet activation, and coronary thrombosis. Further activation occurs during exogenous thrombolysis. Thrombin appears to be the most important stimulator of platelet activation. Thrombin-induced platelet aggregation is incompletely inhibited by aspirin. Oral aspirin alone or in combination with parenteral heparin have been shown to improve mortality with or without combined thrombolytic therapy in acute myocardial infarction, probably by enhancing lysis and reducing simultaneous thrombosis and subsequent reocclusion. Therefore, it is recommended that all patients with acute myocardial infarction be considered for anticoagulant and aspirin therapy.

Antithrombotic Therapy in the Absence of Thrombolytic Therapy

Aspirin

The Second International Study of Infarct Survival (ISIS-2) showed conclusively the efficacy of aspirin alone for the treatment of evolving acute myocardial infarction, with a 35-day mortality reduction of 23%. All patients with acute myocardial infarction should receive 160–325 mg of chewable aspirin as soon as possible after suspected acute myocardial infarction. The dose should be repeated daily indefinitely.

Heparin

Overviews of parenteral heparin therapy in myocardial infarction show reduction in mortality by 17–22%, stroke by 50%, reinfarction by 22%, and pulmonary embolus by 54%.[102] Intravenous heparin and nitroglycerin therapy without lytic therapy resulted in patency of the infarct-related artery in 75% of patients after 10–14 days.[174] This suggests that all patients with ST elevation (evolving Q-wave myocardial infarction should receive heparin therapy (aPTT 60–85 s) for the duration of the hospitalization. Results of the ATACS trial in patients with unstable angina and non-Q-wave myocardial infarction suggest that all patients should receive heparin plus aspirin (160 mg loading plus 80 mg daily thereafter) throughout the hospitalization.[121] Patients with anterior Q-wave infarction and at increased risk of systemic or pulmonary embolism should receive therapeutic-dose heparin treatment throughout hospitalization (aPTT 1.5–2.0 times control) and oral anticoagulation may be given for up to 3 months in those with apical akinesis or dyskinesis.

Antithrombotic Therapy in the Presence of Thrombolytic Therapy

Most large trials demonstrating a reduction of mortality with thrombolytic therapy using streptokinase or rt-PA have also shown a beneficial effect of adjunctive therapy with heparin and/or aspirin. Angiographic data indicate that immediate heparin and aspirin is required to reduce simultaneous thrombosis and consequent reocclusion. To maximize endogenous lysis of residual thrombus with therapy currently available, continuing heparin infusion (aPTT 2–3 times control or 60–85 s) along with aspirin throughout hospitalization maximizes antithrombotic therapy.

Aspirin

All patients without contraindications should receive aspirin 160 mg per day, starting immediately on presentation and continuing indefinitely at 80–160 mg per day.

Heparin

Heparin should be given as a bolus of 5000 u with the lytic agent and followed immediately by an infusion of 1000 u hour^{-1}. The standard dose of 1000 u hour^{-7} results in aPTT values <1.5 times control in nearly half of patients and thus should be monitored at 4–6, 8–12, and 24 hours to bring into range at 60–85 s.[175] The aPTT may be prolonged during thrombolysis. Thus during the first 12 hours of the heparin infusion the dosage of heparin should be adjusted only if the aPTT is low. The heparin infusion should subsequently be adjusted to maintain the aPTT at two to three times the control value (aPTT 60–85 s) for 3–5 days, followed by subcutaneous heparin (minimum 12 500 u, average 17 000 u every 12 hours) to prolong the aPTT 1.5–3.0 times control (60–85 s) for the remainder of hospitalization. Patients receiving streptokinase may be treated with subcutaneous heparin from the beginning of thrombolytic therapy, but need an intravenous bolus of at least 5000 u to achieve immediate therapeutic levels. Less than 50% will achieve adequate anticoagulation with an aPTT >1.5 times control if 12 500 u every 12 hours is given as a fixed dose.

Oral anticoagulants

Switching heparin to warfarin and overlapping for 3–5 days until the prothrombin time is within therapeutic range (INR 2.0–3.5) and continuing with aspirin may maximize potential for endogenous lysis of residual thrombus and a maximal reduction of coronary events[121] but needs testing in prospective trials in patients with acute myocardial infarction. Patients with severe residual stenosis or angiographically identified thrombus after thrombolysis are at particular risk for reocclusion and should be empirically anticoagulated with warfarin for 2–3 months to minimize residual stenosis and reocclusion. While on warfarin, the aspirin dosage should be reduced to 80 mg per day. Patients who develop recurrent angina or ischemia, heart failure, or a positive exercise test are candidates for coronary angiography and possible revascularization.

Antithrombotic Therapy for Patients with a High Thromboembolic Risk

Patients with anterior Q-wave myocardial infarction are at risk for arterial thrombo-embolism, benefit from a patent infarct-related artery, and should receive heparin titrated to prolong aPTT 1.5–2.0 times the control value (60–85 s) throughout hospitaliza-tion, regardless of whether left ventricular thrombus is evident by echocardiography. Although the in-hospital period carries the greatest risk for embolism, patients should probably be then anticoagulated with warfarin to prolong the prothrombin time to an INR of 2.5–3.5 for the next 2–3 months (especially those with apical akinesis or dyskinesis).

All patients with acute myocardial infarction are at risk for venous thromboembolism. Those at high risk, such as patients with large infarcts or heart failure, should be fully anticoagulated with heparin throughout hospitalization. Early mobilization reduces venous thrombosis and embolism. Those patients not fully anticoagulated should receive low-dose heparin (5000 u two or three times daily) prior to mobilization.

More potent inhibitors of platelets and the coagulation cascade, such as specific thrombin inhibitors, show considerable promise for the future and may improve the rate and extent of thrombolysis, incidence of reperfusion, and incidence of normal (TIMI grade 3) blood flow with thrombolytic therapy (TIMI-9 and GUSTO II). A new approach of combining aspirin and warfarin is currently being tested in the ongoing CARS study. Until newer therapy is fully evaluated, heparin and aspirin have an established and important role in the acute management of myocardial infarction.

References

1. Falk, E. (1985) Unstable angina with fatal outcome: dynamic coronary thrombosis leading to infarction and/or sudden death. Autopsy evidence of recurrent mural thrombosis with peripheral embolization culminating in total vascular occlusion. *Circulation*, **71**, 699–708.
2. Richardson, P.D., Davies, M.J. and Born, G.V.R. (1989) Influence of plaque configuration and stress distribution on fissuring of coronary atherosclerotic plaques. *Lancet*, **ii**, 941–4.
3. Fuster, V., Badimon, L., Badimon, J.J. *et al.* (1992) The pathogenesis of coronary artery disease and the acute coronary syndromes. *N. Engl. J. Med.*, **326**, 242–50.
4. Fuster, V., Badimon, L., Badimon, J.J. *et al.* (1992) The pathogenesis of coronary artery disease and the acute coronary syndromes. *N. Eng. J. Med.*, **326**, 310–18.
5. Davies, M.J. (1990) A macro and micro view of coronary vascular insult in ischemic heart disease. *Circulation*, **82** (suppl. II), II-38–II-46.
6. Chesebro, J.H., Webster, M.W.I., Zoldhelyi, P. *et al.* (1992) Antithrombotic therapy and progression of coronary artery disease. Antiplatelets versus antithrombins. *Circulation*, **86** (Suppl. III), III-100–III-110.
7. Parsons, T.J., Haycroft, D.L., Hoak, J.C. *et al.* (1986) Interaction of platelets and purified collagens in a laminar flow model. *Thromb. Res.*, **43**, 435–43.
8. Mayne, R. (1986) Collagenous proteins of blood vessels. *Arteriosclerosis*, **6**, 585–93.
8A. Fernandez-Ortiz, A., Badimon, J.J., Falk, E. *et al.* (1994) Characterization of the relative thrombogenicity of atherosclerotic plaque components: implications for consequences of plaque rupture. *J. Am. Coll. Cardiol.*, **23**, 1562–9.
9. Heras, M., Chesebro, J.H., Penny, W.J. *et al.* (1989) Effects of thrombin inhibition on the development of acute platelet-thrombus deposition during angioplasty in pigs: heparin versus recombinant hirudin, a specific thrombin inhibitor. *Circulation*, **79**, 657–65.
10. Heras, M., Chesebro, J.H., Webster, M.W.I. *et al.* (1990) Hirudin, heparin, and placebo during deep arterial injury in the pig: The *in vivo* role of thrombin in platelet-mediated thrombosis. *Circulation*, **82**, 1476–84.
11. Badimon, L., Badimon, J.J., Galvez, A. *et al.* (1986) Influence of arterial damage and wall shear rate on platelet deposition. *Ex vivo* study in a swine model. *Arteriosclerosis*, **6**, 312–20.
12. Badimon, L. and Badimon, J.J. (1989) Mechanisms of arterial thrombosis in nonparallel streamlines: platelet thrombi grow on the apex of stenotic severely injured vessel wall. Experimental study in the pig model. *J. Clin. Invest.*, **84**, 1134–44.
12A. Sherman, C.T., Litvack, F., Grundfest, W. *et al.* (1986) Coronary angioscopy in patients with unstable angina pectoris. *N. Engl. J. Med.*, **315**, 913–9.
13. Mizuno, K., Satomura, K., Miyamoto, A. *et al.* (1992) Angioscopic evaluation of coronary-artery thrombi in acute coronary syndromes. *N. Engl. J. Med.*, **326**, 287–91.

14. Schmid, J.H., Jackson, D.P. and Conley, C.L. (1962) Mechanism of action of thrombin on platelets. *J. Clin. Invest.*, **41**, 543–53.
15. Hubbel, J.A. and McIntire, L.V. (1986) Platelet active concentration profiles near growing thrombi. *Biophys. J.*, **50**, 937–45.
16. Markwardt, F., Kaiser, B. and Novak, G. (1989) Studies on antithrombotic effects of recombinant hirudin. *Thromb. Res.*, **54**, 377–88.
17. Badimon, L., Badimon, J.J., Cohen, M. *et al.* (1991) Vessel wall-related risk factors in acute vascular events. *Drugs*, **42** (Suppl. 5), 1–9.
18. Scott, J. (1989) Lipoprotein (a). Thrombogenesis linked to artherogenesis at last? *Nature*, **341**, 22–3.
19. Fay, W.P. and Owen, W.G. (1989) Platelet plasminogen activator inhibitor: purification and characterization of interaction with plasminogen activators and activated protein C inhibitor. *Biochemistry*, **28**, 5773–8.
20. Cosgrove, D.M., Heric, B., Lytle, B.W. *et al.* (1992) Aprotinin therapy for reoperative myocardial revascularization: A placebo-controlled study. *Ann. Thorac. Surg.*, **54**, 1031–6.
21. Broze, G.L. and Meletich, J.P. (1987) Characterization of the inhibition of tissue factor in serum. *Blood*, **69**, 150–5.
22. Meyer, B. J., Badimon, J.J., Mailhac, A. *et al.* (1994) Therapeutic probes to inhibit thrombus growth on fresh mural thrombus: role of thrombin inhibition. *Circulation*, **90**, (in press).
23. Webster, M.W.I., Chesebro, J.H. and Fuster, V. (1990) Antithrombotic therapy in acute myocardial infarction: enhancement of thrombolysis, reduction of reocclusion and prevention of thromboembolism. In: Gersh, B.G. and Rahimtoola, S. (eds) *Management of Acute Myocardial Infarction*, pp. 333–348. New York: Elsevier.
24. Weitz, J.I. and Hudoba, M. (1988) Mechanism by which clot-bound thrombin is protected from inactivation by fluid-phase inhibitors. *Circulation*, **78** (Suppl. II), II-119.
25. Mruk, J.S., Chesebro, J.H. and Webster, M.W.I. (1990) Platelet aggregation and interaction with the coagulation system: implications for antithrombotic therapy in arterial thrombosis. *Coronary Artery Dis.*, **1**, 149–58.
26. Lam, J.Y.T., Chesebro, J.H., Steele, P.M. *et al.* (1987) Is vasospasm related to platelet deposition? *In vivo* relationship in a pig model of arterial injury. *Circulation*, **75**, 243–8.
27. Lam, J.Y.T., Chesebro, J.H. and Fuster, V. (1988) Platelets, vasoconstriction, and nitroglycerin during arterial wall injury: a new antithrombotic role for an old drug. *Circulation*, **78**, 712–16.
28. Penny, W.J., Chesebro, J.H., Heras, M. *et al.* (1988) *In vivo* identification of normal and damaged endothelium by quantitative coronary angiography and infusions of acetylcholine and bradykinin in pigs. *J. Am. Coll. Cardiol.*, **11**, 29A.
29. Webster, M.W.I., Chesebro, J.H., Heras, M. *et al.* (1989) Acetylcholine infusion identifies regrowth after porcine coronary endothelial denudation. *Circulation*, **80** (Suppl. II), II-648.
30. Boulanger, C. and Luscher, T.F. (1990) Release of endothelin from the porcine aorta. Inhibition by endothelium-derived nitric oxide. *J. Clin. Invest.*, **85**, 587–90.
31. Fischell, T.A., Derby, G., Tse, T.M. *et al.* (1988) Coronary artery vasoconstriction routinely occurs after percutaneous transluminal coronary angioplasty. *Circulation*, **78**, 1323–34.
32. Webster, M.W.I., Chesebro, J.H., Mruk, J.S. *et al.* (1991) Hypercholesterolemia induces abnormal coronary vasomotion *in vivo*. *J. Am. Coll. Cardiol.*, **17**, 173A.
33. Lerman, A., Webster, M.W.I., Chesebro, J.H. *et al.* (1993) Circulating and tissue endothelin immunoreactivity in hypercholesterolemic pigs. *Circulation*, **88**, 2923–8.
34. Diodati, J., Theroux, P., Latour, J.G. *et al.* (1990) Effects of nitroglycerin at therapeutic doses on platelet aggregation in unstable angina pectoris and acute myocardial infarction. *Am. J. Cardiol.*, **66**, 683–8.
35. Braunwald, E. (1993) The open-artery theory is alive and well again. *N. Engl. J. Med.*, **329**, 1650–52.
36. The GUSTO Angiographic Investigators (1993) The effects of tissue plasminogen activator, streptokinase, or both on coronary-artery patency, ventricular function, and survival after acute myocardial infarction. *N. Eng. J. Med.*, **329**, 1615–22.
36A. Cuccia, C., Volterrani, M., Volpini, M. *et al.* (1992) Relationship between anticoagulation level, ischemic events and angiographic characteristics of infarct-related artery following streptokinase in patients with acute myocardial infarcton (abstract). *J. Am. Coll. Cardiol.*, **19**, 92A.
37. Anderson, J.L., Karagounis, L.A., Becker, L.C. *et al.* (1993) TIMI perfusion grade 3 but not grade 2 results in improved outcome after thrombolysis for myocardial infarction. Ventriculographic, enzymatic, and electrocardiographic evidence form the TEAM-3 study. *Circulation*, **87**, 1829–39.
38. Gibson, C.M., Cannon, C.P., Piana, R.N. *et al.* (1993) Consequences of TIMI grade 2 vs 3 flow at 90 minutes following thrombolysis. *J. Am. Coll. Cardiol.*, **21**, 348A.
39. Chesebro, J.H., Knatterud, G., Roberts, R. *et al.* (1987) Thrombolysis in Myocardial Infarction (TIMI) trial, phase I: a comparison between intravenous tissue plasminogen activator and intravenous streptokinase. *Circulation*, **76**, 142–54.
40. Neuhaus, K.-L., von Essen, R., Tebbe, U. *et al.* (1992) Improved thrombolysis in acute myocardial infarction with front-loaded administration of alteplase: Results of the rt-PA–APSAC patency study (TAPS). *J. Am. Coll. Cardiol.*, **19**, 885–91.
41. Califf, R.M., Topol, E.J., Stack, R.S. *et al.* (1991) Evaluation of combination thrombolytic therapy and timing of cardiac catheterization in acute myocardial infarction: Results of thrombolysis and angioplasty in myocardial infarction–phase 5 randomized trial. *Circulation*, **83**, 1543–56.
42. Neuhaus, K., Tebbe, U., Gottwik, M. *et al.* (1988) Intravenous recombinant tissue plasminogen activator (rt-PA) and urokinase in acute myocardial infarction: Results of the German Activator Urokinase Study (GAUS). *J. Am. Coll. Cardiol.*, **12**, 581–7.

43. Neuhaus, K.L., Feuerer, W., Jeep-Tebbe, S. *et al.* (1989) Improved thrombolysis with a modified dose regimen of recombinant tissue-type plasminogen activator. *J. Am. Coll. Cardiol.*, **14**, 1566–9.
44. Ellis, S.G., Topol, E.J., George, B.S. *et al.* (1989) Recurrent ischemia without warning. Analysis of risk factors for in-hospital ischemic events following successful thrombolysis with intravenous tissue plasminogen activator. *Circulation*, **80**, 1159–65.
45. Kaplan, K., Davison, R., Parker, M. *et al.* (1987) Role of heparin after intravenous thrombolytic therapy for acute myocardial infarction. *Am. J. Cardiol.*, **59**, 241–4.
46. Arnout, J., Simoons, M., de Bono, D. *et al.* (1992) Correlation between level of heparinization and patency of the infarct-related coronary artery after treatment of acute myocardial infarction with alteplase (rt-PA). *J. Am. Coll. Cardiol.*, **20**, 513–19.
47. Topol, E.J., Califf, R.M., Vandormael, M. *et al.* (1992) A randomized trial of late reperfusion therapy for acute myocardial infarction. *Circulation*, **85**, 2090–9.
48. Meijer, A., Verheught, F.W.A., Werter, C.J. *et al.* (1993) Coumadin versus aspirin in the prevention of reocclusion after successful thrombolysis, a prospective placebo-controlled angiographic study. *Circulation*, **87**, 1524–30.
49. Fitzgerald, D.J., Catella, F., Roy, L. *et al.* (1988) Marked platelet activation *in vivo* after intravenous streptokinase in patients with acute myocardial infarction. *Circulation*, **77**, 142–50.
50. Gash, A.K., Spann, J.F., Sherry, S. *et al.* (1986) Factors influencing reocclusion after coronary thrombolysis for acute myocardial infarction. *Am. J. Cardiol.*, **57**, 175–7.
51. Weitz, J.I., Hudoba, M., Massel, D. *et al.* (1990) Clot-bound thrombin is protected from inhibition by heparin–antithrombin III but is susceptible to inactivation by antithrombin III-independent inhibitors. *J. Clin. Invest.*, **86**, 385–91.
52. Merlini, P.A., Bauer, K.A., Ottrona, L. *et al.* (1994) Persistent activation of coagulation mechanism in unstable angina and myocardial infarction. *Circulation*, **90**, 61–8.
53. Gold, H.K., Leinbach, R.C., Garabedian, H.C. *et al.* (1986) Acute coronary reocclusion after thrombolysis with recombinant human tissue-type plasminogen activator: prevention by a maintenance infusion. *Circulation*, **73**, 347–52.
54. Francis, C.W., Markham, R.E. Jr. and Marder, V.J. (1984) Demonstration of *in situ* fibrin degradation in pathologic thrombi. *Blood*, **63**, 1216–24.
55. Lee, C.D. and Mann, K.G. (1989) Activation/inactivation of human factor V by plasmin. *Blood*, **73**, 185–90.
56. Eisenberg, P.R. and Miletich, J.P. (1989) Induction of marked thrombin activity by pharmacologic concentrations of plasminogen activators in nonanticoagulated whole blood. *Thromb. Res.*, **55**, 635–43.
57. Kerins, D.M, Roy, L., Fitzgerald, G.A. *et al.* (1989) Platelet and vascular function during coronary thrombolysis with tissue-type plasminogen activator. *Circulation*, **80**, 1718–25.
58. Fitzgerald, D.J., Catella, F., Roy, L. *et al.* (1988) Marked platelet activation *in vivo* after intravenous streptokinase in patients with acute myocardial infarction. *Circulation*, **77**, 142–50.
59. Vaughan, D.E., Van Houtte, E., Declerck, P.J. *et al.* (1989) Prevalence and mechanism of streptokinase-induced platelet aggregation. *Circulation*, **80** (Suppl. II), II-218.
60. Owen, J., Friedman, K.D., Grossman, B.A. *et al.* (1988) Thrombolytic therapy with tissue plasminogen activator or streptokinase induces transient thrombin activity. *Blood*, **72**, 616–20.
61. Eisenberg, P.R., Sherman, L.A. and Jaffe, A.S. (1987) Paradoxic elevation of fibrinopeptide A after streptokinase: evidence for continued thrombosis despite intense fibrinolysis. *J. Am. Coll. Cardiol.*, **10**, 527–9.
62. Rapold, H.J., de Bono, D., Arnold, A.E.R. *et al.* (1992) Plasma fibrinopeptide A levels in patients with acute myocardial infarction treated with alteplase. Correlation with concomitant heparin, coronary artery patency, and recurrent ischemia. *Circulation*, **85**, 928–34.
63. Rapold, H.J. (1990) Promotion of thrombin activity by thrombolytic therapy without simultaneous anticoagulation. *Lancet*, **335**, 481–2.
64. Gulba, D.C., Barthels, M., Reil, G.-H. *et al.* (1988) Thrombin/antithrombin-III complex level as early predictor of reocclusion after successful thrombolysis. *Lancet*, **ii**, 97.
65. Gulba, D.C., Barthels, M., Westhoff-Bleck, M. *et al.* (1991) Increased thrombin levels during thrombolytic therapy in acute myocardial infarction. Relevance for the success of therapy. *Circulation*, **83**, 937–44.
66. Cercek, B., Lew, A.S. and Hod, H. (1986) Enhancement of thrombolysis with tissue-type plasminogen activator by pretreatment with heparin. *Circulation*, **74**, 583–7.
67. Tomaru, T., Uchida, Y., Nakamura, F. *et al.* (1989) Enhancement of arterial thrombolysis with native tissue type plasminogen activator by pretreatment with heparin or batroxobin: An angioscopic study. *Am. Heart J.*, **117**, 275–81.
68. Fitzgerald, D.J., Wright, F. and Fitzgerald, G.A. (1988) Thrombin-mediated platelet activation during coronary thrombolysis. *Circulation*, **78** (suppl. II), II-120.
69. Tamao, Y., Yamamoto, T., Kikumoto, R. *et al.* (1986) Effect of a selective thrombin inhibitor MCI-9038 on fibrinolysis *in vitro* and *in vivo*. *Thromb. Haemost.*, **56**, 28–34.
70. Jang, I.K., Gold, H.K., Leinbach, R.C. *et al.* (1990) *In vivo* thrombin inhibition enhances and sustains arterial recanalization with recombinant tissue-type plasminogen activator. *Circ. Res.*, **67**, 1552–61.
71. Haskel, E.J., Adams, S.P., Feigen, L.P. *et al.* (1989) Prevention of reoccluding platelet-rich thrombi in canine femoral arteries with a novel peptide antagonist of platelet glycoprotein IIb/IIIa receptors. *Circulation*, **80**, 1775–82.
72. Fitzgerald, D.J., Wright, F. and Fitzgerald, G.A. (1989) Increased thromboxane biosynthesis during coronary thrombolysis. Evidence that platelet activation and thromboxane A_2 modulate the response to tissue-type plasminogen activator *in vivo*. *Circ. Res.*, **65**, 83–94.

73. Gold, H.K., Coller, B.S., Yasuda, T. *et al.* (1988) Rapid and sustained coronary artery recanalization with combined bolus injection of recombinant tissue-type plasminogen activator and monoclonal antiplatelet GPIIb/IIIa antibody in an canine preparation. *Circulation*, **77**, 670–7.
74. Yasuda, T., Gold, H.K., Fallon, J.T. *et al.* (1988) Monoclonal antibody against the platelet glycoprotein (GP) IIb/IIIa receptor prevents coronary artery reocclusion after reperfusion with recombinant tissue-type plasminogen activator in dogs. *J. Clin. Invest.*, **81**, 1284–91.
75. Mickelson, J.K., Simpson, P.J., Cronin, M. *et al.* (1990) Antiplatelet antibody [7E3 F(ab')₂] prevents rethrombosis after recombinant tissue-type plasminogen activator-induced coronary artery thrombolysis in a canine model. *Circulation*, **81**, 617–27.
76. Golino, P., Ashton, J.H. and McNatt, J. (1989) Simultaneous administration of thromboxane A₂- and serotonin S₂-receptor antagonists markedly enhances thrombolysis and prevents or delays reocclusion after tissue-type plasminogen activator in a canine model of coronary thrombosis. *Circulation*, **79**, 911–19.
77. Golino, P., Ashton, J.H., Glas-Greenwalt, P. *et al.* (1988) Mediation of reocclusion by thromboxane A₂ and serotonin after thrombolysis with tissue-type plasminogen activator in a canine preparation of coronary thrombosis. *Circulation*, **77**, 678–84.
78. Haskel, E.J., Prager, N.A., Sobel, B.E. *et al.* (1991) Relative efficacy of antithrombin compared with antiplatelet agents in accelerating coronary thrombolysis and preventing early reocclusion. *Circulation*, **83**, 1048–56.
78A. Chesebro, J.H. and Fuster, V. (1991) Dynamic thrombosis and thrombolysis: role of antithrombins. *Circulation*, **83**, 1815–7.
79. Coller, B.S. (1990) Platelets and thrombolytic therapy. *N. Eng. J. Med.*, **322**, 33–42.
80. Patrignani, P., Filabozzi, P. and Patrono, C. (1982) Selective cumulative inhibition of platelet thromboxane production by low-dose aspirin in healthy subjects. *J. Clin. Invest.*, **69**, 1366–72.
81. Reilly, I.A.G. and Fitzgerald, G.A. (1987) Inhibition of thromboxane formation *in vivo* and *ex vivo*; implications for therapy with platelet inhibitory drugs. *Blood*, **69**, 180–6.
82. ISIS-2 (Second International Study of Infarct Survival) Collaborative Group (1988) Randomized trial of intravenous streptokinase, oral aspirin, both, or neither among 17 187 cases of suspected acute myocardial infarction: ISIS-2 *Lancet*, **ii**, 349–60.
83. Baigent, C. and Collins, R. for the ISIS Collaborative Group (1993) ISIS-2: 4-year mortality follow-up of 17 187 patients after fibrinolytic and antiplatelet therapy in suspected acute myocardial infarction. *Circulation*, **88** (Suppl. I), I-291.
84. Roux, S., Christeller, S. and Ludin, E. (1992) Effects of aspirin on coronary reocclusion and recurrent ischemia after thrombolysis: A meta-analysis. *J. Am. Coll. Cardiol.*, **19**, 671–7.
85. Lewis, H.D., Davis, J.W. and Archibald, D.G. (1983) Protective effects of aspirin against acute myocardial infarction and death in men with unstable angina: results of a Veterans Administration Cooperative Study. *N. Eng. J. Med.*, **309**, 396–403.
86. Cairns, J.A., Gent, M., Singer, J. *et al.* (1985) Aspirin, sulfinpyrazone, or both in unstable angina. *N. Engl. J. Med.*, **313**, 1369–75.
87. Theroux, P., Ouimet, H., McCans, J. *et al.* (1988) Aspirin, heparin, or both to treat acute unstable angina. *N. Eng. J. Med.*, **319**, 1105–11.
88. Theroux, P., Waters, D., Shiqiang, Q. *et al.* (1993) Aspirin versus heparin to prevent myocardial infarction during the acute phase of unstable angina. *Circulation*, **88**, 2045–8.
89. Hirsh, J. (1991) Heparin. *N. Engl. J. Med.*, **324**, 1565–74.
90. Petitou, M., Lormeau, J.C., Perly, B. *et al.* (1988) Is there a unique sequence in heparin for interaction with heparin cofactor II? Structural and biological studies of heparin-cofactor II. *J. Biol. Chem.*, **263**, 8685–90.
91. Tollefsen, D.M., Majerus, D.W. and Blank, M.K. (1982) Heparin cofactor II. Purification and properties of thrombin in human plasma. *J. Biol. Chem.*, **257**, 2162–9.
92. Maimone, M.M. and Tollefsen, D.M. (1988) Activation of heparin cofactor II by heparin oligosaccharides. *Biochem. Biophys. Res. Commun.*, **152**, 1056–61.
93. Hurst, R.E., Poon, M.C. and Griffith, M.J. (1983) Structure–activity relationships of heparin. Independence of heparin charge density and antithrombin binding domains in thrombin inhibition by antithrombin and heparin cofactor II. *J. Clin. Invest.*, **72**, 1042–5.
94. Sie, P., Petitou, M., Lormeau, J.C. *et al.* (1988) Studies on the structural requirements of heparin for the catalysis of thrombin inhibition by heparin cofactor II. *Biochem. Biophys. Acta*, **966**, 188–95.
95. Jang, I.K., Gold, H.K., Ziskind, A.A. *et al.* (1990) Prevention of platelet-rich arterial thrombosis by selective thrombin inhibition. *Circulation*, **81**, 219–25.
96. Bar-Shavit, R., Eldor, A. and Vlodavsky, I. (1989) Binding of thrombin to subendothelial extracellular matrix. *J. Clin. Invest.*, **84**, 1096–104.
97. Bock, P.E., Luscombe, M., Marshall, S.E. *et al.* (1980) The multiple complexes formed by the interaction of platelet factor 4 with heparin. *Biochem. J.*, **191**, 769–76.
98. Zoldhelyi, P., Chesebro, J.H., Mruk, J.S. *et al.* (1992) Failure of aspirin compared with heparin or hirudin to enhance lysis by rt-PA of platelet-rich thrombus after deep arterial injury in the pig. *J. Am. Coll. Cardiol.*, **19** (Suppl. A), 91A.
99. Chalmers, T.C., Matta, R.J., Smith, H. *et al.* (1977) Evidence favoring the use of anticoagulants in the hospital phase of acute myocardial infarction. *N. Engl. J. Med.*, **297**, 1091–6.
100. Yusuf, S., Slieght, P., Held, P. *et al.* (1990) Routine medical management of acute myocardial infarction. *Circulation*, **82** (Suppl. II), II-117–II-134.

101. Lau, J., Antman, E.M., Jimenez-Silva, J. et al. (1992) Cumulative meta-analysis of therapeutic trials for myocardial infarction. N. Eng. J. Med., **327**, 248–54.
102. MacMahon, S., Collins, R., Knight, C. et al. (1988) Reduction in major morbidity and mortality by heparin in acute myocardial infarction. Circulation, **78** (Suppl. II), II-98.
103. Topol, E.J., George, B.S., Kereiakes, D.J. et al. (1989) A randomized controlled trial of intravenous tissue plasminogen activator and early intravenous heparin in acute myocardial infarction. Circulation, **79**, 281–6.
104. De Bono, D.P., Simoons, M.L., Tijssen, J. et al. (1992) Effect of early intravenous heparin on coronary patency, infarct size, and bleeding complications after alteplase thrombolysis: results of a randomized double blind European Cooperative Study Group trial. Br. Heart J., **67**, 122–8.
105. Hsai, J., Hamilton, W.P., Kleiman, N. et al. (1990) A comparison between heparin and low-dose aspirin as adjunctive therapy with tissue plasminogen activator for acute myocardial infarction. Heparin–Aspirin Reperfusion Trial (HART) Investigators. N. Eng. J. Med., **323**, 1433–7.
106. Bleich, S.D., Nichols, T., Schumacher, R. et al. (1989) The role of heparin following coronary thrombolysis with tissue plasminogen activator (t-PA). Circulation, **80** (Suppl. II), II-113.
107. Thompson, P.L., Aylward, P.E., Federman, J. et al. (1991) A randomized comparison of intravenous heparin with oral aspirin and dipyridamole 24 h after recombinant tissue-type plasminogen activator for acute myocardial infarction. Circulation, **83**, 1534–42.
108. Hsai, J., Kleiman, N., Aguirre, F. et al. (1992) Heparin-induced prolongation of partial thromboplastin time after thrombolysis: Relation to coronary artery patency. J. Am. Coll. Cardiol., **20**, 31–5.
109. Gruppo Italiano per lo Studio della Sopravivenza nell'Infarto Miocardico (1990) GISSI-2: A factorial randomized trial of alteplase versus streptokinase and heparin versus no heparin among 12 490 patients with acute myocardial infarction. Lancet, **336**, 65–71.
110. The International Study Group (1990) In-hospital mortality and clinical course of 20 891 patients with suspected acute myocardial infarction randomized between alteplase and streptokinase with or without heparin. Lancet, **336**, 71–5.
111. ISIS-3 (Third International Study of Infarct Survival) Collaborative Group (1992) ISIS-3: a randomized comparison of streptokinase vs tissue plasminogen activator vs anistreplase and of aspirin plus heparin vs aspirin alone among 41 299 cases of suspected acute myocardial infarction. Lancet, **339**, 753–70.
112. SCATI (Second International Study of Infarct Survival) Collaborative Group (1989) Randomized trial of intravenous streptokinase, oral aspirin, both or neither among 17 187 cases of suspected acute myocardial infarction: ISIS-2. Lancet, **ii**, 182–6.
113. Delanty, N. and Fitzgerald, D.J. (1992) Subcutaneous heparin during coronary thrombolysis. 'Too little, too late'. Circulation, **86**, 1636–8.
114. Kroon, C., ten Hove, W.R., de Boer, A. et al. (1990) Highly variable anticoagulant response after subcutaneous administration of high dose (12 500 IU) heparin in patients with myocardial infarction and healthy volunteers. Circulation, **86**, 1370–5.
115. Ohman, E.M. Califf, R., Topol, E.J. et al. (1990) Consequences of reocclusion after successful reperfusion therapy in acute myocardial infarction. Circulation, **82**, 781–91.
116. The Gusto Investigators (1993) An international randomized trial comparing four thrombolytic strategies for acute myocardial infarction. N. Eng. J. Med., **329**, 673–82.
116A. The GUSTO IIa Investigators (1994) A randomized trial of intravenous heparin versus recombinant hirudin for acute coronary syndromes. Circulation (in press).
116B. Antman, E.M. for the TIMI 9A Investigators (1994) Hirudin in acute myocardial infarction: safety report from the thrombolysis and thrombin inhibition in myocardial infarction (TIMI) 9A trial. Circulation (in press).
117. Smith, P., Arnesen, H. and Holme, I. (1990) The effect of warfarin on mortality and reinfarction after myocardial infarction. N. Engl. J. Med., **323**, 147–52.
118. Report of the 60+ Reinfarction Study Research Group (1980) A double-blind trial to assess long-term anticoagulant therapy in elderly patients after myocardial infarction. Lancet, **ii**, 989–94.
119. Nakagawa, S., Hanada, Y. and Koiwaya, Y. (1988) Angiographic features in the infarct-related artery after intracoronary urokinase followed by prolonged anticoagulation. Role of ruptured atheromatous plaque and adherent thrombus in acute myocardial infarction in vivo. Circulation, **78**, 1335–44.
120. Turpie, A.G.G., Gent, M., Laupacis, A. et al. (1993) A comparison of aspirin with placebo in patients treated with warfarin after heart-valve replacement. N. Engl. J. Med., **329**, 524–9.
121. Cohen, M., Adams, P.C., Parry, G. et al. (1994) Combination antithrombotic therapy in rest unstable angina and non-Q wave infarction in non-prior aspirin users. Primary end points analysis from the ATACS trial. Circulation, **89**, 81–8.
122. Cannon, C.P., McCabe, C.H., Henry, T.D. et al. (1994) A pilot trial of recombinant desulfatohirudin compared with heparin in conjunction with tissue-type plasminogen activator and aspirin for acute myocardial infarction: results of the thrombolysis in myocardial infarction (TIMI) 5 Trial. J. Am. Coll. Cardiol., **23**, 993–1003.
123. Zoldhelyi, P., Webster, M.W.I., Fuster, V. et al. (1993) Recombinant hirudin in patients with chronic, stable coronary artery disease. Safety, half-life and effect of coagulation parameters. Circulation, **88**, 2015–22.
124. Verstraete, M., Nurmohamed, M., Kienast, J. et al. (1993) Biologic effects of recombinant hirudin (CGP 39 393) in human volunteers. J. Am. Coll. Cardiol., **22**, 1080–8.
125. Neuhaus, K.L., Niederer, W., Wagner, J. et al. (1993) HIT (hirudin for the improvement of thrombolysis): results of a dose escalating study. Circulation, **88** (Suppl. I), I-292.
126. Markwardt, F. (1991) Hirudin and derivatives as anticoagulant agents. Thromb. Haemost., **66**, 141–52.

127. Zoldhelyi, P., Fuster, V. and Chesebro, J.H. (1992) Antithrombins as conjunctive therapy in arterial thrombolysis. *Coronary Artery Dis.*, **3**, 1003–9.
128. Zoldhelyi, P., Bichler, J., Owen, W.G. *et al.* (1994) Persistent thrombin generation in humans during specific thrombin inhibition with hirudin. *Circulation* (in press).
129. Rigel, D.F., Olson, R.W. and Lappe, R.W. (1993) Comparison of hirudin and heparin as adjuncts to streptokinase thrombolysis in a canine model of coronary thrombosis. *Circ. Res.*, **72**, 1091–102.
130. Lidon, R.-M., Theroux, P., Juneau, M. *et al.* (1993) Initial experience with a direct antithrombin, hirulog, in unstable angina. Anticoagulant, antithrombotic, and clinical effects. *Circulation*, **88**, 1495–501.
131. Topol, E.J., Fuster, V., Harrington, R.A. *et al.* (1994) Recombinant hirudin for unstable angina pectoris: A multicenter, randomized angiographic trial. *Circulation*, **89**, 1557–66.
132. Kleiman, N.S., Ohman, M., Califf, R. *et al.* (1993) Profound inhibition of platelet aggregation with monoclonal antibody 7E3 Fab after thrombolytic therapy. Results of the Thrombolytic and Angioplasty in Myocardial Infarction (TAMI) 8 Pilot Study. *J. Am. Coll. Cardiol.*, **22**, 381–9.
133. Tcheng, J.E., Topol, E.J., Kleinmann, N.S. *et al.* (1993) Improvement in clinical outcomes of coronary angioplasty by treatment with the GPIIb/IIIa inhibitor chimeric 7E3: Multivariate analysis of the EPIC study. *Circulation*, **88** (Suppl. II), II-506.
134. Keren, A., Goldberg, S., Gottlieb, S. *et al.* (1990) Natural history of left ventricular thrombi: their appearance and resolution in the posthospitalization period of acute myocardial infarction. *J. A. Coll. Cardiol.*, **15**, 790–800.
135. Asinger, R.W., Mikell, F.L., Elsperger, J. *et al.* (1981) Incidence of left ventricular thrombosis after acute transmural myocardial infarction: Serial evaluation by two-dimensional echocardiography. *N. Eng. J. Med.*, **305**, 297–302.
136. Galema, T.W., Meijer, A., Kamp, O. *et al.* (1992) Relation between early development of left ventricular thrombus and coronary patency after acute myocardial infarction. *Circulation*, **86** (Suppl. I), I-48.
137. Hochman, J.S., Platia, E.B. and Bulkey, B.H. (1984) Endocardial abnormalities in left ventricular aneurysms: a clinicopathologic study. *Ann. Intern. Med.*, **100**, 29–35.
138. Domenicucci, S., Bellotti, P., Chiarella, F. *et al.* (1987) Spontaneous morphologic changes in left ventricular thrombi: a prospective two-dimensional echocardiographic study. *Circulation*, **75**, 737–43.
139. Domenicucci, S., Chiarella, F., Bellotti, P. *et al.* (1990) Early appearance of left ventricular thrombi after anterior myocardial infarction: a marker of higher in-hospital mortality in patients not treated with antithrombotic drugs. *Eur. Heart J.*, **11**, 51–8.
140. Hilden, R., Iversen, K., Rasaschou, F. *et al.* (1961) Anticoagulants in acute myocardial infarction. *Lancet*, **ii**, 327–31.
141. Veterans Administration Cooperative Investigators (1973) Anticoagulants in acute myocardial infarction: Results of a cooperative clinical trial. *JAMA*, **225**, 724–9.
142. Ezekowitz, M.D., Wilson, D.A., Smith, E.O., *et al.* (1982) Comparison of indium-111 platelet scintigraphy and two-dimensional echocardiography in the diagnosis of left ventricular thrombi. *N. Engl. J. Med.*, **306**, 1509–13.
143. Asinger, R.W., Mikell, F.L., Sharma, B. *et al.* (1981) Observations on detecting left ventricular thrombus with two-dimensional echocardiography: Emphasis on avoidance of false positive diagnoses. *Am. J. Cardiol.*, **47**, 145–56.
144. Visser, C.A., Kan, G., David, G.K. *et al.* (1983) Two-dimensional echocardiography in the diagnosis of left ventricular thrombus: A prospective study of 67 patients with anatomic validation. *Chest*, **83**, 228–32.
145. Turpie, A.G.G., Robinson, J.H., Doyle, D.J. *et al.* (1989) Comparison of high-dose with low-dose subcutaneous heparin to prevent left ventricular mural thrombosis in patients with acute transmural anterior myocardial infarction. *N. Engl. J. Med.*, **320**, 352–7.
146. Nordrehaug, J.E., Johannessen, K.A. and Von Der Lippe, G. (1985) Usefulness of high-dose anticoagulants in preventing left ventricular thrombus in acute myocardial infarction *Am. Heart J.*, **55**, 1491–3.
147. Arvan, S. and Boscha, K. (1987) Prophylactic anticoagulation for left ventricular thrombi after acute myocardial infarction: A prospective randomized trial. *Am. Heart J.*, **113**, 688–93.
148. Davis, M.J.E. and Ireland, M.A. (1986) Effect of early anticoagulation on the frequency of left ventricular thrombi after anterior wall acute myocardial infarction. *Am. J. Cardiol.*, **57**, 1244–7.
149. Gueret, P., Dubourg, O., Ferrier, A. *et al.* (1986) Effects of full-dose heparin anticoagulation on the development of left ventricular thrombosis in acute myocardial infarction. *J. Am. Coll. Cardiol.*, **8**, 419–26.
150. Vecchio, C., Chiarella, F., Lupi, G. *et al.* (1991) Left ventricular thrombus in anterior acute myocardial infarction after thrombolysis. A GISSI-2 connected study. *Circulation*, **84**, 512–19.
151. Vaitkus, P.T. and Barnathan, E.S. (1993) Embolic potential, prevention and management of mural thrombus complicating anterior myocardial infarction: a meta-analysis. *J. Am. Coll. Cardiol.*, **22**, 1004–9.
152. Report of the Working Party on Anticoagulant Therapy in Coronary Thrombosis to the Medical Research Council (1969) Assessment of short-term anticoagulant administration after cardiac infarction. *BMJ*, **1**, 335–42.
153. Kouvaras, G., Chronopoulos, G., Soufras, G. *et al.* (1990) The effects of long-term antithrombotic treatment on left ventricular thrombi in patients after an acute myocardial infarction. *Am. Heart J.*, **119**, 73–8.
154. Tramarin, R., Pozzoli, M., Febo, O. *et al.* (1986) Two-dimensional echocardiographic assessment of anticoagulant therapy in left ventricular thrombosis early after acute myocardial infarction. *Eur. Heart J.*, **7**, 482–92.
155. Funke Kupper, A.J., Verheugt, F.W.A., Peels, C.H. *et al.* (1989) Left ventricular thrombus incidence and behavior studied by serial two-dimensional echocardiography in acute anterior myocardial infarction: Left ventricular wall motion, systemic embolism and oral anticoagulation. *J. Am. Coll. Cardiol.*, **13**, 1514–20.
156. Jugdutt, B.I., Sivaram, C.A., Wortman, C. *et al.* (1989) Prospective two-dimensional echocardiographic evaluation of left ventricular thrombus and embolism after acute myocardial infarction. *J. Am. Coll. Cardiol.*, **13**, 554–64.
157. Johannessen, K.A., Nordrehaug, J.E. and Von Der Lippe, G. (1987) Left ventricular thrombi after short-term high-dose anticoagulants in acute myocardial infarction. *Eur. Heart J.*, **8**, 975–80.

158. Lapeyre, A.C., Steel, P.M., Kazmier, F.J. *et al.* (1985) Systemic embolism in chronic left ventricular aneurysm: Incidence and the role of anticoagulation. *J. Am. Coll. Cardiol.*, **6**, 534–8.

159 Funke Kupper, A.J., Verheugt, F.W.A., Peeis, C.H. *et al.* (1989) Effect of low dose acetylsalicylic acid on the frequency and hematologic activity of left ventricular thrombus in anterior wall acute myocardial infarction. *Am. J. Cardiol.*, **63**, 917–20.

160. Johannessen, K.A., Stratton, J.R., Taulow, E. *et al.* (1989) Usefulness of aspirin plus dipyridamole in reducing left ventricular thrombus formation in anterior wall acute myocardial infarction. *Am. J. Cardiol.*, **63**, 101–2.

161. Nicolaides, A.N., Kakkar, V.V., Renney, J.T.G. *et al.* (1971) Myocardial infarction and deep-vein thrombosis. *BMJ*, **1**, 432–4.

162. Maurer, B.J., Wray, R. and Shillingford, J.P. (1971) Frequency of venous thrombosis after myocardial infarction. *Lancet*, **ii**, 1385–7.

163. Flanc, C., Kakkar, V.V. and Clarke, M.B. (1968) The detection of venous thrombosis of the legs using ^{125}I-labelled fibrinogen. *Br. J. Surg.*, **55**, 742–7.

164. Kakkar, V.V., Howe, C.T., Flanc, C. *et al.* (1969) Natural history of postoperative deep-vein thrombosis. *Lancet*, **ii**, 230–3.

165. Ygge, J. (1970) Changes in blood coagulation and fibrinolysis during the postoperative period. *Am. J. Surg.*, **119** 225–32.

166. Miller, R., Lies, J.E., Caretta, R.F. *et al.* (1976) Prevention of lower extremity venous thrombosis by early mobilization: Confirmation in patients with acute myocardial infarction by ^{125}I-fibrinogen uptake and venography. *Ann. Intern. Med.*, **84**, 700–3.

167. Emerson, P.A., Teather, D. and Handley, A.J. (1974) The application of decision theory to the prevention of deep vein thrombosis following myocardial infarction. *Q. J. Med.*, **43**, 389–98.

168. Gallus, A.S., Hirsh, J., Tuttle, R.J. *et al.* (1973) Small subcutaneous doses of heparin in prevention of venous thrombosis. *N. Engl. J. Med.*, **288**, 545–51.

169. Warlow, C., Beattie, A.G., Terry, G. *et al.* (1973) A double-blind trial of low doses of subcutaneous heparin in the prevention of deep-vein thrombosis after myocardial infarction. *Lancet*, **ii**, 934.

170. Emerson, P.A. and Marks, P. (1977) Preventing thromboembolism after myocardial infarction: Effect of low-dose heparin or smoking. *BMJ*, **1**, 18.

171. Hull, R.D., Rascob, G.E., Pineo, G.F. *et al.* (1992) Subcutaneous low-molecular-weight heparin compared with continuous intravenous heparin in the treatment of proximal vein thrombosis. *N. Eng. J. Med.*, **326**, 975–82.

172. Hull, R.D., Rascob, G.E., Pineo, G.F. *et al.* (1993) A comparison of subcutaneous low-molecular-weight heparin with warfarin sodium for prophylaxis against deep vein thrombosis after hip or knee implantation. *N. Eng. J. Med.*, **329**, 1370–6.

173. Heras, M., Chesebro, J.H., Webster, M.W.I. *et al.* (1992) Antithrombotic efficacy of low-molecular-weight heparin in deep arterial injury. *Arterioscler. Thromb.*, **12**, 250–5.

174. Rentrop, K.P., Feit, F. and Blanke, H. (1984) Effects of intracoronary streptokinase and intracoronary nitroglycerin infusion on coronary angiographic patterns amd mortality in patients with acute myocardial infarction. *N. Eng. J. Med.*, **311**, 1457–63.

175. Bovill, E.G., Granger, C.B., Ross, A. *et al.* (1993) Thrombin inhibition is more closely related to PTT than to heparin level after thrombolysis and heparin therapy. *J. Am. Coll. Cardiol.*, **21**, 137A.

β-Blockers and Calcium Antagonists

D. Chamberlain

β-Adrenoceptor Antagonists (β-blockers)

Basic Pharmacology

The first clear suggestion by Ahlquist[1] in 1948 that receptors for sympathetic stimulation could be divided into α and β subtypes attracted little immediate attention until the development of the β-adrenoceptor antagonist (β-blocker) dichloroisoprenaline (DCI)[2] provided both proof of the hypothesis and a powerful pharmacologic tool. Some clinicians,[3] and more importantly some pharmaceutical companies, realized the potential of β-adrenoceptor blockade for the treatment of cardiac disorders. But exploitation of the concept awaited the introduction of compounds that were capable of blocking the receptors without themselves providing a strong component of stimulation (agonist activity) – a property that made the parent DCI unsuitable for clinical use. The management of myocardial infarction provided the principal motive for Sir James Black to synthesize pronethalol (Nethalide): the first papers in a clinical journal appeared in 1962.[4,5] Possible oncogenic properties led to this drug being abandoned. Propranolol was available almost immediately to take its place. Surprisingly, sotalol had already been synthesized[6] but its potential as a therapeutic agent was not fully appreciated and clinical investigation was greatly delayed.

There followed an explosion of interest in β-adrenoceptor antagonists through the 1960s and 1970s. Progress in the pharmacodynamics of the new class of drugs was accompanied by the introduction of novel compounds by many pharmaceutical companies. Whilst the new compounds had in common the class properties of blockade of β-receptors, they showed considerable diversity in their properties, both in relation to the effects on receptors and, to a much lesser degree, to nonspecfic properties. The latter include membrane (or quinidine) effects.[7] Although these become important only at high concentrations, the volume of distribution of propranolol[8] suggests that intracellular concentrations may routinely be much higher than plasma levels would suggest, in keeping with evidence that membrane-stabilizing action may contribute to the antiarrhythmic effects of propranolol at least at high therapeutic doses.[9]

The diverse pharmacologic actions relate in part to the further subdivision of β-receptors into those categorized as β_1 (predominantly stimulatory cardiac effects) and β_2 (predominantly inhibitory effects such as bronchodilatation and vasodepression but also influencing some ion transport mechanisms). The human heart is unusual, however, in

Table 7.1 Pharmacology of β-Blockers

	β₁ selectivity	Agonist activity	Membrane effects	α-Blockade	Vasodilatation	Log partition coeffecient of octanol/water	Elimination half-life (h)
Acebutolol	+/−	+	+	−	−	1.87	2–3
Alprenolol	−	+	+	−	−	2.61	2–3
Atenolol	+	−	−	−	−	0.23	6–9
Bisoprolol	+	−	−	−	−	2.6	10–12
Celiprolol	+	+(β₂)	−	−	+	0.6–0.9	4.5
Esmolol	+	−	−	−	−	(water sol.)	0.15
Labetalol	−	+(β₂)	+	α₁	+	3.09†	4
Metoprolol	+	−	+/−	−	−	2.15	3–4
Nadolol	−	−	−	−	−	0.17	14–20
Oxprenolol	−	+	+	−	−	2.18	1–4
Pindolol	−	++	+	−	−	1.75	2–5
Practolol*	+	+	−	−	−	0.79	10–13
Propranolol	−	−	+	−	−	3.65	2–5
Sotalol	−	−	−	−	−	0.79	7–18
Timolol	−	−	+	−	−	2.50	2–5

†Theoretical value; *no longer available.
Modified from Hjalmarson, Å., Hugenholtz, P.G., and Julian, D.G. (eds) *β-blockers in Acute Myocardial Infarction*, (p. 74). New Zealand: Adis Press.

that 30% of the β-receptors are of the β₂ subtype.[10] The familiar agents of clinical importance block either β₁ receptors predominantly or block both receptor subtypes. In addition, the β-blockers vary in their degree of agonist activity. One agent that is available for clinical use (labetalol) combines some α-receptor blockade with β-blockade, whilst others (e.g. celiprolol) have direct vasodilator properties. Variation in water or fat solubility (hydrophilic or lipophilic) are determinants of the route of excretion and influence central nervous system effects. Finally, rapid metabolism of some compounds *in vivo* confers an ultra-short half-life that is of considerable clinical importance: esmolol is best known. Table 7.1 summarizes the important variable properties of the agents that are commonly available now or that contibuted in the past to our understanding of the role of β-blockade in the management of myocardial infarction.

At the cellular level the adrenergic antagonists block activity by occupying receptor sites and preventing the activation of the intracellular second messengers. With normal function, receptor activity is mediated when agonists attach to G proteins on cell membranes and thereby release the membrane bound enzymes adenylate cyclase and guanylate cyclase that convert adenosine triphosphate and guanosine triphosphate respectively to the corresponding adenosine cyclic nucleotides adenosine-3', 5'-monophosphate (cyclic AMP) and guanosine-3', 5'-monophosphate (cyclic GMP): these are the so-called second messengers. β-Adrenoceptor stimulation acts principally through the adenosine system to promote phosphorylation of specific substrates. Cyclic AMP does not persist in the cell: it is metabolized by phosphodiesterase which can also be regulated pharmacologically. Phosphodiesterase inhibitors increase cyclic AMP concentrations and have gained prominence as agents to improve myocardial perform-ance in infarction with effects that resemble those of catecholamines and tend to have opposite effects to β-blockers. Phosphodiesterase inhibitors (that include aminophylline as an older agent and milrinone and ethoximone as newer ones) should be mentioned in the present context because they act beyond the site of β-blockade. Thus, they have some value in restoring diminished levels of cyclic AMP if β-blockade has unforseen hemody-namic consequences that pose a serious threat to the patient.

The principal and most fundamental actions of β-blockade on the heart at a clinical level can be deduced by considering the four major ways in which physiologic stimulation of β-receptors modifies cardiac performance. These are: enhanced automaticity of the sinus node, enhanced automaticity of subsidiary pacemakers, enhanced conductivity through the atrioventricular (AV) node, and enhanced contractility of both the atrial and ventricular myocardium. The converse effects of β-blockade are most prominent when sympathetic stimulation is heightened under physiologic or pathophysiologic conditions of stress including exercise, excitement and the conditions such as heart failure that provide a compensatory increase in sympathetic tone.

Other consequences follow that are of a particular importance in the context of myocardial infarction and in some of its complications. Both a fall in heart rate and a decrease in contractility after β-blockade reduce myocardial metabolic requirements. But the effects are complex. For example, the fall in heart rate and decrease in contractility lead also to an increase in ventricular size,[11] and therefore, following the law of Laplace, to increased wall stress. This partly counters any potential fall in metabolic requirement, especially in patients with incipient or overt heart failure. Again, decrease in heart rate may enhance coronary flow in epicardial arteries by prolonging diastolic time, but the benefit is eroded to a degree because the duration of each systole is prolonged.

The overall hemodynamic consequences of β-blockade are complicated further by vascular effects both on the coronary arteries and peripherally. The nature of the direct action on coronary vessels has been controversial but is less important than the physiologic adjustment that balances myocardial oxygen supply to altered metabolic demand:[12] thus, coronary flow usually falls with β-blockade. Lower peripheral resistance, together with a decrease in cardiac output, reduces blood pressure, a desired effect in hypertension but not always in coronary disease where a fall in perfusion pressure may outweigh in importance the further reduction in metabolic requirements. Coronary perfusion pressure may also be slightly reduced by a small increase in atrial pressure after β-blockade.

β-Blocking agents may influence any tendency to arrhythmia in subjects with coronary or other types of heart disease. The reduction in oxygen requirement lessens ischemia and protects the electrical stability of the heart by influencing the substrate of some malignant rhythm disorders. They also counter some of the potentially arrhythmogenic effects of catecholamines, notably the increase in the slope of phase 4 depolarization in Purkinje fibers that can produce repetitive firing[13] and the dispersion of refractoriness that increases the tendency to ventricular tachycardia or fibrillation.[14] The reduction in conductivity through the atrioventricular node may curtail intranodal reentry arrhythmias. On the other hand, the slowing of sinus rate can encourage the emergence of arrhythmias that have been suppressed by a faster dominant rhythm. Receptor subtypes also have importance in the vulnerability to arrhythmias. Thus, $β_2$ stimulation causes a decrease in plasma potassium concentration, due to enhanced transport of the ion across the cell membrane and, thus, augments intracellular potassium within sketetal muscle[15] and red cells. Any consequent hypokalemia may be arrhythmogenic in susceptible individuals.[16] The nonselective $β_1$ blockers offer no protection against this mechanism. Indeed, cardiac $β_2$ receptors may be sensitized by an effect on their G proteins by $β_1$ blockade.[17] The possibility exists, therefore, that whilst nonselective blockers may be protective, the selective $β_1$ blockers may increase risk from this particular hazard, and as a consequence be less effective overall in their protection against malignant arrhythmias.[18] Finally, the antiarrhythmic effects of β-blockade may be enhanced by nonspecific membrane effects with some drugs, e.g. propranolol in high doses, and may also be enhanced by a class III effect in the case of sotalol.

Thus the possible benefits of β-blockade in myocardial infarction depend at least in part on the sparing of metabolic demand that may curtail some of the symptoms and reduce the signs of an evolving infarct, and in the complex antiarrhythmic effects that reduce the tendency to malignant rhythm disorders. The effects are variable, influenced by the degree of myocardial dysfunction and the possible compensatory role of sympathetic drive, and by the pharmacokinetic properties of the drug that is used. With all β-blockers, heart failure and low output states can be aggravated, but proarrythmia is not perceived to be a major problem. If it exists, it is masked by concomitant protective effects. But the precise mechanism of some benefits that are discussed below remain uncertain.

Experimental Background

The balance between myocardial metabolic supply and demand becomes critical in the ischemic myocardium and, during the evolution of acute myocardial infarction, may influence the proportion of myocardium that becomes irreversibly necrotic.[19] β-Adrenoceptor stimulation increases the major determinants of myocardial oxygen consumption[20] and thereby increases infarct size in experimental models.[21] Thus, blocking stimulation during infarction would be expected to reduce oxygen requirement and to decrease infarct size. But the benefits are more complex. Some β-receptor anatagonists have also been shown to increase blood supply to ischemic areas of myocardium[22] and to favor flow to the more vulnerable subendocardial zones.[23] The drugs also have metabolic effects independent of the simple supply and demand equation. They inhibit the rise in free fatty acids stimulated by catecholamines and in consequence increase myocardial glucose extraction.[24] The increase in the respiratory quotient and more effective utilization of oxygen may be reflected in a change in lactate balance across an ischemic coronary vascular bed from substantial production to a more normal pattern of extraction.[25]

β-Blocking drugs seem, therefore, to have an ideal profile for limiting myocardial damage during the evolving phase of myocardial infarction and, indeed, have been shown to do so experimentally.[26] Histologic differences gained credence from additional evidence: there may be more favorable electrocardiographic evolution after infarction with decreased ST elevation[27] and restricted formation of Q waves,[26] and also less enzyme release.[28] But the expectation that such findings could predicate equally impressive results in clinical practice was optimistic: experimentally the process of infarction is usually well advanced within 3 hours of coronary occlusion,[29] and evidence based on thrombolysis suggests that the potential for limiting infarct size even with restoration of blood flow has usually passed after the first 90 min from the onset of major symptoms.[30] Although there is marked individual variation in the time course of the evolution of myocardial infarction,[31] the usual time frame offers little scope for benefit to most patients. The question also arises of whether β-blockade has the potential for benefits that are additive to those of thrombolysis. This too has been addressed experimentally, and further limitation in necrosis has indeed been demonstrated.[32,33] A study in closed chest dogs[34] did suggest, however, that the recovery of systolic function was evanescent: when metoprolol was given after coronary occlusion but before thrombolysis the benefit detected at 24 hours was lost at 1 week.

The potential for antiarrhythmic activity by β-blockade has been discussed above, and is supported experimentally. Thus some of the ventricular tachyarrhythmias that are usually induced by coronary ligation can be prevented by treatment with adrenoceptor antagonists.[35]

The Clinical Use of β-blockade After Myocardial Infarction

The clinical effects of β-blockade in patients who have suffered myocardial infarction are not restricted to reduction in infarct size and antiarrhythmic effects. The various benefits are not fully understood, but may depend partly on the time of administration relative to the onset of symptoms. A full review of all postinfarction trials is beyond the scope of this chapter. But an insight into potential clinical benefits can be obtained by considering in detail the major trials under two headings: those that involved intravenous administration during the first few hours after hospital admission, and others that were restricted to oral administration that began in the convalescent phase of acute infarction but continued long term. The therapeutic implications of other trials that may not necessarily fit into these categories will also be highlighted as necessary and have been included in the major reviews published previously.[36,37]

Intravenous administration of β-blockade in the early hours of myocardial infarction

The value of β-blockade given intravenously early in the course of myocardial infarction has been addressed in over 30 trials involving about 29 000 patients. These trials, of varying size and with disparate entry criteria and primary endpoints, have been reviewed in detail elsewhere.[36,37] Only a minority of trials have contributed in isolation to our appreciation of the role of intravenous β-blockade, but the few large trials and the total data base have yielded important information that can provide some guide to good clinical practice. The major reservation is that only one trial was restricted to patients who had already received thrombolysis. This treatment that became popular only in the 1980s was not used at all in the majority of trials.

Effect on cardiac pain during infarction. Most clinicians who used intravenous β-blockers acutely in infarction noted the symptomatic relief that sometimes followed almost immediately upon their administration. Formal reports of this symptomatic benefit relate to metoprolol,[38,39] to atenolol[40] and to propranolol.[41] The mechanism of this effect is believed to be similar to that in angina: a sparing of myocardial oxygen requirement from decreased heart rate, blood pressure, and contractility leading to an improvement in the balance between myocardial metabolic demand and supply. An evolving infarct has an area of myocardium that is destined to become necrotic but also an adjoining area of ischemia.[42] Pain relief from an area of ischemic but viable myocardium does not necessarily imply, however, that the process of infarction has been aborted or that a reduction in infarct size will necessarily occur.

Effect on infarct size. Reduction in infarct size by therapeutic regimens has long been an area of controversy,[43] and will remain so until a satisfactory and practical method exists to quantify muscle necrosis in clinical practice. Many techniques have been used as a measure of infarct size including scintigraphy, vectorcardiography, and precordial mapping. But the favorite techniques have been based on enzyme release and on the evolution of electrocardiographic changes. All methods have limitations.

The 1985 review of β-blockade in myocardial infarction by Yusuf and colleagues[36] listed 20 trials that had, by then, reported the effects of various intravenous agents on cumulative enzyme release: this included prepublication data from the MIAMI trial.[44] Most patients had been treated within 6 hours of pain. Three studies showed an increase in enzyme release, five showed no difference, and the remaining 12 showed a reduction that averaged about 20% at least for patients enrolled within a few hours of pain (detailed information was not provided by all authors). An analysis by the MIAMI group[45] showed that the average delay from onset of symptoms to treatment was critical in determining whether or not a reduction in enzyme release was found. The median delay in that study was 7 hours. A significant reduction in enzyme release was found for those treated within 7 hours, but none for the cohort treated later than that. The negative findings of the MILIS[46] trial of the effect of propranolol on infarct size are consistent with this observation: of the 269 patients in the study less than 2% were treated within 4 hours of the onset of symptoms, and only 22% within 6 hours. The primary endpoint of infarct size measured as plasma MB creatine kinase (CK-MB) activity was virtually identical in the two groups, and peak enzyme levels were similar. Moreover, no significant difference was observed between the propranolol and placebo groups in the change in left ventricular ejection fraction, the pyrophosphate uptake, or R-wave loss. Whilst the MILIS study does not deny the likelihood of reduction of infarct size when patients are treated very promptly, it does indicate that in usual clinical practice the potential for myocardial salvage from β-blockade must be very limited. But time to treatment may not be the only factor that influences the potential for limiting infarct size. Both the MIAMI group and others have suggested that the effect on heart rate is an important determinant.[47] Whatever the mechanism, the reasonably consistent evidence[36] for a potential but limited improvement in one yardstick of infarct size relates to a broad spectrum of agents, suggesting that it represents a class effect. The relevance of the method is, however, open to question.[48] β_1-Receptors in the coronary arteries mediate vasodilatation when stimulated:[49] the possibility exists, therefore, that opposition by β-blockade under the conditions of infarction may slow egress of enzymes, although under normal conditions the coronary arteries respond to autoregulatory control. Most enzymes released during evolving infarction are destroyed *in situ* and do not enter the circulation.[50] Although autopsy studies have confirmed a reasonable correlation between enzyme release and histologic measurements of infarct size,[51] this relationship may be less secure after intervention by acute β-blockade. Moreover, limitation of infarct size would be expected to cause a mortality reduction measured in months as well as hours or days, yet no significant late mortality benefit was shown in the two largest trials of β-blockade given intravenously in the acute stage of infarction.[44,52]

The evidence from electrocardiographic evolution is of two types, the first relating to the ST segment and the second to the QRS complex. The reduction of ST segment elevation has been shown after the acute administration of at least three β-blockers.[36] Although this seems to relate to a reduction in ischemia which can also be reflected in pain relief (see above), it does not correlate reliably with eventual infarct size.[53] The preservation of R waves noted with atenolol[54] and the reduction in the development of Q waves reported after timolol[55] and propranolol[56] is more persuasive. To achieve such results, it seems likely that β-blockade must be given very early in the course of the illness. This may sometimes represent the prevention of infarction within a phase of an acute coronary syndrome that may still be regarded as unstable angina.

Effect on threatened infarction. In five randomized trials data have been provided on the outcome of treatment with intravenous β-blockade with suspected infarction in terms of final diagnosis.[52,54,56–58] Clearly the potential for benefit may well be greatest before diagnostic accuracy is complete; these controlled data therefore offer some insight into the possibility that the early pathophysiology of infarction may sometimes be aborted. Although the evidence cannot be regarded as firm, the reduction in progression to definite infarction of about 25% (based primarily on enzyme changes) is at least suggestive. The evidence was not confirmed by ISIS-1,[52] but in this trial no firm criteria were laid down for the timing of enzyme confirmation of infarction. As suggested above, aborted infarction may account for much of the electrocardiographic evidence on limitation of infarct size. How it is regarded is largely a matter of semantics.

Effect on mortality. A meta-analysis[36] of small trials available to early 1985 showed no appreciable change in mortality as a result of intravenous β-blockers in acute infarction. Many clinicians concluded that the therapeutic strategy had no clinical value. Opinions had to be revised, however, in the light of the two largest studies that were published subsequently. In the Swedish-led metoprolol MIAMI study[44,59] a total of 5778 patients aged 75 years or younger were randomized within 24 hours of the onset of symptoms of infarction. The median delay was 7 hours and 25% were included within 4 hours. They received placebo (2901) or treatment with metoprolol (2877), which began with intravenous loading of 15 mg (given as three 5-mg doses at 2 min intervals) followed by an oral regimen of 200 mg daily for 15 days after the day of randomization. This study population was drawn from a larger group of 26 439 patients who were considered for inclusion. The most common reason for exclusion was current treatment with either *β*-blockers or calcium channel blockers. Other reasons were: heart rate slower than 65 beats min^{-1}, systolic pressure less than 105 mmHg, left ventricular failure, AV conduction disorder, asthma, and miscellaneous causes for about 10% of those not entered. At 15 days, 142 deaths had occurred in the placebo group (4.9%) compared with 123 deaths in the metoprolol group (4.3%). The 13% difference was not significant; confidence limits range from an 8% excess to 33% reduction in mortality. A tendency was observed, as in some of the convalescent phase trials, for a more pronounced difference in subgroups with a higher-than-average placebo mortality. Indeed, the cohort of over half the study group judged to be at low risk on the basis of risk predictors showed no tendency to mortality reduction, with all the benefit restricted to the 35% in the high-risk group where it amounted to 29%. An analysis was undertaken of the causes of death in the placebo and metoprolol groups. Heart failure was the principal cause in both but no significant difference was observed between them in the proportions with failure, from arrhythmias or sudden circulatory collapse. Rupture confirmed by autopsy occurred in 39 patients who had placebo and 32 who received metoprolol.

ISIS-1[52] was an appreciably larger study with 16 027 patients randomized to an open control group (7990 patients) or to a group receiving atenolol 5–10 mg intravenously followed by 100 mg orally for 7 days (8037 patients). The eligibility criteria were similar to those of MIAMI though a little less restrictive, and there was no age limit. The hypothesis that motivated the trial was an expected difference in infarct size that would reduce mortality over months and years. A mortality reduction of 15% was observed in the atenolol group ($2P < 0.05$) when full data had been analyzed, but this occurred almost wholly during day 0 (randomization) to day 1. As the primary hypothesis had not been confirmed by the results, the clinical results of patients who died on days 0–1 were examined.[60] This subsequent study was confined to 193 of the 217 patients from the UK, Ireland, and Scandinavia whose records were readily available. Of these, 114 had been allocated to placebo and 79 to atenolol, but these details were not known to the cardiologists who examined the records. The major difference in deaths related to confirmed rupture or electromechanical dissociation likely to have been caused by rupture (54 vs 20 in all). A small and non-significant excess of fatal bradycardia or asystole in the atenolol group was balanced by a similar reduction in fatal ventricular fibrillation. The numbers dying of mechanical failure were similar in the two management allocations.

The suggestion that protection from rupture accounts for much of the reduction in mortality accorded by *β*-blockers in acute infarction must be viewed with caution. This mechanism did not form part of the original hypothesis and is purely retrospective. No convincing confirmation is yet available. But the Gothenburg metoprolol study of intravenous followed by oral metoprolol[61] included death from rupture in 15 control patients and 10 who had been allocated to metoprolol, with figures of 39 vs 32 for the MIAMI trial. The TIMI-IIB trial[62] of conservative vs interventional treatment of infarction after thrombolysis also has subsets of 720 patients randomly allocated to intravenous then oral metoprolol (started within 2 hours of initiation of recombinant tissue-type plasminogen activator (rt-PA) and 714 patients allocated to oral metoprolol deferred for 6 days. This study was said to offer no support to the rupture hypothesis for mortality reduction. But in TIMI-IIB only seven deaths occurred from rupture within the first 48 hours (the time frame for mortality reduction in ISIS-1). Four were in metoprolol-treated patients and three had had placebo. These data are too few for any judgment to be made on the issue. An additional large trial would have to be conducted if the hypothesis were to be confirmed or refuted.

Effect on arrhythmias. Although mortality from arrhythmias was not reduced appreciably in the two large trials of intravenous therapy,[44,52] an important effect on the incidence of arrhythmias has been demonstrated in some studies. Two randomized trials have used continuous tape monitoring to assess the effects of intravenous β-blockade on arrhythmias after myocardial infarction. Atenolol[63] led to a threefold reduction in ventricular extrasystoles and R-on-T extrasystoles. Treatment with metoprolol[64] was not associated with any decrease overall in the numbers of ventricular extrasystoles, but ventricular fibrillation was less common, with 17 instances in a control group compared with six in the group with active treatment. In two studies using respectively practolol[65] and atenolol,[54] a reduction in atrial fibrillation has been noted.

The effects of β-blockade on malignant and potentially lethal ventricular arrhythmias are of prime concern. One result with metoprolol has been mentioned above.[64] In the MIAMI trial[44] little difference was noted in the incidence of ventricular fibrillation in the first few days, but from day 6 to the end of the trial on day 15 the total number of episodes was reduced from 54 with placebo to 24 with metoprolol. The Göteborg metoprolol study group[66] reported 17 placebo-treated patients with 41 episodes of ventricular fibrillation against six metoprolol-treated patients with one episode each. In another metoprolol trial[64] using oral therapy, a significant reduction was observed in the incidence of ventricular fibrillation during the hospital phase (17 of 698 controls vs 6 of 697 treated), whilst in PREMIS[18] an even greater effect was observed after intravenous propranolol (14 of 371 controls vs 2 of 364 treated). Suggestions have been made that selective β-antagonists may be less protective because they could fail to prevent or even predispose to arrhythmias that are potentiated by potassium shifts across the cell membrane (see p. 195) and thereby mask other antiarrhythmic effects.[13,17] No good evidence exists for such a distinction in the acute phase of myocardial infarction, although intravenous timolol has been shown to prevent an adverse effect on plasma potassium concentration as a result of diuretic therapy in the first 24 hours of treatment.[67] One of the small trials gave some support to the notion that protection from atenolol might be comparable to that provided by the non-selective agents (10 vs 3 cases).[54] The failure of ISIS-1[52] to find any significant reduction in ventricular fibrillation can be ascribed wholly to the small number of events and indeed did show a favorable trend (13 vs 5). A meta-analysis of almost 30 trials of all intravenous β-blockade suggests a decrease in potentially lethal arrhythmias of 15%.[37] It is important to remember that clinical trials are generally conducted in circumstances that permit immediate defibrillation, so that ventricular fibrillation is not then usually lethal. But the reduction in ventricular fibrillation may be translated into a reduction of mortality under other clinical conditions in which immediate defibrillation may be less readily available. Thus the results of clinical trials relating to intravenous β-blockade for myocardial infarction may slightly underestimate the potential for preventing arrhythmic death in the generality of medical practice.

Oral administration of β-blockade starting in the convalescent phase of acute myocardial infarction and continuing long term

The principal rationale for starting β-blockade as quickly as possible after the onset of myocardial infarction (and therefore by intravenous administration) was limitation of infarct size, though this may have been a somewhat simplistic view. The trials with oral therapy were driven principally by an awareness of the antiarrhythmic action of the drugs mediated in part by effects on the electrical system of the heart and in part by protection from acute ischemia.

The design of most of the major long-term trials involved a delay before treatment was started so that the hazards of compounding heart failure or critically low cardiac output could be minimized. The strategy of using β-blockers long term was encouraged initially by promising results of the first trial conducted over a few weeks by Snow,[68] although the number of patients was very small and the results in reality did not provide any reliable guide. But the numbers recruited in other trials over subsequent years were large. Twelve long-term trials of exclusively oral therapy that enrolled more than 500 subjects have been reported.[69–81] Almost as many smaller trials were conducted. The review by Yusuf and colleagues[36] provides detailed data from all studies available by 1983. The overall total mortality fell from 986 of 9860 patients (10%) to 827 of 10 452 (7.9%). This represents a 21% decrease. Appreciable differences in the effects on mortality of β-blockade are evident. Important matters for consideration are whether the mortality findings are relevant to current practice; whether the observed variations in efficacy of the regimens are real and if so whether they were related to differences in the properties of the drugs that were used; what was the mechanism of the decreased mortality in the postive trials; whether there are important benefits apart from mortality; how far the benefit is general and how far it may be concentrated in identifiable subgroups; and what are the practical clinical implications of all these points.

Mortality reduction: relevance to current practice. That β-blockade is capable of decreasing the risk of death after myocardial infarction is no longer in doubt. A lower incidence of recurrent infarction was also observed in the trials (see below). The scale of benefit in the most successful trials in this group[71,74,81] was appreciable in relation to mortality alone, and the average result for all trials remains impressive. Yet no consensus exists on the routine or even selective use of the drugs after acute myocardial infarction. Many physicians use them only very infrequently, and wide geographic variations exist in prescribing habits both for their long-term use after infarction and for intravenous use in the acute phase.[82] The reluctance to prescribe β-blockers for secondary prevention seems to rest on several perceptions. The introduction of thrombolytic therapy is widely regarded as having moved the goal posts in postinfarction management, and the relevance of any trial in the prethrombolytic era is doubted. But no *a priori* reasons exist for believing that the same benefits will not accrue as far as β-blockade is concerned. Indeed, β-blockade may even have special relevance after thrombolysis if protection against rupture, suggested by the ISIS-1 workers, is confirmed; for rupture is part of the early hazard of thrombolysis and tends to occur sooner than it does after conventional treatment.[83] The TIMI-IIB trial[62] provided experience of intravenous and oral β-blockade in patients who had all received thrombolysis. But all of them received β-blockade, with immediate vs delayed treatment (for 6 weeks) being the only variable. No firm conclusions can therefore be drawn on mortality benefits even with the trend to lower mortality (7 vs 10) in favor of early administration. This issue can be resolved with certainty only if another large-scale trial is performed. But it is not unreasonable to believe in a continuing impact from long-term β-blockade on the proportion of deaths that can be postponed, even if the absolute numbers are reduced by thrombolysis. Other objections that have been raised include cost, adverse effects on quality of life from the burden of side-effects and complex tablet regimens, and the possibility that long-term harm from metabolic effects may erode the benefits of early mortality reduction. These issues will be considered later.

The difference in mortality between trials. Even a reduction in mortality as large as 20% can be demonstrated reliably only in large trials. With 2000 patients included, chance could easily determine whether 100 vs 80 deaths occurred (plausible figures that reflect overall trial results) or 90 vs 90 deaths. Since most trials were smaller than this, random variation would be expected. No statistically significant heterogeneity exists for the chance of mortality reduction about the pooled relative risk of treatment.[36] But it may be unwise to ignore the important differences between β-blocking drugs, especially those differences that are known to have a bearing on factors that influence vulnerability. Two important variable properties have been widely discussed in this regard: partial agonist activity and β_1 selectivity.

Partial agonist activity offers a pharmacokinetic method of preserving some cardiac adrenergic drive, of value in some respects particularly for patients who require *some* adrenergic support because of chronotropic or inotropic impairment. Dose titration does not offer a practical alternative. The advantage in terms of relative preservation of heart rate and contractility may be outweighed after infarction, however, if there is a gradation of decreasing hazard from other complications (arrhythmias for example) to the vulnerable patient as sympathetic activity ranges from full to almost none. Agonist activity may then be an unsuitable property for most patients after myocardial infarction. In an analysis updated from that of Yusuf and colleagues[36] 12 trials of drugs with agonist activity[69,72,77,79,80,85–91] gave a pooled odds ratio of 0.9 (95% confidence limits 0.77–1.05) compared with a pooled odds ratio of 0.69 (confidence limits 0.61–0.79) for trials of drugs with no agonist activity. These findings are consistent with the seemingly reasonable hypothesis that the mortality reduction after β-blockade varies with the degree of residual adrenergic drive: drugs without agonist activity may offer a more suitable profile than those with agonist activity for secondary prevention after myocardial infarction. On present evidence this can be regarded only as a hypothesis, for considerable caution is necessary in interpreting treatment effects in subgroups[84] either within trials or within meta-analyses.

No trial evidence exists that selectivity influences the efficacy of β-blockade either in the acute phase or prophylactically in the convalescent phase. For trials that were continued long-term the selective drugs metoprolol,[78,80,92–94] atenolol,[95] practolol,[69,85] and acebutalol[81] achieved in total a 25% reduction in mortality, consistent with the results for all agents. The actions of β-blockers are complex, so that these results do not exclude the possibility of an adverse effect from selectivity that is masked by other benefits.

The mechanisms of decreased mortality. The evidence is at least suggestive that β-blockade instituted within a very few hours after the onset of symptoms of infarction may limit infarct size (see p. 198), though any such effect can be expected to occur only in a small minority of patients. Any reduction in infarct size will have long-term benefits not only in individual cardiac performance but also in the average survival time. The mechanisms for improved survival after β-blockade are, however, both manifold and complex. If a component in a few individuals depends on myocardial salvage, it must be small and cannot be recognized or distinguished from other greater sources of benefit.

One powerful pointer indicates that an antiarrhythmic effect must be important. At least 11 trials[61,69,71,73,74,78,88,89,92,94] showed a reduction in the incidence of sudden cardiac death (mean of 31%) as a result of β-blockade involving five different agents (for odds ratios[96,97] see Figure 7.1). This class effect therefore exceeds in degree the overall reduction in mortality in the studies with oral agents started in the convalescent phase, and must be the major component of survival benefit. It is an extrapolation, but a reasonable one, to argue that this avoidance of sudden cardiac death (despite its variable definition) represents an antiarrhythmic or specifically an antifibrillatory effect. A lower incidence of ventricular fibrillation was indeed claimed for one of the trials.[92] Moreover, β-blockers have an appropriate profile of activity for antiarrhythmic potential in man[33–35] (and see p. 200). Proof that protection from ventricular fibrillation is the principal mechanism of protection from sudden cardiac death may be unattainable, but clinical trials do lend some support to the concept of an antiarrhythmic effect. A subset of 53 patients in the MIAMI Trial[98] had long-term electrocardiographic tracings that showed a

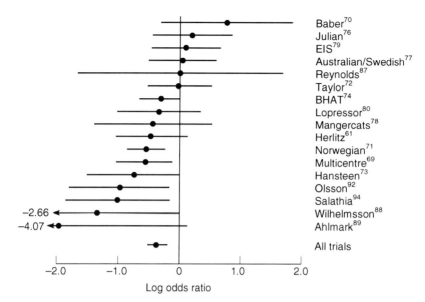

Figure 7.1   Change in incidence of sudden cardiac death as a result of β-blockade. Odds ratios.

significant reduction in premature ventricular complexes as a result of treatment with metoprolol both in the acute phase and long term. The increase in the number and complexity of ventricular extrasystoles that occurs after discharge can also be reversed or blunted by metoprolol.[99] The effect may be less pronounced with agents that have agonist activity[100] though no direct comparisons have been attempted. In general terms ventricular extrasystoles are a poor marker of vulnerability to sudden cardiac death, but a relation does exist after myocardial infarction. Thus in BHAT,[101] multivariant analysis confirmed a relationship between ventricular ectopic activity and sudden death. Both were reduced by propranolol but the relationship remained. Thus, at least some β-blockers have an antiarrhythmic effect after infarction and their benefit is more pronounced in those who have arrhythmias compared with those who do not.[102] If ventricular ectopic activity is taken as a yardstick of antiarrhythmic effect, then β-blockers are only moderately efficacious. It has been argued from this that the antiarrhythmic effect was not the sole mechanism of protection.[103] Probably it is not, but the argument is flawed: trials with antiarrhythmics have demonstrated that reduction in ventricular ectopic activity is a poor measure of protection against ventricular fibrillation.[104] Other mechanisms for reduction in sudden death may depend on protection against reinfarction which was demonstrated in many of the trials.

Other benefits: protection against reinfarction. Data on nonfatal reinfarction are available from 15 trials that were large enough to have 10 or more recurrent episodes in the control groups. In 13 of them, nonfatal reinfarction occurred less frequently in the groups allocated to β-blockade. The others showed no appreciable change with none having an excess in the actively treated patients (for odds ratios see Figure 7.2). In total, reinfarction occurred in 7.7 % allocated control and 5.9 % allocated β-blockade using alprenolol,[88,89] practolol,[69,85] pindolol,[77] oxprenolol,[72,79] sotalol,[76] metoprolol,[78,92,93] propranolol,[70,73,75] or timolol.[71] The protection is therefore a class effect, and powerful.

The protection against reinfarction may have been even greater than the impressive figures suggest. A decrease in overall mortality and in sudden death have already been

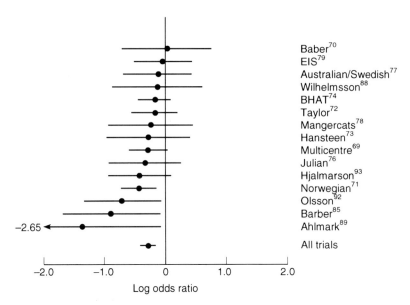

Figure 7.2 Change in incidence of non-fatal reinfarction as a result of β-blockade. Odds ratios.

noted. Some of those who died (suddenly or otherwise) will have done so as a result of fresh infarction which should have left an excess of non fatal reinfarction in the survivors. This unknown figure would have to be added to the reduction that was observed to give a true measure of protection against reinfarction.

Remarkably, the mechanisms for the prevention of reinfarction by β-blockade are unknown or at least incomplete and speculative. Arguments have been put forward that ischemia alone can set in train processes that may lead to infarction with arterial thrombosis as a secondary event.[105] Although the theory is untenable as a general statement following the angiographic observations of DeWood and colleagues on the evolution of events during acute infarction,[105a] it may conceivably account for some cases. Any such tendency may be influenced by β-blockade which appreciably reduces the burden of ischemia. Antiplatelet effects may also be relevant. Increased platelet aggregation has a role in precipitating infarction. In the presence of ischemia (or at least angina) increased platelet aggregability occurs perhaps because of an imbalance between prostacyclin release and hemodynamic changes, but this is prevented by metoprolol.[106] An antiaggregatory effect on platelets is not limited to selective β_1 antagonists: propranolol, for example, also has this property – at least *in vitro* – but without increasing synthesis of prostacyclin.[107] Effects mediated by modification of platelets can hardly play a major role, however, for prevention of reinfarction by more potent antiplatelet agents is by comparison relatively modest.

Nor is the effect on blood coagulation of some β-blockers, mediated by inhibiting the rise in factor VIII with adrenergic stimulation,[108] likely to be a key issue. It is tempting to suppose that the major effect must be mediated by decreasing plaque rupture, the trigger for most acute coronary events. Some observations support this concept. Plaque rupture is believed to be precipitated by acute changes in coronary vasomotor tone. Angiographic studies on patients with classical angina have shown that exercise produces paradoxical constriction of stenosed coronary arteries, and that this can be prevented by propranolol given directly into the coronary tree to avoid systemic effects.[109] The suggested mechanisms for this action are class effects that may well occur with oral β-blockade and thus protect vulnerable plaques. The hypothesis is reasonable and also attractive for offering a unified concept for the prevention of reinfarction and some instances of sudden cardiac death.

Benefit in identifiable subgroups. The major hazards of β-blockade are found in patients with severely impaired myocardial function and in patients with important electrical disorders involving impulse formation or conduction. It is therefore anomalous that patients who can be identified as having mechanical or electrical complications may benefit most from β-blockade given in the convalescent phase of acute myocardial infarction. A careful retrospective analysis of patients (who were less than 70 years old) in BHAT addressed this issue.[102] In 866 randomized patients who had electrical complications (ventricular fibrillation or tachycardia, AV block, or new atrial fibrillation) the relative risk after propranolol was decreased to 0.43. With mechanical complications (shock, compensated or mild heart failure, or hypotension before randomization) the relative risk as a result of propranolol was 0.57. Those who had neither type of complication derived very little benefit from β-blockade with a relative risk of 0.94. Further pooled information is available from an analysis of nine major long-term trials[110] using seven different β-blockers and involving 13 679 patients, including those in BHAT mentioned above. Subgroups with high placebo mortality (patients with a history of previous myocardial infarction, angina pectoris, mechanical or electrical complications, and digitalis usage) benefited particularly well from the treatment of β-blockade. These findings were consistent in the nine trials.

The data with regard to recurrence of heart failure after β-blockade are also reassuring. A history of congestive heart failure before randomization characterized 19% of the placebo group, and 18% in the propranolol group of BHAT.[111] In patients with a history of congestive failure before randomization, 12.6% in placebo-treated patients and a very similar 14.8% in the propranolol group developed congestive failure over an average of 25 months of follow-up. Those specifically with heart failure (as opposed to other mechanical complications defined above) experienced the same percentage decrease in mortality with β-blockade but more benefit in absolute numbers, whereas the decrease in sudden cardiac death was over three times greater after β-blockade in this group. Similar reassuring data to indicate that β-blockade in patients with compensated failure can be continued long term without undue hazard overall were seen in the placebo arm of the Multicentre Diltiazem Post-Infarction Trial,[112] and in two metoprolol trials.[113,114]

One important subgroup, comprising up to one-third of patients with infarction, having a distinctive natural history is that of non-Q-wave infarction. Patients with this condition can be seen as the other end of the spectrum of immediate risk from those with large infarcts and mechanical or electrical complications. As such, they would not be expected to derive major benefit in terms of mortality reduction. This was confirmed in BHAT[115] in which no advantage was obtained with propranolol either in terms of total mortality, sudden cardiac death, or reinfarction. Timolol also failed to reduce reinfarction rate with non-Q-wave infarction.[71] There were symptomatic advantages for patients with angina, however; they comprise another subgroup for which treatment has special value irrespective of mortality, though for most of these, other criteria will determine treatment policy.

When the decision on whether to use β-blockade or not is considered marginal on account of doubts about benefit or risk, considerations relating to side-effects assume greater importance. The most immediate problems arise from lowered cardiac output, cold peripheries from redistribution of blood flow, and the nonspecific symptoms that add to lassitude and rapid exhaustion. Possible long-term sequelae as a result of changes in blood lipids[116] should be mentioned, in particular the increase in triglycerides by all β-blockers and the reduction in HDL cholesterol by all except those with agonist activity.[117] But if this consideration is worthy of attention at all it can only be in patients on very long-term treatment for conditions that pose no immediate threat to life.

Practical implications: who should be treated, with what drug, and for how long

β-Blockade has the potential to reduce mortality and perhaps to limit infarct size when given in the acute stage of myocardial infarction. It has a potential for an even greater reduction in mortality (especially from sudden cardiac death) and for the prevention of reinfarction when used orally very early in the convalescent phase. But it is clear from the trial results and from the wide experience in the use of these drugs that not all patients should be treated. Unfortunately, however, there is no strong consensus on the most appropriate patients to select for treatment.

Early treatment with intravenous β-blockade. Enthusiasm for the use of intravenous β-blockade very early in acute myocardial infarction has been tempered by fear of inducing heart failure or a critical low output state during a hemodynamically unstable phase. The greater potential benefit from intravenous thrombolysis has also distracted attention from β-blockers. Moreover, no proof is available that the benefits of these two strategies is additive or complementary. Although the evidence is not compelling, β-blockers given in the first hour or two after the onset of pain may limit infarct size (see above), with a time-window for myocardial salvage similar to that of thrombolytic therapy.[30] But because the mechanisms are different, it is likely that advantages can be gained by both treatment modalities. Of more practical concern is the possible benefit of intravenous β-blockade given several hours after the onset of symptoms. The relevance of the major positive trials in the thrombolytic era could only be proved by a new study, but evidence currently available provides justification for those who choose to follow thrombolysis with intravenous atenolol (5 mg followed by a further 5 mg after 10 min before oral treatment) or intravenous metoprolol (three 5-mg injections at 2-min intervals before oral treatment) in the absence of contraindications. Exclusion criteria were not closely defined in ISIS-1, but in the metoprolol trials included heart rate less than 65 beats min^{-1}, systolic pressure below 105 mmHg, left ventricular failure, poor peripheral circulation, and severe chronic obstructive airways disease.

An attempt to limit infarct size or improve early prognosis are not the only possible indications for intravenous β-blockade in acute myocardial infarction. An additional valid indication is continuing or recurrent cardiac pain after adequate initial analgesia. This treatment can be convincingly effective in some individuals.

Treatment with oral β-blockade from the convalescent phase. The evidence for initiating long-term secondary prevention with β-blockers during the early convalescent stage of acute myocardial infarction remains strong. But not all patients should be regarded as candidates for treatment. The most importance exclusions depend on the unwanted effects.[118] Patients may not tolerate β-blockers because of severely impaired myocardial function, conduction disorders, asthma or, less importantly, peripheral vascular disease or diabetes. These will account for approximately 30% of patients admitted to hospital with infarction. Inevitably some patients will fall into a group for whom the risk of β-blockade cannot be accurately defined. On the one hand, mechanical and electrical complications that increase risk of death can be taken as an indication for β-blockade because patients with these problems have the greatest prognostic gain. On the other hand, greater severity of the same complications can make the treatment itself more hazardous than the disease and will then constitute an important contraindication. A carefully supervised trial of therapy in hospital may be needed to place a patient in the appropriate category to receive or not receive β-blockade in the early convalescent phase of acute myocardial infarction. An ultra-short-acting β-blocker may be used to make this assessment quickly and safely, but as yet experience in this strategy is limited.[119] Even those treated appropriately will suffer nonspecific side effects that may have an important impact on the quality of life – a fact to weigh against the average statistic that every death postponed necessitates 24 patient years of treatment even with the most successful regimen.[120] Benign side-effects are not an issue if angina is relieved by β-blockade, but in asymptomatic patients after infarction new symptoms should not be added to the burden of disease unless there is an acceptable gain in prognosis to balance any loss in quality of life.[121] The penalty in terms of quality of life exacted by β-blockade is, however, variable. One double-blind randomized study[122] showed an improvement in a composite index that included not only mortality and morbidity but also functional state and side-effects. But individuals may differ in how the components of the index should be weighted.

Defining a group for whom treatment is not indicated on account of low risk is more contentious than defining the group who cannot tolerate β-blockade. The measurement of ejection fraction seems to be a single test that can have excellent prognostic value,[123] but this is not always available. Simple clinical criteria can also be used with acceptable reliability.[124,125] Even if the risk of death is so small that protection against it at the cost of obtrusive side-effects may not be justified, there is also the consideration of protection against reinfarction. The BHAT experience,[115] however, suggests that patients with low risk of death may also have low risks of reinfarction, so that the same arguments may apply. In addition to the 30% of patients after infarction who may not tolerate β-blockade, it may be reasonable to define another group of approximately similar size for whom β-blockade is not indicated on grounds of good prognosis.[124,125]

Choice of drug. β-Adrenergic blocking agents have diverse pharmacokinetic and ancillary properties. The results of trials, particularly the long-term ones, also suggest heterogeneity of benefit that may reflect these differences. The prudent physician may therefore seek to copy as far as possible the regimen used in the most successful trials in order to have the best prospects of reproducing their benefits. This implies the use of metoprolol or atenolol intravenously in the acute stage of infarction, and the use of timolol 10 mg twice daily, propranolol 80 mg three times daily, or metoprolol 100 mg twice daily in the convalescent phase. For high-risk patients acebutalol 100 mg twice daily has good evidence of benefit, and the extrapolation of this result to all patients who merit treatment may be thought reasonable. The nonspecific side-effects that can be very troublesome to patients must also be a consideration in the choice of drug. Most difficulties relate to the influence of β-blockers on the central nervous system. Entry into the brain depends on many factors,[126] not all of which are fully understood. The concentration gradient between plasma and cerebrospinal fluid must be important, but the relation between dosage and plasma levels is not always predictable, with variations in metabolism and excretion that depend on pharmacodynamic factors. Only free drug equilibrates with the cerebrospinal fluid and this depends on the degree of protein binding, which hinders transfer. Propranolol, for example is 90% protein bound, whereas the average figure for metoprolol is 10%. But equilibration with the cerebro-spinal fluid and subsequently with the brain is aided by lipophilicity, which is high for propranolol and appreciably less for metoprolol and atenolol. The washout effect is also relevant. In general, central nervous side-effects tend to be worse with the lipophilic agents, but there are large individual variations and selection for those troubled by side-effects is often best handled by therapeutic trial. Many patients who have difficulty tolerating the drugs have been treated with smaller doses than those used in the trials. It must be remembered that any such modification of the treatment regimen is of unproven benefit. A more appropriate clinical decision at least initially would be a trial with another proven agent in full recommended dosage.

Duration of treatment. The long-term trials of β-blockade with positive results showed benefit for as long as observations were made. This extended for up to 3 years for timolol.[71] The implication can be drawn that treatment may reduce risk for as long as it is continued. Certainly there seems little point in withdrawing treatment at some arbitrary time if unwanted effects are not burdensome. But if patients do complain of iatrogenic symptoms, consideration may be given to continuing treatment for a limited period. The rationale is based on the natural history of myocardial infarction: risk of death is highest in the early months after the acute attack, and amounts to about 10% in the first year falling to approximately 4% per annum after a few years. Even if the percentage benefit shows no fall with time, more lives in absolute terms will be saved by treatment earlier rather than later. Many patients who do have side-effects to contend with may accept treatment for 6 months after myocardial infarction even if they are reluctant to accept indefinite treatment. In most cases it would be appropriate to discuss these issues with the patients themselves before any decision is reached.

The cost implications of long-term treatment with β-blockade after myocardial infarction

Discussion of the merits of starting long-term β-blockade in the convalescent phase of acute infarction cannot be complete without reference to cost-effectiveness and cost–benefit. An analysis of pooled data published in 1988[127] suggested a 25% reduction in mortality annually for years 1–3, and a 7% reduction annually for years 4–6 after the initial event. On this basis the estimated cost of 6 years of treatment to save an additional year of life ranged from $US23 400 in low-risk patients to $US3600 in high-risk patients if there is no further benefit after 6 years. If the benefit wears off progressively over the next 9 years these figures are reduced respectively to $US13 000 and $US2400. This is clearly a very favorable cost-effectiveness ratio yet takes no account of morbidity benefit. A study based on the Stockholm metoprolol trial[128] confirmed that readmissions were fewer and sick leave or early retirement were reduced. Allowing for these factors the authors suggested that active treatment led to an average saving of kr. 19 000 (£1930 or $US2895) per patient over 3 years.

Calcium Antagonists (Calcium Channel Blockers)

Basic Pharmacology

The functions of excitable cells that are fundamental to the cardiovascular system are governed in part by the behavior of the semipermeable hydrophobic membranes that envelop them. These membranes control the movement of some ions into and out of the cells against their concentration gradients by ion pumps (for example Na^+, K^+ ATPase), by ion exchangers (for example Na^+: Ca^{2+} ion exchangers), and by ion-carrying channels that can open in response to transmembrane potential difference or ligand binding.[129,130] Ion-carrying channels may be relatively specific for sodium, for potassium, or for calcium. Calcium flux is controlled by all three mechanisms, but the calcium-selective voltage-sensitive channels provide the route for calcium entry that is ultimately responsible for excitation–contraction coupling and also form the principal site of action for calcium antagonists. One channel allows up to 10 million ions to enter a cell each second. Each cell has numerous channels, perhaps one per micrometer of cell surface, so the mechanism forms a very active entry route. The calcium that enters myocardial and other smooth muscle cells acts as the major trigger for release of more calcium from the major internal reservoir in the sarcoplasmic reticulum, which is then directly active in cardiac excitation–contraction coupling.[131] The channels permitting the release of calcium from the sarcoplasmic reticulum are influenced by ischemia: this may increase the probability of their remaining open,[132] resulting in damaging calcium overload with the risk of contractile dysfunction. But they are affected by calcium antagonists only indirectly

Table 7.2 The relative tissue selectivity of some widely used calcium antagonists

Calcium antagonists	Myocardium	Vasculature	Conducting and nodal tissue	Skeletal muscle
Amlodipine	+	++++	−	−
Diltiazem	+	+	+	−
Felodipine	+	++++	−	−
Gallopamil	+	+	+	−
Nifedipine	+	++	−	−
Nimodipine	+	++++	−	−
Nisoldipine	+	++++	−	−
Nitrendipine	+	+++	−	−
Verapamil	+	+	+	−

(From Ref. 130. (Adapted from Ref. 133) with permission.)

through variation in the availability of the triggering calcium cations that cross the specific channels of the cell membrane.

The specific calcium channels act as ion-selective pores on the cell membrane. They can be subdivided into four main varieties, designated L, T, N, and P types. The calcium anatagonists affect only L-type calcium channels which are widely distributed, have the Largest (hence 'L') ion-carrying capacity, and inactivate relatively slowly. Their complex structure is described in detail by Nayler.[130] The central pore of the channel is known as the α_1 subunit. The subunit on myocardial cells, which differs chemically and functionally from that on skeletal muscle, binds the three principal classes of calcium antagonists at different receptor sites, which accounts for their diverse effects. Thus there are dihydropyridine recognition sites with nifedipine as the prototype drug, phenylalkylamine recognition sites with verapamil as the prototype drug, and bezothiazepine recognition sites with diltiazem as the prototype drug. All three drug classes have second-generation agents, but most experience in the context of myocardial infarction has been limited to the prototypes: discussion will therefore largely be restricted to them. They differ from each other principally in tissue selectivity because of variations in receptor binding. At one end of the spectrum verapamil is almost devoid of selectivity and blocks the L-type calcium channel receptors in myocardial cells as well as in blood vessels. Verapamil therefore shares with β-blockers a powerful negative inotropic effect, but it achieves this by a completely different mechanistic route to the final common path of intracellular calcium release. Nifedipine has selectivity for dilatation of blood vessels, although the second-generation dihydropyridines have appreciably more. Diltiazem resembles verapamil in its pharmacologic profile but has differences that follow from distinct receptor binding, which include less negative inotropic effect and greater vascular (and specifically coronary) dilatation. Both verapamil and diltiazem slow AV conduction. Clinically, therefore, diltiazem can be regarded as a drug with a profile somewhere intermediate between that of nifedipine and verapamil, though the concept represents an oversimplification in pharmacodynamic terms. Selectivity of all the common calcium channel blocking agents is shown in Table 7.2.

Experimental Background

Myocardial ischemia sets in train a series of hemodynamic and biochemical events that compound the insult resulting from any imbalance between metabolic supply and demand. Thus stimuli that would be expected to cause vasodilatation may lead to paradoxical constriction of coronary arteries.[134] At a cellular level, a rise in cytosolic calcium[135] and the generation of free oxygen radicals[136] hinder myocardial relaxation and increase end-diastolic pressure, increase energy consumption, disrupt membrane structure, and interfere with intracellular enzyme systems. These processes accelerate cell necrosis. Calcium antagonists, however, have the potential to prevent or mitigate some of these processes. They are coronary vasodilators;[137] they dilate systemic vessels and thereby reduce afterload; as with β-blockers their negative inotropic effects spare metabolic demand; they reduce calcium flux through calcium channels at the time of reperfusion thereby ameliorating stunning;[138] mitochondrial function is protected during ischemia and afterwards;[139] diastolic dysfunction can be improved in the presence of coronary artery disease;[140] some limit lipid peroxidation induced by free radicals;[141] they reduce platelet aggregation[142] and thromboxane production;[143] and they can protect against cardiac arrhythmias induced by several mechanisms with a spectrum that includes ventricular fibrillation generated by ischemia.[144] Moreover, animal studies have shown a reduction of infarct size with verapamil,[145,146] with diltiazem as a sole agent[147] or with propranolol,[32] and with nifedipine given either before or after coronary occlusion.[148,149] Second-generation agents including amlodipine also have protective effects experimentally when the drug is used prophylactically.[150,151.]

The Clinical Use of Calcium Antagonists after Myocardial Infarction

The pharmacologic and experimental profile of calcium antagonists strongly suggested that clinical application for vascular diseases would carry appreciable benefit. In addition to their exploitation for the management of hypertension and angina, a promise which was largely fulfilled, many trials were undertaken for patients with established or threatened myocardial infarction. But in this sphere most results to date have been disappointing.

Effect on mortality

Mortality data by treatment allocation are available for at least 23 trials. Most of them were short term, small, and not designed with survival as a primary endpoint. The 1989 overview by Held and colleagues[152] included all but the latest of them. By that time more than 17 000 patients had been included in controlled trials of calcium channel blockers for the management of acute myocardial infarction for prophylaxis afterwards. In three trials mortality was lower in the group allocated to calcium blockers, five trials reported no difference, but in 13 trials mortality was higher in patients who received active therapy. None of the differences was significant, but the failure of any favorable trend to emerge provided an important conclusion. Overall 9.8% of those allocated to active treatment died compared with 9.3% allocated to placebo. The trial that was not included in the review (DAVIT II) did, however, suggest that verapamil may reduce mortality in selected patients; it is discussed in detail below. In a more recent review[153] that included available data from all trials, the odds ratios and confidence limits for mortality changes were presented not only in total but also separately for verapamil, nifedipine, diltiazem and lidoflazine. No significant benefit was found in any of these meta-analyses.

Three studies designed specifically to address mortality effects have been conducted with nifedipine tested against placebo. In the Trent[154] study 4491 patients with suspected infarction received nifedipine 10 mg four times a day or placebo starting immediately after admission and continued for 28 days. Mortality rates were respectively 10.2% and 9.3%. The Israeli SPRINT study group enrolled 2276 survivors of acute infarction and randomized them at 7 days.[155] By 21 days, mortality was 5.8% with nifedipine 30 mg per day compared with 5.7% with placebo. In SPRINT II,[156] nifedipine was started immediately after admission but the trial was discontinued because a harmful trend was observed in those treated with the active drug.

The sole diltiazem mortality study[157] was also negative. Entry of 2466 patients was 3–15 days after the onset of myocardial infarction. They received either 240 mg diltiazem each day or placebo during a follow-up period averaging a little over 2 years. Mortality rates were almost identical in the two groups, but the investigators claimed a significant bidirectional interaction between diltiazem and early radiologic pulmonary congestion. The primary endpoint had been changed after the first year of trial from mortality to first recurrent cardiac event (cardiac death or nonfatal reinfarction). The hazard ratio with this index was 0.77 for the majority of patients without pulmonary congestion and 1.41 for those with pulmonary congestion. This finding emerged from retrospective data analysis. Though plausible both on a priori grounds and by analogy to findings with verapamil (see later), it must treated with considerable caution unless it is confirmed by a prospective trial. Indeed, a previous study had suggested that diltiazem was safe even in the presence of heart failure.[158] One potentially confounding factor deserves mention. No less than 55% of patients in the trial were taking a β-blocking agent throughout. This would have added to the hazard of patients with poor myocardial function and decreased the prospects of achieving a positive result. A reduction in mortality over and above that which could be achieved by β-blockers would be difficult to demonstrate, and the trial design was optimistic in this regard.

Two major mortality studies have been carried out by a Danish cooperative group using verapamil. In the first of these, known as DAVIT,[159] randomization of 3498 patients took place immediately after admission, with exclusion criteria comprising cardiogenic shock, heart failure, hypotension, conduction blocks, and other potentially confounding variables. Because limitation of infarct size[145,146] was a principal motive for the trial, treatment began using the intravenous route; it continued for 6 months with 360 mg oral verapamil per day or matching placebo. Patients were withdrawn after 1 week if the inclusion criteria for infarction were not met after full hospital evaluation, leaving 1436 patients to continue in the trial. Death rates at 6 months were 12.8% on verapamil and 13.9% on placebo, with heart failure and AV block more frequent in the verapamil group. Contrary to the hypothesis that inspired the trial, very early intervention showed no benefit, but a retrospective analysis showed a significant reduction in mortality in the group first treated 6–24 hours after onset of symptoms. The investigators postulated that very early entry, which prevented accurate identification of many destined to develop heart failure, may have precluded a positive result and were also aware of the need to test any revised hypothesis with a new prospective trial. This was planned and executed under the acronym DAVIT II.[160] The design was similar to the earlier verapamil trial, with 1775 patients less than 76 yearsof age randomized between verapamil 360 mg daily and placebo, but treatment started in the second week of hospital admission and continued for an average of 16 months. Despite the problems with the earlier trial, exclusion criteria were not very restrictive. Those who had heart failure could be included if they were controlled on 160 mg frusemide per day or less, and if abnormalities of conduction resolved within 3 days of the infarct. The primary endpoints were total mortality and first major event (death and nonfatal reinfarction). These occurred respectively in 95 and 146 patients in the verapamil group compared with 119 and 180 patients in the placebo group. The reduction of 16.7% in major events at 18 months was significant ($P = 0.03$). No mortality reduction occurred in the cohort who had had failure. In patients who had remained free of heart failure in the cardiac care unit the mortality rates were 7.7% in the verapamil group and 11.8% in the placebo group ($P = 0.02$). The seemingly impressive reduction was not based on a prior hypothesis. But neither was it strictly data derived because a decision to perform subgroup analyses was made before breaking the code: these were based on age, previous myocardial infarction, cardiac arrest in the cardiac care unit, atrial fibrillation, angina pectoris, type and location of infarct, and the presence of heart failure at any time. Little additional credence can be claimed because so many subgroups were examined independently: chance alone would offer a reasonable prospect of a seemingly impressive result in one or other of them. Nevertheless there is a consistency that commands attention in the apparent hazard of using diltiazem or verapamil for secondary prevention in patients with heart failure after infarction. And if this be accepted as plausible then the corollary follows of the likelihood of impressive benefit in the remainder.

Prevention of reinfarction

The effect of calcium channel blockers on calcium flux at cellular level, on systemic and coronary vasodilatation and, in the case of diltiazem and verapamil, on heart rate and contractility that were postulated to reduce mortality after infarction may also protect against reinfarction. This may be especially true of non-Q-wave infarction in which coronary vascular tone is believed to be especially important.[161,162] A meta-analysis for trials involving the three prototype drugs and for all trials showed a favorable trend (Figure 7.3).[153] If trials with nifedipine were excluded, the possibility of benefit would be persuasive.

Two large trials were set up specifically to explore the hypothesis that reinfarction may be prevented in patients with non-Q-wave infarction by diltiazem, which may be more suitable than the other prototype calcium antagonists for this indication. In addition to experimental evidence for a selective action on coronary vasomotor tone and beneficial effects in vasospastic angina, prevention of coronary vasoconstriction has been demonstrated during dynamic exercise in patients with coronary artery disease. In this regard it resembles at least one of the β-blockers that also prevents reinfarction.[109] In the first multicenter trial[163] a subset of 576 patients with non-Q-wave infarction was selected from a total of 1603, with exclusion criteria based principally on conduction disorders, shock,

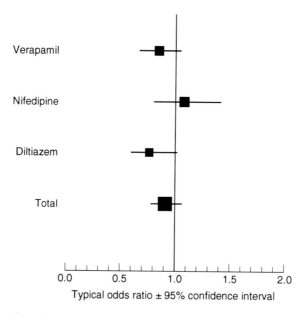

Figure 7.3 Meta-analysis for trials on prevention of reinfarction involving the three prototype drugs. (From Ref. 37 with permission.)

severe noncoronary disease, or perceived need for treatment with calcium channel blockers. Treatment was started 24–72 hours after admission using diltiazem with one dose at 30 mg, one dose at 60 mg, then 90 mg at 6-hourly intervals for 14 days or until the patient was discharged from hospital or withdrawn from the trial. The primary endpoint was an increase of 50% or more in CK-MB activity above the previous baseline. Reinfarction by this definition occurred in 27 patients (9.3%) in the placebo group and in 15 patients (5.2%) in the diltiazem group. The event rate in the two groups diverged from 5 days onwards, and unusually the results were expressed as a reinfarction *rate* at 14 days for which a 51.2% reduction was claimed ($P < 0.03$). A life-table type of analysis and the choice of a one-tailed significance test both seem inappropriate and perhaps misleading.[164] Not unexpectedly, patients on diltiazem had less postinfarction angina. When the difference in prespecified endpoints of refractory angina necessitating withdrawal and reinfarction were combined, the result was expressed in a more familiar manner as a simple reduction in incidence that amounted to 49% and achieved conventional significance ($P < 0.05$). A subsequent study[165] of 514 patients with non-Q-wave infarction followed long term for 25 months showed a highly significant reduction in reinfarction during the first 6 months of follow-up (17 vs 2 patients, $P < 0.001$) but no difference in the period 6 months to the end of the trial (13 vs 14 patients). Bearing in mind the very short follow-up period of the earlier trial the conclusions are clear. There is no evidence for long-term protection with diltiazem in patients with non-Q-wave infarction, but at least suggestive evidence for short-term protection, perhaps over several months, that may be useful between the index event and full prognostic evaluation. One small trial did suggest that nifedipine reduces the incidence of myocardial infarction in patients undergoing coronary bypass grafting.[166] The pathophysiology of this type of infarct may differ considerably from usual infarction, and no general conclusions can be drawn. Experience of calcium channel blockers in unstable angina is limited and indeed was discouraged by the results of the HINT study,[167] but nifedipine at least did not show any promise in an early trial[168] in this category of patients who may be regarded as most vulnerable to the early development of myocardial infarction.

The Potential for Calcium Antagonists after Myocardial Infarction

Studies available at the present time are disappointing with regard to the modification of clinical endpoints by calcium antagonists in patients with acute infarction. Nevertheless the promise inherent in the experimental profile of the drugs should not be overlooked. General class effects are not a major consideration with drugs that exhibit so much receptor selectivity. The diversity of drug effects imply that individual drugs are likely to have very specific indications. The hints of benefit and of hazard indicated or suggested by trials suggest ways in which existing agents may be used to greater effect and new agents should be explored in the future. However, progress may be impeded by the discouragement born of existing experience.

The risk of worsening heart failure with diltiazem and verapamil is real. Even nifedipine, which has little effect on myocardial contractility and achieves afterload reduction, seems risky in susceptible subjects because of the activation of endogenous neurohumoral systems[169] and perhaps also because of interference with the release of atrial natriuretic peptides from the atria that depend on calcium ions.[169] Results might have been more encouraging if these considerations had been better understood when early trials were being planned. The prospects for limiting infarct size that prompted some trials[170–175] are probably illusory, although diltiazem may improve coronary perfusion and even some hemodynamic variables.[174,176] No benefit of clinical value has been demonstrated in rhythm abnormalities as a result of calcium blockers after myocardial infarction, with only minor reductions in the incidence of some transient ventricular arrhythmias.[174,177] As with most studies, results are necessarily restricted to the short and medium term. If the observation that nifedipine can retard the progression of coronary artery disease[178] is confirmed, important in degree, sustained, and general to calcium antagonists then this unique effect should have long-term clinical implications for the survivors of myocardial infarction. A similar trial with nicardipine,[179] however, offered little encouragement to the hope of a useful class effect.

Where are we now? The calcium channel blocker used with greatest confidence after myocardial infarction may be verapamil, prescribed to reduce late mortality in patients who have never had overt evidence of heart failure. Diltiazem is also a contender for a favored position as part of a short or middle-term strategy to prevent reinfarction in patients with non-Q-wave infarction. All calcium channel blockers may find an appropriate role in the management of postinfarction angina, although the dihydropyridines cannot at present be recommended as drugs of choice because the balance of benefit against risk after infarction is more problematical with these than other agents in the class. Any reservations on the use of nifedipine should not, however, impede investigation of second-generation dihydropyridines such as amlodipine, because they show important differences from the prototype drug in their pharmacodynamic profiles. The cost implications of the long-term use of calcium channel blockers has not been analyzed in any published study, but the considerations for prophylaxis with verapamil will be similar to those relating to β-blockers. Other calcium antagonists will be used appropriately only short term or for symptomatic reasons: cost–benefit is then based on different criteria.

Much remains to be learnt about the potential value of calcium antagonists in patients with myocardial infarction, but opportunities for progress may be inappropriately few. The major interests of clinicians and the pharmaceutical industry have moved to other fields and judgments may continue to be made on evidence that is available at the present time.

β-Blockers and Calcium Antagonists in the Management of Acute Myocardial Infarction

β-Adrenoceptor antagonists and calcium channel blockers are of clinical value for a substantial minority of patients in the hospital phase of acute myocardial infarction, and for many of them it is appropriate to continue with the treatment long-term.

As agents for symptomatic relief, β-blockers may be used for refractory or recurrent cardiac pain, especially in the presence of a tachycardia that is not induced by overt heart failure. β-Blockers alone or in combination with calcium anatagonists are of value in the management of postinfarction angina, though usually for only a limited time because this symptom should generally be regarded as an indication for coronary angiography and intervention. Patients admitted with possible infarction that is subsequently diagnosed as unstable angina remain at risk of infarction, and in some of these β-blockade may not only relieve pain but also help to arrest or minimize progression to muscle necrosis.

A persuasive case can be made for the prophylactic use of intravenous β-blockade in the acute stage of myocardial infarction for three reasons: if administered within an hour or so it may contribute, with thrombolysis, to the strategy of limiting infarct size by myocardial salvage; its value in preventing myocardial rupture is not proven but the hypothesis may be considered strong enough at least to support other indications for early use; and the protection against malignant arrhythmias that has been demonstrated with reasonable certainty in trials may underestimate the benefit in the generality of medical practice where the potential for successful defibrillation is variable. Whatever the mechanisms, a reduction in mortality has been demonstrated and the notion that it may no longer be relevant in the era of thrombolysis is one that requires the justification of proof that many would consider unlikely to be forthcoming. Evidence is best for atenolol and for metoprolol. No indication exists for the routine intravenous use of any calcium channel blocker in the context of acute myocardial infarction.

Prophylaxis against late death should always be considered in patients during the hospital phase of myocardial infarction. The five classes of drugs that may be of benefit – antiplatelet agents, oral anticoagulants, angiotensin-converting enzyme (ACE) inhibitors, *β*-blockers, and calcium channel blockers – are not all mutually exclusive and up to three may find an appropriate role in any one patient. All physicians agree that antiplatelet agents should be used in all who have no important contraindications. Present evidence supports the use of ACE inhibitors only for patients with large infarcts and important residual damage (see Chapters 10 and 15). The role of anticoagulants is less well agreed, and discussion of their role is outside the scope of this chapter, but few patients are so treated at the present time.

The selection of patients for prophylactic *β*-blockade has been discussed above (see p. 206). Arguments have been put forward against their routine use in all who are able to tolerate them because the potential benefit in identifiable low-risk patients may not justify the burden of unwanted effects and the cost. One specific group with low initial risk, identified by the occurrence of a non-Q-wave infarction, requires protection against reinfarction, and the short- or medium-term use of diltiazem may appropriately be considered even in the absence of strict scientific proof of efficacy for this indication. The evidence of benefit from diltiazem is better than for *β*-blockers. At the other end of the spectrum of immediate risk, patients who have suffered heart failure that cannot readily be controlled, or who have persistent important anomalies of impulse formation or conduction, are not potential candidates for *β*-blockade or for calcium antagonists. But the intermediate group with damage that may herald long-term risk yet can tolerate the hemodynamic effects of *β*-blockade are usually appropriate candidates for long-term prophylaxis with one of these drugs. As the trials showed considerable variation in efficacy and the drugs have disparate pharmacodynamic properties, there is at least a possibility that some agents are more effective than others. The careful physician may therefore feel it best to copy the recipe of one of the most successful trials and thus decide to use timolol, propranolol, acebutalol, or metoprolol in the doses for which positive data are available. But this recommendation based solely on hemodynamic considerations has a proviso. *β*-Blockade may still be contraindicated on account of asthma, peripheral vascular disease, or nonspecific unwanted effects that are unacceptable to the patient even for a limited period that spans the time of greatest risk. For these patients verapamil should be considered because the evidence for benefit is good, yet not strong enough to make it an alternative to *β*-blockade when either might be equally well tolerated.

References

1. Ahlquist, R.P. (1948) A study of adrenotropic receptors. *Am. J. Physiol.*, **153**, 586–600.
2. Powell, C.E. and Slater, I.H. (1958) Blockade of inhibitory adrenergic receptors by a dichloro analog of isoproterenol. *J. Pharmacol. Exp. Ther.*, **122**, 480–8.
3. Cruickshank, J.M. and Prichard, B.N.C. (eds) (1988) *Beta-blockers in Clinical Practice*, p. 3. Edinburgh: Churchill Livingstone.
4. Black, J.W. and Stephenson, J.S. (1962) Pharmacology of a new adrenergic beta-receptor-blocking compound (Nethalide). *Lancet*, **ii**, 311–14.
5. Dornhorst, A.C. and Robinson, B.F. (1962) Clinical pharmacology of a beta-adrenergic-blocking agent (Nethalide). *Lancet*, **ii**, 314–16.
6. Shanks, R.G. (1984) The discovery of beta adrenoceptor blocking drugs. In: Parnham, M.J. and Bruinvels, J. (eds) *Discoveries in Pharmacology, Volume 2: Haemodynamics, Hormones & Inflammation*, p. 68. Amsterdam: Elsevier Science Publishers.
7. Smith, H.J. (1982) The need to redefine membrane stabilizing activity of beta-adrenergic receptor antagonists. *J. Mol. Cell. Cardiol.*, **14**, 495–500.

8. Kornhauser, D.M., Wood, A.J.J., Vestal, R.E. *et al.* (1978) Biological determinants of propranolol disposition in man. *Clin. Pharmacol. Ther.*, **23**, 165–74.

9. Woosley, R.L., Kornhauser, D., Smith, R. *et al.* (1979) Suppression of chronic ventricular arrhythmias with propranolol. *Circulation*, **60**, 819–27.

10. Lands, A.M., Arnold, A., McAuliff, J.P. *et al.* (1967) Differentiation of receptor systems activated by sympathetic amines. *Nature*, **214**, 597–8.

11. Chamberlain, D.A. (1966) Effects of beta adrenergic blockade on heart size. *Am. J. Cardiol.*, **18**, 321–5.

12. Lombardo, T.A., Rose, L., Taeschler, M. *et al.* (1953) The effect of exercise on coronary blood flow, myocardial oxygen consumption and cardiac efficiency in man. *Circulation*, **7**, 71–8.

13. Hoffman, B.F. and Cranefield, P.F. (1964) The physiological basis of cardiac arrhythmias. *Am. J. Med.*, **37**, 670–84.

14. Han, J. (1969) Mechanisms of ventricular arrhythmias associated with myocardial infarction. *Am. J. Cardiol.*, **24**, 800–13.

15. Clausen, T. and Flatman, J.A. (1980) β_2-adrenoceptors mediate the stimulating effect of adrenaline on active electrogenic Na-K-transport in rat soleus muscle. *Br. J. Pharmacol.*, **68**, 749–55.

16. Brown, M.J., Brown, D.C. and Murphy, M.B. (1983) Hypokalemia from beta$_2$-receptor stimulation by circulating epinephrine. *N. Engl. J. Med.*, **309**, 1414–19.

17. Hall, J.A., Ferro, A., Dickerson, J.E.C. and Brown, M.J. (1983) β adrenoceptor subtype cross regulation in the human heart. *Br. Heart J.*, **69**, 332–7.

18. Norris, R.M., Brown, M.A., Clarke, E.D. *et al.* (1984) Prevention of ventricular fibrillation during acute myocardial infarction by intravenous propranolol. *Lancet*, **ii**, 883–6.

19. Braunwald, E., and Maroko, P.R. (1974) The reduction of infarct size – an idea whose time (for testing) has come. *Circulation*, **50**, 206–9.

20. Sonnenblick, E.H. (1962) Implications of muscle mechanics in the heart. *Fed. Proc.*, **21**, 975–90.

21. Maroko, P.R., Kjekshus, J.K., Sobel, B.E. *et al.* (1971) Factors influencing infarct size following experimental coronary artery occlusions. *Circulation*, **43**, 67–82.

22. Pitt, B. and Craven, P. (1970) Effect of propranolol on regional myocardial blood flow in acute ischaemia. *Cardiovasc. Res.*, **4**, 176–9.

23. Becker, L.C., Fortuin, N.J. and Pitt, B. (1971) Effect of ischemia and antianginal drugs on the distribution of radioactive microspheres in the canine left ventricle. *Circ. Res.*, **28**, 263–9.

24. Opie, L.H. and Thomas M. (1976) Propranolol and experimental myocardial infarction: substrate effects. *Postgrad. Med. J.*, **52** (suppl. 4), 124–32.

25. Religa, A., Mueller, H., Evans, R. and Ayres, S. (1973) Metabolic effect of propranolol on ischemic tissue in human and experimental infarction (abstract). *Clin. Res.*, **21**, 954.

26. Reimer, K.A., Rasmussen, M.M. and Jennings, R.B. (1976) On the nature of protection by propranolol against myocardial necrosis after temporary coronary occlusion in dogs. *Am. J. Cardiol.*, **37**, 520–7.

27. Libby, P., Maroko, P.R., Covell, J.W. *et al.* (1973) The effect of practolol on the extent of myocardial ischaemic injury after experimental coronary occlusion and its effects on ventricular function in normal and ischaemic heart. *Cardiovasc. Res.*, **7**, 167–73.

28. Nayler, W.G., Yepez, C.E., Fassold, E. and Ferrari, R. (1978) Prolonged protective effect of propranolol on hypoxic heart muscle. *Am. J. Cardiol.*, **42**, 217–25.

29. Reimer, K.A., Lowe, J.E., Rasmussen, M.M. and Jennings, R.B. (1977) The wavefront phenomenon of ischemic cell death. 1. Myocardial infarct size vs duration of coronary occlusion in dogs. *Circulation*, **56**, 786–94.

30. Linderer, T., Schröder, R., Arntz, R. *et al.* (1993) Prehospital thrombolysis; beneficial effects of very early treatment on infarct size and left ventricular function. *J. Am. Coll. Cardiol.*, **22**, 1304–10.

31. Yusuf, S., Lopez, R., Maddison, A. and Sleight, P. (1981) Variability of electrocardiographic and enzyme evolution of myocardial infarction in man. *Br. Heart J.*, **45**, 271–80.

32. Bush, L.R., Buja, L.M., Tilton, G. *et al.* (1985) Effects of propranolol and diltiazam alone and in combination on the recovery of left ventricular segmental function after temporary coronary occlusion and long-term reperfusion in conscious dogs. *Circulation*, **72**, 413–30.

33. Lange, R., Kloner, R.A. and Braunwald, E. (1983) First ultra-short-acting beta-adrenergic blocking agent: its effect on size and segmental wall dynamics of reperfused myocardial infarcts in dogs. *Am. J. Cardiol.*, **51**, 1759–67.

34. Van de Werf, F., Vanhaecke, J., Jang, I.K. *et al.* (1987) Reduction in infarct size and enhanced recovery of systolic function after coronary thrombolysis with tissue-type plasminogen activator combined with beta-adrenergic blockade with metoprolol. *Circulation*, **75**, 830–6.

35. Jewitt, D.E. and Singh, R.N. (1974) The role of β-adrenergic blockade in myocardial infarction. *Prog. Cardiovasc. Dis.*, **16**, 421–38.

36. Yusuf, S., Peto. R., Lewis, J. *et al.* (1985) Beta blockade during and after myocardial infarction: an overview of the randomized trials. *Prog. Cardiovasc. Dis.*, **27**, 335–71.

37. Held, P.H. and Yusuf, S. (1993) Effects of β-blockers and calcium channel blockers in acute myocardial infarction. *Eur. Heart J.*, **14** (suppl. F): 18–25.

38. Waagstein, F. and Hjalmarson, Å.C. (1975) Double-blind study of the effect of cardioselective beta-blockade on chest pain in acute myocardial infarction. *Acta Med. Scand. (Suppl.)*, **587**, 201–8.

39. Herlitz, J., Hjalmarson, Å., Holmberg, S. *et al.* (1984) Effect of metoprolol on chest pain in acute myocardial infarction. *Br. Heart J.*, **51**, 438–44.

40. Ramsdale, D.R., Faragher, E.B., Bennett, D.H. *et al.* (1982) Ischemic pain relief in patients with acute myocardial infarction by intravenous atenolol. *Am. Heart J.*, **103**, 459–67.
41. Gold, H.K., Leinbach, R.C. and Maroko, P.R. (1976) Propranolol-induced reduction of signs of ischemic injury during acute myocardial infarction. *Am. J. Cardiol.*, **38**, 689–95.
42. Cox, J.L., McLaughlin, V.W., Flowers, N.C. and Horan, L.G. (1968) The ischemic zone surrounding acute myocardial infarction. Its morphology as detected by dehydrogenase staining. *Am. Heart J.*, **76**, 650–9.
43. Poole-Wilson, P.A. (1983) Reduction of infarct size; a misleading concept? *Postgrad. Med. J.*, **59** (suppl. 3), 95–6.
44. The MIAMI Trial Research Group (1985) Metoprolol in acute myocardial infarction (MIAMI). A randomised placebo-controlled international trial. *Eur. Heart J.*, **6**, 199–226.
45. The MIAMI Trial Research Group (1985) Enzymatic estimation of infarct size. *Am. J. Cardiol.*, **56**, 27G–29G.
46. Roberts, R., Croft, C., Gold, H.K. *et al.* and the MILIS Study Group (1984) Effect of propranolol on myocardial-infarct size in a randomized blinded multicenter trial. *N. Engl. J. Med.*, **311**, 218–25.
47. Kjekshus, J. (1986) Importance of heart rate in determining beta-blocker efficacy in acute and long-term acute myocardial infarction intervention trials. *Am. J. Cardiol.*, **57**, 43F–49F.
48. Roe, C.R., Cobb, F.R. and Starmer, C.F. (1977) The relationship between enzymatic and histologic estimates of the extent of myocardial infarction in conscious dogs with permanent coronary occlusion. *Circulation*, **55**, 438–49.
49. Lewis, M.J., Griffith, T.M. and Hendersen, A.H. (1983) β-blockade and coronary arteries. *Drugs*, **25** (suppl. 2), 247–9.
50. Bleifeld, W., Mathey, D., Hanrath, P. *et al.* (1977) Infarct size estimated from serial serum creatine phosphokinase in relation to left ventricular hemodynamics. *Circulation*, **55**, 303–11.
51. Grande, P. Hansen, B.F., Christiansen, C. and Naestoft, J. (1982) Estimation of acute myocardial infarct size in man by serum CK-MB measurements. *Circulation*, **66**, 756–64.
52. ISIS-1 (First International Study of Infarct Survival) Collaborative Group (1986) Randomised trial of intravenous atenolol among 16 027 cases of suspected acute myocardial infarction: ISIS-1. *Lancet*, **ii**, 57–66.
53. Holland, R.P. and Arnsdorf, M.R. (1977) Solid angle theory and the electrocardiogram: physiologic and quantitative interpretations. *Prog. Cardiovasc. Dis.*, **19**, 431–57.
54. Yusuf, S., Sleight, P., Rossi, P. *et al.* (1983) Reduction in infarct size, arrhythmias and chest pain by early intravenous beta blockade in suspected acute myocardial infarction. *Circulation*, **67** (suppl. 1), I-32–I-41.
55. International Collaborative Study Group (1984) Reduction of infarct size with the early use of timolol in acute myocardial infarction. *N. Engl. J. Med.*, **310**, 9–15.
56. Norris, R.M., Clarke, E.D., Sammel, N.L. *et al.* (1978) Protective effect of propranolol in threatened myocardial infarction. *Lancet*, **ii**, 907–9.
57. Herlitz, J., Emanuelsson, H., Swedberg, K. *et al.* (1984) Göteborg metoprolol trial: enzyme-estimated infarct size. *Am. J. Cardiol.* **53**, 15D–21D.
58. The MIAMI Trial Research Group (1985) Development of myocardial infarction. *Am. J. Cardiol.*, **56**, 23G–26G.
59. Hjalmarson, A. (ed.) (1985) MIAMI: Metoprolol in acute myocardial infarction (supplement). *Am. J. Cardiol.*, **56**, 1G–57G.
60. ISIS-1 (First International Study of Infarct Survival) Collaborative Group (1988) Mechanisms for the early mortality reduction poroduced by beta-blockade started early in myocardial infarction; ISIS-1. *Lancet*, **i**, 921–3.
61. Herlitz, J., Elmfeldt, D., Holmberg, S. *et al.* (1984) Göteborg metoprolol trial: mortality and causes of death. *Am. J. Cardiol.*, **53**, 9D–14D.
62. Roberts, R., Rogers, W.J., Mueller, H.S. *et al.* for the TIMI Investigators. (1991) Immediate versus deferred β-blockade following thrombolytic therapy in patients with acute myocardial infarction. Results of the Thrombolysis In Myocardial Infarction (TIMI) II-B study. *Circulation*, **83**, 422–37.
63. Rossi, P.R.F., Yusuf, S., Ramsdale, D. *et al.* (1983) reduction of ventricular arrhythmias by early intravenous atenolol in suspected acute myocardial infarction. *BMJ*, **286**, 506–10.
64. Rydén, L., Ariniego, R., Arnman, K. *et al.* (1983) A double-blind trial of metoprolol in acute myocardial infarction: effects on venticular tachyarrhythmias. *N. Eng. J. Med.*, **308**, 614–18.
65. Evemy, K.L. and Pentecost, B.L. (1978) Intravenous and oral practolol in the acute stages of myocardial infarction. *Eur. J. Cardiol.*, **7**, 391–8.
66. Herlitz, J., Edvardsson, N., Holmberg, S. *et al.* (1984) Göteborg metoprolol trial: effects on arrhythmias. *Am. J. Cardiol.*, **53**, 27D–31D.
67. Nordrehaug, J.E., Johannessen, K.-A., Von der Lippe, G. *et al.* (1985) Effect of timolol on changes in serum potassium concentration during acute myocardial infarction. *Br. Heart J.*, **53**, 388–93.
68. Snow, P.J.D. (1965) Effect of propranolol in myocardial infarction. *Lancet*, **ii**, 551–3.
69. Multicentre International Study: Supplementary Report (1977) Reduction in mortality after myocardial infarction with long-term beta-adrenoceptor blockade. *BMJ*, **ii**, 419–21.
70. Baber, N.S., Evans, D.W., Howitt, G. *et al.* (1980) Multicentre post-infarction trial of propranolol in 49 hospitals in the United Kingdom, Italy andYugoslavia. *Br. Heart J.*, **44**, 96–100.
71. The Norwegian Multicenter Study Group (1981) Timolol-induced reduction in mortality and re-infarction in patients surviving acute myocardial infarction. *N. Engl. J. Med.*, **304**, 801–7.
72. Taylor, S.H., Silke, B., Ebbutt, A. *et al.* (1982) A long-term prevention study with oxprenolol in coronary heart disease. *N. Engl. J. Med.*, **307**, 1293–301.
73. Hansteen, V., Møinichen, E., Lorentsen, E. *et al.* (1982) One year's treatment with propranolol after myocardial infarction: preliminary report of Norwegian multicentre trial. *BMJ*, **284**, 155–60.

74. Beta-blocker Heart Attack Trial Research Group (1982) A randomised trial of propranolol in patients with acute myocardial infarction: I. Mortality results. *JAMA*, **247**, 1707–14.
75. Beta-blocker Heart Attack Trial Research Group (1983) A randomised trial of propranolol in patients with acute myocardial infarction: II. Morbidity results. *JAMA*, **250**, 2814–19.
76. Julian, D.G., Prescott, R.J., Jackson, F.S. and Szekely, P. (1982) Controlled trial of sotolol for one year after myocardial infarction. *Lancet*, **i**, 1142–7.
77. Australian and Swedish Pindolol Study Group (1983) The effect of pindolol on the two years mortality after complicated myocardial infarction. *Eur. Heart J.* **4**, 367–75.
78. Manger Cats, V., van Capelle, F.J.L., Lie, K.I. and Durrer, D. (1983) Effect of treatment with 2×100 mg metoprolol on mortality in a single-center study with low placebo-mortality rate after infarction (abstract). *Circulation*, **68**, (suppl. 3): 181. (Also The Amsterdam metoprolol trial. *Drugs*, 1985, suppl. 1, p. 8.)
79. European Infarction Study Group (1984) European infarction study (E.I.S.): a secondary prevention study with slow-release oxprenolol after myocardial infarction: morbidity and mortality. *Eur. Heart J.*, **5**, 189–202.
80. Lopressor Intervention Trial Research Group (1987) The Lopressor intervention trial: multicentre study of metoprolol in survivors of acute myocardial infarction. *Eur. Heart J.*, **8**, 1056–64.
81. Boissel, J.-P., Leizorovicz, A., Picolet, H. and Peyrieux, J.-C. for the APSI investigators (1990) Secondary prevention after high-risk acute myocardial infarction with low-dose acebutolol. *Am. J. Cardiol.*, **66**, 251–60.
82. Collins, R. *et al.* ISIS-4 (In press)
83. Cowan, M.J., Reichenbach, D., Turner, P. and Thostenson, C. (1991) Cellular response of the evolving myocardial infarction after therapeutic coronary artery reperfusion. *Hum. Pathol.*, **22**, 154–63.
84. Yusuf, S., Wittes, J., Probstfield, J. and Tyroler, H. (1991) Analysis and interpretation of treatment effects in subgroups of patients in randomized clinical trials. *JAMA*, **266**, 93–8.
85. Barber, J.M., Boyle, D.McC., Chaturvedi, N.C. *et al.* (1976) Practolol in acute myocardial infarction. *Acta Med. Scand. (Suppl.)*, **587**, 213–19.
86. Andersen, M.P., Bechsgaard, P., Frederiksen, J. *et al.* (1979) Effect of alprenolol on mortality among patients with definite or suspected acute myocardial infarction. *Lancet*, **ii**, 865–7.
87. Reynolds, J.L. and Whitlock, R.M.L. (1972) Effects of a beta-adrenergic receptor blocker in myocardial infarction treated for one year from onset. *Br. Heart J.*, **34**, 252–9.
88. Wilhelmsson, C., Vedin, J.A., Wilhelmsen, L. *et al.* (1974) Reduction of sudden deaths after myocardial infarction by treatment with alprenolol. *Lancet*, **ii**, 1157–60.
89. Ahlmark, G., Saetre, H. and Korsgren, M. (1974) Reduction of sudden deaths after myocardial infarction (letter). *Lancet*, **ii**, 1563.
90. Coronary Prevention Research Group (1981) An early intervention secondary prevention study with oxprenolol following myocardial infarction. *Eur. Heart J.*, **2**, 389–93.
91. Wilcox, R.G., Rowley, J.M., Hampton, J.R. *et al.* (1980) Randomised placebo-controlled trial comparing oxprenolol with disopyramide phosphate in immediate treatment of suspected myocardial infarction. *Lancet*, **ii**, 765–9.
92. Olsson, G., Rehnqvist, N., Sjögren, A. *et al.* (1985) Long-term treatment with metoprolol after myocardial infarction: effect on 3 year mortality and morbidity. *J. Am. Coll. Cardiol.*, **5**, 1428–37.
93. Hjalmarson, Å., Elmfeldt, D., Herlitz, J. *et al.* (1981) Effect on mortality of metoprolol in acute myocardial infarction. *Lancet*, **ii**, 823–7.
94. Salathia, K.S., Barber, J.M., McIlmoyle, E.L. *et al.* (1985) Very early intervention with metoprolol in suspected acute myocardial infarction. *Eur. Heart. J.*, **6**, 190–8.
95. Wilcox, R.G., Roland, J.M., Banks, D.C. *et al.* (1980) Randomised trial comparing propranolol with atenolol in immediate treatment of suspected myocardial infarction. *BMJ*, **280**, 885–8.
96. Breslow, N.E. and Day, N.E. (1980) *Statistical Methods in Cancer Research*, Vol. 1. The analysis of case-control studies (p.124). Lyons: IARC Scientific Publications.
97. Fleiss, J.L. (1993) The statistical basis of meta-analysis. In: Pocock S. (ed) *Statistical Methods in Medical Research*. Sevenoaks: Edward Arnold.
98. Rehnqvist, N., Olsson, G., Erhardt, L. and Ekman, A.-M. (1987) Metoprolol in acute myocardial infarction reduces ventricular arrhythmias both in the early stage and after the acute event. *Int. J. Cardiol.*, **15**, 301–8.
99. Olsson, G. and Rehnqvist, N. (1984) Ventricular arrhythmias during the first year after acute myocardial infarction: influence of long-term treatment with metoprolol. *Circulation*, **69**, 1129–34.
100. Bethge, K.-P., Andresen, D., Boissel, J.-P. *et al.* (1985) Effect of oxprenolol on ventricular arrhythmias: the European infarction study experience. *J. Am. Coll. Cardiol.*, **6**, 963–72.
101. Kostis, J.B., Wilson, A.C., Sanders, M.R. and Byington, R.P., for the BHAT Study Group (1988). Prognostic significance of ventricular ectopic activity in survivors of acute myocardial infarction who receive propranolol. *Am. J. Cardiol.*, **61**, 975–8.
102. Furberg, C.D., Hawkins, C.M. and Lichstein, E. for the Beta-Blocker Heart Attack Trial Study Group (1984) Effect of propranolol in postinfarction patients with mechanical or electrical complications. *Circulation*, **69**, 761–5.
103. Friedman, L.M., Byington, R.P., Capone, R.J. *et al.* for the Beta-Blocker Heart Attack Trial Research Group (1986) Effect of propranolol in patients with myocardial infarction and ventricular arrhythmias. *J. Am. Coll. Cardiol.*, **7**, 1–8.
104. The Cardiac Arrhythmia Suppression Trial (CAST) Investigators (1989) Preliminary report: effect of encainide and flecainide on mortality in a randomized trial of arrhythmia suppression after myocardial infarction. *N. Engl. J. Med.*, **321**, 406–12.

105. Baroldi, G., Radice, F., Schmid, G. and Leone, A. (1974) Morphology of acute myocardial infarction in relation to coronary thrombosis. *Am. Heart J.*, **87**, 65–75.

105a. DeWood, M.A., Spores, J., Notske, R. *et al.* (1980) Prevalence of total coronary occlusion during the early hours of transmural myocardial infarction. *N. Engl. J. Med.*, **303**, 897–902.

106. Winther, K. and Rein, E. (1990) Exercise-induced platelet aggregation in angina and its possible prevention by $β_1$-selective blockade. *Eur. Heart J.* **11**, 819–23.

107. Callahan, K.S., Johnson, A.R. and Campbell, W.B. (1985) Enhancement of the antiaggregatory activity of prostacyclin by propranolol in human platelets. *Circulation*, **71**, 1237–46.

108. Brommer, E.J.P. and Loeliger, E.A. (1981) Timolol after myocardial infarction (letter). *N. Engl. J. Med.*, **305** 406–7.

109. Gaglione, A., Hess, O.M., Corin, W.J. *et al.* (1987) Is there coronary vasoconstriction after intracoronary beta-adrenergic blockade in patients with coronary artery disease? *J. Am. Coll. Cardiol.*, **10**, 299–310.

110. The Beta-Blocker Pooling Project Research Group (1988) The Beta-Blocker Pooling Project (BBPP); subgroup findings from randomized trials in post infarction patients. *Eur. Heart J.*, **9**, 8–16.

111. Chadda, K., Goldstein, S., Byington, R. and Curb, J.D. (1986) Effect of propranolol after acute myocardial infarction in patients with congestive heart failure. *Circulation*, **73**, 503–10.

112. Lichstein, E., Hager, W.D., Gregory, J.J. *et al*, for the Multicenter Diltiazem Post-Infarction Research Group (1990) Relation between beta-adrenergic blocker use, various correlates of left ventricular function and the chance of developing congestive heart failure. *J. Am. Coll. Cardiol.*, **16**, 1327–32.

113. Herlitz, J., Hjalmarson, Å., Holmberg, S. *et al.* (1984) Development of congestive heart failure after treatment with metoprolol in acute myocardial infarction. *Br. Heart J.*, **51**, 539–44.

114. Olsson, G. and Rehnqvist, N. (1986) Effect of metoprolol in postinfarction patients with increased heart size. *Eur. Heart J.*, **7**, 468–74.

115. Gheorghiade, M., Schultz, L., Tilley, B. *et al.* (1990) Effects of propranolol in non-Q-wave acute myocardial infarction in the beta blocker heart attack trial. *Am. J. Cardiol.*, **66**, 129–33.

116. Ames, R.P. (1986) The effects of antihypertensive drugs on serum lipids and lipoproteins II. Non-diuretic drugs. *Drugs*, **32**, 335–57.

117. Roberts, W.C. (1989) Recent studies on the effects of beta blockers on on blood lipid levels. *Am. Heart J.*, **117**, 709–14.

118. Chamberlain, D.A. (1983) Beta adrenoceptor antagonists after myocardial infarction – where are we now? *Br. Heart J.*, **49**, 105–10.

119. Kirshenbaum, J.M., Kloner, R.F., McGowan, N. and Antman, E.M. (1988) Use of ultrashort-acting beta-receptor blocker (esmolol) in patients with acute myocardial ischemia and relative contraindications to beta-blockade therapy. *J. Am. Coll. Cardiol.*, **12**, 773–80.

120. Rose, G. (1982) Prophylaxis with *β*-blockers and the community. *Br. J. Clin. Pharmacol.*, **14**, 45S–48S.

121. Smith, S.E. (1982) Personal view. *BMJ*, **284**, 818.

122. Olsson, G., Lubsen, J., van Es, G.-A. and Rehnqvist, N. (1986) Quality of life after myocardial infarction: effect of long term metoprolol on mortality and morbidity. *BMJ*, **292**, 1491–3.

123. Sanz, G., Castañer, A., Betriu, A. *et al.* (1982) Determinants of prognosis in survivors of myocardial infarction. *N. Engl. J. Med.*, **306**, 1065–70.

124. Lau, Y.K., Smith, J., Morrison, S.L. and Chamberlain, D.A. (1980) Policy for early discharge after acute myocardial infarction. *BMJ*, **280**, 1489–92.

125. Parsons, R.W., Jamrozik, K.D., Hobbs, M.S.T. and Thompson, D.L. (1984) Early identification of patients at low risk of death after myocardial infarction and potentially suitable for early hospital discharge. *BMJ*, **308**, 1006–10.

126. McLeod, A. and Chamberlain, D. (1985) Beta adrenoceptor antagonists: developments in pharmacology and therapy. In: Yu, P.N. and Goodwin, J.F. (eds) *Progress in Cardiology 13*, pp. 145–78. Philadelphia: Lea and Febiger.

127. Goldman, L. Benjamin, S.T., Cook, E.F. *et al.* (1988) Costs and effectiveness of routine therapy with long-term beta-adrenergic antagonists after acute myocardial infarction. *N. Engl. J. Med.*, **319**, 152–7.

128. Olsson, G., Levin, L.-Å. and Rehnqvist, N. (1987) Economic consequences of postinfarction prophylaxis with *β* blockers: cost effectiveness of metoprolol. *BMJ*, **294**, 339–42.

129. Nayler, W. G. (1988) *Calcium Antagonists*. London: Academic Press.

130. Nayler, W. G. (1993) *Amlodipine*. Berlin: Springer-Verlag.

131. Cleemann, L. and Morad, M. (1991) Role of Ca^{2+} channel in cardiac excitation–contraction coupling in the rat: evidence from Ca^{2+} transients and contraction. *J. Physiol.*, **432**, 283–312.

132. Holmberg, S.R.M. and Williams, A.J. (1989) Single channel recordings from human cardiac sarcoplasmic reticulum. *Circ. Res.*, **65**, 1445–9.

133. Kern, M.J. (1992) Perspective: the cellular influences of calcium antagonists on systemic and coronary hemodynamics. *Am. J. Cardiol.*, **69**, 3B–7B.

134. Gage, J.E., Hess, O.M., Murakami, T. *et al.* (1986) Vasoconstriction of stenotic coronary arteries during dynamic exercise in patients with classical angina pectoris: reversibility by nitroglycerin. *Circulation*, **73**, 865–76.

135. Steenbergen, C., Murphy, E., Levy, L. and London, R.E. (1987) Elevation in cytosolic free calcium concentration early in myocardial ischaemia in perfused rat heart. *Circ. Res.*, **60**, 700–7.

136. Weisfeldt, M.L. (1987) Reperfusion and reperfusion injury. *J. Clin. Res.*, **35**, 13–20.

137. Fleckenstein, A. (1977) Specific pharmacology of calcium in myocardium, cardiac pacemakers and vascular smooth muscle. *Ann. Rev. Pharmacol. Toxicol.*, **17**, 149–66.

138. Przyklenk, K., Ghafari, G.B., Eitzman, D.T. and Kloner, R.A. (1989) Nifedipine administered after reperfusion ablates systolic contractile dysfunction of postischemic 'stunned' myocardium. *J. Am. Coll. Cardiol.*, **13**, 1176–83.

139. Naylor, W.G., Ferrari, R. and Williams, A. (1980) Protective effect of pretreatment with verapamil, nifedipine and propranolol on mitochondrial function in the ischemic and reperfused myocardium. *Am. J. Cardiol.*, **46**, 242–8.

140. Walsh, R.A. (1989) The effects of calcium entry blockade on normal and ischemic ventricular diastolic function. *Circulation*, **80** (suppl. IV): IV-52–IV-58.

141. Mak, I.T., Boehme, P. and Weglicki, W.B. (1992) Antioxidant effects of calcium channel blockers against free radical injury in endothelial cells. Correlation of protection with preservation of glutathione levels. *Circ. Res.*, **70**, 1099–103.

142. Takahara, K., Kuroiwa, A., Matsushima, T. *et al.* (1985) Effects of nifedipine on platelet function. *Am. Heart J.*, **109**, 4–8.

143. Nakashima, Y., Kawashima, T., Nandate, H. *et al.* (1990) Sustained-release nifedipine (nifedipine-L) suppresses plasma thromboxane B_2 and 6-ketoprostaglandin $F_{1\alpha}$ in both young male smokers and nonsmokers. *Am. Heart J.*, **119**, 1267–73.

144. Levy, M. N. (1989) Role of calcium in arrhythmogenesis. *Circulation*, **80** (suppl. IV): IV-23–IV-30.

145. Reimer, K.A., Lowe, J.E. and Jennings, R.B. (1977) Effect of the calcium antagonist verapamil on necrosis following temporary coronary artery occlusion in dogs. *Circulation*, **55**, 581–7.

146. Yellon, D.M., Hearse, D.J., Maxwell, M.P. *et al.* (1981) Sustained limitation of myocardial necrosis 24 hours after coronary artery occlusion: verapamil infusion in dogs with small myocardial infarcts. *Am. J. Cardiol.*, **51**, 1409–13.

147. Klein, H.H., Schubothe, M., Nebendahl, K. and Kreuzer, H. (1984) The effect of two different diltiazem treatments on infarct size in ischemic, reperfused porcine hearts. *Circulation*, **69**, 1000–5.

148. Melin, J.A., Becker, L.C. and Hutchins, G.M. (1984) Protective effect of early and late treatment with nifedipine during myocardial infarction in the conscious dog. *Circulation*, **69**, 131–41.

149. Selwyn, A.P., Welman, E., Fox, K. *et al.* (1979) The effects of nifedipine on acute experimental myocardium ischemia and infarction in dogs. *Circ. Res.*, **44**, 16–23.

150. Hoff, P.T., Tamura, Y. and Lucchesi, B.R. (1989) Cardioprotective effects of amlodipine in the ischemic-reperfused heart. *Am. J. Cardiol.*, **64**, 101-I–116-I.

151. Nayler, W.G. (1989) Amlodipine pretreatment and the ischemic heart. *Am. J. Cardiol.*, **64**, 651–701.

152. Held, P.H., Yusuf, S. and Furberg, C.D. (1989) Calcium channel blockers in acute myocardial infarction and unstable angina: an overview. *BMJ*, **299**, 1187–92.

153. Held, P.H. and Yusuf, S. (1993) Effects of β-blockers and calcium channel blockers in acute myocardial infarction. *Eur. Heart J.*, **14** (suppl. F): 18–25.

154. Wilcox, R.G., Hampton, J.R., Banks, D.C. *et al.* (1986) Trial of early nifedipine in acute myocardial infarction: the Trent study. *BMJ*, **293**, 1204–8.

155. The Israeli SPRINT study group (1988) Secondary Prevention Reinfarction Israeli Nifedipine Trial (SPRINT). A randomized intervention trial of nifedipine in patients with acute myocardial infarction. *Eur. Heart J.*, **9**, 354–64.

156. The Israeli SPRINT study group (1988) The Secondary Prevention Reinfarction Israeli Nifedipine Trial (SPRINT II): design and methods, results. *Eur. Heart J.*, **9** (suppl. 1): 350A.

157. The Multicenter Diltiazem Postinfarction Trial Research Group (1988) The effect of diltiazem on mortality and reinfarction after myocardial infarction. *N. Engl. J. Med.*, **319**, 385–92.

158. Walsh, R.W., Porter, C.B., Starling, M.R. and O'Rourke, R.A. (1984) Beneficial hemodynamic effects of intravenous and oral diltiazem in severe congestive heart failure. *J. Am. Coll. Cardiol.*, **3**, 1044–50.

159. The Danish Study Group on Verapamil in Myocardial Infarction (1984) Verapamil in acute myocardial infarction. *Eur. Heart J.*, **5**, 516–28.

160. The Danish Study Group on Verapamil in Myocardial Infarction (1990) Effect of verapamil on mortality and major events after acute myocardial infarction (The Danish Verapamil Infarction Trial II–DAVIT II). *Am. J. Cardiol.*, **66**, 779–85.

161. Gibson, R.S., Beller, G.A., Gheorghiade, M. *et al.* (1986) The prevalence and clinical significance of residual myocardial ischemia 2 weeks after uncomplicated non-Q wave infarction: a prospective natural history study. *Circulation*, **73**, 1186–98.

162. Willerson, J.T., Campbell., W.B., Winniford, M.D. *et al.* (1984) Conversion from chronic to acute artery disease: speculation regarding mechanisms. *Am. J. Cardiol.*, **54**, 1349–54.

163. Gibson, R.S., Boden, W.E., Theroux, P. *et al.* and the Diltiazem Reinfarction Study Group (1986) Diltiazem and reinfarction in patients with non-Q-wave myocardial infarction. *N. Engl. J. Med.*, **315**, 423–9.

164. Reeves, R.A. (1987) Diltiazem in non-Q-wave myocardial infarction (letter). *N. Engl. J. Med.*, **316**, 220.

165. Wong, S.-C., Greenberg, H., Hager, W.D. and Dwer, E.M. (1992) Effects of diltiazem on recurrent myocardial infarction in patients with non-Q wave myocardial infarction. *J. Am. Coll. Cardiol.*, **19**, 1421–5.

166. Seitelberger, R., Zwölfer, W., Huber, S. *et al.* (1991) Nifedipine reduces the incidence of myocardial infarction and transient ischemia in patients undergoing coronary bypass grafting. *Circulation*, **83**, 460–8.

167. The HINT Research Group (1987) Nifedipine and metoprolol in suspected unstable angina (HINT). *Eur. Heart J.*, **8** (suppl. H).

168. Muller, J.E., Turi, Z.G., Pearle, D.L. *et al.* (1984) Nifedipine and conventional therapy for unstable angina pectoris: a randomized, double-blind comparison. *Circulation*, **69**, 728–39.

169. Opie, L.H. (1993) Calcium antagonists for congestive heart failure: is it really one bridge too far to cross? *Cardiovasc. Drugs Ther.*, **7**, 93–4.

170. Muller, J.E., Morrison, J., Stone, P.H. *et al.* (1984) Nifedipine therapy for patients with threatened and acute myocardial infarction: a randomized, double-blind, placebo-controlled comparison. *Circulation*, **69**, 740–7.

171. Sirnes, P.A., Overskeid, K., Pedersen, T.R. *et al.* (1984) Evolution of infarct size during the early use of nifedipine in patients with acute myocardial infarction: The Norwegian Nifedipine Multicenter Trial. *Circulation*, **70**, 638–44.
172. Gottlieb, S.O., Becker, L.C., Weiss, J.L. *et al.* (1988) Nifedipine in acute myocardial infarction: an assessment of left ventricular function, infarct size and infarct expansion. *Br. Heart J.*, **59**, 411–8.
173. Branagan, J.P., Walsh, K., Kelly, P. *et al.* (1986) Effect of early treatment with nifedipine in suspected acute myocardial infarction. *Eur. Heart J.*, **7**, 859–65.
174. Zannad, F., Amor, M., Karcher, G. *et al.* (1988) Effect of diltiazem on myocardial infarct size estimated by enzyme release, serial thallium-201 single-photon emission computed tomography and radionuclide angiography. *Am. J. Cardiol.*, **61**, 1172–7.
175. Thuesen, L., Jørgensen, J.R., Kvistgaard, H.J. *et al.* (1983) Effect of verapamil on enzyme release after early intravenous administration in acute myocardial infarction; double-blind randomised trial. *BMJ*, **286**, 1107–8.
176. Ghio, S., De Servi, S., Ferrario, M. *et al.* (1988) Acute haemodynamic effects of diltiazem in patients with recent Q-wave myocardial infarction. *Eur. Heart J.*, **9**, 740–5.
177. Walker, L.J.E., MacKenzie, G. and Adgey, A.A.J. (1988) Effect of nifedipine on arrhythmias in the acute phase of myocardial infarction. *Eur. Heart J.*, **9**, 471–8.
178. Lichtlen, P.R., Hugenholtz, P.G., Rafflenbeul, W. *et al.* and the INTACT Group Investigators (1990) *Lancet*, **335**, 1109–13.
179. Walters, D., Lespérance, J., Francetich, M. *et al.* (1990) A controlled clinical trial to assess the effect of a calcium channel blocker on the progression of coronary atherosclerosis. *Circulation*, **82**, 1940–53.

8

Arrhythmias

R. W. F. Campbell

Introduction

Acute myocardial infarction (AMI) is common and lethal. Although long recognized by its clinical presentation,[1] it required technical advances in electrocardiography and the vision of a few individuals to highlight that the not so insubstantial mortality of the condition was due to ventricular fibrillation (VF).[2,3]. Until 1947, VF could not be treated but in that year, Beck and colleagues,[4] reported the first successful human defibrillation. Since then, defibrillators have been considerably refined such that safe, reliable, compact and easily used equipment is now widely available.

Coronary care units (CCUs) were established in the 1960s with the earliest reports by Julian et al.,[5] Day et al.,[6] and Brown et al.[7] CCUs brought patients at risk of VF into a care environment that offered continuous ECG monitoring and the ready availability of defibrillators. In the first years of CCU management, VF complicated up to 10% of infarct events.[7,8] Comparisons of hospital mortality rates for those managed in purpose-designed CCUs with those managed in conventional medical wards showed the former to offer substantial benefit.[9] These benefits remain to this day[10] despite the steady improvements in hospital mortality rates for infarction.[11]

CCUs have evolved in their 30 years of existence but there is still a considerable emphasis on the detection of arrhythmias. ECG monitoring of patients with infarction reveals a remarkable prevalence of arrhythmias in the earliest phases of the condition.[12] With VF presenting a none too infrequent emergency, it was natural that effort be spent on finding a predictor for the occurrence of VF. Premonitory arrhythmias, particularly ventricular ectopic beats (VEBs), seemed likely candidates and were intensively investigated. VEBs whatever their pattern however, are neither sensitive nor specific for VF.[13-15]. Perhaps surprisingly, VF remains an unpredictable event.[15]

Enthusiasm for the detection and suppression of VEBs has been tempered by the results of research but there is still a strong emotional distrust of VEBs. As is often the case in medicine, such emotion has modified clinical care. In many CCUs, VEBs are still treated despite the evidence that little or nothing is gained. In other CCUs, all but immediately hemodynamically important arrhythmias are ignored with the management emphasis being on speedy reperfusion. Thrombolysis is obviously important but it is premature to abandon interest in arrhythmias. Although VF may now be less important as a cause of hospital mortality, this arrhythmia still claims lives in even the best-equipped centers and it is responsible for the considerable out-of-hospital mortality of AMI.[16,17] Were VF predictable and preventable a significant advance in AMI care would have been achieved.

As the outlook for those with AMI has improved, more attention is being paid to other than immediately lethal events. Arrhythmias such as ventricular tachycardia (VT) and atrial fibrillation (AF) are commonly detected in CCU patients but little is known of their immediate or late implications and there is little consensus on how they should be managed. Given the many years of CCU monitoring, such problems should have been answered long ago. Belatedly, they are now receiving attention.

Mechanisms and Modulators of Arrhythmias in Acute Myocardial Infarction.

The human heart has a series of safety mechanisms that contrive to prevent arrhythmias. They include the system of hierarchical pacemakers with the most dominant (i.e. fastest) suppressing those that are slower; the organization of action potential durations to achieve a near synchronous return of electrical excitability to the ventricular myocardium; the unidirectional gating mechanism at the His–Purkinje–myocardial junctions; and the disparity between the refractory period of the His–Purkinje network and the ventricular myocardium which discourages retrograde penetration of the system. AMI can disrupt these mechanisms to create arrhythmias but the pathologic process can also add new arrhythmogenic factors as, for instance, when rapid ectopic generators are created.

Reentry

During acute myocardial ischemia, the action potential duration of the ischemic tissue shortens. This disrupts the normally near homogeneous conditions for the return of ventricular excitability and creates an electrical milieu that can support VF. Membrane instability in the ischemic region may also reach threshold in some cells to produce an ectopic pacemaker. R-on-T VEBs are evidence of this. These beats interrupt the T wave of the preceding sinus beat. That they propagate indicates that they must arise from an area of myocardium which has recovered excitability and their interruption of the T wave is a clear demonstration of the inhomogeneity of recovery of excitability. VEBs in themselves disturb recovery of excitability to produce the electrical conditions which would support VF.[18] VF is generally considered to be due to random reentry, a process in which each individual myocyte obeys the normal rules of activation but the coherent process of wavespread through the myocardium is lost.[19] The electrical wavefront spreads in various directions to depolarize any myocardium that can be activated. It is deflected by areas of myocardium that have yet to recover their excitability. VF seldom starts instantaneously as an irregular rapid incoherent waveform; as a minimum, there is usually an identifiable initiating VEB or a run of organized ventricular tachycardia from which it subsequently degenerates. This observation has been the basis for much of the interest in the relationship of ventricular arrhythmias to VF.

The potential for random reentry is a feature of the ischemic conditions that exist in acute phase myocardial infarction. As these conditions are in a state of constant flux, it is not surprising that the pattern and the risk of random reentry varies from moment to moment. Moreover there are important modulating factors of which the most important is the effect of the automatic nervous system. High levels of sympathetic drive decrease the threshold for arrhythmias, particularly VF.[20]

Fixed circuit micro or macro reentry is not a feature of the first 48 hours of myocardial infarction. This type of arrhythmia mechanism depends upon the creation of a fixed anatomic substrate around which the reentrant wavefront can circulate. The dynamic conditions caused by myocardial ischemia in the earliest phases of acute infarction are not those that create this arrhythmogenic substrate. Fixed circuit reentry is manifest classically as sustained monomorphic VT.[21] This arrhythmia is an important late complication of infarction, presenting typically between 2 weeks and 1 year after the original event and has a strong but not exclusive association with the presence of a left ventricular aneurysm.[22]

Altered Automaticity

Altered automaticity undoubtedly plays a part in the arrhythmias of AMI but proving such is difficult. This mechanism has been well established in animal models of infarction but is assumed rather than proven in humans. It is likely that at least a proportion of isolated VEBs are due to this mechanism and reflect acute membrane instability. As cells die during the first 12–24 hours of infarction, VEBs become progressively less common. Their subsequent increase in the late rehabilitation phase of infarction may be related to catecholamine levels, to wall tension abnormalities, or to continuing ischemia.

Triggered Automaticity

Triggered automaticity is an important arrhythmia mechanism. Until recently, it was debated whether it had relevance for humans but there is increasing circumstantial evidence that it is the basis of torsade de pointes.[23] It may also be responsible for the brief polymorphic episodes of VT that complicate heart failure and which may arise by myocardial stretch.[24] AMI is also complicated by VT in its earliest hours. This is not sustained monomorphic VT but brief runs of irregular, often polymorphic, VT. These may arise from single ectopic pacemaker sites with variable conduction patterns through the surrounding myocardium or, more likely, a cascade of pacemakers activated by the previous one. Triggered automaticity has not been proven as a mechanism of these VTs but it is a plausible contender mechanism.

Parasystole

Parasystolic rhythms are a feature of late phase infarction[25] and are unlikely to be a mechanism of early phase arrhythmias.

Damage to Specific Structures

The process of infarction may damage specific structures and thereby create arrhythmias. The atrioventricular (AV) node is the most important vulnerable structure. Its blood supply, which is usually from the right coronary artery, may be jeopardized when occlusion of this artery produces acute inferior infarction.[26] The problem is not usually serious. It owes much to associated high levels of parasympathetic tone and in many instances can be controlled by parenteral atropine. As the problem is principally within the upper autonomically innervated areas of the AV node it is usual for relatively stable subsidiary pacemakers to appear.

Serious damage to the lower parts of AV node and to the His–Purkinje system are associated with anterior myocardial infarction. Such interference with the normal conducting system usually signifies a substantial infarction and through this mechanism, in part, the feature has poor prognostic associations.[27,28] Mortality might be expected to be linked with myocardial failure or a risk of asystole, but somewhat unexpectedly, the pattern of anteroseptal infarction and bundle branch block has been identified as a risk factor for late VF. The VF risk, however, seems contained to a 6 week period from the onset of the infarction.[29]

Infarct damage to the sinus node may also occur but is rare. Subsidiary pacemakers would be expected to maintain a stable rhythm at a reasonable rate.

Autonomic Tone

Almost all arrhythmogenic processes are aggravated by high levels of adrenergic tone. This condition prevails in the early phase of AMI[30] although, due to the multifactorial mechanism of most arrhythmias, it is difficult to incriminate sympathetic tone as other than a modulator. For example, large infarcts are associated with high levels of sympathetic drive and with arrhythmias but the arrhythmias may owe their genesis as much to the extent of the myocardial damage as to autonomic tone.

High levels of parasympathetic tone are associated with some inferior infarcts and can be causal in the appearance of all degrees of AV block. As might be expected, this block is at AV nodal level and it usually responds well to atropine administration.

Potassium and Magnesium Levels

Low serum potassium levels have been reported in patients resuscitated from in-hospital cardiac arrest[31,32] and hypokalemia is well recognized as an arrhythmogenic factor.[33–35] The relation of hypokalemia and VF has been examined in some detail. There is an association of low serum potassium and VF.[35–37] The relation may not be based merely on disturbances of cardiac electrophysiology. Hypokalemia is associated with large infarcts and with sympathetic activation, the latter causing peripheral potassium uptake. Despite the statistically significant relationship of hypokalemia and VF,[35–37] the finding is of only modest practical value. Hypokalemia is neither a specific nor a sensitive predictor of VF[37] (Figure. 8.1), and there is no evidence that VF is prevented by normalizing potassium values. It is possible that more detailed knowledge of the arrhythmogenic problem of the sympathetic nervous system interaction with electrolytes will come from examination of red blood cell ionic transport kinetics.[38]

Magnesium has received much less attention than potassium in respect to its arrhythmogenic potential.[34,37] In a large prospective study no relationship of hypomagnesemia to VF was found[37] (Figure. 8.1).

Myocardial Lipid Substrate

Work has suggested that the change of cardiac metabolic substrate that occurs in AMI may in itself be arrhythmogenic; the risk of serious ventricular arrhythmias has been linked to adipose tissue fatty acid composition.[39]

Prevalence and Pattern of Arrhythmias

The most prominent and the most important arrhythmia to complicate AMI is VF. It does not occur randomly during the course of the infarct. It has its highest incidence in the earliest minutes of AMI and appears to decline exponentially thereafter.[40] This pattern would fit with the hypothesis that it is the acute ischemic disruption of myocardial electrophysiology that is responsible for the arrhythmia rather than the chance play of events or the consequence of specific structural damage.

In the early 1960s, ECG monitoring of patients with infarction suggested that some specific VEB patterns might predict the occurrence of VF.[8] From this emerged the concept of warning arrhythmias. These arrhythmias were grouped in a hierarchical

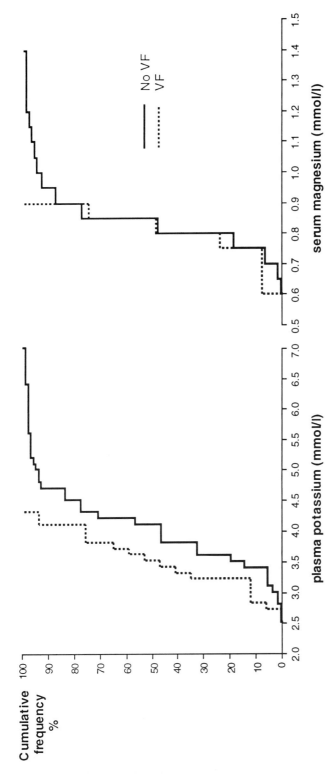

Figure 8.1 Cumulative frequency distributions of plasma potassium and serum magnesium concentrations in patients with acute myocardial infarction with or without ventricular fibrillation. (From Ref. 37 by permission of Oxford University Press.)

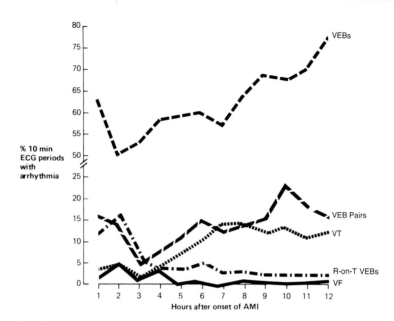

Figure 8.2 Prevalence of specific ventricular arrhythmias plotted as the percentage of 10 min ECG analysis period containing the arrhythmia. Prevalence is shown related to time from the onset of symptoms of myocardial infarction. (From Ref. 15 with permission of BMJ Publishing Group.)

scheme of increasing importance with respect to their putative risk association with VF. It was suggested that with the energetic treatment of these arrhythmias, VF could be forestalled. The practice of VEB suppression was universally adopted and the need to detect and treat these so-called warning events shaped much of CCU practice for the next two decades. There were, however, concerns. Some patients developed VF without warning arrhythmias while others developed VF despite suppression of warning arrhythmias.[41]

There is a relationship of VEBs, particularly R-on-T VEBs, to VF but the relationship is neither sensitive nor specific and it has no practical value for the management of patients with AMI. [15] All ventricular arrhythmias are common in the early phase of myocardial infarction (Figure. 8.2). Primary VF and R-on-T VEBs have their highest incidence in the first 3 hours and therein lies their interrelationship. Both probably reflect the existence of a sizeable area of myocardium that is still electrically excitable but has characteristics of electrical recovery which create inhomogeneity. The R-on-T VEB exposes that hetero-geneity by its interruption of the T wave of the preceding beat while VF is evidence of conditions that would support random reentry. Thus these two arrhythmias are tem-porally and mechanistically related. R-on-T VEBs are very frequent both in patients who will and who will not develop VF. The majority of incidents of primary VF are initiated by an R-on-T VEB but only a very small minority of R-on-T VEBs are associated with VF.[42]

If VF cannot be foretold on the basis of ECG monitoring, it might reasonably be asked why rhythm monitoring is still performed. ECG monitoring will provide the earliest identification of VF, a rhythm for which speedy resuscitation is of the essence. It will also reveal asymptomatic but potentially important events such as AV block, VT and atrial fibrillation (AF). Whilst perhaps the need to count and detect individual VEBs has passed, ECG monitoring remains a vital element in the management of the infarct patient.

Sinus bradycardia[43] and sinus tachycardia[44] have been suggested as associated with the development of primary VF. The former might reflect protective high vagal tone but

Table 8.1 Selected studies using continuous ECG analysis to determine the prevalence (%) of specific arrhythmias during the acute phase of myocardial infarction

Study	Year	Primary VF	Secondary VF	R-on-T VEB	VT	VEBs >30 hour⁻¹	First-degree AVB	Second-degree AVB	Third-degree AVB
Julian et al.[5]	1964	10		–	6	–	13	10	8
Meltzer and Kitchell[47]	1966	10	–	–	14	–	9	4	4
Sloman[48]	1969	23	–	–	15	–	–	–	12
Brown et al.[49]	1969	20	–	–	19	–	–	–	11
Lie et al.[13]	1974	9	–	–	6	–	–	–	–
Campbell et al.[15]	1981	5	–	52	67	–	–	–	–
Yusuf et al.[50]	1983	–	–	–	–	–	14	3	4
Ryden et al.[51]	1983	2	–	–	26	22	–	–	–
Dubois et al.[52]	1986	5	3	–	–	–	–	–	–

AVB, atrioventricular block; VEBs, Ventricular ectopic beats; VF, ventricular fibrillation; VT, ventricular tachycardia.

when there is variability of R–R interval, e.g. long–short–long sequences, electrophysiologic stability of the myocardium may be compromised. There is no evidence that atropine is useful in VF prevention in this circumstance; indeed atropine can provoke VF.[45] Sinus tachycardia may reflect high sympathetic tone, which almost certainly is a risk factor for the development of ventricular arrhythmias including VF.

Primary VF complicated about 10% of all AMIs in the 1960s[46] but over the years the pattern has changed. Now VF complicates about 5% of patients hospitalized for AMI.[46] It is tempting but dangerous to read too much into this change in arrhythmia expression. Patients are being brought to hospitals earlier, more are being attended by out-of-hospital paramedics, more are surviving out-of-hospital cardiac arrest and, in hospital, the use of drugs has changed dramatically. Isolated VEBs, VEB pairs and VT are very common in acute AMI but their peak incidence is several hours after the acute event, at a time when it would be expected that most of the threatened myocardium has died and become electrically inactive.[15] It may be that these arrhythmias arise from stretch-related phenomena in normal myocardium, from activity in surviving His–Purkinje cells, or perhaps from damaged but electrically active cells at the border of the infarct. Whatever the source, these arrhythmias appear to depend on abnormal automatic activity and not on reentry.

Continuous ECG monitoring reveals that all patients with AMI will have VEBs at some time in the first 12 hours of infarction, that many will have at least one R-on-T VEB, and that up to two-thirds of patients will have VT (at least satisfying a technical definition of three or more consecutive VEBs at a rate equal to or greater than 120 beats min⁻¹ (Table 8.1).[5,13,15,47–52]

Primary Ventricular Fibrillation

Primary VF (VF in the absence of shock or cardiac failure) is the most important arrhythmic complication of AMI.[53] It occurs in the earliest hours of infarction and, if corrected promptly, resuscitated patients have a reasonably good prognosis.[54,55] There has been debate about the prognostic implications of the arrhythmia with some reports suggesting that the event conferred no significant adverse effect[56] and others suggesting the resuscitated survivors faced a 30% mortality risk in the next year if the VF had complicated an acute anterior MI.[57] It seems remarkable that such an important problem has not been definitively investigated. The variable findings must reflect patient selection and relatively small numbers. Primary VF is associated with larger infarcts but in general, if promptly treated, there is a very good chance that it can be converted to sinus rhythm.

Immediate Therapy

DC cardioversion is the only accredited management for primary VF. Depending upon local protocols, the initial DC shock should be of 200 or 400 J. There is little evidence to support repetition of an initially unsuccessful 200 J DC shock. The salvage from such would have to be high to justify the time lost in recharging the defibrillator.

When VF is not reverted by defibrillation, a variety of adjunctive agents have been suggested as of benefit. None has been proven so. Fashionable adjunctive agents have included adrenaline,[58] lidocaine,[59] bretylium,[60] and bicarbonate.[61] None of these have been subjected to rigorous scientific scrutiny; many have been recommended on the basis of promising animal experiments. Many organizations involved in advanced life support have endorsed these adjunctive agents but in so doing they imply proven benefit. Management guidelines are necessary but they should not overpromote questionable interventions, particularly when changes to guidelines can have considerable medicolegal and training implications. Adjunctive agents should be offered as no more than suggestions for therapy when DC shocks have failed to restore sinus rhythm. If the insecure scientific basis of their use is made clear then continuing research is encouraged and subsequent guideline changes are more easily and readily assimilated into practice. In practice at present there is little to encourage the use of adjunctive agents; failure to restore sinus rhythm by DC shock alone indicates a very poor prognosis.

It is naive to expect that all apparent primary VF can be returned to sinus rhythm. Some incidents may be a consequence of fresh coronary occlusion with loss of contractile myocardium to the extent that the VF is merely a final electrical pathway of demise. Current estimates are that primary VF in the hospital setting has an immediate mortality of 5%.[10]

Prophylaxis

Primary VF can be lethal and it is an unexpected and unpredictable complication of AMI. A method for either its prediction or its prevention would have an important and useful impact on the management of AMI. With time, refined algorithms may identify high-risk patients for primary VF. They likely would include not only aspects of VEB patterns but also features reflecting electrical recovery such as QT dispersion.[62] For the present no reliable algorithm does exist and primary VF is managed either expectantly or by the prescription of prophylactic therapy.

Lidocaine

The apparent association of primary VF with antecedent VEB patterns and the relatively powerful VEB-suppressant effect of lidocaine was the basis for the first tests of antiarrhythmic prophylaxis of VF by lidocaine. Numerous small studies have been performed but none had sufficient power to be reliable. Three larger studies have reported statistically significant benefits of prophylactic lidocaine.[63–65]

In the first,[63] patients were randomized to receive lidocaine or a saline placebo. The endpoint was sudden death. This was significantly lower in those who received the active therapy (2% vs 7%) and the benefit was assumed to be by prevention of VF. This interesting study was flawed by a preponderance of those receiving lidocaine; it emerged that some trial participants may have unblinded the therapy by tasting the solutions and identifying the local anesthetic.

In a study reported by Lie *et al.*,[64] high-dose intravenous lidocaine therapy was compared to placebo in 212 patients with acute infarction. The 0% VF rate in those receiving lidocaine was significantly lower than the 10.5% rate observed in patients receiving placebo; 15% of patients administered lidocaine experienced unwanted effects. Despite the positive effect of lidocaine against VF, the study was small and provided little information on the risks of lidocaine given to those suspected of having an AMI but in whom the diagnosis was later not proven.

The definitive study was reported in 1985.[65] A negative VF prophylactic study of intramuscular lidocaine (300 mg) had been previously reported in 1978[66] (4% VF in lidocaine group vs 3% placebo) but in Koster and Dunning's study,[65] the intramuscular lidocaine dose was increased to 400 mg. VF prophylaxis was tested in an out-of-hospital situation. Patients suspected by paramedics of having an AMI randomly received either lidocaine or placebo. The endpoint was the VF rate between 15 and 60 min after drug administration. This time period was chosen to allow for the lag of 15 min expected before a therapeutic plasma concentration of lidocaine would have been achieved. VF was significantly reduced (0.06% vs 0.4%; $P < 0.01$) but the incidence of asystole was significantly increased (0.9% vs 0.4%; $P < 0.05$). The study thus confirms an anti-VF effect of lidocaine but it reveals that this benefit comes at the risk of asystole. In hospital practice this risk–benefit ratio is not attractive and most CCUs have abandoned the use of prophylactic lidocaine. The regimen may still have a place in some special situations as, for instance, when patients are seen remote from a defibrillator and when someone can stay with the patient to provide cardiac massage in the event that asystole occurs.

Other Class I drugs

A variety of small studies have attempted to prevent primary VF with other Class I antiarrhythmic drugs. Most have shown reductions in VEBs but none has shown an effect against VF. Not even the close structural analogs of lidocaine, mexiletine[67] and tocainide,[68] have affected VF rates.

β-Blockers

Lidocaine is not the only intervention shown to reduce the rate of VF in AMI. β-blockers have also proved effective. In one of the earliest interventional studies in AMI, Snow reported mortality benefits from the use of propranolol.[69] This finding was not substantiated by later work.[70] β-Blockers were identified as having suppressive effects on ventricular arrhythmias[71–74] but it was not until the report of Norris *et al.*[75] that there was clear evidence of an action against VF. In that study, intravenous and oral propranolol reduced the incidence of VF from 4% to 0.5%. Subsequently the ISIS-1 Study[76] confirmed a similar effect for intravenous atenolol. When pooled with 27 other intravenous β-blocker studies, a statistically significant reduction of VF was evident (2.6% reduced to 2.2%; $P < 0.05$).[76]

There has been great variation in enthusiasm for the use of β-blockers in AMI. Clearly if their anti-VF effect is to be of use they need to be deployed early and parenterally. Concern about their depression of hemodynamic performance has led many to eschew the use of these agents until after the first 24 hours of infarction, when any benefit against VF would be lost.

Magnesium

At one time it seemed that intravenous magnesium might play an important antiarrhythmic role in AMI. Several early studies suggested antiarrhythmic benefit.[77–81] That effect was further supported by meta-analyses[82,83] but was not substantiated by subsequent larger investigations.[84,85] Indeed, even in the early studies, the effect had been against a collective endpoint of arrhythmias rather than a specific effect against VF. There is no evidence to support routine use of magnesium in AMI but it has a role for the control of torsade de pointes.[86] Torsade de pointes is not a feature of myocardial infarction but may arise as a consequence of drug toxicity. It has been especially associated with drugs such as Class I drugs (sodium channel blockers).[87]

Spontaneous Termination

Classically, primary VF is considered to be manageable only by DC conversion; there are only very isolated reports of medical conversion.[88] Spontaneous conversion of primary VF to sinus rhythm does occur and was first documented in 1949[89] and was observed in one of the earliest studies of rhythm in AMI.[5] In a more recent report, 12 of 57 VF-like events in AMI were self-terminating VF.[90] The events ranged in duration from 5 to 50 seconds and 3 of the 12 subsequently developed 'nonself-terminating' VF. Whether the self-terminating events were indeed true VF is impossible to prove but regardless they raise considerable problems for diagnosis and classification.

Primary VF is not as disorganized an arrhythmia as has been thought.[91,92] Sophisticated signal analysis suggests a considerable degree of electrical organization during the event that persists for a considerable time. This relatively newly recognized feature may, in future, have therapeutic implications.

Prevention of Recurrences of Primary Ventricular Fibrillation

When primary VF has been DC converted to sinus rhythm, the electrophysiologic milieu that created the initial event probably is still present. With an appropriate trigger, VF may recur. It has been customary to give intravenous lidocaine to such patients in an attempt to control this problem. Data supporting this approach are sparse; no randomized controlled trial has been performed, but in one review of the antiarrhythmic strategy 22% of lidocaine-treated patients redeveloped VF. This would suggest that lidocaine has relatively limited efficacy.[93] In a study of metoprolol,[94] patients receiving this drug had fewer late occurrences of VF than their placebo-treated counterparts.

There are no data to establish an optimal management strategy to prevent VF recurrences but the following should be considered after DC version of the first event: normalize acid–base and electrolyte status; administer β-blockers (particularly if there has been evidence of high sympathetic tone–sinus tachycardia); administer intravenous lidocaine (bearing in mind its questionable efficacy). There is no information about alternative strategies, e.g. magnesium, amiodarone, etc.

Secondary Ventricular Fibrillation

Secondary VF[53] has the same ECG appearance as primary VF. It is distinguished by occurring in the setting of shock and/or heart failure. As such it has a poor immediate prognosis.[95] Less than 20% of patients can be returned to sinus rhythm, although it may be that the outlook for those in whom defibrillation is successful may have a better late prognosis than has been generally recognized.[95]

Ventricular Tachycardia

VT occurs in up to 67% of patients in the acute phase of MI[15] but most events at this time are short-lived and pass unnoticed by the patient. They undoubtedly have some

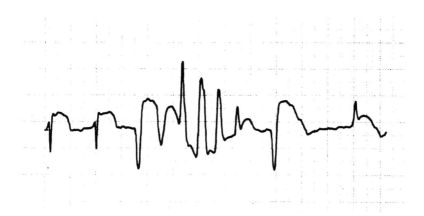

Figure 8.3 A typical short-lived run of ventricular ectopic beats occurring in the acute phase of myocardial infarction. The rate is irregular and the morphology varies. The incident satisfies a technical definition of ventricular tachycardia.

immediate hemodynamic effect but their brevity renders them near asymptomatic. These events are often irregular and polymorphic suggesting either multiple sources or different activation routes through the myocardium (Figure 8.3). Sustained monomorphic VT is not a typical arrhythmia at this phase of infarction. VT is not a predictor of VF and in itself it appears not to be of prognostic importance.

Only those VT episodes with immediate hemodynamic impact merit treatment. Occasionally such VT reflects electrolyte imbalance; levels should be checked and corrected if appropriate. Lidocaine is the safest and most effective pharmacologic option and should be the drug of first choice.

When VT does not respond to lidocaine and is not a consequence of electrolyte imbalance, the optimal second-line therapy is not generally agreed. Many anti-arrhythmic agents are available and most will have some potential for VT control. However, most can depress left ventricular contractility[96–98] and many can aggravate the existing arrhythmia or create a new arrhythmia (arrhythmogenesis or proarrhythmia). Drug-refractory hemodynamically significant VT is a serious problem. Small studies have reported a benefit of most agents in particular and specific situations. Intravenous amiodarone (given via a central line) is an attractive option.[99] This agent is well tolerated in acute infarction and its antiarrhythmic profile is different from that of the Class I agents of which lidocaine is a member. Small studies would support its use as a second-line agent but sadly the definitive study has yet to be performed.

R-on-T Ventricular Ectopic Beats

R-on-T VEBs are a feature of the earliest hours of AMI and they demonstrate that there is inhomogeneity of electrical recovery within the myocardium. They have been linked with the genesis of primary VF and they often are the initiating complex of that event. However, they occur in at least 50% of patients with AMI (Table 8.1) and most have no untoward consequences. There is no case for their suppression but their presence should warn of the existence of the electrophysiologic conditions that support primary VF.

Ventricular Ectopic Beats

VEBs are ubiquitous in AMI. Neither their form nor their frequency has prognostic significance.[100] They may arise by a variety of mechanisms and they follow a pattern of expression that varies over follow-up. There is no mandate for their active treatment. It is most unusual that they are perceived by the patient during the acute phase of the MI.

Atrial Fibrillation

AF is a neglected arrhythmia that is only now receiving the attention that it deserves. In its paroxysmal form, it complicates up to 20% of acute infarctions.[95,101,102] It is associated with either atrial infarction[103,104] or with large ventricular infarcts with hemodynamic decompensation[95,101,102,105] particularly those involving the right ventricle.[106] AF compli- cating AMI thus has adverse prognostic implications. There is no reason to expect that prognosis would be ameliorated by treating AF: the arrhythmia seems to be merely a marker of a phenomenon which in itself carries the prognostic burden. Patients whose AMI is complicated by AF may, even in the absence of therapy, have ventricular response rates that are virtually normal; they often tolerate the arrhythmia well and need no treatment other than close monitoring for hemodynamic deterioration. Most AF events last little longer than a few hours and spontaeous termination can be awaited. For other patients, AF causes significant hemodynamic compromise.[107] Treatment is indicated and may take one of two approaches: ventricular rate control or restoration of sinus rhythm. It is unclear whether it is loss of atrial transport or irregularity of the consequent ventricular response rate that creates the greatest problem.[108]

Restoration of sinus rhythm is the ideal. Cardioversion will restore rhythm in most patients but, as the initiating factors are usually still present, the relapse rate is high. Drug restoration of sinus rhythm is possible with agents such as flecainide[109] and propafe- none[110] but as these may be poorly tolerated by patients with infarction they are not recommended as first-line agents in this situation. Intravenous amiodarone, given by a central line, is a much more attractive approach. It can both control rate and encourage restoration of sinus rhythm[111] and can do so within a relatively short time period. For ventricular rate control, digoxin has traditionally been the drug of choice but it is unlikely to restore sinus rhythm and it may take hours before rate control is achieved. Cautious concomitant β-blockade may be given with digoxin, particularly if the AF reflects atrial infarction and high sympathetic tone rather than cardiac decompensation. When AF complicating acute infarction seems due to hemodynamic compromise, it is rarely possible to restore sinus rhythm until heart failure is ameliorated. This has become an important situation in which to use angiotensin-converting enzyme (ACE) inhibition therapy,[112] although as yet, the effect of these agents on AF is unknown.

Reperfusion Arrhythmias

Early animal experiments of acute reperfusion following coronary artery ligation re- vealed that ventricular arrhythmias including VF were commmonly produced.[113] Reper- fusion by thrombolysis produced similar arrhythmogenic effects in some experimental models and, for a time, it was believed that arrhythmia provocation would seriously restrict the clinical use of thrombolytic agents.[114] In the event, humans behave differently from animals: reperfusional arrhythmias, although common,[115–117] are typically non- lethal[118] and include accelerated idioventricular rhythm (Figure 8.4) and salvoes of VEBs.[119–121] Accelerated idioventricular rhythms occur throughout the first 12 hours of AMI and for this reason the occurrence of the arrhythmia is not specific as a marker of successful reperfusion.[122] In a variety of large well-controlled investigations of thrombo- lytic therapy,[123–125] VF rates have, if anything, been slightly lower in those receiving active therapy. This is probably attributable to two phenomena: an absence of acute reperfusional VF and a reduction of subsequent VF by successful and substantial

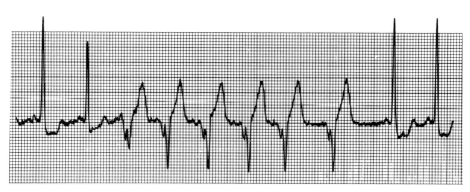

Figure 8.4 A 6-beat run of accelerated idioventricular rhythm attending successful reperfusion of ventricular myocardium. The patient had been treated with streptokinase and was unaware of this change in cardiac rhythm. The arrhythmia decelerates and is replaced by sinus rhythm.

myocardial salvage. In one study, however, very early thrombolytic therapy was associated with a higher incidence of VF than when similar therapy was given later.[126]

There is growing evidence of the electrophysiologic benefits of early reperfusion. Several studies have demonstrated reduced signal-averaged abnormalities,[127–129] reduced spontaneous ventricular arrhythmias,[129–131] reduced AF,[132] and reduced VT inducibility by programmed stimulation[133] in those successfully treated with thrombolytic agents. Whilst most of these benefits relate to the late phase of infarction, myocardial salvage and the attendant restoration of normal or near normal electrophysiology is a powerful antiarrhythmic strategy.

Spontaneous reperfusion occurs in a proportion of patients with infarction but clinical recognition of such is difficult. Based on the pattern of enzyme release, it seems unlikely that spontaneous reperfusion accounts for other than rare incidents of VF in humans.[134]

The brief time frame of occurrence and the relatively innocuous types of ventricular arrhythmias associated with reperfusion all but dismiss a need for treatment. At worst, reperfusion is attended by a very short-lived 'electrical storm' that subsides within seconds. As such events are rare, there is no justification for prophylactic therapy, although there have been some clinical assessments of classical antiarrhythmic agents. In limited studies, lidocaine appears ineffective against reperfusional ventricular arrhythmias.[135,136] There is still considerable ignorance of the mechanisms of reperfusional arrhythmias, although animal evidence might suggest an important role for α-adrenergic tone.[137] In the future, β-blockers[138] and free radical scavengers like superoxide dismutase[139–141] may also prove to have a useful clinical antiarrhythmic role.

Out-of-Hospital Ventricular Fibrillation

Despite advances in the management of AMI, the condition still has a substantial mortality, principally through out-of-hospital VF. Paramedic services and community resuscitation programs have had an impact on the problem but the sudden unexpected nature of coronary artery occlusion, the substantial rural population, and the often solitary conditions of work and recreation ensure that a considerable proportion of patients will die without medical, paramedic or even bystander intervention.

Early reports of the arrhythmias recorded from victims of out-of-hospital cardiac arrest suggested that asystole and bradyarrhythmias might be at least as important as VF.[142] As access time to these victims shortened, however, the proportion found to be in VF rose.[142] There is now no doubt that VF is the major lethal arrhythmic event associated with acute coronary ischemia. VF may be the first sign of ischemia and, if help is not available, will be manifest as sudden unexpected death.

In a high proportion of those resuscitated from out-of-hospital VF, AMI is not confirmed.[143] They usually have severe coronary artery disease and probably have suffered an acute temporary coronary occlusion (transient thrombosis with or without spasm). Contrary to initial belief, the prognosis for such patients is poorer than for those in whom VF is associated with completed infarction. In the former group, the circumstances that produced VF are still present and the risk of recurrence is high. In the latter group, the infarction both creates and subsequently destroys the electrophysiologic milieu that supported VF.

Post Acute Phase Arrhythmias

The arrhythmias of the first 24 hours of acute myocardial infarction largely reflect the acute unstable electrophysiology of ischemia. The arrhythmias usually subside rapidly, but in some patients, late arrhythmias are a problem. Most, if not all, patients will have ventricular ectopic beats. These are of little immediate impact but when frequent (more than 10 per hour) they have prognostic implication.[123] There is no mandate for the suppression; Class 1 drugs can do this but at a risk of increased mortality. Management should address the underlying disease using interventions accredited with prognostic improvements (for example beta-blockers, aspirin, ACE inhibitors, revascularization). In a few patients, sustained monomorphic ventricular tachycardia occurs. This is due to macro re-entry[21,22] and is likely to be a recurrent threat. Drug therapy can be evaluated by programmed stimulation, but for those who are drug refractory, an implanted cardioverter–defibrillator or antiarrhythmic surgery may be needed. Finally, in those with severe left ventricular dysfunction, atrial fibrillation may be a problem that further impairs cardiac output.[24,102] Atrial fibrillation and indeed the other post-acute-phase arrhythmias, including monomorphic VT, are becoming less common with the aggressive use of thrombolytic therapy[132,133] and perhaps with ACE inhibitors.

References

1. Herrick, J.B. (1912) Clinical features of sudden obstruction of the coronary arteries. *JAMA*, **46**, 2015–20.
2. Julian, D.G. (1961) Treatment of cardiac arrest in acute myocardial ischemia and infarction. *Lancet*, **ii**, 840–4.
3. Beck, C.F., Weckesser, E.C. and Barry, F.M. (1956) Fatal heart attack and successful defibrillation: new concepts in coronary artery disease. *JAMA* **161**, 434–6.
4. Beck, C.F., Pritchard, W.H. and Feil, H.S. (1947) Ventricular fibrillation of long duration abolished by electric shock. *JAMA*, **135**, 985–6.
5. Julian, D.G., Valentine, P.A. and Miller, G.G. (1964) Disturbances of rate, rhythm and conduction in acute myocardial infarction. *Am. J. Med.*, **37**, 915–27.
6. Day, H.W. (1963) An intensive coronary care area. *Dis. Chest*, **44**, 423–7.
7. Brown, K.W.G., MacMillan, R.L., Forbatt, N. *et al.* (1963) Coronary unit. An intensive care centre for acute myocardial infarction. *Lancet*, **ii**, 349–52.
8. Lown, B., Fakhro, A.M., Hood, W.B. and Thorn, G.W. (1967) The coronary care unit. New perspectives and directions. *JAMA*, **19**, 188–98.
9. Julian, D.G. (1968) Coronary care and the community. *Ann. Intern. Med.*, **68**, 607–13.
10. Karlson, B.W., Herlitz, J., Wiklund, O. *et al.* (1992) Characteristics and prognosis of patients with acute myocardial infarction in relation to whether they were treated in the coronary care unit or in another ward. *Cardiology*, **81**, 134–44.
11. Hopper, J.L., Pathik, B., Hunt, D. and Chan, W.W.C. (1989) Improved prognosis since 1969 of myocardial infarction treated in a coronary care unit: lack of relation with changes in severity. *BMJ*, **299**, 892–6.
12. Julian, D.G., Valentine, P.A. and Miller, G.G. (1964) Routine electrocardiographic monitoring in acute myocardial infarction. *Med. J. Aust.*, **1**, 433–6.
13. Lie, K.I., Wellens, H.J.J. and Durrer, D. (1974) Characteristics and predictability of primary ventricular fibrillation. *Euro. J. Cardiol.*, **1**, 379–84.
14. El-Sherif, N., Myerburg, R.J., Scherlag, B.J. *et al.* (1976) Electrocardiographic antecedents of primary ventricular. *Br. Heart J.*, **38**, 415–22.
15. Campbell, R.W.F., Murray, A. and Julian, D.G. (1981) Ventricular arrhythmias in first 12 hours of acute myocardial infarction. Natural history study. *Br. Heart J.*, **46**, 351–7.

16. Liberthson, R.R., Nagel, E.L., Hirschman, J.C. and Nussenfeld, S.R. (1974) Pre-hospital ventricular defibrillation. Prognosis and follow up course. *N. Engl. J. Med.*, **291**, 317–21.

17. Schaffer, W.A. and Cobb, L.A. (1975) Recurrent ventricular fibrillation and modes of death in survivors of out-of-hospital ventricular fibrillation. *N. Engl. J. Med.*, **293**, 259–62.

18. Day, C.P., McComb, J.M. and Campbell, R.W.F. (1992) QT dispersion in sinus beats and ventricular extrasystoles in normal hearts. *Br. Heart J.*, **67**, 39–41.

19. Josephson, M.E., Spielman, S.R., Greenspan, A.M. and Horowitz, L.N. (1979) Mechanism of ventricular fibrillation in man. *Am. J. Cardiol.*, **44**, 623–31.

20. McAlpine, H.M., Morton, J.J., Leckie, B. *et al.* (1988) Neuroendocrine activation after acute myocardial infarction. *Br. Heart J.*, **60**, 117–24.

21. Josephson, M.E., Horowitz, L.N., Farshidi, A. and Kastor, J.A. (1978) Recurrent sustained ventricular tachycardia: I mechanisms. *Circulation*, **57**, 431–9.

22. De Bakker, J.M.T., Van Capelle, F.J.L., Janse, M.J. *et al.* (1988) Reentry as a cause of ventricular tachycardia in patients with chronic ischemic heart disease: electrophysiologic and anatomic correlation. *Circulation*, **77**, 589–606.

23. Kadish, A.H. and Morady, F. (1991) Torsade de Pointes. In: D.P. Zipes and J. Jalliffe, (eds) *Cardiac Electrophysiology–From Cell to Bedside*, pp.605–10. W.B. Saunders, Philadelphia.

24. Dean, J.W. and Lab, M.J. (1989) Arrhythmia in heart failure: role of mechanically induced changes in electrophysiology. *Lancet*, **i**, 1309–12.

25. Vellani, C.W., Murray A. and Neilson, J.M. (1979) Coupling interval, exit block and periodicity of ventricular parasystolic rhythm. *Cardiovasc. Res.*, **13**, 320–9.

26. Sutton, R. and Davies, M. (1968) The conduction system in acute myocardial infarction complicated by heart block. *Circulation*, **38**, 987–92.

27. Godman, M.J., Alpert, B.A. and Julian, D.G. (1971) Bilateral bundle-branch block complicating acute myocardial infarction. *Lancet*, **ii**, 345–7.

28. Hauer, R.N.W., Lie, K.I., Liem, K.L. and Durrer, D. (1982) Long term prognosis in patients with bundle branch block complicating acute anteroseptal infarction. *Am. J. Cardiol.*, **449**, 1581–5.

29. Lie, K.I., Liem, K.L., Schuilenberg, R.M. *et al.* (1978) Early identification of patients developing late in-hospital ventricular fibrillation after discharge from the coronary care unit. A 5.5 year retrospective study of 1897 patients. *Am. J. Cardiol.*, **41**, 674–7.

30. Harris, A.S., Otero, H. and Bocage, A.J. (1971) The induction of arrhythmias by sympathetic activity before and after occlusion of a coronary artery in the canine heart. *J. Electrocardiol.*, **4**, 34–43.

31. Beck, O.A. and Hochrein, H. (1977) Initial serum potassium level in relation to cardiac arrhythmias in acute myocardial infarction. *Z. Kardiol.*, **66**, 187–90.

32. Friedensohn, A., Faibel, H.E., Bairey, O. *et al.* (1991) Malignant arrhythmias in relation to values of serum potassium in patients with acute myocardial infarction. *Int. J. Cardiol.*, **32**, 331–8.

33. Duke, M. (1978) Thiazide-induced hypokalemia. Association with acute myocardial infarction and ventricular fibrillation. *JAMA*, **239**, 43–5.

34. Kafka, H., Langevin, L. and Armstrong, P.W. (1987) Serum magnesium and potassium in acute myocardial infarction. Influence on ventricular arrhythmias. *Arch. Intern. Med.*, **147**, 465–9.

35. Nordrehaug, J.E., Johannessen, K.A. and Van der Lippe, G. (1985) Serum potassium concentration as a risk factor of ventricular arrhythmias early in acute myocardial infarction. *Circulation*, **71**, 645–9.

36. Dyckner, T., Helmers, C., Lundman, T. and Wester, P.O. (1975) Initial serum potassium level in relation to early complications and prognosis in patients with acute myocardial infarction. *Acta Med. Scand.*, **197**, 207–10.

37. Higham, P.D., Adams, P.C., Murray, A. and Campbell, RWF. (1993) Plasma potassium, serum magnesium and ventricular fibrillation: a prospective study. *Q. J. Med.*, **86**, 609–17.

38. Borgia, M.C., Borgia, C., Betto, P. *et al.* (1994) Early detection of the catecholamine-induced sodium, potassium pump-dependent genesis of arrhythmias in acute myocardial infarction. *Curr. Ther. Res. Clin. Exp.*, **4**, 823–31.

39. Abraham, R., Riemersma, R.A., Wood D. *et al.* (1989) Adipose fatty acid composition and the risk of serious ventricular arrhythmias in acute myocardial infarction. *Am. J. Cardiol.*, **63**, 269–72.

40. Adgey, A.A.J., Allen, J.D., Geddes, J.S. *et al.* (1971) Acute myocardial infarction. *Lancet*, **ii**, 501–4.

41. Lawrie, D.M., Higgins, M.R., Godman, M.J. *et al.* (1968) Ventricular fibrillation complicating acute myocardial infarction. *Lancet*, **ii**, 523–8.

42. Surawicz, B. (1986) R on T phenomenon: dangerous and harmless. *J. Appl. Cardiol.*, **1**, 39–61.

43. Pantridge, J.F. and Geddes, J.S. (1966) Cardiac arrest after myocardial infarction. *Lancet*, **i**, 807–8.

44. Lie, K.I., Wellens, H.J., Downar, E. and Durrer, D. (1975) Observations on patients with primary ventricular fibrillation complicating acute myocardial infarction. *Circulation*, **52**, 755–9.

45. Massumi, R.A., Mason, D.T., Amsterdam, E.A., DeMaria, A., Miller, R.R., Scheinman, M.M. and Zelis, R. (1972) Ventricular fibrillation and tachycardia after intravenous atropine for treatment of bradycardias. *N. Engl. J. Med.*, **287**, 336–8.

46. Antman, E.M. and Berlin, J.A. (1992) Declining incidence of ventricular fibrillation in myocardial infarction. *Circulation*, **86**, 764–73.

47. Meltzer, L.E and Kitchell, J.B. (1966) The incidence of arrhythmias associated with acute myocardial infarction. *Prog. Cardiovasc. Dis.*, **9**, 50–63.

48. Sloman, G. (1969) Changing concepts in the care of patients with acute myocardial infarction. *Med. J. Aust.*, **1**, 1157–65.

49. Brown, R., Hunt, D. and Sloman, J.G. (1969) The natural history of atrioventricular conduction defects in acute myocardial infarction. *Am. Heart J.*, **78**, 460–6.

50 Yusuf, S., Sleight, P., Rossi, P. *et al.* (1983) Reduction in infarct size, arrhythmias and chest pain by early intravenous beta blockade in suspected myocardial infarction. *Circulation*, **67** (suppl. I), 32–45.

51. Ryden, L., Ariniego, R., Arnman, K. *et al.* (1984) A double-blind trial of metoprolol in acute myocardium infarction: Effect on ventricular tachyarrythmias. *N. Engl. J. Med.*, **308**, 614–18.

52. Dubois, C., Smeets, J.P., Demoulin, C. *et al.* (1986) Incidence, clinical significance and prognosis of ventricular fibrillation in the early phase of myocardial infarction. *Eur. Heart J.*, **7**, 945–51.

53. Oliver, M.F., Julian, D.G. and Donald K.W. (1967) Problems in evaluating coronary care units. Their responsibility and their relation to the community. *Am. J. Cardiol.*, **20**, 465–74.

54. Kushnir, B., Fox, K.M., Tomlinson. I.W. *et al.* (1975) Primary ventricular fibrillation and resumption of work, sexual activity and driving after first acute myocardial infarction. *BMJ*, **4**, 609–13.

55 Geddes, J.S., Adgey, A.A.J. and Pantridge, J.F. (1969) Prognosis after recovery from ventricular fibrillation complicating ischemic heart-disease. *Lancet*, **ii**, 273–5.

56. Nicod, P., Gilpin, E., Dittrich, H. *et al.* (1988) Late clinical outcome in patients with early ventricular fibrillation after myocardial infarction. *J. Am. Coll. Cardiol.*, **11**, 464–70.

57. Schwartz. P.J., Zara, A., Grazi, S. *et al.* Effects of ventricular fibrillation complicating acute myocardial infarction on long term prognosis. Influence of site of infarction. *Am. J. Cardiol.*, **57**, 384–9.

58 Linder, K.H., Ahnefeld, F.W. and Bowdler, I.M. (1988) The effect of epinephrine on hemodynamics, acid–base status and potassium during spontaneous circulation and cardiopulmonary resuscitation. *Resuscitation*, **16**, 251–61.

59. Weaver, W.D., Fahrenbruch, C.E., Johnson, D.D., Hallstrom, A.P., Cobb, L.A. and Copass, M.K. (1990) Effect of epinephrine and lidocaine therapy on outcome after cardiac arrest due to ventricular fibrillation. *Circulation*, **82**, 2027–34.

60. Haynes, R.E., Chinn, T.L., Copass, M.K. and Cobb, L.A. (1981) Comparison of bretylium tosylate and lidocaine in management of out of hospital ventricular fibrillation: A randomized clinical trial. *Am. J. Cardiol.*, **48**, 353–6.

61. Guerci, A.D., Chandra, N., Johnson, E. *et al.* (1986) Failure of sodium bicarbonate to improve resuscitation from ventricular fibrillation in dogs. *Circulation*, **74** (suppl. IV), 75–79.

62. Higham, P.D., Furniss, S.S. and Campbell, R.W.F. (1994) QT dispersion and components of the QT interval in ischaemia and infarction. *Br. Heart J.*, (in press)

63. Valentine, P.A., Frew, J.L., Mashford, M.L. and Sloman, J.G. (1974) Lidocaine in the prevention of sudden death in the pre-hospital phase of acute infarction. *N. Engl. J. Med.*, **291**, 1327–31.

64. Lie, K.I., Wellens, H.J.J., Von Capeele, F.J. and Durrer, D. (1974) Lidocaine in the prevention of primary ventricular fibrillation. *N. Engl. J. Med.*, **29**, 1324–6.

65. Koster, R.W. and Dunning, A.J. (1985) Intramuscular lidocaine for prevention of lethal arrhythmias in the prehospitalisation phase of acute myocardial infarction. *N. Engl. J. Med.*, **313**, 1105–10.

66. Lie, K.I., Liem, K.L., Louridtz, W.L. *et al.* (1978) Efficacy of lignocaine in preventing ventricular fibrillation within 1 hour after a 300 mg intramuscular injection. A double blind randomised study of 300 hospitalised patients with acute myocardial infarction. *Am. J. Cardiol.*, **42**, 486–8.

67. Achuff, S.C., Campbell, R.W.F., Pottage, A. *et al.* (1977) Mexiletine in the prevention of ventricular arrhythmias in acute myocardial infarction. *Postgrad. Med. J.*, **53** (suppl. 1), 163–64.

68. Campbell, R.W.F., Hutton, I., Elton, R.A. *et al.* (1983) Prophylaxis of primary ventricular fibrillation with tocainide in acute myocardial infarction. *Br. Heart J.*, **49**, 557–63.

69. Snow, P.J.D. (1965) Effect of propranolol in myocardial infarction. *Lancet*, **ii**, 551–3.

70. Multicentre Trial Investigators. (1966) Propranolol in acute myocardial infarction. *Lancet*, **ii**, 1435–8.

71. Ahumada, G.G., Karlsberg, R.P., Jaffe, A.S. *et al.* (1979) Reduction of early ventricular arrhythmia by acebutolol in patients with acute myocardial infarction. *Br. Heart J.*, **41**, 654–9.

72. Rossi, P.R.F., Yusuf, S., Ramsdale, D. *et al.* (1983) Reduction of ventricular arrhythmias by early intravenous atenolol in suspected acute myocardial infarction. *BMJ*, **286**, 506–10.

73. Rehnqvist, N., Olsson, G., Erhardt, L. and Ekman, A.M. (1987) Metoprolol in acute myocardial infarction reduces ventricular arrhythmias both in the early stage and after the acute event. *Int. J. Cardiol.*, **15**, 301–8.

74. Ramsdale, D.R., Llewellyn, M.J., Pidgeon, J. *et al.* (1988) Effects of intravenous sotalol on the QT interval and incidence of ventricular arrhythmias early in acute myocardial infarction. *Am. J. Noninv. Cardiol.*, **2**, 52–8.

75. Norris, R.M., Barnaby, P.F., Brown, M.A. *et al.* (1984) Prevention of ventricular fibrillation during acute myocardial infarction by intravenous propranolol. *Lancet*, **ii**, 883–6.

76. ISIS-I (First Study of Infarct Survival) Collaborative Group. (1986) Randomised trial of intravenous atenolol among 16 027 cases of suspected acute myocardial infarction. *Lancet*, **ii**, 57–66.

77. Smith, L.F., Heagerty, A.M., Bing, R.F. and Barnett, D.B. (1986) Intravenous infusion of magnesium sulphate after acute myocardial infarction: effects on arrhythmias and mortality. *Int. J. Cardiol.*, **12**, 175–80.

78. Rasmussen, H.S., McNair, P., Norregard, P. *et al.* (1986) Intravenous magnesium in acute myocardial infarction. *Lancet*, **ii**, 234–6.

79. Nattel, S., Turmel, N., Macleod, R. and Solymoss, B.C. (1991) Actions of intravenous magnesium on ventricular arrhythmias caused by myocardial infarction. *J. Pharmacol. Exp. Ther.*, **259**, 939–46.

80. Abraham, A.S., Rosenmann, D., Kramer, M. *et al.* (1987) Magnesium in the prevention of lethal arrhythmias in acute myocardial infarction. *Arch. Intern. Med.*, **147**, 753–5.

81. Shechter, M., Hod, H., Marks, N. *et al.* (1990) Beneficial effect of magnesium sulfate in acute myocardial infarction. *Am. J. Cardiol.*, **66**, 271–4.

82. Horner, S.M. (1992) Efficacy of Intravenous magnesium in acute myocardial infarction in reducing arrhythmias and mortality: meta-analysis of magnesium in acute myocardial infarction. *Circulation*, **86**, 774–9.

83. Teo, K.K., Yusuf, S., Collins, R. *et al.* (1991) Effects of intravenous magnesium in suspected acute myocardial infarction: overview of randomised trials. *BMJ*, **303**, 1499–503.

84. Woods, K.L., Fletcher, S., Roffe, C. and Haider, Y. (1992) Intravenous magnesium sulphate in suspected acute myocardial infarction: results of the second Leicester intravenous magnesium intervention trial (LIMIT-2). *Lancet*, **339**, 1553–8.

85. Collins, R. (1993) ISIS-4 results. Communication at the American Heart Association, Atlanta, November 1993.

86. Banai, S. and Tzivoni, D. (1993) Drug therapy for torsade de pointes. *J. Cardiovasc. Electrophysiol.*, **2**, 206–10.

87. Ohe, T., Kurita, T., Aihara, N., Kamakura, S., Matsuhisa, M. and Shimomura, K. (1990) Electrocardiographic and electrophysiologic studies in patients with torsades de pointe – role of monophasic action potentials. *Jap. Circulation. J.*, **54**, 1323–30.

88. Sanna, G. and Arcidicacono, R. (1973) Chemical ventricular defibrillation of the human heart with bretylium tosylate. *Am. J. Cardiol.*, **32**, 982–7.

89. Priest, W.M. (1949) Ventricular fibrillation recorded 10 hours before death from myocardial infarction. *Lancet*, **ii**, 699–700.

90. Clayton, R.H., Murray, A., Higham, P.D. and Campbell, R.W.F. (1993) Self-terminating ventricular tachyarrhythmias – a diagnostic dilemma. *Lancet*, **341**, 93–5.

91. Bayly, P.V., Johnson, E.E., Wolf, P.D. *et al.* (1993) A quantitative measurement of spatial order in ventricular fibrillation. *J. Cardiovasc. Electrophysiol.*, **4**, 533–46.

92. Clayton, R.H., Murray, A. and Campbell, R.W.F. (1991). Changes in the surface ECG frequency spectrum during the onset of ventricular fibrillation. In: Murray, A. and Ripley, K.L. (eds) *Computers in Cardiology 1990*, pp. 515–18. Los Alamitos, California: IEEE Comp. Soc. Press.

93. Kertes, P. and Hunt, D. (1984) Prophylaxis of primary ventricular fibrillation in acute myocardial infarction. The case against lignocaine. *Br. Heart J.*, **52**, 241–47.

94. Herlitz, J. Edvardsson, N., Holmberg, S., Ryden, L., Waagstein, F., Waldenström, A., Swedberg, K. and Hjalmarson, A. (1984) Göteborg Metoprolol Trial: effects on arrhythmias. *Am. J. Cardiol.*, **53**, 27D–31D.

95. Behar, S., Reicher Reiss, H., Schechter, M. *et al.* (1993) Frequency and prognostic significance of secondary ventricular fibrillation complicating acute myocardial infarction. *Am. J. Cardiol.*, **71**, 152–6.

96. Touboul, P., Moleur, P., Mathieu, M.P. *et al.* (1988) A comparative evaluation of the effects of propafenone and lidocaine on early ventricular arrhythmias after acute myocardial infarction. *Eur. Heart J.*, **9**, 1188–93.

97. Silke B., Frais, M.A., Verma, S.P. *et al.* (1986) Comparative haemodynamic effects of intravenous lignocaine, disopyramide and flecainide in uncomplicated acute myocardial infarction. *Br. J. Clin. Pharmacol.*, **22**, 707–714.

98. Ronnevik, P.K., Gundersen, T. and Abrahamsen, A.M. (1987) Tolerability and antiarrhythmic efficacy of disopyramide compared to lignocaine in selected patients with suspected acute myocardial infarction. *Eur. Heart. J.*, **8**, 19–24.

99. Wolfe, C.L., Nibley, C., Bhandari, A. *et al.*, Polymorphous ventricular tachycardia associated with acute myocardial infarction. *Circulation*, **84**, 1543–51.

100. Hong, M., Peter, T., Peters, W. *et al.* (1991) Relation between acute ventricular arrhythmias, ventricular late potentials and mortality in acute myocardial infarction. *Am. J. Cardiol.*, **68**, 1403–9.

101. Sugiura, T., Iwasaka, T., Takahashi, N. *et al.* (1991) Factors associated with atrial fibrillation in Q wave anterior myocardial infarction. *Am. Heart J.*, **121**, 1409–12.

102. Kobayashi, Y., Katoh, T., Takano, T. and Hayakawa, H. (1992) Paroxysmal atrial fibrillation and flutter associated with acute myocardial infarction: hemodynamic evaluation in relation to the development of arrhythmias and prognosis. *Jpn. Circ. J.*, **56**, 1–11.

103. Nielsen, F.E., Andersen, H.H., GramHansen, P. *et al.* (1992) The relationship between ECG signs of atrial infarction and the development of supraventricular arrhythmias in patients with acute myocardial infarction. *Am. Heart J.*, **123**, 69–72.

104. Kyriakidis, M., Barbetseas, J., Antonopoulos, A. *et al.* (1992) Early atrial arrhythmias in acute myocardial infarction: role of the sinus node artery. *Chest*, **101**, 944–7.

105. Hod, H., Lew, A.S., Keltai, M. *et al.* (1987) Early atrial fibrillation during evolving myocardial infarction: a consequence of impaired left atrial perfusion. *Circulation*, **75**, 146–50.

106. Rechavia, E., Strasberg, B., Mager, A. *et al.* (1992) The incidence of atrial arrhythmias during inferior wall myocardial infarction with and without right ventricular involvement. *Am. Heart J.*, **124**, 387–91.

107. Sugiura, T., Iwasaka, T., Ogawa, A., Shiroyama, Y., Tsuji, H., Onoyama, H. and Inada, M. (1985) Atrial fibrillation in acute myocardial infarction. *Am. J. Cardiol.*, **56**, 27–9.

108. Naito, M., David, D., Michelson, E.L., Íchaffenburg, M. and Dreifus, L.S. (1983) The hemodynamic consequences of cardiac arrhythmias: evaluation of the relative roles of abnormal atrioventricular sequencing, irregularity of ventricular rhythm and atrial fibrillation in a canine model. *Am. Heart J.*, **106**, 284–91.

109. Borgeat, A., Goy, J.J., Maendly, R. *et al.* (1986) Flecainide versus quinidine for conversion of atrial fibrillation to sinus rhythm. *Am. J. Cardiol.*, **58**, 496–8.

110. Porterfield, J.G. and Porterfield, L.M. (1989) Therapeutic efficacy and safety of oral propafenone for atrial fibrillation. *Am. J. Cardiol.*, **63**, 114–16.

111. Cowan, J.C., Gardiner, P., Reid, D.S. *et al.* (1986) Amiodarone in the management of atrial fibrillation complicating myocardial infarction. *Br. J. Clin. Pract.*, **40**, 155–61.

112. Hall, A.S., Winter, C., Bogle, S.M., Mackintosh, A.F., Murray, G.D. and Ball, S.G. (1991) The Acute Infarcton Ramipril Efficacy (AIRE) Study: rationale, design, organization, and outcome definitions. *J. Cardiovasc. Pharmacol.*, **18** (Suppl 2), S105–S109.

113 Jennings, R.B., Sommers, H.M. and Smyth, G.A. (1960) Myocardial necrosis induced by temporary occlusion of a coronary artery in the dog. *Arch. Pathol.*, **70**, 68–78.

114. Burney, R.E., Walsh, D., Kaplan, L.R. *et al.* (1989) Reperfusion arrhythmia: myth or reality? *Ann. Emerg. Med.*, **18**, 240–3.
115. Gressin, V., Louvard, Y., Pezzano, M. and Lardoux, H. (1992) Holter recording of ventricular arrhythmias during intravenous thrombolysis for acute myocardial infarction. *Am. J. Cardiol.*, **69**, 152–9.
116. Cercek, B., Lew, A.S., Laramee, P. *et al.* (1987) Time course and characteristics of ventricular arrhythmias after reperfusion in acute myocardial infarction. *Am. J. Cardiol.*, **60**, 214–18.
117. Gore, J.M., Ball, S.P., Corrao, J.M. and Goldberg, R.J. (1988) Arrhythmias in the assessment of coronary artery reperfusion following thrombolytic therapy. *Chest*, **94**, 727–30.
118. Hackett, D., McKenna, W., Davies, G. and Maseri, A. (1990) Reperfusion arrhythmias are rare during acute myocardial infarction and thrombolysis in man. *Int. J. Cardiol.*, **29**, 205–13.
119. Miller, F.C., Krucoff, M.W., Satler, L.F. *et al.* (1986) Ventricular arrhythmias during reperfusion. *Am. Heart. J.*, **112**, 928–32.
120. Solomon, S.D., Ridker, P.M. and Antman, E.M. (1994) Ventricular arrhythmias in trials of thrombolytic therapy for acute myocardial infarction. *Circulation* (in press).
121. Zehender, M., Utzolino, S., Furtwangler, A. *et al.* (1991) Time course and interrelation of reperfusion-induced ST changes and ventricular arrhythmias in acute myocardial infarction. *Am. J. Cardiol.*, **68**, 1138–42.
122. Six, A.J., Louwerenburg, J.H., Kingma, J.H. *et al.* (1991) Predictive value of ventricular arrhythmias for patency of the infarct-related coronary artery after thrombolytic therapy. *Br. Heart J.*, **66**, 143–6.
123. Maggioni, A.P., Zuanetti, G., Franzosi, M.G. *et al.* (1993) Prevalence and prognostic significance of ventricular arrhythmias after acute myocardial infarction in the fibrinolytic era. GISSI-2 results. *Circulation*, **87**, 312–22.
124. Volpi, A., Cavalli, A., Santoro, E. and Tognoni, G. for the Gruppo Italiano per lo Studio della Streptochinasi nell'Infarto Miocardico (1990). Incidence and prognosis of secondary ventricular fibrillation in acute myocardial infarction. Evidence for a protective effect of thrombolytic therapy. *Circulation*, **82**, 1279–88.
125. ISIS-2 (Second International Study of Infarct Survival). Collaborative Group (1988). Randomised trial of intravenous streptokinase, oral aspirin, both, or neither among 17 187 cases of suspected acute myocardial infarction. *Lancet*, **ii**, 349–60.
126. The European Myocardial Infarction Project Group (EMIP) (1993). Prehospital thrombolytic therapy in patients with suspected acute myocardial infarction. *N. Engl. J. Med.*, **329**, 383–9.
127. Makijarvi, M., Heikkila, J., Montonen, J. *et al.* (1992) The effects of thrombolytic therapy on the high-resolution electrocardiogram after myocardial infarction. *Eur. Heart J.*, **13**, 1046–52.
128. Vatterott, R.J., Hammill, S.C., Bailey, K.R. *et al.* (1991) Late potentials on signal-averaged electrocardiograms and patency of infarct-related artery in survivors of acute myocardial infarction. *J. Am. Coll. Cardiol.*, **17**, 330–7.
129. Turitto, G., Risa, A.L., Zanchi, E. and Prati, P.L. (1990) The signal-averaged electrocardiogram and ventricular arrhythmias after thrombolysis for acute myocardial infarction. *J. Am. Coll. Cardiol.*, **15**, 1270–6.
130. Wilcox, R.G., Eastgate, J., Harrison, E. and Skene, A.M. (1991) Ventricular arrhythmias during treatment with alteplase (recombinant tissue plasminogen activator) in suspected acute myocardial infarction. *Br. Heart J.*, **65**, 4–8.
131. Alexopoulos, D., Collins, R., Adamopoulos, S. *et al.* (1991) Holter monitoring of ventricular arrhythmias in a randomised controlled study of intravenous streptokinase in acute myocardial infarction. *Br. Heart J.*, **65**, 9–13.
132. Nielson, F.E., Sorensen, H.T., Christensen, J.H. *et al.* (1991) Reduced occurrence of atrial fibrillation in acute myocardial infarction treated with streptokinase. *Eur. Heart J.*, **12**, 1081–3.
133. Bourke, J.P., Young, A.A., Richards, D.A.B. and Uther, J,B. (1990) Reduction in incidence of inducible ventricular tachycardia after myocardial infarction by treatment with streptokinase during infarct evolution. *J. Am. Coll. Cardiol.*, **16**, 1703–10.
134. Cowan, J.C., Been, M. and Gibb, I. (1987) Lack of evidence of spontaneous reperfusion when ventricular fibrillation complicates early myocardial infarction. *Am. J. Cardiol.*, **59**, 1419–20.
135. Ruano Marco M., Lacueva, M.V., Garcia, P. *et al.* (1989) Lignocaine prophylaxis for reperfusion arrhythmias during treatment with streptokinase in acute myocardial infarction. *Lancet*, **ii**, 872–3.
136. Kuck, K.H., Scofer, J., Schulter, M. *et al.* (1985) Reperfusion arrhythmias in man; influence of intravenous lidocaine. *Eur. Heart. J.*, **6** (suppl. E), 163–7.
137. Corr, P.B. and Witkowski, F.X. (1983) Potential electrophysiologic mechanisms responsible for dysrhythmias associated with reperfusion of ischemic myocardium. *Circulation*, **68**, 116–24.
138. Hohnloser, S.H., Zabel, M., Olschewski, M. *et al.* (1992) Arrhythmias during the acute phase of reperfusion therapy for acute myocardial infarction: effects of beta-adrenergic blockade. *Am. Heart J.*, **123**, 1530–35.
139. Murohara, Y., Yui, Y., Hattori, R. and Kawai, O. (1991) Effects of superoxide dismutase on reperfusion arrhythmias and left ventricular function in patients undergoing thrombolysis for anterior wall acute myocardial infarction. *Am. J. Cardiol.*, **67**, 765–8.
140. Mehta, J.L., Nichols, W.W., Saldeen, T.G.P. *et al.* (1990) Superoxide dismutase decreases reperfusion arrhythmias and preserves myocardial function during thrombolysis with tissue plasminogen activator. *J. Cardiovasc. Pharmacol.*, **16**, 112–20.
141. Nejima, J., Knight, D.R., Fallon, J.T. *et al.* (1989) Superoxide dismutase reduces reperfusion arrhythmias but fails to salvage regional function or myocardium at risk in conscious dogs. *Circulation*, **79**, 143–53.
142. Wennerblom, B., Ekstrom, L. and Holmberg, S. (1984) Resuscitation of patients in cardiac arrest outside hospital. Comparison of two different organizations of mobile coronary care in one community. *Eur. Heart J.*, **5**, 21–6.
143. McLaran, C.J., Gersh, B.J., Sugrue, D.D. *et al.* (1987) Out-of-hospital cardiac arrest in patients without clinically significant coronary artery disease; comparison of clinical, electrophysiological and survival characteristics with those in similar patients who have clinically significant coronary artery disease. *Br. Heart J.*, **58**, 583–91.

9

Nitrates

L. Wilhelmsen

Background and Significance

The use of a nitrate preparation, amyl nitrite, in myocardial ischemia was first reported in 1867.[1] Somewhat later it was found that nitroglycerin produced similar effects to those of amyl nitrite,[2] but the effects of both preparations were very short-lasting. The more long-acting isosorbide dinitrate was first reported from Sweden in 1946,[3] and this was followed by pentaerythritol tetranitrate and erythritol tetranitrate. These drugs are all organic nitrate esters, which contain —ONO_2 groups. In the following discussion, they will be referred to as nitrates. In recent years, long-acting nitrates have become available in a variety of formulations including sublingual sprays and solutions for parenteral use. Beneficial effects in angina pectoris are long established, even though there have been serious doubts concerning the effectiveness of long-acting compounds, not least due to the development of tolerance.

The use of nitrates in acute myocardial infarction (AMI) was considered to be contraindicated until the early 1970s according to, for example, Friedberg's textbook.[4] The reason was chiefly the expected risk of excessive nitrate-induced hypotension. During the 1970s nitrates began to be used with great caution to control ischemia and improve hemodynamics in AMI.[5-8] Subsequent experimental[9] and clinical findings[10-14] have confirmed their great usefulness in acute coronary occlusion.

Today, these agents have become first-line therapy in the management of acute myocardial ischemia because of their beneficial effects on chest pain, myocardial perfusion, central hemodynamics, and mortality in AMI. Thus, nitrates have become of increasing interest. However, there are also drawbacks such as risks of hypotension, development of tolerance, and the unsolved questions regarding their proper indications in the thrombolytic era.

Characteristics of Nitrates

Biochemical

Several mechanisms for the smooth muscle relaxation by nitrates have been proposed, and the following describes the most widely accepted at present. Cyclic guanosine monophosphate (cGMP) plays a major role in vascular smooth muscle relaxation. Activation of a cGMP-dependent protein kinase results in the phosphorylation of the light chain of myosin. Interaction between actin and myosin is thus blocked and smooth

241

muscle relaxation and vasodilatation ensues.[15–17] It is believed that the cGMP-dependent protein kinase activates a calcium-dependent ATPase, which reduces intracellular calcium concentration and myosin light-chain kinase activity.[17] It was found that intact endothelium was needed to elicit vascular dilatory capacity (by, for example, acetylcholine and bradykinin)[18] and this factor was termed endothelium-derived relaxant factor (EDRF). There is now convincing evidence that EDRF is nitric oxide (NO).[19] Nitric oxide is thus released from vascular endothelium, reacts with heme in hemoglobin and forms a nitrosyl–heme complex, and NO–hemoglobin. This complex in turn activates guanylate cyclase and forms cGMP. Organic nitrates and a variety of other compounds appear to induce vascular smooth muscle relaxation through NO-induced activation of cGMP.[16,20,21] Thus, these drugs may be considered as prodrugs, which are metabolized to NO in the smooth muscle cell. Nitric oxide is normally widely distributed throughout the body, and has different biologic effects. Coronary atherosclerosis leads to endothelial dysfunction and abnormal vasodilatory capacity of the coronary arteries. It is believed that nitrates have special effects in the coronary vessels in this situation. It seems as if nitrates have unique effects in their ability to dilate abnormal coronary vessels with depressed endothelial function. In human coronary artery disease the sensitivity, but not the maximal response, to nitroglycerin is reduced.[22]

Hemodynamics

All physiologic effects of nitrates can be explained by their dilatory effects on veins, arteries, and arterioles. The effects on the various vascular beds are, however, nonuniform and dose related.[23] Venodilatation is produced at very low blood concentrations, and at these doses there is pooling of blood in the systemic capacitance vessels, which causes decreased venous return to the heart, and decreased ventricular filling volumes and pressure. Due to these effects, wall tension and heart size also decrease. Both systemic, splanchnic, and pulmonary veins seem to be involved in this venodilatation.[24,25]

Arterial conductance vessels are dilated at lower doses of nitrates whereas arteriolar dilatation requires higher doses. High doses result in decreased blood pressure, diminished afterload, as well as decreased systemic vascular resistance. A measurable decrease of systemic blood pressure does not, however, seem to be necessary to achieve a decreased afterload.[26]

Venodilatation reduces preload and consequently myocardial oxygen demand. The ensuing reduction in diastolic ventricular pressure would most probably result in improved coronary blood flow, in particular to the subendocardial region. These effects should prevent ischemia and relieve angina pectoris. The pulmonary congestion following acute and chronic left ventricular failure due to ischemia give symptoms such as dyspnea at rest or on exertion as well as orthopnea and are considerably relieved by the actions of nitrates.

The effects on arteries and arterial conductance vessels, which are accomplished at higher doses, decrease afterload, which also contributes to unloading of the heart and improved balance between myocardial oxygen supply and demand. However, a fall in systemic blood pressure occurring at higher nitrate doses may result in baroreceptor-mediated stimulation of the sympathetic nervous system with ensuing tachycardia and regional (or systemic) vasoconstriction. This may have serious undesired effects. Unfortunately, neither cardiac output nor peripheral vascular resistance accurately reflect the regional distribution of blood flow in this situation. Without very extensive monitoring of the various vascular beds it is difficult adequately to determine these effects. In the clinical situation, it is advisable to avoid too excessive effects on the arterial bed by careful monitoring of hemodynamics. As further discussed below, this need not involve complicated monitoring procedures.

In addition to the above effects, nitrates are potent dilators of coronary vessels including collateral channels. It should be stressed that coronary perfusion pressure is a major determinant of collateral blood flow, and if blood pressure is allowed to fall excessively collateral flow may in fact decrease.[27,28] The clinical effects of nitrates on collateral vessels in patients with multivessel disease have varied in different studies from being increased[29] to unchanged.[30] These different results can be explained by varying effects on coronary perfusion pressure and on coronary collateral blood flow.

Of great importance is the fact that nitrates have been shown to cause favorable redistribution of flow from nonischemic to ischemic areas,[29,31] and nitrates improve regional perfusion despite a minimal change in total flow.[32] However, as with the peripheral hemodynamic effects, excessive doses of nitroglycerin cause hypotension and reflex tachycardia and result in loss of the beneficial effect on collateral flow.[9]

An important sequela to coronary occlusion and myocardial infarction is ventricular remodeling.[33] Necrotic myocardium is prone to stretching and thinning due to the distending intracavitary forces, and this will cause outward bulging of the infarct zone as well as intramural traction of contractile adjacent myocardium together with increased wall stress. This process initiates a vicious circle of ineffective contraction, decreased systolic ejection, decreased cardiac output, and more cardiac dilatation with resulting cardiac failure.[34] These effects can be limited by nitrates by way of their reduction of preload, wall stress, cavity size, and limitation of infarct size. This has also been documented in clinical studies.[14]

Antiplatelet Effects

The first report on inhibition of platelet function was published in 1967.[35] However, very high doses were used. Loscalzo showed in 1985 that by maintaining intracellular reduced thiol equivalents, both nitroglycerin and nitroprusside inhibited platelet aggregation at pharmacologically achievable concentrations *in vivo*.[36] The platelet inhibition was associated with an increase in cGMP levels. It was found that platelet inhibition was accompanied by inhibition of calcium flux and reduction of fibrinogen binding to the glycoprotein IIb/IIIa receptor. Fibrinogen binding is essential for platelet aggregation and its inhibition appears to be the critical mechanism by which platelet function is impaired by nitrates.[37] It is possible that these effects on thrombocytes are involved in their apparent positive effects in acute coronary syndromes.

Effects of Different Nitrate Preparations

The elimination half-life of nitroglycerin is quite short, about 1–3 min,[38] and this rapid elimination is of value when administering nitroglycerin intravenously so that the blood concentration can be adjusted rapidly. Sublingual nitroglycerin has a somewhat longer half-life, about 4–5 min.[39] There has been a search for longer-acting compounds for treatment of angina pectoris and congestive heart failure. Isosorbide dinitrate and isosorbide 5-mononitrate have been developed and have come into use for these indications, particularly in Europe.[40] Other long-acting compounds are pentaerythritol tetranitrate and erythritol tetranitrate. According to the need for rapid adjustment of doses, the long-acting nitrates have little place in the acute treatment of AMI. For long-term use, however, some of them have an established place in therapy.

Tolerance

Tolerance to nitrates has gained progressive attention during recent years.[41] Tolerance is seen as an attenuation of the hemodynamic and clinical response, usually after chronic use of relatively high doses in congestive heart failure. However, tolerance is considered to be relatively rare among patients with coronary heart disease.[42] The most probable cause of nitrate tolerance is a reduction of the activity of guanylate cyclase leading to a decrease of cGMP and a loss of the vasodilatory effects. Sulfhydryl groups are needed for the organic nitrates to activate guanylate cyclase. These groups are subjected to continuous interaction with nitrates, and when there is a lack of reduced sulfhydryl groups guanylate cyclase cannot be activated. However, availability of reduced sulfhydryl groups may facilitate the vasodilating action of nitrates, but development of tolerance is not necessarily a result of sulfhydryl depletion. Tolerance can be remedied by nitrate-free intervals, for example during night time. Sulfhydryl donors can at least bring about partial reversal of nitrate tolerance, but there is a lack of potent such donors that can be used in the clinical setting. N-Acetylcysteine and methionine need to be administered at very high doses if any clinical effect is to be seen.[43] It is interesting that angiotensin-converting enzyme (ACE) inhibitors either containing sulfhydryl groups, such as captopril, or not , such as enalapril, have beneficial interactions with nitrates and are able to counteract the tolerance development.[44] The full theoretic explanation and clinical handling of nitrate tolerance is, however, not solved.[45] With low to moderate intravenous nitrate doses in AMI partial tolerance was found in 24% of patients.[46] Accordingly, tolerance to acute treatment with intravenous nitrate in AMI does not seem to be a major problem.

Observational Data

The first group to start studying the effects of intravenous nitroglycerin in patients with AMI were the cardiologists at the Johns Hopkins Hospital in Baltimore.[6] In their first studies, precordial ST-segment monitoring was used to monitor that regional myocardial ischemia did not worsen with the treatment. The mean blood pressure decreased by only 7 mmHg, while there was a significant lowering of left ventricular filling pressure, as well as a reduction in some of the precordial ST-segment voltages.[6] In their continued studies even greater reductions in mean arterial pressure (15–30 mmHg) resulted, but beneficial antiischemic effects were still observed in patients both with and without left ventricular failure. In accordance with other authors, previously cited in this chapter, they found that stepwise titration of the intravenous infusion of nitroglycerin led to venodilatation at lower infusion rates, which decreased left ventricular filling pressure by a mean of 10 mmHg, but little effect on mean arterial pressure was seen. At higher infusion rates, more balanced venous and arterial dilating effects were observed. In association with a similar lowering of left ventricular filling pressure (52%), a 20% lowering of mean arterial pressure was observed. Effects on left ventricular hemodynamics varied with the degree of underlying left ventricular failure. Thus, patients without hemodynamic evidence of left ventricular failure demonstrated both a decrease in stroke volume and a decrease in the left ventricular filling pressure, providing evidence of the predominant preload lowering or 'diuretic-like effect' induced by venodilatation. In contrast, patients with mild left ventricular failure, as evidenced by an elevated left ventricular filling pressure but a normal stroke volume, demonstrated a lowering of left ventricular filling pressure but with maintenance of stroke volume, suggesting that nitroglycerin was inducing a degree of afterload lowering as well. Patients with hemodynamic evidence of a more severe degree of left ventricular failure, with both an elevated filling pressure and reduced stroke volume, demonstrated the most beneficial hemodynamic effects.[47] A differential effect of nitroglycerin on stroke volume is most likely due to differences in arterial impedance being of greater importance for stroke volume among patients with severe left ventricular dysfunction. The arterial–arteriolar actions of nitroglycerin are particularly useful in subjects with impaired left ventricular contractile function. Of great importance , as mentioned by Flaherty and collaborators as well as others, is the careful upward titration of the infusion rate whereby the beneficial antiischemic and hemodynamic effects can be obtained without excessive lowering of coronary pressure and without inducing reflex tachycardia. In fact, heart rate was lower in many patients during intravenous nitroglycerin therapy.

Nitroprusside has also been tested in experimental infarcts in animals and AMI in patients. There is a strong suggestion that nitroprusside may induce a coronary steal phenomenon; this may explain why the effects are less positive than with nitroglycerin. In an experimental study, Chiarello *et al.*[48] found that myocardial blood flow distal to a ligated left anterior descending coronary artery was found to decrease, and epicardial ST-segment elevations to increase, during nitroprusside infusion. This was in contrast to the nitroglycerin infusion, which caused increased flow and decreased epicardial ST-segment elevations. This was taken as evidence for an increase in intercoronary collateral blood flow on nitroglycerin treatment, and conversely a decrease in collateral flow on nitroprusside infusion. Similar findings with other techniques have been reported by Mann *et al.*,[49] Capurro *et al.*[50] and Marcho and Vatner.[51]

In summary, these findings from nonrandomized studies indicate beneficial effects of intravenous nitroglycerin in AMI. As a consequence of the reduced myocardial oxygen demand and increased coronary flow, nitrate therapy may limit infarct size.[52,53]

Clinical Trials

Acute Phase Treatment

An overview of the randomized trials of intravenous nitrates or nitroprusside in the acute phase of an AMI has been published by Yusuf *et al.*[54] Most of the trials were small and only three of them showed significant results on mortality with either nitroprusside or nitroglycerin.[11,55,56] Even so, in all but one of the randomized trials mentioned in this overview[13] there were trends towards lower mortality among the nitrate-allocated patients as compared to the controls. The overview of the 10 randomized trials involving a total of about 2000 patients showed a significant result on mortality of the treatment[10,12,57–60] (Figure 9.1). There was a trend in favor of active treatment both in nitroglycerin and nitroprusside treatments; however, the largest trial with 812 patients showed a tendency to increased mortality on nitroprusside. The early treatment benefit seemed also to persist during an extended follow-up. The overall reduction of mortality was between 1/6 and 1/2 (mean 35%) among the randomized patients, who were at relatively high risk of death. It should be emphasized that the overview was small compared to most other overviews, and the effect may well be overestimated. These trials also demonstrated reductions in cardiac enzyme release with treatment, suggesting infarct size limitation.[11,55,56,58–60] Findings from one of the randomized clinical trials are shown in Table 9.1, indicating reductions of creatine kinase (CK) enzyme release, global left ventricular ejection fraction, as well as left ventricular end-diastolic volume.[14] Many clinicians have appreciated the trial results as convincing enough to apply intravenous nitrates in AMI, and the joint guidelines by the Task Forces of the American College of Cardiology and the American Heart Association recommended this therapy in 1990.[61]

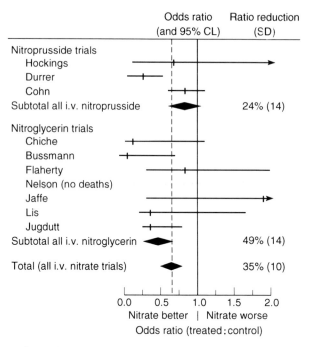

Figure 9.1 Apparent effects of intravenous nitroprusside and nitroglycerin on mortality in the random-ized trials of the treatment of AMI. Vertical stroke, odds ratio. Horizontal line, 95% CI; a 95% CI that does not include 1.0 indicates a statistically significant difference (2P <0.05) in mortality between the treatment groups; broken line, 'typical' odds ratio indicated by an overview of all intravenous nitrate trials. (From Ref. 54 with permission; © by The Lancet Ltd.)

It should be emphasized that the above-mentioned trials were all performed before the widespread use of thrombolytics. The latter treatment has definitely decreased in-hospital mortality in AMI, and it is possible that the effects of nitrates may be somewhat smaller in patients treated with thrombolytics. However, there are no indications that there is any adverse interaction between the two treatments as long as fall in blood pressure (which is a well-known side-effect of both treatments) is monitored appropriately.

Table 9.1 Effects of intravenous nitroglycerin versus placebo in patients with acute myocardial infarction according to Jugdutt and Warnica[14]

Outcome measure	Nitroglycerin ($n = 154$)	Placebo ($n = 156$)	P value
Infarct size (CK release, gEq)	41 ± 35	55 ± 42	<0.001
Global LVEF (%) (day 10)	51 ± 9	42 ± 9	<0.05
LVEV (ml) (day 10)	112 ± 5	138 ± 5	<0.05

LVEF, left ventricular ejection fraction; LVEV, left ventricular end-diastolic volume.

Long-Term Nitrate Therapy

Nitrates have been in use for many years for relieving angina, and to some extent also silent ischemia in the long-term management of patients with and without a previous AMI. The aforementioned effects of nitrate on hemodynamics and thrombocytes would be valuable also with regard to healing after an AMI. Such healing takes place up to 6 months in humans.[62,63] The infarcted area undergoes expansion with stretching, thinning, and dilatation. The mechanisms of this remodeling remain elusive despite considerable recent attention. They probably involve a combination of mechanical factors and specific trophic substances.[64] The remodeling is progressive and can go on for about 6 weeks, leading to cardiac dilatation and even rupture.[62] Further remodeling after the infarct healing can go on up to 4–6 months. There are good experimental and clinical reasons for early prophylactic therapy to prevent such remodeling. Nitroglycerin, with its favorable hemodynamic effects without any known negative effects on the infarct collagen deposition, would be ideal to prevent such remodeling. In a recent experimental report it was also shown that long-term oral nitrate therapy in dogs attenuated the early and late manifestations of ventricular remodeling after experimental myocardial damage.[65] The hemodynamic analyses suggested that the drug-induced preload or afterload reduction did not completely explain the favorable nitrate effects. Beneficial effects on ventricular remodeling have been demonstrated also with captopril.[66] In addition to direct hemodynamic effects, nitrates may be valuable also because of their antiplatelet/antithrombotic effects.

Studies in humans have been performed by the Jugdutt group.[67] After an initial period of intravenous nitrate, buccal nitrates were given with intervals to avoid tolerance. More than 50% of their patients had received thrombolytic therapy together with intravenous nitroglycerin. The prolonged nitrate therapy resulted in further limitation of remodeling, further improvement of left ventricular function, limitation of left ventricular dilatation, and decreased frequency of aneurysm formation, and the positive effects persisted up to 1 year. The effects seemed to be similar to those of captopril on this remodeling process. Confirmation by studies in other groups is needed.

Interestingly, Pipilis *et al.*[68] demonstrated reduced incidence of ventricular arrhythmias by mononitrate within the first 24 hours of AMI among 100 patients randomized to mononitrate, captopril or placebo.

Effects on mortality with long-term nitrate treatment have been studied in the large multicenter trials GISSI-3 and ISIS-4. In GISSI-3, 19 394 patients were randomized to either 6 weeks of oral lisinopril or open control, or to intravenous nitrates followed by transdermal nitroglycerin or to open control.[69] Oral administration of lisinopril either alone or in combination with transdermal nitrates produced statistically significant reductions in overall mortality as well as in the combined outcome measure of mortality and severe ventricular dysfunction compared with placebo. However, the administration of transdermal nitrates did not show any independent effect on the same outcome measures. In this study, 44% of patients received intravenous nitroglycerin during the first day, 72% received thrombolysis acutely, 31% intravenous β-blockade, and aspirin was given to 84%. ISIS-4 completed randomization of 58 000 patients in early autumn 1993. In the factorial design of this trial 50% of the patients were given an oral mononitrate (Imdur) and 50% placebo, but patients in both groups were randomized to either captopril or its placebo or, in the acute phase, to magnesium infusion or control. The main findings were presented at the meeting of the American Heart Association in November 1993.[70] The mononitrate was given for 1 month and mortality during the first 5 weeks was not significantly altered as compared to placebo. The drug was well tolerated in relatively hypotensive patients and, in addition, the incidence of hypotension-related clinical events were in fact lower with the nitrate than with captopril. In summary, these two large trials do not support any beneficial effects of long-term, oral nitrate treatment after AMI. It may be that significant effects are only to be expected among patients with impaired left ventricular function and during longer term treatment, as has been demonstrated with captopril[71] and ramipril,[72] but such an effect ought to have been detected to some degree in these major trials. Furthermore, oral or transdermal administration may not be as effective immediately as the intravenous nitroglycerin given in the earlier trials.

Practical Implications

Trial results suggest that intravenous nitrates may have beneficial effects on mortality even when invasive monitoring of central hemodynamics is not used. The dosage employed in the various trials have differed, with an actual dose range between 5 and $250\,\mu g\,min^{-1}$. The moderate dose therapy as proposed by Jugdutt[14] for 24–48 hours seems recommendable. According to this author the drug is titrated to decrease the mean blood pressure by 10% for normotensive patients and by 30% for hypertensive patients (blood pressure >140/90 mmHg) and never below a systolic blood pressure of 90 mmHg. This simple noninvasive monitoring by standard sphygmomanometry can be used in all coronary care units. The regimen consists of starting an intravenous nitroglycerin infusion at $5\,\mu g\,min^{-1}$ and increasing the rate by $5–20\,\mu g\,min^{-1}$ every 5 min during the first 30 min until the target decremental cut-off, or a dose of $200\,\mu g\,min^{-1}$ is reached. Infusions are slowed or temporarily discontinued when the mean blood pressure drops below 80 mmHg or the systolic blood pressure drops below 90 mmHg. Infusions are gradually tapered after 48 hours in decremental steps of $5–10\,\mu g\,min^{-1}$ every 5 min.[73]

It is generally appreciated that there is no fixed dose of intravenous nitroglycerin that can be adopted for all patients with AMI. This is due to several factors. Patients with AMI differ markedly regarding hemodynamics and there is a wide variation in their responsiveness to intravenous nitroglycerin. Concomitant drug therapy with thrombolytics and β-blockers has to be taken into consideration. Patients in hypovolemia and those with inferior wall or right ventricular infarction seem to be more sensitive, as well as elderly patients, and for these patients special caution is needed. As previously stated, development of tolerance does not seem to be a major problem in the acute phase treatment of AMI. However, if patients develop marked early tolerance, one may have to try nitrate-free intervals or an ACE inhibitor.

There are reasons to believe that all interventions in the acute phase, as well as long term, will not be additive regarding their effects. Thus, it is probable that in patients in whom a major part of the myocardium has been saved due to early thrombolytic treatment, intravenous nitroglycerin (as well as ACE inhibitors) will be of less importance than in those with large transmural infarctions. The apparent beneficial effects of nitrates in addition to those of ACE inhibitors in the GISSI-3 trial will have to be further evaluated. At least nitrate therapy did not appear to complicate treatment with long-term ACE inhibitors in the ISIS trial.[70] So far, ACE inhibitors are to be preferred for the postinfarction treatment in selected cases.

In summary, future treatment of AMI will most probably have to be tailored according to the size of the AMI as well as various criteria for left ventricular remodeling and clinical signs of heart failure during the first months of follow-up. Hargreaves et al.[74] have recently questioned the use of vasodilator treatment with both ACE inhibitors and nitrates after AMI especially in those treated with thrombolytics, but their study was quite small (in total 105 patients randomized to three treatment arms), and there are still reasons to expect positive effects also in the thrombolytic era. Nobody has questioned the beneficial effects of nitrates with the aim of relieving ischemia and associated chest pain.

References

1. Brunton, T.L. (1867) *Lectures on the Actions of Medicines*. New York: MacMillan.
2. Murrell, W. (1979) Nitroglycerin as a remedy for angina pectoris. *Lancet*, **i**, 80, 113, 225, 284, 642–6.
3. Goldberg, L. and Porjé, I.G. (1946) En studie över sorbid-nitratets kärleffekt (A study of the vascular effects of sorbide dinitrate). *Nordisk Medicin*, **29**, 190–3.
4. Friedberg, C.K. (1966) Acute coronary occlusion and myocardial infarction. In: Friedberg, C.K. (ed.) *Diseases of the Heart*, 3rd edn, pp. 913–14. Philadelphia: W.B. Saunders.
5. Gold, H.K., Leinbach, R.C. and Sanders, C.A. (1972) Use of sublingual nitroglycerin in congestive heart failure following acute myocardial infarction. *Circulation*, **46**, 839–45.
6. Flaherty, J.T., Reid, P.R., Kelly, D.T. *et al.* (1975) Intravenous nitroglycerin in acute myocardial infarction. *Circulation*, **51**, 132–9.
7. Epstein, S.E., Kent, K.M., Goldstein, R.E. *et al.* (1975) Reduction of ischemic injury by nitroglycerin during acute myocardial infarction. *N. Engl. J. Med.*, **292**, 29–35.
8. Armstrong, P.W., Walker, D.C., Burton, J.R. and Parker, J.O. (1975) Vasodilator therapy in acute myocardial infarction. A comparison of sodium nitroprusside and nitroglycerin. *Circulation*, **52**, 1118–22.
9. Jugdutt, B.I. (1983) Myocardial salvage by intravenous nitroglycerin in conscious dogs. Loss of beneficial effect with marked nitroglycerin-induced hypotension. *Circulation*, **68**, 673–84.
10. Chiche, P., Baligadoo, S.J. and Derrida, J.P. (1979) A randomized trial of prolonged nitroglycerin infusion in acute myocardial infarction (abstract). *Circulation*, **59/60** (suppl. II), II-165.
11. Bussman, W.D., Passek, D., Seidel, W. and Kaltenbach, M. (1981) Reduction of CK and CK-MB indexes of infarct size by intravenous nitroglycerin. *Circulation*, **63**, 615–22.
12. Flaherty, J.T., Becker, L,C., Bulkley, B.H. *et al.* (1983) A randomized prospective trial of intravenous nitroglycerin in patients with acute myocardial infarction. *Circulation*, **68**, 576–88.
13. Jaffe, A.S., Geltman, E.M., Tiefenbrunn, A.J. *et al.* (1983) Reduction of infarct size in patients with inferior infarction with intravenous glyceryl trinitrate. A randomized study. *Br. Heart J.*, **49**, 452–60.
14. Jugdutt, B.I. and Warnica, J.W. (1988) Intravenous nitroglycerin therapy to limit myocardial infarct size, expansion, and complications. Effect of timing, dosage, and infarct location. *Circulation*, **78**, 906–19.
15. Murad, F. (1986) Cyclic guanosine monophosphate as a mediator of vasodilation. *J. Clin. Invest.*, **78**, 1–5.
16. Waldman, S.A. and Murad, F. (1987) Cyclic GMP synthesis and function. *Pharmacol. Rev.*, **39**, 163–96.
17. Rapoport, R.M., Draznin, M.B. and Murad, F (1983) Endothelium-dependent vasodilator and nitrovasodilator-induced relaxation may be mediated through cyclic GMP formation and cyclic GMP-dependent protein phosphorylation. *Trans. Assoc. Am. Physicians*, **96**, 19–30.
18. Furchgott, R.F. and Zawadzki, J.V. (1980) The obligatory role of endothelial cells in the relaxation of arterial smooth muscle by acetylcholine. *Nature*, **288**, 373–6.
19. Palmer, R.M.J., Ferrige, A.G. and Moncada, S. (1987) Nitric oxide release accounts for the biological activity of endothelium-derived relaxing factor. *Nature*, **327**, 524–6.
20. Murad, F., Arnold, W.P., Mittal, C.K. and Braughler, J.M. (1979) Properties and regulation of guanylate cyclase and some proposed functions for cyclic GMP. *Adv. Cyclic Nucleotide Res.*, **11**, 175–204.
21. Ignarro, L.J. and Kadowitz, P.J. (1985) The pharmacological and physiological role of cyclic GMP in vascular smooth muscle relaxation. *Annu. Rev. Pharmacol. Toxicol.*, **25**, 171–91.
22. Förstermann, U., Mugge, A., Bode, S.M. and Frölich, I.C. (1988) Response of human coronary arteries to aggregating platelets: Importance of endothelium-derived relaxing factor and prostanoids. *Circulation*, **63**, 306–12.
23. Imhof, P.R., Ott, B., Frankhauser, P. *et al.* (1980) Difference in nitroglycerin dose-response in the venous and arterial beds. *Eur. J. Clin. Pharmacol.*, **18**, 455–60.
24. Miller, R.R., Fennell, W.H., Young, J.B. *et al.* (1982) Differential systemic arterial and venous actions and consequent cardiac effects of vasodilator drugs. *Prog. Cardiovasc. Dis.*, **24**, 353–74.
25. Smith, E.R., Smiseth, O.A., Kingma, I. *et al.* (1984) Mechanism of action of nitrates. Role of changes in venous capacitance and in the left ventricular diastolic pressure volume relation. *Am. J. Med.*, **76**, 14–21.
26. Kelly, R.P., Gibbs, H.H., O'Rourke, M.F. *et al.* (1990) Nitroglycerin has more favorable effects on left ventricular afterload than apparent from measurement of pressure in a peripheral artery. *Eur. Heart J.*, **11**, 138–44.
27. Kattus, A.A. and Gregg, D.E. (1959) Some determinants of coronary collateral blood flow in the open-chest dog. *Circ. Res.*, **7**, 628-42.
28. Maroko, P.R., Libby, P., Covell, J.W. *et al.* (1972) Precordial ST segment mapping: A method for assessing alterations in the event of myocardial ischemic injury: The effects of pharmacologic and hemodynamic interventions. *Am. J. Cardiol.*, **29**, 223–30.
29. Horowitz, L.D., Gorlin, R., Taylor, W.J. and Kemp, H.G. (1971) Effects of nitroglycerin on regional myocardial blood flow in coronary artery disease. *J. Clin. Invest.*, **50**, 1578–84.
30. Goldstein, R.E., Stinson, E.B., Scherer, J.L. *et al.* (1974) Intraoperative coronary collateral function in patients with coronary occlusive disease: Nitroglycerin responsiveness and angiographic correlations. *Circulation*, **49**, 298–308.
31. Fuchs, R.M., Brinker, J.A., Guzman, P.A. *et al.* (1983) Regional coronary blood flow during relief of pacing-induced angina by nitroglycerin: Implications for mechanism of action. *Am. J. Cardiol.*, **51**, 19–23.
32. Gorlin, R., Brachfeld, N., MacLeod, C. and Bopp, P. (1959) Effect of nitroglycerin on the coronary circulation in patients with coronary artery disease or increased left ventricular work. *Circulation*, **19**, 705–18.

33. Pfeffer, M.A. and Braunwald, E. (1990) Ventricular remodeling after myocardial infarction. Experimental observations and clinical implications. *Circulation*, 81, 1161–72.
34. Jugdutt, B.I. (1990) The use of intravenous nitroglycerin and ACE-inhibitors for ventricular remodeling after myocardial infarction. *Life Sci. Adv. Phamacol.*, 9, 698–716.
35. Hampton, J.R., Harrison, A.J., Honour, A.J. and Mitchell, J.R. (1967) Platelet behavior and drugs used in cardiovascular disease. *Cardiovasc. Res.*, 1, 101–6.
36. Loscalzo, J. (1985) *n*-Acetylcysteine potentiates inhibition of platelet aggregation by nitroglycerin. *J. Clin. Invest.*, 76, 703–8.
37. Loscalzo, J. (1992) Antiplatelet and antithrombotic effects of organic nitrates. *Am. J. Cardiol.*, 70, 18B–22B.
38. Fung, H. (1987) Pharmacokinetics and pharmacodynamics of organic nitrates. *Am. J. Cardiol.*, 60, 4H–9H.
39. Blumenthal, H.P., Fung, H.L., McNiff, E.F. and Yap, S.K. (1977) Plasma nitroglycerin levels after sublingual, oral, and topical administration. *Br. J. Clin. Pharmacol.*, 4, 241–2.
40. Bogaert, M.G. (1983) Clinical pharmacokinetics of organic nitrates. *Clin. Pharmacokinet.*, 8, 410–21.
41. Flaherty, J.T. (1987) Transdermal nitroglycerin: Is intermittent therapy the answer to tolerance? *Pract. Cardiol.*, 13, 49–61.
42. Abrams, J. (1991) The mystery of nitrate resistance. *Am. J. Cardiol.*, 68, 1393–6.
43. Packer, M., Lee, W.H., Kessler, P.D. *et al.* (1987) Prevention and reversal of nitrate tolerance in patients with congestive heart failure. *N. Eng. J. Med.*, 317, 799–804.
44. Katz, R.J., Levy, W.S., Buff, L. and Wasserman, A.G. (1991) Prevention of nitrate tolerance with angiotensin converting enzyme inhibitors. *Circulation*, 83, 1271–7.
45. Packer, M. (1990) What causes tolerance to nitroglycerin? The 100 year old mystery continues. *J. Am. Coll. Cardiol.*, 16, 932–5.
46. Jugdutt, B.I. and Warnica, J.W. (1989) Tolerance with low dose intravenous nitroglycerin therapy in acute myocardial infarction. *Am. J. Cardiol.*, 64, 581–7.
47. Flaherty, J.T. (1992) Role of nitrates in acute myocardial infarction. *Am. J. Cardiol.*, 73, 73B–81B.
48. Chiariello, M., Gold, H.K., Leinbach, R.C. *et al.* (1976) Comparison between the effects of nitroprusside and nitroglycerin on ischemic injury during acute myocardial infarction. *Circulation*, 54, 766–73.
49. Mann, T., Cohn, P.F., Holman, B.L. *et al.* (1978) Effect of nitroprusside on regional myocardial blood flow in coronary disease: results in 25 patients and comparison with nitroglycerin. *Circulation*, 57, 732–8.
50. Capurro, N.L., Kent, K.M. and Epstein, S.E. (1977) Comparison of nitroglycerin, nitroprusside and phentolamine induced changes in coronary collateral function in dogs. *J. Clin. Invest.*, 60, 295–301.
51. Macho, P. and Vatner, S.F. (1981) Effects of nitroglycerin and nitroprusside in large and small coronary vessels in conscious dogs. *Circulation*, 64, 1101–7.
52. Franciosa, J.A., Gulha, N.H., Limas, C.J. *et al.* (1972) Improved left ventricular function during nitroprusside infusion in acute myocardial infarction. *Lancet*, i, 650–4.
53. Rude, R.E., Muller, J.E. and Braunwald, E. (1981) Efforts to limit the size of myocardial infarcts. *Ann. Intern. Med.*, 95, 736–61.
54. Yusuf, S., Collins, R., MacMahon, S. and Peto, R. (1988) Effect of intravenous nitrates on mortality in acute myocardial infarction. An overview of randomized trials. *Lancet*, i, 1088–92.
55. Durrer, J.D., Lie, K.I., van Capelle, F.J.P. and Durrer, D. (1982) Effect of sodium nitroprusside on mortality in acute myocardial infarction. *N. Engl. J. Med.*, 306, 1121–8.
56. Jugdutt, B.I., Sussex, B.A., Tymchak, W.J. and Warnica, J.W. (1989) Intravenous nitroglycerin in the early management of acute myocardial infarction. *Cardiovasc. Rev. Rep.*, 10, 29–35.
57. Hockings, B.E.F., Cope, G.D., Clarke, G.M. and Taylor R.R. (1981) Randomized controlled trial of vasodilator therapy after myocardial infarction. *Am. J. Cardiol.*, 48, 345–51.
58. Cohn, J.N., Franciosa, J.A. and Francis, G.S. (1982) Effect of short-term infusion of sodium nitroprusside on mortality rate in acute myocardial infarction complicated by left ventricular failure. Results of a VA Cooperative Study. *N. Engl. J. Med.*, 306, 1129–35.
59. Nelson, G.I.C., Silke, B., Ahuja, R.C. *et al.* (1983) Haemodynamic advantages of isosorbide dinitrate over furosemide in acute heart-failure following myocardial infarction. *Lancet*, i, 730–3.
60. Lis, Y., Bennett, D., Lambert, G. and Robson, D. (1984) A preliminary double-blind study of IV nitroglycerin in acute myocardial infarction. *Intensive Care Med.*, 10, 179–84.
61. Gunnar, R.M. and Fisch, C. (1990) Special Report: ACC/AHA Guidelines for the early management of patients with acute myocardial infarction. *Circulation*, 82, 664–707.
62. Jugdutt, B.I. and Michorowski, B.L. (1987) Role of infarct expansion in rupture of the ventricular septum after acute myocardial infarction: a two-dimensional echocardiographic study. *Clin. Cardiol.*, 10, 641–52.
63. Olivetti, G., Capasso, J.M., Meggs, L.G. *et al.* (1991) Cellular basis of chronic ventricular remodeling after myocardial infarction in rats. *Circ. Res.*, 68, 856–69.
64. Morgan, H.E. and Baker, K.M. (1991) Cardiac hypertrophy. Mechanical, neural and endocrine dependence. *Circulation*, 83, 13–25.
65. McDonald, K.M., Francis, G.S., Matthews, J.*et al.* (1993) Long-term oral nitrate therapy prevents chronic ventricular remodeling in the dog. *J. Am. Coll. Cardiol.*, 21, 514–22.
66. Pfeffer, J.M., Pfeffer, M.A. and Braunwald, E. (1985) Influence of chronic captopril therapy on the infarcted left ventricle of the rat. *Circ. Res.*, 57, 84–95.
67. Jugdutt, B.I. (1992) Role of nitrates after acute myocardial infarction. *Am. J. Cardiol.*, 70, 82B–87B.

68. Pipilis, A., Flather, M., Collins, R. *et al.* (1993) Hemodynamic effects of captopril and isosorbide mononitrate started early in acute myocardial infarction: a randomized placebo-controlled study. *J. Am. Coll. Cardiol.*, **21**, 73–9.
69. Gruppo Italiano per lo Studio della Sopravvivenza nell'Infarto Miocardico (1994) GISSI-3: Effects of lisinopril, of transdermal nitroglycerin and of their association on six-week mortality and ventricular function among 19 394 patients with acute myocardial infarction. *Lancet*, **343**, 1115–22.
70. ISIS Collaborative Group (1993) ISIS-4: Randomised study of oral isosorbide mononitrate in over 50 000 patients with suspected acute myocardial infarction. *Circulation*, **88**, I-394.
71. Pfeffer, M.A., Braunwald, E., Moyé, L. *et al.* on behalf of the SAVE Investigators (1992) Effect of captopril on mortality and morbidity in patients with left ventricular dysfunction after myocardial infarction. Results of the Survival and Ventricular Enlargement Trial. *N. Engl. J. Med.*, **327**, 669–77.
72. The Acute Infarction Ramipril Efficacy (AIRE) Study Investigators (1993) Effect of ramipril on mortality and morbidity of survivors of acute myocardial infarction with clinical evidence of heart failure. *Lancet*, **342**, 821–8.
73. Jugdutt, B.I. (1993) Nitrates in unstable angina and acute myocardial infarction. In: Rezakovic, D.Z.E. and Alpert, J.S. (eds) *Nitrate Therapy and Nitrate Tolerance. Current Concepts and Controversies*, p. 137. Basel: Karger.
74. Hargreaves, A.D., Kolettis, T., Jacob, A.J. *et al.* (1992) Early vasodilator treatment in myocardial infarction: appropriate for the majority or minority? *Br. Heart J.*, **68**, 369–73.

10

The Role of Angiotensin-converting Enzyme Inhibitors during the Early Phase

B. Pitt

Angiotensin-converting enzyme (ACE) inhibitors have been shown to be effective when administered during the convalescent stage of acute myocardial infarction (commencing more than 3 days after the onset of symptoms) in patients with a left ventricular ejection fraction (LVEF) ≤40%, whether symptomatic or not,[1] and in patients with clinical evidence of manifest heart failure post infarction.[2] As described in Chapter 15 the administration of these drugs during the healing phase of the infarction and thereafter reduces long-term morbidity and mortality. The mechanism for the effectiveness of ACE inhibitors in acute myocardial infarction is thought to be related to their ability to prevent ventricular dilatation and remodeling as well as compensatory ventricular hypertrophy associated with extensive myocardial damage.[3-5] This benefit in preventing progressive ventricular dilatation can be seen even in asymptomatic patients with a large infarct (LVEF ≤35%) treated several years post infarction. The SOLVD Prevention Trial[6] showed that asymptomatic patients with compromised ventricular systolic function, approximately 80% of whom had a history of a prior myocardial infarction, when treated with enalapril had a significant reduction in the development of new-onset heart failure and hospitalization for heart failure, although not mortality.

On the basis of the SAVE[1] and AIRE[2] trials, in patients randomized to an ACE inhibitor during the convalescent stage of an acute myocardial infarction (≥3 days), and the CONSENSUS I,[7] SOLVD Treatment,[8] V-HeFT II,[9] and SOLVD Prevention trial,[6] in patients with chronic heart failure, most of whom had a history of myocardial infarction as the cause of their left ventricular dysfunction and/or manifest heart failure, the following recommendations for clinical practice appear reasonable. Patients with an acute myocardial infarction and clinical evidence of heart failure who are hemodynamically stable on the second or third day post infarction should be started on an ACE inhibitor. Patients with myocardial infarction whose heart failure is controlled on medical therapy such as diuretics, digoxin, and/or nitroglycerin, as well as asymptomatic patients with an LVEF ≤40%, should also be started and maintained on an ACE inhibitor if hemodynamically stable during the convalescent phase of myocardial infarction, unless contraindicated because of hyperkalemia, a history of angioedema, or inability to tolerate an ACE inhibitor because of first dose hypotension, intractable cough, or progressive renal dysfunction. If a patient with a history of myocardial infarction and compromised left ventricular systolic function (LVEF ≤35%) has not been started on an ACE inhibitor during the convalescent phase of their infarction (after the third day) they should be started on an ACE inhibitor as an outpatient even up to several years post infarction unless contraindicated or not tolerated, regardless of symptoms, age, gender, New York Heart Association Class, or baseline medication. The rationale for these recommendations, including the preclinical and clinical trials supporting the use of ACE inhibitors in patients with acute or chronic left ventricular systolic dysfunction, are reviewed by Richard Gorlin in Chapter 15.

One area of remaining uncertainty is the role of ACE inhibitors during the early phase (0–24 hours) of acute myocardial infarction. This chapter will review the rationale for the use of ACE inhibitors during this early phase, the available clinical data, and make a recommendation based upon these data for their clinical use. The potential importance of early ACE inhibition can be seen from the fact that one-third to one-half of all deaths during the first month post infarction occur during the first or second day after admission to the hospital for myocardial infarction.[11,12] Efforts to further reduce this mortality are therefore justified. It should, however, be pointed out that despite numerous preclinical and clinical studies in over 75 000 patients in randomized trials of ACE inhibitors during the early phase of acute myocardial infarction that our understanding of the role of the renin–angiotensin–aldosterone system (RAAS) in the pathophysiology of acute myocardial infarction remains incomplete, as does our insight into the benefits and risks of blocking this system during the early phase of acute myocardial infarction.

Background for the Use of Early-Phase (0–24 hours) ACE Inhibitors in Acute Myocardial Infarction

Ventricular Remodeling

The process of ventricular remodeling in humans and its prevention by ACE inhibitors in experimental and clinical studies[13–18] have been reviewed by Gorlin.[10] It should however be emphasized that remodeling begins within the early hours of acute infarction.[13,19,20] Within the early hours after infarction there is expansion of the infarct zone due to slippage of myocytes.[21] Dilatation of the noninfarct zone occurs later, but much of the dilatation occurs in the early days after infarction. At 1 week post infarction left ventricular end systolic volume may be 80% above normal.[15] The degree of ventricular dilatation appears dependent upon infarct size and patency of the infarct-related artery.[16,22] The increase in myocardial wall stress as a result of ventricular dilatation has been thought to activate the plasma renin–angiotensin system.[23–25] More recent data suggest however that there may be local activation of the renin–angiotensin system in the noninfarcted remaining viable portion of the postinfarct ventricle.[26–28] This local increase in angiotensin II production has been shown to precede the changes in ventricular volume following infarction and may not be associated with an increase in serum angiotensin II levels.[28] An early local increase in angiotensin II through autocrine or paracrine mechanisms could play an important role in the development of compensatory left and right ventricular hypertrophy, vascular changes after infarction, subsequent pathophysiology, and natural history of the postinfarction patient.[29,30]

Neuroendocrine Changes

In a study of patients with acute myocardial infarction, at risk for ventricular dilatation, randomized to captopril or placebo 6–24 hours postinfarction, Ray et al. found that the concentration of renin and angiotensin II rose from admission to the third postinfarct day, even in the absence of diuretic therapy, which would tend to activate the RAAS.[31]

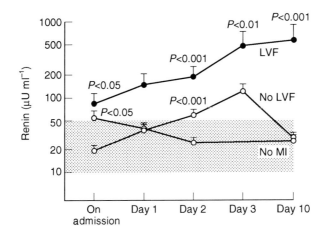

Figure 10.1 Changes in mean renin concentration post-infarction. (From Ref. 32.)

Plasma levels of norepinephrine and atrial natriuretic factor were also elevated. Captopril caused a rise in serum renin concentration and a significant decrease in angiotensin II levels confirming the effectiveness of the blockade of the ACE. There was however no effect on serum norepinephrine, atrial natriuretic factor, or vasopressin levels. Similar findings of a reduction in serum angiotensin II levels after administration of an ACE inhibitor in acute myocardial infarction have been seen by some but not all investigators.[32–36] In contrast to norepinephrine, which tends to be elevated during the earlier hours of onset of symptoms of acute myocardial infarction, angiotensin II levels tend to rise more gradually reaching a peak around 72 hours[32] (Figure 10.1). In patients with myocardial infarction and clinical evidence of heart failure angiotensin II levels may be elevated during the early hours of infarction and continue to increase from these levels reaching a peak at 72–96 hours.[32] The degree of activation of the RAAS in this phase of acute infarction is however variable[31–36] and may account for the variable degree of ACE inhibitor-induced hypotension during the early phase of myocardial infarction.

The importance of an increase in plasma and tissue angiotensin II levels during the early postinfarction phase relates to the finding that angiotensin II is an important mitogen, stimulating various growth factors such as platelet-derived growth factor and transforming growth factor β, which could play a role in the compensatory hypertrophy of the left and right ventricles as well as the hyperplasia of the infarct-related and other coronary vessels.[29,30,37] Angiotensin II causes the release of endothelin,[38] which depending upon pathophysiologic circumstances may cause coronary vasoconstriction. Angiotensin II is also an independent coronary and peripheral vasoconstrictor, which could increase preload, afterload, and myocardial oxygen demands. Angiotensin II has also been shown to cause the release of plasminogen activator inhibitor (PAI-1).[39] Increased levels of PAI-1 could impair intrinsic fibrinolysis and might therefore predispose to reocclusion after spontaneous or pharmacologically induced fibrinolysis. Angiotensin II has been suggested to play a role in the development of endothelial dysfunction.[40–42]

Angiotensin II also plays a role, along with aldosterone, in collagen production,[43,44] which is important both in scar healing and in the compensatory ventricular hypertrophy of the noninfarcted areas of myocardium. Aldosterone production, stimulated in part by angiotensin II, has recently been shown to cause a release of norepinephrine from the myocardium.[45] Similarly, angiotensin II itself may cause a release of norepinephrine from its nerve terminals.[46,47] These changes in norepinephrine concentration would be expected to predispose to an increase in myocardial oxygen demands, ischemia, ventricular arrhythmias, and possibly myocardial cell death. The importance of activation of the RAAS in situations with catecholamine release can be seen, for example, in a patient with pheochromocytoma.[48] In this patient with a pheochromocytoma an ACE inhibitor, but not a β-adrenergic receptor blocking agent, was shown to reduce catecholamine levels and the patient's symptoms. Treatment of pheochromocytoma with a β-blocker has been shown to be associated with worsening heart failure due to unopposed α-adrenergic stimulation.[49,50]

The Effect of ACE Inhibitors in Experimental Myocardial Infarction

In experimental studies ACE inhibitors as well as specific angiotensin II type I receptor antagonists have been shown to exert a beneficial hemodynamic effect when given in the early phase after infarction, as manifested by a significant decrease in left ventricular end-diastolic pressure and volume.[51] ACE inhibitors have also been shown to reduce experimental infarct size and reperfusion injury.[52–55] The reduction in infarct size has in part been attributed to ACE inhibitor-induced prevention of bradykinin degradation.[55] Bradykinin has a number of important effects that suggest it would have a beneficial effect during the acute phase of infarction and/or reperfusion. Bradykinin causes the stimulation of prostaglandins as well as the release of nitric oxide from the endothelium.[56] The demonstration that the beneficial effects of ACE inhibitors in limiting infarct size can in part be negated by the specific bradykinin antagonist HOE-140[55] supports the hypothesis that the beneficial effects of ACE inhibitors in acute myocardial infarction are due to bradykinin.

It may be premature to reach a final conclusion regarding the role of bradykinin in the beneficial effects on ACE inhibitors in infarction in humans. There are important species differences in bradykinin production, but more importantly bradykinin is an endothelial-dependent vasodilator.[57] Patients with coronary atherosclerosis as well as those with heart failure have been shown to have diffuse endothelial dysfunction.[58–61] Both angiographically abnormal as well as normal coronary vessels have been shown to exhibit endothelial dysfunction, in that they fail to show a vasodilator response to intracoronary acetylcholine while retaining a vasodilator response to nitroglycerin.[58] Bradykinin when administered directly into the coronary arteries of patients with angiographic evidence of coronary artery disease fails to cause coronary vasodilatation, whereas these vessels vasodilate in response to intracoronary nitroglycerin.[57] These observations suggest that in patients with coronary artery disease the effect of ACE inhibitor-induced bradykinin formation may not be as important as inferred from animal experiments. Endothelial dysfunction, may, however, not be diffuse in patients with coronary artery disease.[62] The response to intracoronary acetylcholine in patients with coronary artery disease is variable: some angiographically normal segments retain a vasodilator response to intracoronary acetylcholine while others do not.[62] One should therefore be hesitant to extrapolate the beneficial effects of ACE inhibitors on infarct size and reperfusion injury as well as the importance of ACE inhibitor-induced bradykinin formation in animal models of myocardial infarction to the clinical situation without further clinical confirmation.

ACE inhibitors have been shown to have a favorable effect on compensatory ventricular hypertrophy following experimental myocardial infarction or damage.[63] After experimental myocardial infarction there is a compensatory hypertrophy of the noninfarcted areas of the left ventricle as well as the right ventricle.[64] This hypertrophy has been shown to be associated with a reduction in coronary flow reserve.[64] McDonald et al. have shown that ACE inhibitors can prevent the development of ventricular hypertrophy of the remaining viable areas of the left ventricle as well as preventing ventricular dilatation following experimental myocardial damage.[63] Recent evidence suggests that the increase in ventricular hypertrophy may not be necessarily related to ventricular dilatation but may be due to local tissue angiotensin II formation and stimulation of myocardial and vascular growth factors.[28]

ACE inhibitors have been shown to prevent reperfusion arrhythmias during experimental myocardial infarction and reperfusion.[66–68] The decrease in reperfusion arrhythmias has been attributed in part to the effect of ACE inhibitors in preventing norepinephrine release,[67] prevention of ventricular dilatation, increase in bradykinin levels,[69] and in part to the antioxidant effects of SH-containing ACE inhibitors, such as captopril[70] although nonsulfhydryl ACE inhibitors have also been found to prevent ischemic and reperfusion-induced arrhythmias.[67] However, the effect of ACE inhibitors on ventricular arrhythmias in the major randomized studies in patients with acute myocardial infarction and chronic heart failure has been variable.[7–9]

Although experimental animal studies suggest a beneficial effect of ACE inhibitors in the acute phase of myocardial infarction there may also be some adverse effects that deserve comment. Patients with acute infarction and activation of the RAAS may be dependent upon angiotensin II-induced peripheral vasoconstriction. Administration of an ACE inhibitor under such circumstances could result in systemic hypotension, which could predispose to an increase in the extent of subendocardial ischemia, infarct size, and circulatory compensation resulting in more extensive myocardial damage. Of greater concern is the finding that angiotensin II and aldosterone are important for collagen formation[43,44] and that ACE inhibitors might interfere with scar formation and healing if administered during the early phase of acute myocardial infarction. Infarct scar healing has been suggested to be compromised when ACE inhibitors are given during the early hours of experimental infarction.[71] Interference with myocardial scar formation and healing could have important consequences on myocardial functional reserve, exercise, or stress-induced ventricular performance and long-term survival. It is possible that administration of an ACE inhibitor during the early phase of acute myocardial infarction, before collagen deposition and scar formation, could have a different effect than when administered during the convalescent phase, when scar formation is more complete but ventricular dilatation still progressive.

The Effects of ACE Inhibitors in Patients with Acute Myocardial Infarction

The effects of ACE inhibitors administered during the early phase (0–24 hours) from onset of symptoms of acute myocardial infarction have been explored in several small studies in which the majority of patients did not receive thrombolytic therapy[31,34,36,72–75] and in those that did.[33,76,77] The question of reperfusion therapy is of potential importance since it has been suggested that successful reperfusion and a patent infarct-related artery are important factors in limiting infarct expansion.[22,78] Since infarct expansion and ventricular remodeling as well as dilatation are important risk factors for death post infarction[10] it could be argued that ACE inhibitors might be less efficacious in patients undergoing successful reperfusion. However, pilot studies in patients with acute myocardial infarction who did, and those who did not, undergo reperfusion have for the most part shown that the administration of an ACE inhibitor such as captopril is effective in inhibiting the formation of angiotensin II and an increase in left ventricular end-diastolic volumes with a variable effect upon systemic blood pressure.[31,33,34] For the most part these pilot studies were carried out in patients with large or anterior myocardial infarctions,[31,33] with the assumption that the major benefit of ACE inhibitors would be the prevention of infarct expansion; and that the benefit of ACE inhibitors in the experimental studies and large randomized patient studies of acute infarction such as

SAVE[1] and AIRE,[2] where ACE inhibitors were administered during the convalescent phase of myocardial infarction (after the third day), could be further extended if given in the early phase of acute infarction.

Effect of ACE Inhibitors during the Acute Phase of Myocardial Infarction in Large-scale Placebo-controlled Randomized Studies

The CONSENSUS II trial

In the CONSENSUS II trial,[79] intravenous enalaprilat 1 mg or placebo was administered as an infusion to patients with acute myocardial infarction within 24 hours of onset of symptoms. This was followed by 2.5 mg on day 2, 5 mg on day 3 and then 10 mg, followed by 10 mg twice a day of enalapril or placebo. The mean time of administration of intravenous enalaprilat from onset of symptoms was 15 hours. Of patients in CONSEN-SUS II 57% underwent thrombolysis, and approximately 41% of patients had an anterior infarction. The trial was prematurely terminated after an enrollment of 6090 patients out of a planned 9000 patients because of the finding, given the data available at that time, that it was unlikely that enalapril would be found to have a significant beneficial effect, along with the likelihood that it was having a detrimental effect in some subsets such as elderly females.

The failure of enalapril to produce a beneficial effect in this study despite the previous beneficial effects of oral enalapril in patients with chronic heart failure,[7–9] the effects of ACE inhibition in experimental infarction,[80] and small pilot studies of patients with acute infarction[31,33] is not entirely clear. One explanation may relate to the use of intravenous enalaprilat. It was noticed that intravenous enalaprilat produced severe hypotension in some patients that could not be predicted by baseline parameters.[79] First-dose hypotension occurred in 10.5% of the enalapril-treated patients vs 2.5% of the placebo group; 25.3% of enalapril-treated patients had hypotension compared to 9.6% of placebo-treated patients ($P < 0.001$). The occurrence of hypotension was significantly associated with an adverse outcome in elderly females. The occurrence of hypotension could produce subendocardial ischemia and a coronary 'steal'. In patients with angina pectoris ACE inhibitors have in some instances exacerbated myocardial ischemia.[81] Experimental studies have suggested that in contrast to low doses of ACE inhibitors high doses[82] do not decrease experimental infarct size. Another explanation could be that, as shown in the neuroendocrine substudy of CONSENSUS II,[35] intravenous enalaprilat followed by the oral dosing regimen of 2.5 mg increasing to 10 mg b.i.d. by the fifth day, despite the significant reduction in plasma ACE activity, did not result in significant inhibition of angiotensin II formation over the first several days for the group as a whole compared to placebo, and only partially in those with a first myocardial infarction. It would appear that complete suppression of plasma angiotensin II formation was not achieved for the group as a whole despite the initial adverse effects of intravenous enalaprilat-induced hypotension.

An escape of aldosterone production despite suppression of plasma ACE activity during the early phase of acute myocardial infarction was noted by Borghi *et al.*[36] They noticed that while the ACE inhibitor zofinopril administered during the early hours of acute myocardial infarction almost completely blocked plasma ACE activity, aldosterone production was not completely inhibited. Paradoxically a further increase in the dose of zofinopril led to an increase in aldosterone production and blood pressure. They found that the increased dose of the ACE inhibitor stimulated plasma renin and angiotensin I levels. Under these circumstances a residual small but physiologically important amount of activity of ACE could have led to production of angiotensin II and aldosterone. An increase in angiotensin II and aldosterone production might also be due to non-ACE-dependent mechanisms. Angiotensin II can be produced within the ventricular myocardium and vascular wall independently of ACE by chymase-dependent mechanisms.[83] Aldosterone can also be produced independently of ACE-mediated angiotensin II formation in response to adrenocorticotropic hormone (ACTH), hypokalemia, hypomagnesemia, and other factors.[84,85] However, it is likely that the incomplete suppression of plasma levels of angiotensin II and aldosterone seen by Sigurdsson *et al.*[35] and Borghi *et al.*[36] are the result of residual ACE-dependent rather than non-ACE-dependent angiotensin II and aldosterone production. Production of angiotensin II and aldosterone despite an ACE inhibitor and partial suppression of plasma ACE activity could account for the variable results noted in some of the pilot studies of ACE inhibition during the early phase of acute myocardial infarction.[31,33,35,36]

The finding of suppression of angiotensin II levels during the early phase of an acute infarction by captopril[31,33] but not zofinopril[36] raises important issues as to the relative effectiveness of various ACE inhibitors in these circumstances. It has been suggested that the sulfhydryl-containing ACE inhibitors such as captopril might be more effective in preventing reperfusion injury and in improving recovery of ventricular function than nonsulfhydryl-containing ACE inhibitors such as enalapril.[70] Although there may be a benefit of sulfhydryl containing ACE inhibitors when used in the early phase of acute infarction and reperfusion, this is unlikely to be the entire or even the correct explanation since a nonsulfhydryl ACE inhibitor, lisinopril, has also been shown to be effective in reducing mortality when administered during the early phase of acute infarction.[86] More information is needed on the effective doses of various ACE inhibitors to suppress both plasma and tissue angiotensin II and aldosterone formation during the early phase of acute infarction, as well as a direct comparison of various ACE inhibitors, both sulfhydryl and nonsulfhydryl, during the early phase of acute infarction in humans before we can understand the failure of enalapril to result in a reduction in mortality in CONSENSUS II.[35]

Yet another explanation could relate to trial design in that intravenous enalapril was administered to all patients with infarcts regardless of extent. Previous studies[22] have shown that patients with modest to small infarcts do not undergo progressive left ventricular dilatation and their ventricular volume may actually decrease. One might therefore speculate that a portion of the patients, i.e. those with a large infarct and an increase in plasma angiotensin II levels, may have received some benefit from enalapril whereas in those with a relatively small infarct without elevation of plasma angiotensin II levels or the potential of infarct expansion that the possibly adverse effects of intravenous enalapril-induced hypotension and infarct healing may have outweighed the potential beneficial effects. Against this hypothesis was the finding in the CONSENSUS II trial that the results of enalapril administered to patients with Q-wave anterior infarction were not different from other types of infarctions.[35]

The ISIS-IV and GISSI-III trials

The available data do not allow a firm conclusion as to which if any of the above speculations are valid to explain the failure of enalapril to exert a beneficial effect when administered during the early phase of acute infarction in CONSENSUS II.[35] The role of ACE inhibitors in the early phase of acute infarction has, however, in part been clarified by the results of the large-scale ISIS-IV[86] and GISSI-III trials.[87] In the ISIS-IV trial,[86] 54 000 patients with acute infarction were administered oral captopril or placebo during the early phase of acute infarction. Approximately 70% of these patients underwent thrombolysis. As in the CONSENSUS II trial,[35] patients with both large and small infarcts were eligible for randomization. In the GISSI-III trial[87] the effects of oral lisinopril were studied in 40 000 patients during the early phase of acute infarction. As in the CONSEN-SUS II[35] and ISIS-IV[86] trials inclusion was not restricted to patients with evidence of a large infarct. The ISIS-IV study[86] found a small, statistically significant (6–7%) reduction in short-term 35-day mortality in patients randomized to oral captopril. A similar 11% significant reduction in 6-week mortality was found in patients randomized to oral lisinopril in the GISSI-III trial.[87] These results along with the results of a Chinese study,[88] as yet incompletely reported, the results of seven previous small randomized studies of early ACE inhibition in the acute phase of myocardial infarction, as well as the CONSENSUS II study,[35] have been included in a meta-analysis (H. White, personal communication) showing a $6 \pm 2\%$ statistically significant reduction in mortality in patients randomized to an ACE inhibitor during the early phase of acute infarction. There were 3563 deaths out of 47 404 patients (7.5%) in the control group compared to 3363 deaths out of 47 403 patients (7.1%) randomized to an ACE inhibitor ($2P = 0.01$). The test for heterogeneity failed to reveal a significant difference between the results of the various trials.

Although subgroup analysis is hazardous it appears that the benefits of ACE inhibitors in the ISIS-IV[86] and GISSI-III[87] studies tended to be greater in those with a previous infarct, evidence of heart failure, tachycardia, and an anterior location of their infarction. In the GISSI-III trial[87] lisinopril was significantly more effective in reducing mortality in patients who are randomized greater than 6 hours from onset of symptoms. Also of interest in the GISSI-III trial[87] was the finding that although nitrates alone were not significantly effective in reducing mortality during the acute phase of infarction, when added to lisinopril nitrates were more effective than lisinopril alone. In a previous small study by Hargreaves *et al.*[76] the administration of captopril and nitrates to patients undergoing thrombolysis was not associated with a reduction in ventricular volumes compared to placebo. The majority of the patients in this trial had inferior rather than an anterior infarction and the mean LVEF at the fifth week of follow-up was greater than 35% in the placebo as well as in the captopril and nitrate group. Nabel *et al.*[33] on the other hand gave intravenous captopril followed by oral captopril and noted a significant reduction in ventricular dilatation compared to placebo in patients with an acute anterior infarction receiving thrombolysis with tissue-type plasminogen activator (t-PA). In the ISIS-IV trial[86] captopril was effective both in patients undergoing thrombolysis and in those who did not, suggesting that ACE inhibition was beneficial despite the potential advantage of thrombolysis-induced patency of the infarct-related artery and prevention of ventricular dilatation. A more precise statement and speculation on the relative benefits of administration of ACE inhibitors during the acute phase of myocardial infarction must, however, await publication of detailed subgroup analyses derived from a meta-analysis of all ACE inhibitor trials during the acute phase of infarction.

In the ISIS-IV[86] and GISSI-III[87] trials the mortality curves of those assigned to ACE inhibitor or placebo diverged rather early and the 35-day or 6-week mortality was significantly reduced, whereas in the SAVE study,[1] carried out in patients all of whom had an LVEF <40%, the survival curves of those assigned to captopril or placebo after the third day did not diverge for almost 1 year. The early divergence of the mortality curves in ISIS-IV[86] and GISSI-III[87] suggest a beneficial effect of ACE inhibitors administered within the early phase of acute infarction. Although there was an early divergence of the mortality curves in the AIRE study,[2] in which patients with clinical evidence of heart failure were randomized to ramipril during the convalescent phase of acute infarction, this experience was only in a high-risk group while the SAVE patients[1] were in a moderate-risk group; in ISIS-IV[86] and GISSI-III[87] both low- and high-risk patients were included. To answer the question as to the exact timing of administration of an ACE inhibitor to patients with acute infarction will require prospective randomized studies in which patients with acute infarction are randomized to early administration of an ACE inhibitor or an ACE inhibitor administered during the convalescent stage (after 3 days).

Prospective trials designed to answer this question are currently underway and should provide an answer as to the necessity, benefits, and risk of early vs convalescent-phase administration of an ACE inhibitor in acute infarction.[89]

Current Recommendations for ACE Inhibitors in the Acute Phase of Myocardial Infarction

Given the available data what should be the recommendations for the administration of ACE inhibitors in acute myocardial infarction? Although the results of the ISIS-IV, GISSI-III, and meta-analysis of all randomized trials of ACE inhibitors administered during the early phase of acute infarction (0–24 hours) show a significant benefit in favor of ACE inhibition, the magnitude of this effect is relatively small. While acknowledging the hazards of subgroup analysis and extrapolations beyond that shown by the primary analysis and the likelihood that individual clinicians examining the data may reach different conclusions, the following recommendations concerning the use of ACE inhibitors during the early phase of acute infarction appear reasonable.

It has been demonstrated that ACE inhibitors, at least oral captopril and lisinopril,[86,87] can be safely administered to patients during the early phase of acute infarction. However, the current data in patients with or without thrombolytic therapy are not strong enough to mandate the use of oral ACE inhibitors in all patients with acute myocardial infarction at this time. Further data comparing the acute to convalescent phase administration of ACE inhibitors are necessary as well as long-term data on survival and ventricular function both at rest and during stress in patients receiving early vs convalescent-phase ACE inhibition, to rule out the possibility of any adverse effects of early administration of ACE inhibitors on scar formation and myocardial healing. Until further data are available from randomized studies of early vs convalescent-phase administration of ACE inhibitors, it would be reasonable to administer an oral ACE inhibitor such as captopril or lisinopril to patients at high risk of death during the early phase post infarction, such as those with a large infarct, history of a previous infarct, anterior Q-wave infarction, tachycardia, and those with clinical evidence of heart failure if hemodynamically stable over the first 6 hours, whether undergoing reperfusion therapy with a thrombolytic agent or not.

Interaction with Other Drugs

The available evidence suggests that the benefits of ACE inhibition in these patients is additive to that received from β-adrenergic receptor blockade and nitrates. The failure of nitrates alone to reduce mortality in ISIS-IV[86] and GISSI-III[87] suggests that factors other than ventricular remodeling may be important for the beneficial effects of ACE inhibitors when administered during the early phase of acute infarction. Since nitroglycerin has been shown to prevent experimental and clinical infarct expansion similar to that demonstrated for ACE inhibitors,[90] it can be postulated that the beneficial effects of ACE inhibitors during the early phase of acute infarction may relate to the direct effects of angiotensin II and/or bradykinin formation with subsequent prostaglandin stimulation on factors other than ventricular dilatation such as those reviewed above, including the effects on vascular and ventricular growth factors, catecholamine release, and fibrinolysis. Alternatively, it can be speculated that the added effects of nitrates when given with an ACE inhibitor during the acute phase of myocardial infarction might be due to an added effect of ventricular dilatation and possibly prevention of nitrate tolerance.[91]

The finding in the convalescent stage[1,2] and the acute phase[86] of myocardial infarction that the beneficial effects of ACE inhibitors are additive to those of β-adrenergic receptor blocking agents is of clinical importance. β-Adrenergic blocking agents have been shown to be of importance in the early phase of acute infarction in reducing mortality.[11] Although there have been as yet no prospective randomized studies in humans during the early phase of acute myocardial infarction in which the effectiveness of β-adrenergic receptor blockade alone, ACE inhibitors alone, or their combination have been systematically investigated, it would be reasonable based upon the available evidence to recommend that in patients with a large infarct, previous myocardial infarction, or tachycardia without clinical evidence of moderate or severe heart failure that an intravenous β-adrenergic blocking agent be administered on admission along with reperfusion therapy, if appropriate, and that if the patient remains hemodynamically stable over the first several hours that oral ACE inhibition be started, as in ISIS-IV[86] or GISSI-III.[87] Patients with clinical evidence of moderate or severe failure should receive an ACE inhibitor along with other appropriate therapy and an oral β-adrenergic blocking agent be considered during the convalescent stage if clinical evidence of heart failure is absent. Patients without an indication for acute-phase ACE inhibition as reviewed above might be treated with early β-adrenergic blockade, reperfusion therapy if appropriate, and considered for an ACE inhibitor in the convalescent phase of myocardial infarction if they are found to have an LVEF $\leqslant 40\%$.

The situation in regard to the concomitant use of aspirin or nonsteroidal antiinflammatory agents such as indomethacin is somewhat less clear. The beneficial effects of ACE inhibitors in experimental myocardial infarction have been suggested to be due, at least in part, to bradykinin-induced prostaglandin formation. In experimental studies, indomethacin but not L-NAME, an inhibitor of NO production, can block the beneficial effects of ACE inhibition.[92] Aspirin and nonsteroidal antiinflammatory agents have been shown to negate the arterial vasodilatation induced by ACE inhibitors and can cause sodium retention.[93,94] However, aspirin clearly has a beneficial effect in the early hours of acute infarction[12] and may promote spontaneous reperfusion and/or prevent reocclusion after thrombolysis. Until further data are available from prospective randomized studies aspirin should not be withheld from patients receiving ACE inhibitors during the early phase of acute infarction.

Once begun, ACE inhibitors should be continued indefinitely in patients with evidence of persistent left ventricular systolic dysfunction and an LVEF $<35-40\%$. In patients with recovery of ventricular function, such as those with an LVEF $>40\%$ during the late convalescent phase of infarction, as a result of recovery of stunning and/or hibernation, the value of long-term use of an ACE inhibitor is uncertain and might be stopped after the first year. This recommendation is, however, subject to change depending upon the results of ongoing studies of ACE inhibitors in patients with coronary artery disease and preserved left ventricular function (LVEF $\geqslant 40\%$) in whom the effects of ACE inhibitors on the development of progression of atherosclerosis is being evaluated.[95] Should these studies show that ACE inhibitors have a beneficial long-term effect in patients with small infarcts and preserved ventricular function, the above recommendations would need to be revised and further consideration given to the early and long-term use of ACE inhibitors in all patients with acute infarction.

The extrapolation of the results of ISIS-IV and GISSI-III with oral captopril and lisinopril to the use of other oral ACE inhibitors and dosing regimens is speculative. The difference in effects of various dosing regimens of ACE inhibitors to suppress angiotensin II and aldosterone,[31,33,35,36] and the uncertainty as to the clinical importance of tissue ACE activity and the relative effectiveness of different ACE inhibitors in suppressing tissue ACE activity, make it difficult to conclude that the effects of ACE inhibitors in ISIS-IV and GISSI-III are a class effect. Until further data are available on the effective dose of other ACE inhibitors during the early phase of acute infarction, the clinician would be wise to be cautious and not to extrapolate the results of ISIS-IV[86] and GISSI-III[87] obtained with captopril and lisinopril respectively, to other ACE inhibitors for which we do not have evidence for suppression of plasma angiotensin II or clinical effectiveness during the early phase of acute infarction.

Conclusions

Although over 100 000 patients have been studied in randomized trials of ACE inhibitors in acute myocardial infarction, it must be stated that we are only at the beginning rather than at the end of our understanding of their use. Many further questions need to be addressed, such as optimal timing of administration, dose, relative potency, effectiveness in various subsets such as those with large vs small infarcts, concomitant medications such as aspirin, the effects on spontaneous clot lysis, reocclusion after thrombolysis, and duration of therapy. Regardless of the outcome of these studies ACE inhibitors have earned an important place in the therapy of acute infarction and if cautiously and properly applied will result in the saving of many lives, as well as a reduction in the development and costs of the acute therapy of subsequent heart failure in these patients.

References

1. Pfeffer, M.A., Braunwald, E., Moye, L.A. *et al.* on behalf of the SAVE Investigators (1992) Effect of captopril on mortality and morbidity in patients with left ventricular dysfunction after myocardial infarction. Results of the Survival and Ventricular Enlargement Trial. *N. Eng. J. Med.*, **327**, 669–77.
2. The Acute Infarction Ramipril Efficacy (AIRE) Study Investigators (1993) Effect of ramipril on mortality and morbidity of survivors of acute myocardial infarction with clinical evidence of heart failure. *Lancet*, **342**, 812–28.
3. Pfeffer, J.M., Pfeffer, M.A., Mirsky, I. and Braunwald, E. (1982) Regression of left ventricular hypertrophy and prevention of left venticular dysfunction by captopril in the spontaneously hypertensive rat. *Proc. Nat. Acad. Sci. USA*, **79**, 3310–14.
4. Pfeffer, M.A., Lamas, G.A., Vaughan, D.E. *et al.* (1988) Effect of captopril on progressive ventricular dilatation after anterior myocardial infarction. *N. Engl. J. Med.*, **319**, 80–6.
5. Ertl, G., Gaudron, P., Eilles, C. and Kochsiek, K. (1991) Serial changes in left ventricular size after acute myocardial infarction. *Am. J. Cardiol.*, **68**, 116D–120D.
6. The SOLVD Investigators (1992) Effect of enalapril on mortality and the development of heart failure in asymptomatic patients with reduced left ventricular ejection fractions. *N. Engl. J. Med.*, **327**, 685–91.
7. The CONSENSUS Trial Study Group (1987) Effects on enalapril on mortality in severe congestive heart failure: results of the Cooperative North Scandanavian Enalapril Survival Study (CONSENSUS). *N. Engl. J. Med.*, **316**, 1429–35.
8. The SOLVD Investigators (1991) Effect of enalapril on survival in patients with reduced left ventricular ejection fractions and congestive heart failure. *N. Engl. J. Med.*, **325**, 293–302.
9. Cohn, J.N., Johnson, G., Ziesche, S. *et al.* (1991) A comparison of enalapril with hydralazine–isosorbide dinitrate in the treatment of chronic congestive heart failure. *N. Engl. J. Med.*, **324**, 303–10.
10. Gorlin, R. (1994) Late use of angiotensin converting enzyme inhibitors. In: Julian, D.G. and Braunwald, E. (eds) *Management of Acute Myocardial Infarction*, Ch. 15. London: W.B. Saunders.
11. ISIS-1 (First International Study of Infarct Survival) Collaborative Group (1986) Randomised trial of intravenous atenolol among 16 027 cases of suspected acute myocardial infarction: ISIS-1. *Lancet*, **ii**, 57–66.
12. ISIS-2 (Second International Study of Infarct Survival) Collaborative Group (1988) Randomised trial of intravenous streptokinase, oral aspirin, both, or neither among 17 187 cases of suspected acute myocardial infarction: ISIS-2. *Lancet*, **ii**, 349–60.
13. Eaton, L.W., Weiss, J.L., Bulkley, B.H. *et al.* (1979) Regional cardiac dilatation after acute myocardial infarction. Recognition by two-dimensional echocardiography. *N. Engl. J. Med.*, **300**, 57–62.
14. Erlebacher, J.A., Weiss, J.L., Seisfeldg, M.L. and Bulkley, B.H. (1984) Early dilatation of the infarcted segment in acute transmural myocardial infarction: Role of infarct expansion in acute left ventricular enlargement. *J. Am. Coll. Cardiol.*, **4**, 201–8.
15. Sharpe, N., Smith, H., Murphy, J. and Hannan, S. (1988) Treatment of patients with symptomless left ventricular dysfunction after myocardial infarction. *Lancet*, **i**, 256–9.

16. Pfeffer, M.A., Lamas, G.A., Vaughn, D.E. *et al.* (1988) Effect of captopril on progressive ventricular dilatation after anterior myocardial infarction. *N. Engl. J. Med.*, **319**, 80–6.
17. White, H.D. (1992) Remodelling of the heart after myocardial infarction. *Aust. NZ J. Med.*, **22**, 601–6.
18. Jugdutt, B.I. (1993) Prevention of ventricular remodelling post myocardial infarction: Timing and duration of therapy. *Can. J. Cardiol.*, **9**, 103–14.
19. Hutchins, G.M. and Bulkley, B.H. (1978) Infarct expansion versus extension: two different complications of acute myocardial infarction. *Am. J. Cardiol.*, **41**, 1127–32.
20. Kass, D.A., Maughan, L., Ciuffo, A. *et al.* (1988) Disproportionate epicardial dilatation after transmural infarction of the canine left ventricle: acute and chronic differences. *J. Am. Coll. Cardiol.*, **1**, 177–85.
21. Weisman, H.F., Bush, D.E., Mannisi, J.A. *et al.* (1988) Cellular mechanisms of myocardial infarct expansion. *Circulation*, **78**, 186–201.
22. Jeremy, R.W., Hackworthy, R.A., Bautovich, G. *et al.* (1987) Infarct artery perfusion and changes in left ventricular volume in the month after acute myocardial infarction. *J. Am. Coll. Cardiol.*, **9**, 989–95.
23. Rouleau, J.L., Moye, L.A., DeChamplain, J. *et al.* (1991) Activation of neurohumoral systems following acute myocardial infarction. *Am. J. Cardiol.*, **68**, D80–D86.
24. McAlpine, H.M., Morton, J.J., Leckie, B. *et al.* (1988) Neuroendocrine activation after acute myocardial infarction. *Br. Heart J.*, **60**, 117–24.
25. Vaughan, D.E., Lamas, G.E. and Pfeffer, M.A. (1990) Role of left ventricular dysfunction in selective neurohumoral activation in the recovery phase of anterior or wall acute myocardial infarction. *Am. J. Cardiol.*, **66**, 529–32.
26. Weinstock, J.V. (1986) The significance of angiotensin I converting enzyme in granulomatous inflammation: functions of ACE in granulomas. *Sarcoidosis*, **3**, 19–26.
27. Johnston, C.I., Mooser, V., Sun, Y. and Fabris, B. (1990) Changes in cardiac angiotensin converting enzyme after myocardial infarction and hypertrophy in rats. *Clin. Exp. Pharmacol. Physiol.*, **18**, 107–10.
28. Hirsch, A.T., Talsnecs, C.E., Schunkert, H. *et al.* (1991) Tissue specific activation of cardiac angiotensin converting enzyme in experimental heart failure. *Circ. Res.*, **69**, 475–82.
29. Johnston, C.I. (1994) Tissue angiotensin coverting enzyme in cardiac and vascular hypertrophy, repair, and remodeling. *Hypertension*, **23**, 258–68.
30. Dzau, V.J. (1993) Vascular renin–angiotensin system and vascular protection. *J. Cardiovasc. Pharmacol.*, **22**, S1–S9.
31. Ray, S.G., Pye, M., Oldroyd, K.G. *et al.* (1993) Early treatment with captopril after acute myocardial infarction. *Br. Heart J.*, **69**, 215–22.
32. McAlpine, H.M., Morton, J.J., Leckie, B. *et al.* (1988) Neuroendocrine activation after acute myocardial infarction. *Br. Heart J.*, **60**, 117–24.
33. Nabel, E.G., Topol, E.J., Galeana, A. *et al.* (1991) A randomized placebo-controlled trial of combined early intravenous captopril and recombinant tissue-type plasminogen activator therapy in acute myocardial infarction. *J. Am. Coll. Cardiol.*, **17**, 467–73.
34. Gonzalez-Fernandez, R.A., Altieri, P.I., Lugo, J.E. and Fernandez-Martinez, J. (1993) Effects of enalapril on ventricular volumes and neurohumoral status after inferior wall myocardial infarction. *Am. J. Med. Sci.*, **305**, 216–21.
35. Sigurdsson, A., Held, P., Swedberg, K. and Wall, B. (1993) Neurohormonal effects of early treatment with enalapril after acute myocardial infarction and the impact on left ventricular remodelling. *Eur. Heart J.*, **14**, 1110–17.
36. Borghi, C., Boschi, S., Ambrosioni, E. *et al.* (1993) Evidence of a partial escape of renin–angiotensin–aldosterone blockade in patients with acute myocardial infarction treated with ACE inhibitors. *J. Clin. Pharmacol.*, **33**, 40–5.
37. Dzau, V.J., Gibbons, G.H., Cooke, J.P. and Omoigui, N. (1993) Vascular biology and medicine in the 1990s: Scope, concepts, potentials, and perspectives. *Circulation*, **87**, 705–19.
38. Dohi, Y., Hahn, A.W.A., Boulanger, C.M. *et al.* (1992) Endothelin stimulated by angiotensin II augments contractility of spontaneously hypertensive rat resistance arteries. *Hypertension*, **19**, 131–7.
39. Ridker, P.R.M., Gaboury, C.L., Conlin, P.R. *et al.* (1993) Stimulation of plasminogen activator inhibitor *in vivo* by infusion of angiotensin II. Evidence of a potential interaction between the renin–angiotensin system and fibrinolytic function. *Circulation*, **87**, 1969–73.
40. Webb, R.C., Finta, K.M., Fisher, M. *et al.* (1992) Ramipril reverses impaired endothelium dependent relaxation in arteries of rabbit fed an atherogenic diet. *FASEB J.*, **6**, A1458.
41. Becker, R.H.A., Wiemer, G. and Linz, W. (1991) Preservation of endothelial function by ramipril in rabbits on a long-term atherogenic diet. *J. Cardiovasc. Pharmacol.*, **18**, (suppl. 2): S110–S115.
42. Bossaller, C., Auch-Schwelk, W., Gotze, S. *et al.* (1992) Die chronische Behandlung mit Enalapril fuhrt zu einer Zunahme der endohelabhangigen Relaxation. *Z. Kardiol.*, **81** (suppl. 1), 29.
43. Weber, K.T. and Brilla, C.G. (1991) Pathological hypertrophy and cardiac interstitium: Fibrosis and renin–angiotensin–aldosterone system. *Circulation*, **83**, 1849–65.
44. Weber, K.T. and Villareal, D. (1993) Aldosterone and antialdosterone therapy in congestive heart failure. *Am. J. Cardiol.*, **71**, 3A–11A.
45. Barr, C.S., Hanson, J., Kennedy, N. *et al.* (1993) The effect of a mineralocorticoid antagonist on myocardial mIBG uptake in congestive heart failure. *Circulation*, **88**, I-256.
46. Boadle, M.C., Hughes, J. and Roth, R.H. (1969) Angiotensin accelerates catecholamine biosynthesis in sympathetically innervated tissues. *Nature*, **222**, 987–8.
47. Starke, K. (1971) Action of angiotensin on uptake, release, and metabolism of ^{14}C-NE by isolated rabbit hearts. *Eur. J. Pharmacol.*, **14**, 112–23.

48. Salathe, M., Weiss, P. and Ritz, R. (1992) Rapid reversal of heart failure in a patient with phaeochromocytoma and catecholamine-induced cardiomyopathy who was treated with captopril. *Br. Heart J.*, **68**, 527–8.

49. Sloand, E.M. and Thompson, B.T. (1984) Propranolol-induced pulmonary edema and shock in a patient with phaeochromocytoma. *Arch. Intern. Med.*, **144**, 173–4.

50. Wark, J.D. and Larkins, R.G. (1978) Pulmonary oedema after propranolol therapy in two cases of phaeochromocytoma. *BMJ*, **1**, 1395–6.

51. Raya, T.E., Fonken, S.J., Lee, R.W. *et al.* (1991) Hemodynamic effects of direct angiotensin II blockade compared to converting enzyme inhibition in rat model of heart failure. *Am. J. Hypertens.*, **4**, 334S–340S.

52. Ertl, G., Kloner, R.A., Alexander, R.W. and Braunwald, E. (1982) Limitation of experimental infarct size by angiotensin converting enzyme inhibitor. *Circulation*, **65**, 40–8.

53. Ertl, G., Alexander, R.W. and Kloner, R.A. (1983) Interactions between coronary occlusion and the renin–angiotensin system in the dog. *Basic Res. Cardiol.*, **78**, 518–33.

54. DeGraeff, P.A., van Gilst, W.H., Bel, K. *et al.* (1987) Concentration dependent protection by captopril against myocardial damage during ischemia and reperfusion in a closed-chest pig model. *J. Cardiovasc. Pharmacol.*, **9** (suppl. 2): S37–S42.

55. Martorara, P.A., Kettenbach, B., Breipohl, G. *et al.* (1990) Reduction of infarct size by local angiotensin-converting enzyme inhibition is abolished by a bradykinin antagonist. *Eur. J. Pharmacol.*, **182**, 395–6.

56. Weiner, G., Scholkens, B.A., Becker, R.H. and Busse, R. (1991) Ramiprilat enhances endothelial autocoid formation by inhibiting breakdown of endothelium-derived bradykinin. *Hypertension*, **18**, 558–63.

57. Wafflenbeul, W., Bassenge, E. and Lichtlen, P. (1989) Konkurrenz zwischen endothelabhangiger und nitroglycerin-induzierter koronarer vasodilatation. *Z. Kardiol.*, **78** (suppl. 2), 45–7.

58. Werns, S.W., Walton, J.A., Hsia, H.H. *et al.* (1989) Evidence of endothelial dysfunction in angiographically normal coronary arteries of patients with coronary artery disease. *Circulation*, **79**, 287–91.

59. Zeiher, A.M., Drexler, S., Saurbier, B. and Just, H. (1993) Endothelium-mediated coronary blood flow modulation in humans: effects of age, atherosclerosis, hypercholesterolemia, and hypertension. *J. Clin. Invest.*, **92**, 652–62.

60. Creager, M.C., Cooke, J.P., Mendelsohn, M.E. *et al.* (1990) Impaired vasodilation of forearm resistance vessels in hypercholesterolemic humans. *J. Clin. Invest.*, **86**, 228–34.

61. Drexler, H., Hayoz, D., Munzel, T. *et al.* (1993) Endothelial function in congestive heart failure. *Am. Heart J.*, **126**, 761–74.

62. El-Tamimi, H., Mansour, M., Wargovich, T.J. *et al.* (1994) Segmental constrictor and dilator responses to intracoronary acetycholine in patients with coronary artery disease. *J. Am. Coll. Cardiol.*, **23**, 200A.

63. McDonald, K.M., Carlye, P.F., Matthews, J. *et al.* (1990) Early ventricular remodelling after myocardial damage and its attenuation by converting enzyme inhibition. *Trans. Assoc. Am. Physicians*, **103**, 229–35.

64. Karam, R., Healy, B.P. and Wicker, P. (1990) Coronary reserve is depressed in postmyocardial infarction reactive cardiac hypertrophy. *Circulation*, **81**, 238–46.

65. Gerasimou, E.M., Rigling, R.C. and Keller, A.M. (1994) Compensatory hypertrophy in humans following extensive myocardial infarction is discordant with changes in left ventricular volume. *J. Am. Coll. Cardiol.*, **23**, 413A.

66. De Graeff, P.A., van Gilst W.H. and de Langen, C.D.J. (1986) Concentration-dependent protection by captopril against ischemia–reperfusion injury in the isolated rat heart. *Arch. Int. Pharmacodyn.*, **280**, 181–93.

67. Van Gilst, W.H., deGraeff, P.A. and Wesseling, H. (1986) Reduction of perfusion arrhythmias in the ischemic isolated rat heart by angiotensin converting enzyme inhibitors: A comparison of captopril, enalapril, and HOE 498. *J. Cardiovasc. Pharmacol.*, **8**, 722–8.

68. Rochette, L., Ribuot, C., Belichard, P. *et al.* (1987) Protective effect of angiotensin converting enzyme inhibitors (CEI): Captopril and perindopril on vulnerability to ventricular fibrillation during myocardial ischemia and reperfusion in rat. *Clin. Exp. Hypertens.*, **9**, 365–8.

69. Scholkens, B.A., Linz, W. and Konig, W. (1988) Effects of the angiotensin converting enzyme inhibitor, ramipril, in isolated ischemic rat heart are abolished by a bradykinin antagonist. *J. Hypertens.*, **6**, S25–S28.

70. Westlin, W. and Mullane, K. (1988) Does captopril attenuate reperfusion-induced myocardial dysfunction by scavenging free radicals? *Circulation*, **77** (suppl. I), I-30–I-34.

71. Zdrojewski, T., Gaudron, P., Whittaker, P. *et al.* (1994) Divergent effects of ACE-inhibition on hemodynamics and scar healing after myocardial infarction in spontaneously hypertensive rats. *J. Am. Coll. Cardiol.*, **412A**, 958–87.

72. McAlpine, H.M., Morton, J.J., Leckie, B. *et al.* (1987) Haemodynamic effects of captopril in acute left ventricular failure complicating acute myocardial infarction. *J. Cardiovasc. Pharmacol.*, **9** (suppl. 2), 525–30.

73. Mattioli, G., Ricci, S., Rigo, R. *et al.* (1986) Effects of captopril in heart failure complicating acute myocardial infarction and persistence of acute haemodynamic effects in chronic heart failure after three years of treatment. *Postgrad. Med. J.*, **62** (suppl. 1), 164–6.

74. Wenting, G.J., Man in't Veld, Woittiez, A.J. *et al.* (1983) Effects of captopril in acute and chronic heart failure. *Br. Heart J.*, **49**, 65–76.

75. Oldroyd, K.G., Pye, M., Ray, S.G. *et al.* (1991) Effects of early captopril administration on infarct expansion left ventricular remodelling and exercise capacity after acute myocardial infarction. *Am. J. Cardiol.*, **68**, 304–10.

76. Hargreaves, A.D., Kolettis, T., Jacob, A.J. *et al.* (1992) Early vasodilator treatment in myocardial infarction: appropriate for the majority or minority? *Br. Heart J.*, **68**, 369–73.

77. Pipilis, A., Flather, M., Collins, R. *et al.* (1993) Hemodynamic effects of captopril and isosorbide mononitrate started early in acute myocardial infarction: a randomized placebo-controlled study. *J. Am. Coll. Cardiol.*, **22**, 73–9.

78. White, H.D., Cross, D.B., Elliott, J.M. *et al.* (1994) Long-term prognostic importance of patency of the infarct-related coronary artery after thrombolytic therapy for acute myocardial infarction. *Circulation*, **89**, 61–7.

79. Swedberg, K., Held, P., Kjekshus, J. *et al.* on behalf of the CONSENSUS II Study Group (1992) Effects of the early administration of enalapril on mortality in patients with acute myocardial infarction. Results of the cooperative new Scandanavian enalapril survival study II (CONSENSUS II). *N. Engl. J. Med.*, **327**, 678–84.

80. Pfeffer, M.A. and Pfeffer, J.M. (1987) Ventricular enlargement and reduced survival after myocardial infarction. *Circulation*, **75**, (suppl. IV): 93–7.

81. Cleland, J.G., Henderson, E., McLenachan, J. *et al.* (1991) Effect of captopril, an angiotensin-converting enzyme inhibitor, in patients with angina pectoris and heart failure. *J. Am. Coll. Cardiol.*, **17**, 733–9.

82. Daniell, H.G., Carson, R.R., Ballard, K.D. *et al.* (1984) Effects of captopril on limiting infarct size in conscious dogs. *J. Cardiovasc. Pharmacol.*, **6**, 1043–7.

83. Kinoshita, A., Urata, H., Bumpus, F.M. and Husain, A. (1993) Measurement of angiotensin I converting enzyme inhibition in the heart. *Circ. Res.*, **73**, 51–60.

84. Husain, A. (1993) The chymase–angiotensin system in humans. *J. Hypertens.*, **11**, 1155–9.

85. Dzau, V.J. (1992) Vascular renin angiotensin pathways: A new therapeutic target. *J. Cardiovasc. Pharmacol.*, **10** (suppl. 7), S13–S26.

86. ISIS Collaborative Group (1993) ISIS-IV: Randomized study of oral captopril in over 50 000 patients with suspected acute myocardial infarction. *Circulation*, **88**, I-394.

87. Gruppo Italiano per lo studio della sopravvivenza nell 'Infarto Miocardico (1994) GISSI-3: Effects of lisinopril and transdermal glyceryl trinitrate singly and together on 6-week mortality and ventricular function after acute myocardial infarction. *Lancet*, **343**, 1115–22.

88. Chinese ACEI-AMI Clinical Trial Collaborative Group (1992) Effects of captopril on the early mortality and complications in patients with AMI (Pilot Study). *J. Am. Coll. Cardiol.*, **19**, 380A.

89. Pfeffer, M.A. (1994) Angiotensin-converting enzyme inhibition use in myocardial infarction: Current perspective. *Am. J. Cardiol.* (in press).

90. Jugdutt, B.I. (1993) Prevention of ventricular remodelling post myocardial infarction: timing and duration of therapy. *Can. J. Cardiol.*, **9**, 103–14.

91. Katz, R.J., Levy, W.S., Buff, L. and Wasserman, A.G. (1991) Prevention of nitrate tolerance with angiotensin converting enzyme inhibitors. *Circulation*, **18**, 1271–7.

92. Ehring, T., Baumgart, D., Krajcar, M. *et al.* (1994) Attenuation of myocardial stunning by the ACE-inhibitor ramiprilat through a signal cascade of bradykinin and prostaglandins, but not NO. *J. Am. Coll. Cardiol.*, **23**, 199A.

93. Nishimura, A., Kubo, S., Ueyama, M. *et al.* (1989) Peripheral hemodynamic effects of captopril in patients with congestive heart failure. *Am. Heart J.*, **17**, 100–5.

94. Chennavasin, P., Seiwell, R. and Brater, D.C. (1980) Pharmacokinetic–dynamic analysis of the indomethacin–furosemide interaction in man. *J. Pharmacol. Exp. Ther.*, **215**, 77–81.

95. Texter, M., Lees, R.S., Pitt, B. *et al.* (1993) The Quinipril ischemic event trial (QUIET) design and methods: Evaluation of chronic ACE inhibitor therapy after coronary artery intervention. *Cardiovasc. Drugs Ther.*, **7**, 273–82.

11

Management of Cardiogenic Shock

J. S. Hochman and T. LeJemtel

Even in the thrombolytic era, left ventricular systolic dysfunction remains a frequent and serious complication of acute myocardial infarction (MI).[1] Indeed, left ventricular systolic dysfunction leads to left ventricular enlargement, which is the strongest predictor of mortality in patients with MI. Cardiogenic shock and congestive heart failure are the clinical manifestations of left ventricular dysfunction. Overall, the immediate prognosis of patients with left ventricular dysfunction and acute MI depends on the severity of the hemodynamic abnormality[2] (see Figure 2.6, p. 43) which, in turn, reflects the amount of myocardial necrosis.

Background and Significance

Cardiogenic shock represents the most frequent mode of death for patients who are hospitalized with acute MI.[3] Based on a 7% incidence of cardiogenic shock in acute MI and a mortality of 80%, 42 000 deaths are due each year to cardiogenic shock in the USA. The mortality rate remained constant in a study of cardiogenic shock complicating acute MI in the Worcester community from 1975 to 1988[4] when all mechanisms of cardiogenic shock, including mechanical complications were included (Figure 11.1a). The overall in-hospital mortality was 70% in a recent prospective multicenter registry of cardiogenic shock (early 1990s), which also included mechanical causes of shock.[5]

Definition

Cardiogenic shock is characterized by systemic hypotension with end-organ hypoperfusion despite adequate ventricular filling pressures. Shock results from a profound reduction in the cardiac output due to either left or right ventricular dysfunction or mechanical complications (see section on Pathophysiology). Two subsets of cardiogenic shock have been defined:[3] (1) mild shock with a low cardiac index (CI) and elevated end-diastolic filling pressures without frank hypotension; and (2) frank cardiogenic shock with reduced CI, elevated ventricular filling pressures and systemic hypotension, systolic pressure <90 mmHg. Most clinical trials and studies of cardiogenic shock adhere to the latter definition. It is important to note that several reports of cardiogenic shock lack hemodynamic confirmation of elevated pulmonary capillary wedge pressure (PCWP) and depressed CI and rely on hypotension to define shock. Varying definitions, lack of definitions and lack of confirmation of all the criteria for the diagnosis of cardiogenic shock confound this literature.

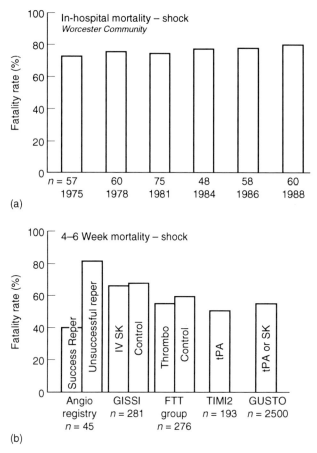

Figure 11.1   (a) The mortality (fatality) rates for cardiogenic shock in the Worcester community appear constant over the 13-year period ending in 1988. Only 7.6% of shock patients received thrombolytics, 7.5% intraaortic balloon pump (IABP), 1.7% percutaneous transluminal coronary angioplasty (PTCA) and 1.1% coronary artery bypass graft (CABG). From Ref. 4 with permission. (b) More recent mortality (fatality) rates in the thrombolytic era (see text for discussion).
Reper, reperfusion; SK, streptokinase; Thrombo, thrombolytic; tPA, tissue-type plasminogen activator.

Incidence

Among patients with MI, the incidence of cardiogenic shock from 1965 to 1970 in a single center was 15–19%.[6,7] The Multicenter Investigation of Limitation of Infarct Size (MILIS) study reported that 7.1% of 845 patients ≤76 years old with acute MI developed cardiogenic shock after hospitalization.[8] The study was in the prethrombolytic period from 1979 to 1983. This incidence does not include those presenting in shock, which is typically 1.5–2.5% of MI patients, and is further underestimated by an upper age limit of 75 years in MILIS. The incidence of shock in the Worcester, Massachusetts community[4] was reported to be constant at approximately 7.5% from 1976 to 1988. Thrombolytic therapy was administered in only 14% of all MI patients[4] during that period.

The incidence of cardiogenic shock diagnosed in the 41 299-patient International Study of Infarct Survival 3 trial (ISIS 3) in 1990, in which all patients received a thrombolytic, was 7%.[9] The rate of development of cardiogenic shock was not significantly different in patients treated with tissue plasminogen activator (tPA) (6.8%), streptokinase (7.1%) and

Table 11.1 Effect of thrombolysis on development of delayed[a] cardiogenic shock

Reference	Thrombolytic (%)	Heparin (%)	P value
APSAC Multicenter Trial Group[12]			
≤24 hours post MI	6.0	7.4	NS
>24 hours post MI	3.2	9.5	0.031
ASSET Study Group[13]	3.8	5.1	<0.05

[a]Shock that develops after hospital presentation
MI, myocardial infarction.

anisoylated streptokinase plasminogen activator complex (APSAC) (7.1%). The Thrombolysis in Myocardial Infarction 2 Study (TIMI 2), which had an upper age limit of 75 years and used tPA and more aggressive anticoagulation with full intravenous heparin, reported cardiogenic shock in 5.1%.[10] The 41 000-patient Global Use of Strategies to Open Occluded Arteries in Acute Coronary Syndromes (GUSTO) trial had an overall incidence of cardiogenic shock of 6.1%.[11] Interestingly, patients treated with front-loaded tPA developed cardiogenic shock less often than those treated with SK (5.1% vs 6.6%, P < 0.05). Two randomized trials of thrombolytics vs heparin alone[12,13] offer the best controlled data on the impact of thrombolytics on the development of cardiogenic shock (Table 11.1). In the first 24 hours in the APSAC Multicenter Trial Group,[12] the incidence of shock was similar in the groups treated with APSAC and heparin alone (6.0% vs 7.4%). However, after the first day, the APSAC-treated group had a significantly lower incidence of cardiogenic shock (3.2% vs 9.5%, P = 0.031). In the ASSET trial,[13] cardiogenic shock developed in 3.8% of the tPA group and 5.1% of the heparin group (P < 0.05).

These data suggest that the incidence of cardiogenic shock *may* have declined over the past 20 years, before thrombolytics and again after thrombolytics. However, the Worcester community study is the only one that specifically examined the incidence of cardiogenic shock, mostly in the prethrombolytic period, in the same community over time with constant criteria for the diagnosis of cardiogenic shock. The randomized trials demonstrating a lower incidence of cardiogenic shock for patients receiving thrombolytic therapy, and possibly even lower with more aggressive lytic and anticoagulation strategies, appear convincing and encouraging.

Patient Profile

The mean age of patients with cardiogenic shock in the Worcester series was significantly older than those without cardiogenic shock (71.4 vs 66.5 years, P < 0.001).[4] A similar finding was reported in the MILIS study (61.4 ± 1.1 vs 56.5 ± 0.4 years, P = 0.0003).[8] Interestingly, women are disproportionately represented among cardiogenic shock patients.[4,7,8,11] The Worcester series reported that 38% of patients without shock were women in contrast to 49% of patients with shock (P < 0.001). In the MILIS study, 38% of patients with shock were women vs 26% of patients without shock (P = 0.04). In GUSTO, similar rates were observed: 37% of patients with shock were women vs 24% of patients without shock (P < 0.001).[11] The SHOCK registry[5] also reported that a large proportion of the cardiogenic shock patients were women (43%) and they were only 3 years older, on average, than the men. Women are disproportionately represented among patients with cardiac rupture, mitral regurgitation (MR) and ventricular septal defect (VSD).[14–16] The pathophysiologic basis for this needs further exploration.

Patients with cardiogenic shock in the Worcester series more frequently had prior MI (43% vs 33%, $P < 0.001$) and Q-wave MI (70% vs 57%, $P < 0.001$) than those without shock.[4] The MILIS study also reported more prior MI in the shock group (39% vs 22%, $P = 0.003$), but similar rates of Q-wave MI.[8] Both studies reported significantly higher peak creatine kinase (CK) in the shock patients as evidence for larger infarcts. Most series[5,7,11,17] reported a similar frequency (50%) of anterior and nonanterior location of MI for patients with cardiogenic shock. This is in contrast to MILIS, which reported that 80% of patients with cardiogenic shock had anterior MI. This percentage was significantly higher than the 65% of patients without shock in MILIS who had anterior MI ($P = 0.03$). Independent predictors for the development of cardiogenic shock in MILIS were age >65 years, left ventricular ejection fraction (LVEF) <35%, peak MB-CK >160 iu l^{-1}, diabetes and prior MI.[8] Patients with all five risk factors had a 54% probability of developing cardiogenic shock.

Pathophysiology

Cardiogenic shock can result from severe left ventricular dysfunction (LV shock), severe right ventricular dysfunction (RV shock) or 'mechanical complications', including papillary muscle infarct with or without rupture of a chord or head of the papillary muscle resulting in severe MR, rupture of the interventricular septum, and cardiac tamponade due to a hemorrhagic effusion with or without cardiac rupture. Right ventricular infarction is discussed in Chapter 14 and mechanical complications are discussed in Chapter 12.

Early shock

Cardiogenic shock can develop early in the course of an acute MI, but it is present on hospital presentation in only 10–30% of patients who develop cardiogenic shock.[6,11] In the prethrombolytic era, the MILIS study reported that when cardiogenic shock developed *after* hospitalization, it was diagnosed ≥24 hours after admission in 50% of the patients (Figure 11.2). In the thrombolytic era, the TIMI 2 trial reported that cardiogenic shock was diagnosed on admission in 25% of all patients who developed shock.[10] In the recent large GUSTO trial of three thrombolytic regimens, only 10% of the patients

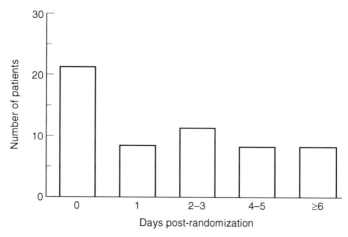

Figure 11.2   Time from randomization into the MILIS study to the onset of in-hospital cardiogenic shock. (From Ref. 8 with permission.)

ultimately diagnosed with cardiogenic shock were in shock on hospital presentation.[11] In patients without prior myocardial damage, the development of cardiogenic shock within hours of the onset of symptoms indicates that a very large amount of myocardium has been damaged.[18,19] This results from total occlusion of a coronary artery supplying a large risk region with no appreciable collateral flow. Multivessel disease is frequently present.[19–22] Autopsies of patients with cardiogenic shock due to acute MI have consistently shown that at least 40% of the total left ventricular mass is infarcted.[18,19] Clinically, this is reflected by marked elevation of CPK values.[4,8]

As discussed above, prior MI is a common finding in cardiogenic shock patients, with an incidence of approximately 40%.[4,8] In patients with prior myocardial damage and borderline left ventricular function, even a small to moderate size MI can lead to severe left ventricular decompensation and cardiogenic shock. A downward spiral of low output leading to increasing myocardial ischemia further compromises myocardial blood flow and thereby promotes myocardial damage and refractory cardiogenic shock.[23,24]

Late shock

The exact cascade of events leading to the development of cardiogenic shock several hours to days after the onset of acute MI is not fully understood. The previously mentioned downward spiral of compromised left ventricular performance due to regional myocardial dysfunction, infarct expansion, increased left ventricular volume, reduction of coronary perfusion pressure, decreased myocardial perfusion, further myocardial ischemia and necrosis is important. Complex and interdependent changes occur in the infarcted and uninfarcted remote myocardium as well as the culprit and nonculprit coronary arteries. Acute infarct expansion and acute left ventricular aneurysm formation have been associated with hemodynamic deterioration.[25,26] Paradoxic systolic bulging of the expanded infarct results in a mechanical disadvantage.[27,28] Additionally, expansion promotes acute left ventricular dilatation, which results in increased wall stress in the uninfarcted as well as infarcted zones. Increased wall stress in the setting of multivessel disease leads to the rapid development of ischemia in the uninfarcted zone and global left ventricular dysfunction. This is further exacerbated by resultant coronary hypoperfusion from hypotension and an elevated left ventricular end-diastolic pressure.[28,29] The resulting reduction in the coronary perfusion pressure gradient contributes to the intensification of ischemia and the hemodynamic deterioration seen in patients with infarct expansion.

Interestingly, even in a model of single-vessel coronary artery disease where coronary flow to the uninfarcted myocardium is demonstrated to be normal, metabolic and functional abnormalities can be demonstrated.[28–30] Hypercontractility of the uninfarcted zone supplied by a normal coronary artery rapidly occurs after remote coronary ligation, and persists over a period of time. However, the ability to maintain hypercontractility is lost over time and this is associated with metabolic changes, which include preferential utilization of glucose over fatty acids, loss of Krebs cycle intermediates, and depletion of substances needed for ATP production and utilization.[28,29] These remote myocardial functional and metabolic abnormalities are intensified when a stenosis, even mild, is present in a nonculprit coronary artery. Failure of initial hypercontractility and a progressive fall in segmental shortening of the uninfarcted zone and decreased stroke work index was demonstrated by Beyersorf *et al.*[28] in a model of mild circumflex stenosis with total left anterior descending coronary artery occlusion. These authors postulate that 'cardiogenic shock ensues when remote muscle fails to develop and maintain the compensatory hypercontractility needed to sustain systemic blood flow'. Hypokinesis of the uninfarcted zones was more frequently observed by two-dimensional echocardiography in patients with cardiogenic shock than in patients with similar infarct sizes without cardiogenic shock.[31]

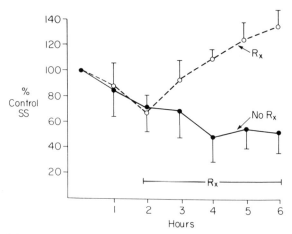

Figure 11.3 Segmental shortening (SS) in remote myocardium during left anterior descending coronary artery (LAD) occlusion and circumflex stenosis. Note: (1) progressive hypocontractility of remote muscle (circumflex distribution) during the first 2 hours of observation; (2) progressive decline in contractility in dogs receiving no treatment (no Rx, solid line); and (3) progressive improvement while intravenous substrate infusion was delivered (hatched line). Substrate infusion contains glutamate, aspartate, glucose, insulin, potassium, coenzyme Q and 2-mercapto-propionyl-glycine. Treatment (Rx) was administered over 4 hours. SE, standard error. (From Ref. 29 with permission.)

Glutamate- and aspartate-enriched solutions also containing coenzyme Q and a sulfhydryl donor have been shown experimentally to improve the functional and metabolic abnormalities in the uninfarcted myocardium in a model of multivessel disease[29] (Figure 11.3). Prior attempts to improve outcome with glucose/potassium/insulin in acute MI were disappointing.[32] However, when combined with reperfusion and/or mechanical circulatory support this approach may be promising for patients with cardiogenic shock. Similarly, although agents that reduce reperfusion injury experimentally[33] have not been demonstrated to benefit patients when used for acute MI, they may be of benefit in the cardiogenic shock subgroup where even a small amount of myocardial salvage instead of further injury may be critical. Clinical promise for substrate-enriched perfusion is discussed in the section on coronary artery bypass graft surgery (CABG).

Infarct extension can occur in the subepicardial and lateral borders of the myocardium at risk by reocclusion of a previously recanalized culprit coronary artery or by propagation of intracoronary clot with new branch occlusion. Both are more likely to occur in the presence of reduced coronary perfusion pressure and flow. Infarct extension may also supervene in a territory distant from the myocardium initially at risk. This can occur due to thrombosis on a critical coronary lesion in the setting of low coronary blood flow and hypercoagulability, to increased metabolic demands secondary to left ventricular dilatation and tachycardia, or merely to the coronary hypoperfusion discussed above. Progressive myocardial damage documented by continuous release of CPK-MB in the circulation of patients who develop cardiogenic shock within 48 hours of admission for acute MI strongly argues that progressive necrosis leads to critical cardiac impairment in patients with late cardiogenic shock.[34] Pathologic examination frequently reveals varying ages of infarction, with extension of necrosis.[18,19] The MILIS study documented reinfarction or infarct extension in 23.3% of 60 patients who developed shock in hospital in contrast to 7.4% in those without shock ($P < 0.0001$).[8] Their criteria for reinfarction were very strict, as extension was only diagnosed by reelevation of CPK-MB $\geq$48 hours after onset of MI; therefore this estimate is conservative. Data from the recent GUSTO trial also demonstrate that recurrence of MI and/or ischemia is more frequent in patients with cardiogenic shock than without cardiogenic shock (29.3% vs 6.1%, $P < 0.05$).[11]

The mechanisms previously discussed are pertinent to the development of shock beginning with a regional myocardial infarct. Global subendocardial infarction/ischemia without acute total occlusion of a culprit vessel can also occur, for example in the presence of left main or critical three-vessel disease, resulting in cardiogenic shock. In the SHOCK registry, 14% of patients with cardiogenic shock had ST depression, nonspecific ST changes or old left bundle branch block with a lack of ST elevation or Q waves.[5] The Worcester community series reported that 30% of patients with shock did not have a Q-wave MI.[4]

In view of the heterogeneity of the pathophysiology of cardiogenic shock complicating acute MI, a uniform therapeutic approach to the management of patients with shock is unlikely to be consistently successfully.

Diagnostic Testing

Once cardiogenic shock is suspected, a fluid challenge is warranted in patients without pulmonary congestion. Right heart catheterization is necessary to confirm the clinical diagnosis of cardiogenic shock or intravascular depletion. The diagnosis of the etiology of cardiogenic shock is critical to management. Cardiogenic shock due to right ventricular MI can be distinguished from shock due to left ventricular systolic dysfunction by documenting elevated (post fluid challenge) right atrial pressure and low PCWP with a low cardiac index. VSD can be diagnosed by a step-up in oxygen saturation from right atrium to right ventricle, and MR suggested but not proven[35] by a large V wave in the PCWP.

Equalization of diastolic pressures usually suggests a diagnosis of tamponade, but similar findings are sometimes fortuitously present in right ventricular MI.[36] Echocardiography with color flow Doppler is extremely useful in distinguishing these etiologies of cardiogenic shock[37] and may be obtained on an emergency basis to diagnose and distinguish among VSD, MR, left or right ventricular failure, and tamponade. However, it cannot assess the adequacy of the ventricular filling pressures, nor can it guide inotropic, vasopressor, and vasodilator therapy.

The indications for a coronary angiogram to assess the coronary anatomy in patients with left ventricular failure are discussed below in relation to the need for revascularization with percutaneous transluminal coronary angioplasty (PTCA) or CABG.

Interventions

General Measures

Metabolic conditions that develop due to severe ventricular dysfunction and systemic hypoperfusion, such as hypoxemia and lactic acidosis, can cause further contractile depression. Correction of hypoxemia, which frequently requires intubation and mechanical ventilation, is extremely important. Hyperventilation may be required to compensate for a metabolic acidosis.

Aspirin, which reduces mortality and reinfarction in acute MI, should be administered routinely, although its efficacy has not been tested in cardiogenic shock. Full heparinization is indicated[3] to reduce the risk of left ventricular thrombus, deep vein thrombosis, and coronary artery thrombus formation/propagation in the setting of low flow, stasis, and hypercoagulability.

Pharmacologic Circulatory Support

Treatment of patients with cardiogenic shock has traditionally focused on support of the systemic circulation with pharmacologic agents, such as inotropes and/or vasopressors. Reversing hypotension with vasopressors (i.e. norepinephrine) leads to improved myocardial perfusion and oxygenation,[38] but mortality is unchanged. Dopamine is most commonly used for inotropic therapy and, in higher doses, to reverse hypotension. Of course, increasing systemic vascular resistance further when it is elevated initially in shock limits improvement in cardiac output[38] and increases cardiac work. Therefore enthusiasm developed for mechanical support devices.

More mild cases of shock, with low CI and high PCWP without frank hypotension, can be managed by vasodilator therapy to improve left ventricular performance.[39] Nitroprusside alone resulted in hemodynamic improvement in patients with cardiogenic shock and mean systemic arterial pressure above 80 mmHg. The use of an arterial vasodilator alone is often limited by systemic hypotension. Agents that produce positive inotropy and vasodilatation, like dobutamine, are frequently used for severe left ventricular systolic dysfunction.

Vasopressors remain the mainstay of first-line temporary therapy to reverse hypotension and maintain vital organ perfusion. Augmentation of coronary perfusion may be extremely important for the success of reperfusion therapies (see below).

Mechanical Circulatory Support

Mechanical devices aimed at supporting the systemic circulation have the major theoretic advantage over pharmacologic agents of being able to improve coronary perfusion and cardiac performance while reducing myocardial ischemia and cardiac work.

Intraaortic balloon pump

Characteristics. Inflation and deflation of an intraaortic balloon pump synchronized with the cardiac cycle results in diastolic blood flow augmentation in the coronary and systemic circulation as well as reduction of afterload and aortic impedance.[40,41] Both mechanisms tend to increase CI and diastolic pressure.[38,42,43] Assessment of myocardial metabolism during intraaortic balloon counterpulsation (IABC) has documented an improvement in lactate extraction and reduction in myocardial oxygen requirements.[38] Such metabolic benefits were not documented during positive inotropic and vasopressor therapy.[38]

Nontrial data. Shortly after it was made clinically available, IABC appeared in nonrandomized studies to lower mortality when compared to historic controls.[44,45] IABC was reported to reverse the shock state. However, many patients became dependent on IABC and died with or without CABG.[42,43]

Trial data. A large cooperative trial was carried out by Scheidt et al.[46] to determine the efficacy of IABC in patients with refractory cardiogenic shock complicating MI. This trial, in the prethrombolytic era, specifically selected patients who were refractory to vasopressor therapy, with persistent systolic blood pressure less than 80 mmHg, and evidence of end-organ hypoperfusion. Most of these patients, who were refractory to pharmacologic therapy, were initially improved by IABC as evidenced by an increase in CI despite a decrease in heart rate, while diastolic arterial pressure and urine flow increased (Figure 11.4). A high percentage of these patients in refractory cardiogenic shock demonstrated improvement of end-organ function (Table 11.2). This cooperative

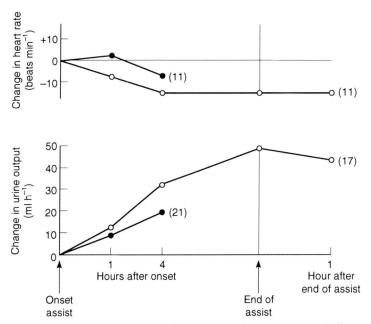

Figure 11.4 Changes in heart rate and urine output (as compared to baseline values before assistance) in patients who survived at least 4 hours of intraaortic balloon counterpulsation. The increase in urine flow is highly significant, although there is no difference in the response of patients who survived (open symbols) and those who died during assistance (closed symbols). Numbers in parenthesis indicate patients in subgroup. (From Ref. 46.)

Table 11.2 Clinical effects of intraaortic balloon counterpulsation in 87 patients

Abnormality before assistance	Patients with abnormality[a]	Improvement to normal during assistance[b]	
		No.	%
Oliguria (urine flow <20 ml hour^{-1}	46	32/46	70
Acidemia (arterial pH <7.35)	32	22/32	69
Cardiac arrhythmia	34	23/34	68
Need for pressor agents	59	38/59	64
Cold, clammy skin	48	28/48	58
Abnormal mental status	57	25/57	44
Need for antiarrhythmic agents	21	9/21	43
Pulmonary congestion	47	16/47	34

From Ref. 46 with permission.
[a]This column reports the number of patients with each abnormality before balloon pump assistance. It includes any patients with complete data before and after at least 1 hour of balloon assistance.
[b]Does not include patients who showed improvement but not completely to normal.

trial clearly demonstrated that patients could be initially stabilized and clinically improved with IABC, even when they had previously been refractory to pharmacologic therapy. A subgroup of patients underwent careful metabolic studies that demonstrated improved myocardial metabolism with reduced lactate production or improved extraction. Unfortunately, the in-hospital mortality was still 83%. In the absence of a control group, it is unknown whether this mortality was any different from patients with shock refractory to medical management who were not supported with IABC. However, it is clear that despite the early stabilization provided by IABC, the overall mortality was extremely high.

A small randomized trial of 30 patients with severe heart failure and cardiogenic shock demonstrated the same in-hospital survival for patients treated with IABP and for those who were not (50% vs 44%).[47] Despite initial enthusiasm for IABC to reduce mortality in cardiogenic shock, current trial data demonstrate that its use without reperfusion therapy, i.e. thrombolysis, PTCA or CABG, does not improve outcome.

Newer support devices

The usefulness of newer techniques that potentially can provide better circulatory support than IABC are currently being investigated.

Left ventricular and biventricular assist devices (LVAD) have been inserted in patients with cardiogenic shock complicating acute MI or CABG.[48] These devices provide a cardiac output ranging from 2.6 to $3.21min^{-1}m^{-2}$. Of six patients with the Norvacor LVAD,[49] three survived with cardiac transplantation. Total artificial hearts have been implanted in patients with cardiogenic shock of varied etiologies as a bridge to cardiac transplantation.[50,51]

Percutaneous cardiopulmonary bypass support has been carried out in patients with cardiogenic shock due to acute MI.[51,52] Shawl *et al.* reported on eight patients in whom support was initiated at an average of 4.4 hours after MI onset. Cardiac output was maintained at $2.2–5.21min^{-1}$ and PTCA was then performed. Seven of eight patients survived.[52] An extracorporeal membrane oxygenator has been used for cardiogenic shock of multiple etiologies, including one patient with acute MI who underwent CABG and died.[53]

The Hemopump is a motor-driven turbine that is placed percutaneously and advanced across the aortic valve retrogradely to the left ventricle. It ejects blood in a nonpulsatile manner, decompresses the left ventricle and can maintain cardiac outputs of up to $3.91min^{-1}$.[51,54] When compared experimentally to IABC in calves, visceral organ perfusion was significantly greater with the Hemopump than IABC.[55] Clinical evaluation, as with the other support devices, is limited. In spite of improvement in cardiac output and ability to perform PTCA with the device in place, patient outcome so far has been poor.[51,54]

In summary, limited information is available on the use of these newer devices to support the circulation in patients with cardiogenic shock complicating acute MI. Future investigation is needed to determine whether the promise of better circulatory support will improve outcome.

Coronary Artery Reperfusion/Revascularization

Early shock. Coronary blood flow to the infarct zone can be restored by pharmacologic coronary reperfusion with thrombolytics or by mechanical revascularization (PTCA or CABG). Both strategies have been proven extremely effective strategies for acute MI. However, the mechanisms that potentially mediate the benefits of restoring blood flow in the infarct-related artery are complex. When cardiogenic shock develops early after coronary occlusion, the region at risk is large and progressive necrosis and ischemia in the region result in severe left ventricular dysfunction. If blood flow can be restored, the wavefront of necrosis[56] is interrupted, and the ultimate infarct size is smaller. When stunned myocardium in the region at risk recovers function, the hemodynamic status of the patient can improve significantly. Potential complications of this strategy, in addition to the usual risks of thrombolysis, PTCA and emergency CABG, are the risks of reperfusion into a large area of infarction. Reperfusion arrhythmias, which are not a problem in uncomplicated MIs, may become a problem in patients with cardiogenic shock. Indeed, treatment of sustained ventricular tachycardia or fibrillation in the setting of hypoxemia, acidosis, severe left ventricular dysfunction, and coronary hypoperfusion is likely to be less successful than in patients with uncomplicated infarction.

Late shock. The pathophysiology of late cardiogenic shock involves multiple mechanisms and the potential benefit of reperfusion/revascularization includes mechanisms other than salvaging myocardium in the region at risk. Infarct expansion and early functional aneurysm formation contribute to the development of late shock. Restoring blood flow, even when the region at risk is no longer viable, can reduce the degree of infarct expansion and left ventricular remodeling.[57,58] The resulting improvement in infarct healing beneficially alters left ventricular remodeling. Additionally, late restoration of blood flow converts the type of injury from coagulation to contraction-band necrosis. This in turn results in immediate reduction in left ventricular size and reduced infarct thinning.[59-61] Decreased paradoxic bulging[27] of the infarcted zone and decreased wall stress in the noninfarcted myocardium improve global left ventricular mechanics. As noted above, abnormalities in the uninfarcted zone, in the presence of either multivessel disease or single-vessel disease, may also play a major role in the pathogenesis of late cardiogenic shock complicating acute MI.

If late shock is due to reinfarction with coronary reocclusion, either silent or clinically evident, restoring blood flow might exert the same benefits as previously reported in patients with early cardiogenic shock. For patients who have single-vessel disease with reinfarction/ischemia or those with multivessel disease with infarction or ischemia at a distance,[62] restoring blood flow potentially relieves ischemia and reverses the vicious cycle of hypoperfusion–ischemia described above.

Bengston *et al.*[17] reported on 200 patients with cardiogenic shock complicating acute MI screened from 1611 patients with acute MI who were entered in 1987 and 1988 in the Duke database. Regardless of whether infarct-artery patency was achieved spontaneously or with thrombolysis or mechanical intervention, it was the variable most highly correlated with in-hospital survival in a logistic regression model. The importance of an open infarct-related artery for acute MI patients not complicated by cardiogenic shock has been extensively demonstrated and is reviewed in Chapter 5.

Thrombolysis

Characteristics. Pharmacologic reperfusion of the infarct-related coronary artery with thrombolytics has markedly reduced mortality associated with MI (see Chapter 3). Early reperfusion reduces infarct size, improves left ventricular function and electrical stability, and lowers mortality. Late reperfusion also exerts beneficial effects on left ventricular remodeling and electrical stability.[63,64] Thrombolytic administration appears to have reduced the incidence of cardiogenic shock development, as discussed above.

Adjunctive therapy has been found to be extremely important for improving the efficacy of thrombolytics. The International Study of Infarct Survival 2 (ISIS 2) trial demonstrated that aspirin and streptokinase together had additive effects on reducing

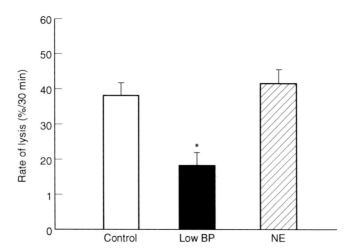

Figure 11.5 The effect of altered blood pressure on the rate of recombinant tissue-type plasminogen activator-induced coronary thrombolysis. Values expressed as mean value ± SE. (From Ref. 70 with permission.) NE, norepinephrine.

mortality.[65] Adjunctive antithrombotics such as heparin are similarly important, particularly for fibrin-specific lytic agents such as tPA.[66,67] Thrombolytic regimens that restore coronary blood flow rapidly appear to result in lower rates of cardiogenic shock than thrombolytic regimens that restore blood flow less rapidly. The front-loaded tPA regimen in the GUSTO study resulted in a lower incidence of cardiogenic shock than streptokinase (5.1% vs 6.6%, $P < 0.05$).[68] However, the ISIS 3 trial, which compared streptokinase, tPA and anisoylated streptokinase plasminogen activator complex (APSAC), reported that the rates of development of cardiogenic shock were similar.[9] This latter finding may be explained by a different tPA regimen with a 3-hour infusion and subcutaneous heparin. Newer thrombolytic agents and newer antithrombotic agents combined with thrombolytics are being investigated for acute MI, and may have particular relevance for the cardiogenic shock population. Improved rates of rapid successful reperfusion for patients presenting in cardiogenic shock may affect outcome. The shock state, with coronary hypoperfusion, poses a particular challenge to the efficacy of thrombolytics. Recanalization rates in shock patients are lower than in nonshock patients.[69] Experimentally, it has been demonstrated that reversing systemic hypotension with either vasopressors or intraaortic balloon counterpulsation significantly increases the rate and extent of thrombolytic-induced reperfusion[70,71] (Figure 11.5). Similarly, diastolic pressure augmentation with IABC enhanced thrombolysis in *non*hypotensive dogs.[72]

Observational data. The Society for Cardiac Angiography Registry of intracoronary streptokinase reported their experience with patients in cardiogenic shock. The recanalization rate for patients in shock was significantly lower than for patients who were in a stable hemodynamic state (43% vs 73%, $P < 0.0001$).[69] The mortality rate for patients in whom the infarct-related artery was recanalized with intracoronary streptokinase was significantly lower than that noted in patients with persistent artery occlusion (42% vs 84%, $P < 0.0005$). These results are very similar to the mortality rates reported for successful vs unsuccessful PTCA, as discussed below. It is appealing to conclude a cause-and-effect relationship, i.e. that opening the infarct-related artery resulted in a lower mortality. However, this was not a randomized trial. Patients in whom intracoronary streptokinase was successful at establishing recanalization were different, by definition, than patients in whom it was unsuccessful. This may be due to more severe coronary artery disease with more plaque and less thrombus, or due to less coronary blood flow and lower coronary perfusion pressure, reducing the efficacy of the thrombolytic in the patients who failed to undergo reperfusion.

Of interest is the relatively low mortality of patients with cardiogenic shock due to acute MI recently reported in two nonplacebo-controlled thrombolytic trials. The TIMI 2B trial, which used rtPA with an aggressive antithrombotic regimen of full intravenous heparin and aspirin, reported a 6-week mortality rate of 51% for patients with cardiogenic shock.[10] Unfortunately, the clinical diagnosis of shock was not confirmed by hemodynamic data in most patients. GUSTO recently reported a 30-day mortality of 55% for patients with shock.[11] The trial had no upper age limit, and all patients received thrombolytics, aspirin and heparin. Although, as described above, the different thrombolytic regimens appeared to result in different rates of development of cardiogenic shock, the 30-day mortality rates were similar for all thrombolytic strategies once shock was diagnosed.

It is unclear whether these relatively lower mortality rates in TIMI 2B and GUSTO compared to 'historic controls' reflect an impact of these combined thrombolytic anticoagulation regimens on mortality or result from case selection. The mortality rates in the Worcester community series, where 14% of all patients received thrombolytics, and the mortality rates in recent thrombolytic trials are shown in Figure 11.1a,b.

Case reports of successful thrombolysis for left main occlusion with cardiogenic shock[73,74] including an unpublished case of ours, and successful lysis for other culprit vessels (R. Prewitt, personal communication) demonstrate dramatic clinical improvement when reperfusion is established by lytics early after MI onset.

Randomized trial data. Controlled trials of thrombolysis have not been carried out in patients with acute MI and cardiogenic shock. Scarce data are available from the large placebo-controlled thrombolytic trials addressing specifically those patients who present in cardiogenic shock. The landmark GISSI trial[75] examined 11 806 patients randomly assigned to either intravenous streptokinase or placebo: 2.5% of the streptokinase-treated patients and 2.3% of the placebo-treated patients presented in Killip class 4. Therefore 281 patients with both ST elevation and ST depression MIs presenting in cardiogenic shock and treated ≤12 hours after MI onset were evaluated. Disappointingly, the mortality of the streptokinase-treated patients (69.9%) was not significantly different from that for patients receiving placebo (70.1%). The overall efficacy of streptokinase without aspirin in the GISSI trial was significantly less than in subsequent trials which used adjunctive aspirin.[65] The Fibrinolytic Therapy Trialist (FTT) Collaborative Group recently pooled data from the large placebo-controlled thrombolytic trials.[76] Although the presence of cardiogenic shock was not specifically reported on hospital presentation, patients with heart rate >100 beats min^{-1} and systolic blood pressure <100 mmHg on admission identified those with severe pump failure. Among this small group, seven lives were saved for every 100 patients treated with thrombolysis [(71/132 (54)% vs 88/144 (61)%)] (Figure 11.1b). It was noted by the FTT Collaborative Group that this absolute mortality reduction was larger than for other patient subgroups treated with thrombolytics.

Mechanical revascularization

Establishing coronary artery patency by mechanical interventions has been shown to be feasible in the setting of cardiogenic shock complicating acute MI. CABG, which restores blood flow to the infarct culprit artery as well as other stenosed vessels, has been performed.[17,43,45,77–91] PTCA of the infarct-related artery has also been used to restore coronary flow to the infarct zone.[51,91–103]

Coronary Artery Bypass Graft Surgery. In 1980 DeWood *et al.*[83] reported on mortality rates in two groups of patients with cardiogenic shock and acute MI: one underwent IABC and CABG and the other group underwent only IABC. Patients were not randomized, but treated according to the different practices of the two clinical groups managing acute MI patients. In-hospital mortality was similar in the two groups (52% vs 42%). Those operated on within 16 hours of MI onset had a lower long-term mortality than those not operated on (25% vs 71%, $P < 0.03$). Other nonrandomized series of CABG have also reported encouraging results compared to historic controls.[82,84–88]

Older nonrandomized reports of CABG with IABC support have not been encouraging.[43,45,78,82] Dunkman *et al.*[104] reported on 15 patients who were dependent of IABC and underwent CABG surgery. Six of the 15 patients (40%) survived the hospitalization. The failure of IABC to reverse cardiogenic shock predicted fatal outcome, whether or not CABG surgery was performed. Pooled data on CABG in cardiogenic shock reported by Bates and Topol[1] are updated and shown in Table 11.3.

Techniques of myocardial preservation during CABG surgery have improved dramatically over the past 20 years. Recently, specially developed cardioplegic solutions have been used with remarkable success. Beyersdorf *et al.* reported on the use of controlled reperfusion using amino acid-enriched (glutamate and aspartate) warm whole blood cardioplegic solution on total vented bypass in 14 patients with perioperative arrest who underwent CABG during arrest with cardiopulmonary resuscitation administered:[105] 13 patients had complete hemodynamic recovery with improved LVEF. Investigators at six institutions reviewed retrospectively their experience with 156 patients who underwent

Table 11.3 Coronary artery bypass graft surgery for cardiogenic shock complicating acute myocardial infarction

Reference	Year	No.	Mortality
Dunkham *et al.*[104]	1972	15	6 (40)
Mundth *et al.*[77]	1973	33	20 (61)
Miller *et al.*[78]	1974	12	7 (58)
Willerson *et al.*[43]	1975	3	2 (67)
Johnson *et al.*[79]	1977	5	3 (60)
Ehrich *et al.*[80]	1977	3	2 (67)
Bardet *et al.*[81]	1977	4	2 (50)
O'Rourke *et al.*[45]	1979	6	4 (67)
Subramanian *et al.*[82]	1980	20	6 (45)
DeWood *et al.*[83]	1980	19	8 (42)
Kirklin *et al.*[84]	1985	4	0 (0)
Phillips *et al.*[85]	1986	34	8 (24)
Laks *et al.*[86]	1986	50	15 (30)
Guyton *et al.*[87]	1987	9	2 (22)
Bolooki[88]	1989	7	3 (43)
Beyersdorf *et al.*[89]	1990	11	6 (55)
Bengston *et al.*[17]	1992	17	2 (12)
Allen *et al.*[90]	1993	66	6 (9)
Quigley *et al.*[a][91]	1993	5	4 (80)
Total		323	103/323 (32)

Modified from Ref. 1.
[a]Left main stenosis $\geq$75%.
Data represent patient numbers. Numbers in parentheses represent percentage.

Table 11.4 Coronary angioplasty for cardiogenic shock complicating acute myocardial infarction

Reference	No.	PTCA success rate	Mortality rate Total	Successful PTCA	Unsuccessful PTCA
O'Neill et al.[92]	27	24/27 (88)	8/27 (30)	6/24 (25)	2/3 (67)
Shani et al.[93]	9	6/9 (67)	3/9 (33)	NA NA	NA NA
Heuser et al.[94]	10	6/10 (60)	4/10 (30)	1/6 (17)	3/4 (75)
Brown et al.[95]	28	17/28 (61)	16/28 (57)	7/17 (42)	9/11 (82)
Laramee et al.[96]	39	33/39 (86)	16/39 (41)	NA NA	NA NA
Lee et al.[21]	24	13/24 (54)	12/24 (50)	3/13 (23)	9/11 (82)
Lee et al.[97]	69	49/69 (71)	31/69 (45)	15/49 (31)	16/20 (80)
Gacioch et al.[51]	25	18/25 (72)	11/25 (44)	4/18 (22)	7/7 (100)
Disler et al.[98]	7	5/7 (71)	4/7 (57)	2/5 (40)	2/2 (100)
Verna et al.[99]	7	7/7 (100)	1/7 (14)	1/7 (14)	0/0 (0)
Meyer et al.[100]	25	22/25 (88)	12/25 (47)	9/22 (41)	3/3 (100)
Hibbard et al.[20]	45	28/45 (62)	20/45 (44)	8/28 (29)	12/17 (71)
Moosvi et al.[22]	38	29/38 (76)	18/38 (47)	11/29 (38)	7/9 (78)
Eltchaninoff et al.[101]	33	25/33 (76)	12/33 (36)	6/25 (24)	6/8 (75)
Yamamoto et al.[102]	26	16/26 (62)	16/26 (62)	7/16 (44)	9/10 (90)
Seydoux et al.[103]	21	18/21 (85)	9/21 (43)	6/18 (33)	3/3 (100)
Total	433	316/433 (73)	193/433 (45)	86/277 (31)	88/108 (81)

Modified from Refs 1 and 106.
Data represent patient numbers. Numbers in parenthesis represent percents.
NA, not available.

surgically controlled reperfusion with this cardioplegic solution; 66 were preoperatively in cardiogenic shock[90] and only six of them (9%) died. These investigators compared this mortality rate for patients in cardiogenic shock to published reports of 'medically uncontrolled reperfusion' with PTCA in which 49 of 114 (43%) patients with preprocedure cardiogenic shock died. They concluded from these nonrandomized data that controlled surgical reperfusion with amino acid-enriched cardioplegic solution is superior to reperfusion with PTCA. Of course this comparison suffers from the same confounding problem present throughout the literature on cardiogenic shock, i.e. comparison of nonrandomized patients, which precludes conclusions about the relative efficacy of CABG vs PTCA or other therapies. Nevertheless, substrates used in the cardioplegic solution may play an important role in protecting ischemic myocardium and reducing reperfusion injury. Improved myocardial preservation with *complete* myocardial revascularization might be the optimal therapy for patients in cardiogenic shock complicating acute MI. With the inherent high risk of open heart surgery in this population, this hypothesis remains to be tested in a randomized trial.

Percutaneous Transluminal Coronary Angioplasty. The pooled data on PTCA for cardiogenic shock complicating acute MI were reviewed by O'Neill[106] and Bates and Topol,[1] and updated data are shown in Table 11.4. Two types of patient series, all retrospective, are reported.

1. All patients diagnosed with cardiogenic shock, whether or not they underwent cardiac catheterization were reviewed. The two groups consisted of patients with successful PTCA vs those who never had cardiac catheterization or PTCA combined with those with failed PTCA.[21,22] Patients who had successful angioplasty had consistently lower in-hospital mortality rates than those with failed angioplasty and those with no angioplasty.

2. All patients with cardiogenic shock in whom PTCA was performed were reviewed. Mortality for those with successful vs unsuccessful PTCA was compared.[92–103]

Lee et al.[21] observed a 50% 30-day survival overall with PTCA vs 17% in patients treated with conventional therapy; 77% survived with successful PTCA vs 18% with unsuccessful PTCA. In a retrospective analysis, Moosvi et al.[22] reported an in-hospital survival of 56% in 32 patients who underwent successful revascularization and a survival of 8% in 49 patients in whom PTCA was either unsuccessful or not performed. The difference in survival between the groups of patients was still present at 22 ± 15 months. In both studies,[21,22] patients in whom PTCA was unsuccessful or not attempted had a greater incidence of previous MI and left ventricular dysfunction as evidenced by increased use of digoxin and diuretic. These patients were less likely to receive IABC and dobutamine, and more likely to require vasopressors than patients who underwent successful PTCA. These different patient characteristics reflect more severe disease in the group not undergoing, or with unsuccessful, PTCA. These reports are distinctly different from other reports of emergency PTCA for cardiogenic shock in the *early* hours after MI. First, the time to cardiogenic shock onset following MI is late, even in those with successful PTCA (58 ± 83 hours;[22] 28 ± 30 hours[21]). Additionally PTCA was performed late (33 ± 66 hours;[22] 20 ± 32 hours[21]) after the onset of cardiogenic shock. In the report by Lee et al.[21] there was no clear relationship between time from MI to revascularization and outcome. This may reflect that PTCA was performed in a selected group, i.e. in patients who had already survived the acute shock state. In contrast, Moosvi et al. noted that PTCA was performed 12.4 ± 16 hours after shock onset in patients who survived and at 58 ± 93 hours in patients who died ($P < 0.05$).[22] As noted, even successful revascularization in survivors was performed in a relatively late time frame in relation to the index MI.

A multicenter retrospective registry of 69 patients undergoing PTCA for cardiogenic shock[98] reported that the improved survival rate noted at 30 days in patients with cardiogenic shock who had undergone an emergency PTCA was maintained for 24 months. The long-term survival rate was 54% for patients who had undergone immediate, successful PTCA and only 11% in patients in whom PTCA had been unsuccessful. In both groups of patients PTCA was attempted early after the diagnosis of cardiogenic shock, i.e. 4 and 5 hours median. Baseline characteristics were similar, except that CI in the unsuccessful group was $1.8 \pm 0.5\,l\,min^{-1}\,m^{-2}$ and $2.2 \pm 0.6\,l\,min^{-1}\,m^{-2}$ ($P = 0.05$) in the successful group. Hibbard et al. reported on the Mayo Clinic experience in 45 patients with cardiogenic shock complicating acute MI who underwent PTCA: 71% survived to hospital discharge when PTCA was successful, whereas 29% survived when it was unsuccessful.[20] The group with unsuccessful PTCA was older than the group with successful PTCA (67 ± 12 years vs 60 ± 11 years, $P = 0.055$). Those with unsuccessful PTCA in this study also had a higher incidence of prior MI (47% vs 18%, $P = 0.036$). A detailed assessment of the extent of coronary artery disease and morphologic features of the vessel undergoing PTCA was performed. Most patients had multivessel disease, and more extensive disease was demonstrated in the group with failed PTCA. Total occlusion of the infarct-related artery was present in 79% of patients, and the prevalence of total occlusion was similar for the groups with successful vs unsuccessful PTCA. Subtotal occlusion was present in an additional 19%. Thus 98% of patients had a total or subtotal occlusion. Of note, thrombolytic agents had been used as primary treatment in only 8 of 45 patients. Lesion characteristics known to affect the ease and success of PTCA were examined, such as the presence of calcium, tortuosity, bends, lesion length and presence of thrombus, and there were no differences between the groups with successful and unsuccessful PTCA. Although there was a trend for the elderly to have a lower PTCA success rate, 43% (6/14) of patients greater than 70 years old had successful PTCA. It

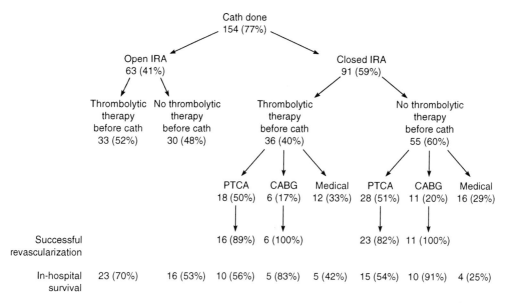

Figure 11.6 Interventions in 200 patients with cardiogenic shock after acute myocardial infarction. Percentages add to 100% across rows except for the bottom two rows, in which percentages are based on therapy received. CABG, coronary artery bypass graft surgery; Cath, cardiac catheterization; IRA, infarct-related artery; PTCA, percutaneous transluminal coronary angioplasty. (From Ref. 17 with permission.)

should be noted that the overall PTCA success rate in cardiogenic shock (73%, Table 11.4) is substantially lower than PTCA success rates when cardiogenic shock is not present.

In the nonrandomized Duke series[17] (Figure 11.6) patients found to have a closed infarct-related artery who underwent successful PTCA had an in-hospital survival of 55%. Those undergoing successful CABG had a remarkable survival of 88%. Patients with closed infarct-related artery who did not undergo revascularization had an in-hospital survival of 33%. Patients with open infarct-related artery after thrombolysis had an in-hospital survival of 70%. The 43 patients in whom cardiac catheterization was not attempted and the status of the infarct-related artery was thus unknown had an in-hospital survival of 16%. This is likely evidence of biased case selection for cardiac catheterization: clinicians can identify those with better prognosis and refer them to cardiac catheterization, and those who are most unstable die before they can undergo cardiac catheterization.

Verna *et al.* confirmed the apparent beneficial effect of immediate and successful PTCA in patients with cardiogenic shock.[99] In addition, these investigators documented immediate improvement in left ventricular performance, as evidenced by a rise in ejection fraction from 27% to 41%, a fall in left ventricular filling pressure from 26 to 18 mmHg, and a systemic systolic arterial pressure increase from 86 to 126 mmHg.[99] Yamamoto *et al.*[102] reported improvement in the CI within 24 hours in those patients with successful PTCA (1.9 ± 0.3 to $2.2 \pm 0.6 \, l \, min^{-1} \, m^{-2}$) and no improvement and significantly lower CI in those with failed PTCA (1.6 ± 0.5 to $1.6 \pm 0.7 \, l \, min^{-1} \, m^{-2}$). Of 18 patients with successful PTCA reported by Seydoux *et al.*,[103] seven patients had a rapid hemodynamic response and five had progressive improvement over 36 hours. All survivors had rapid and marked hemodynamic improvement. In another report, death could be predicted by persistence of a low CI at 12 hours after shock onset, independently of attempts at revascularization.[107]

To examine the spectrum of cardiogenic shock and the percentage of patients who are candidates for an invasive strategy with early revascularization, the first prospective study was recently performed.[5] Nineteen centers *prospectively* registered 251 patients with cardiogenic shock from January 1992 to April 1993. Cardiogenic shock was due to mechanical complication, i.e. VSD or MR, in 19 (8%), isolated right ventricular shock in 6 (2%) and associated with concurrent conditions contributing to the development of shock in 12 (5%). Electrocardiographic tracings revealed old left bundle branch block, ST depressions or nonspecific findings in 14% of patients. The in-hospital mortality was 70%. Patients who were not eligible for emergency revascularization, due to associated medical conditions and for cardiogenic shock of other etiology, had a higher mortality than those who were eligible for emergency revascularization (78% vs 64%, $P = 0.052$). Patients with isolated left ventricular failure who were clinically selected to undergo cardiac catheterization ($n = 120$) had significantly lower in-hospital mortality than those not selected to undergo cardiac catheterization ($n = 88$) (51% vs 85%). Patients not undergoing cardiac catheterization were significantly older (70 ± 12 vs 64 ± 11 years), less often had ST elevation/new left bundle branch block MIs (78% vs 94%) and less often received thrombolytics (33% vs 51%). The time to death/discharge was significantly shorter (2 days vs 11.5 days) in patients not undergoing cardiac catheterization. Age and mortality were significantly correlated. The difference in mortality between those selected and not selected to undergo cardiac catheterization remained significant after correcting for age. Remarkably, the outcome of patients who underwent cardiac catheterization was uniformly better than those who did not undergo cardiac catheterization, regardless of whether revascularization was performed within 24 hours of onset of cardiogenic shock or later, or not attempted. Selection bias is evident, with the most stable patients selected for cardiac catheterization. Age was a significant predictor of death in patients not undergoing early revascularization after the diagnosis of shock. However, no readily available clinical parameter that was associated with survival in patients who underwent early revascularization was discerned, including age, gender, thrombolysis, infarct location, time from MI onset to diagnosis of cardiogenic shock, and time from diagnosis of cardiogenic shock to revascularization.

Recent reports of primary PTCA for thrombolytic eligible patients early after MI onset have demonstrated promising results.[108–110] Patients with cardiogenic shock were either excluded or a very small number included. Their results cannot be extrapolated to shock as (1) the PTCA success rate in cardiogenic shock is lower, (2) the complications of the procedures in shock are greater, (3) multivessel coronary artery disease is most often observed in shock, and (4) most cardiogenic shock develops late after the onset of MI, and therefore PTCA is not performed early after symptom onset.

There are currently no published reports on the use of newer devices such as atherectomy, rotablater, transluminal extraction catheter, laser, and stents for cardiogenic shock. It is possible that these newer devices may improve the primary success rate of catheter intervention above the overall 73% success reported for cardiogenic shock.

Practical Implications, Indications and Contraindications

Five treatment regimens have been widely used in an attempt to reduce the mortality from cardiogenic shock: vasopressors, IABC, thrombolytics, PTCA and CABG. Although vasopressors and IABC alone can maintain coronary perfusion and in some cases postpone death, they do not reduce in-hospital mortality in patients with cardiogenic shock. They do, however, have an important role as adjunctive therapy to the newer, more promising pharmacologic reperfusion and mechanical revascularization strategies. Vasopressors (e.g. dopamine) should be administered immediately to reverse systemic hypotension in patients with cardiogenic shock.

IABC provides excellent initial support in patients with cardiogenic shock and frequently reverses the clinical and hemodynamic patterns of cardiogenic shock. Contraindications to IABC include significant peripheral vascular disease, as the catheter may compromise limb blood flow. The use of sheathless balloons and smaller balloon sizes is promising for reducing this complication. As discussed earlier, only a minority of patients in cardiogenic shock who undergo IABC will ultimately survive without other therapeutic interventions. IABC may allow recovery of stunned myocardium thereby improving left ventricular function and survival. IABC is commonly used for circulatory support in patients who are undergoing CABG surgery or PTCA for cardiogenic shock. With PTCA, not only is stabilization with IABC important for the procedure, but it may result in reduced acute closure after PTCA when used adjunctively.[111]

Thrombolysis alone appears to be of limited efficacy in patients with cardiogenic shock. However, by enhancing coronary perfusion pressure IABC may improve the efficacy of thrombolytic agents in patients with cardiogenic shock. Additionally, this circulatory support may be necessary to sustain patients long enough for stunned myocardium to recover.

The contraindications to thrombolytic therapy are related to the risks of bleeding. Because cardiogenic shock carries a dismal prognosis, only *absolute* contraindications, not relative ones, should preclude use of thrombolytics. Further evaluation is needed of aggressive thrombolytic and anticoagulation regimens combined with augmented systemic arterial pressure by IABC and vasopressors in patients with early cardiogenic shock and in patients who, after rethrombosis, develop late cardiogenic shock.

Some strategy of reperfusion/revascularization for patients with cardiogenic shock due to left ventricular failure is strongly advised whenever cardiogenic shock is diagnosed on presentation or with clinical reocclusion/reinfarction. When thrombolytics are used, they probably should be combined with vasopressors and IABC (inserted cautiously to reduce the risk of bleeding) to attempt to normalize coronary perfusion pressure and facilitate reperfusion.

The data from nonrandomized studies suggest that PTCA and CABG are very promising modalities for reducing mortality in cardiogenic shock complicating acute MI. Contraindications to revascularization with PTCA or CABG include the presence of other terminal conditions, or inadequate vascular access for coronary angiography. An international randomized trial (SHOCK) is currently ongoing to compare, in a prospective randomized fashion, mortality with either immediate direct revascularization with PTCA or CABG surgery to conventional therapy, including thrombolysis, IABC, and late revascularization when clinically indicated. If emergency mechanical revascularization for cardiogenic shock is shown to reduce mortality, the optimal mode of revascularization, i.e. PTCA vs CABG, will need to be better defined.

Pending results of randomized trials, patients should be individually selected for emergency coronary angiography and, based on the coronary anatomy and the experience and skills of the staff, undergo either PTCA or CABG.

The role of adjunctive therapy for myocardial preservation and reduction of reperfusion injury in patients with cardiogenic shock also need further investigation. The optimal device for temporary circulatory support also remains to be determined.

Acknowledgments

We gratefully acknowledge Chris Rembert and Joanne Cioffi for their expert secretarial assistance and Richard Fuchs MD for his thoughtful review of the manuscript.

References

1. Bates, E.R. and Topol, E.J. (1991) Limitations of thrombolytic therapy for acute myocardial infarction complicated by congestive heart failure and cardiogenic shock. *J. Am. Coll. Cardiol.*, **18**, 1077–84.

2. Forrester, J.S., Diamond, G., Chatterjee, K. and Swan, H.J.C. (1976) Medical therapy of acute myocardial infarction by application of hemodynamic subsets. *N. Engl. J. Med.*, **295**, 1356–62.
3. ACC/AHA Task Force Report (1990) Guidelines for the early management of patients with acute myocardial infarction. *J. Am. Coll. Cardiol.*, **16**, 249–92.
4. Goldberg, R.J., Gore, J.M., Alpert, J.S. *et al.* (1991) Cardiogenic shock after acute myocardial infarction. Incidence and mortality from a community-wide perspective, 1975 to 1988. *N. Engl. J. Med.*, **325**, 1117–22.
5. Hochman, J.S., Boland, J., Brinker, J. *et al.* for the SHOCK investigators. (1993) Current spectrum of cardiogenic shock and effect of early revascularization on mortality. Results of an international registry. *Circulation*, **88** (suppl. 4), 1357.
6. Killip, T. and Kimball, J.T. (1967) Treatment of myocardial infarction in a coronary care unit: A two-year experience with 250 patients. *Am. J. Cardiol.*, **20**, 457–64.
7. Scheidt, S., Ascheim, R., Killip III, T. (1970) Shock after acute myocardial infarction. A clinical and hemodynamic profile. *Am. J. Cardiol.*, **26**, 556–64.
8. Hands, M.E., Rutherford, J.D., Muller, J.E. *et al.* (1989) The in-hospital development of cardiogenic shock after myocardial infarction: Incidence, predictors of occurrence, outcome and prognostic factors. *J. Am. Coll. Cardiol.*, **14**, 40–6.
9. ISIS-3 Third International Study of Infarct Survival Collaborative Group (1992) A randomized comparison of streptokinase vs tissue plasminogen activator vs anistreplase and of aspirin plus heparin vs aspirin alone among 41 299 cases of suspected acute myocardial infarction. *Lancet*, **339**, 753–70.
10. Garrahy, P.J., Hazlowa, M.J., Forman, S. and Rogers, W.J. (1989) Has thrombolysis improved survival from cardiogenic shock? Thrombolysis in myocardial infarction (TIMI II) results (abstract). *Circulation Suppl.*, II-623.
11. Holmes, D.R. and Bates, E. for the GUSTO investigators (1993) Cardiogenic shock during myocardial infarction. The GUSTO experience with thrombolytic therapy (abstract). *Circulation*, **88**, I-25.
12. Meinertz, T., Kasper, W., Schumacher, M. and Just, H. for the APSAC Multicenter Trial Group (1988) The German multicenter trial of anisoylated plasminogen streptokinase activator complex versus heparin for acute myocardial infarction. *Am. J. Cardiol.*, **62**, 347–51.
13. Wilcox, R.G., Von Der Lippe, G., Olsson, C.G. *et al.* for the ASSET study group (1988) Trial of tissue plasminogen activator for mortality reduction in acute myocardial infarction. *Lancet*, **ii**, 525–30.
14. Montoya, A., McKeever, L., Scanlon, P. *et al.* (1980) Early repair of ventricular septal rupture after infarction. *Am. J. Cardiol.*, **45**, 345–8.
15. Shapira, I., Isakov, A., Burke, M. and Almong, C.H. (1987) Cardiac rupture in patients with acute myocardial infarction. *Chest*, **92**, 219–23.
16. Becker, A. and Van Mantgem, J.P. (1975) Cardiac tamponade; a study of 50 hearts. *Eur. J. Cardiol.*, **3/4**, 349–58.
17. Bengston, J.R., Kaplin, A.J., Pieper, K.S. *et al.* (1992) Prognosis in cardiogenic shock after acute myocardial infarction in the interventional era. *J. Am. Coll. Cardiol.*, **20**, 1482–9.
18. Page, D.L., Caulfield, J.B., Kastor, J.A. *et al.* (1971) Myocardial changes associated with cardiogenic shock. *N. Engl. J. Med.*, **285**, 133–7.
19. Alonso, D.R., Scheidt, S., Post, M. and Killip, T. (1973) Pathophysiology of cardiogenic shock: Quantification of myocardial necrosis. Clinical pathologic and electrocardiographic correlation. *Circulation*, **48**, 588–96.
20. Hibbard, M.D., Holmes, D.R., Bailey, K.R. *et al.* (1992) Percutaneous transluminal coronary angioplasty in patients with cardiogenic shock. *J. Am. Coll. Cardiol.*, **19**, 639–46.
21. Lee, L., Bates, E.R., Pitt, B. *et al.* (1988) Percutaneous transluminal coronary angioplasty improves survival in acute myocardial infarction complicated by cardiogenic shock. *Circulation*, **78**(6), 1345–51.
22. Moosvi, A.R., Khaja, F., Villaneuva, L. *et al.* (1992) Early revascularization improves survival in cardiogenic shock complicating acute myocardial infarction. *J. Am. Coll. Cardiol.*, **19**, 907–14.
23. Wigger, C.J. (1947) Myocardial depression in shock: Survey of cardiodynamic studies. *Am. Heart J.*, **33**, 633–50.
24. Pasternak, R.C., Braunwald, E. and Alpert, J.S. (1986) Acute myocardial infarction. In: Braunwald, E., Isselbacher, K.J., Petersdorf, R.G. *et al.* (eds) *Harrison's Principles of Internal Medicine*, pp. 986–93. New York: McGraw Hill.
25. Visser, C.A., Kan, G., Meltzer, R.S. *et al.* (1986) Incidence, timing and prognostic value of left ventricular aneurysm formation after myocardial infarction: A prospective serial echocardiographic study of 158 patients. *Am. J. Cardiol.*, **57**, 729.
26. Eaton, L.W., Weiss, J.L., Bulkley, B.H. *et al.* (1979) Regional cardiac dilatation after acute myocardial infarction: Recognition by two-dimensional echocardiography. *N. Engl. J. Med.*, **300**, 57.
27. Parmley, W.W., Chuck, L., Kivowitz, C. *et al.* (1973) *In vitro* length–tension relations of human ventricular aneurysms. Relation of stiffness to mechanical disadvantage. *Am. J. Cardiol.*, **32**, 889–94.
28. Beyersdorf, F., Acar, C., Buckberg, G.D. *et al.* (1989) Studies on prolonged acute regional ischemia: III. Early natural history of simulated single and multivessel disease with emphasis on remote myocardium. *J. Thorac. Cardiovasc. Surg.*, **98**, 368–80.
29. Beyersdorf, F., Acar, C., Buckberg, G.D. *et al.* (1989) Studies on prolonged acute regional ischemia: V. Metabolic support of remote myocardium during left ventricular power failure. *J. Thorac. Cardiovasc. Surg.*, **98**, 567–79.
30. Guth, B.D., White, F.C., Gallagher, K.P. and Bloor, C.M. (1984) Decreased systolic wall thickening in myocardium adjacent to ischemic zones in conscious swine during brief coronary artery occlusion. *Am. Heart J.*, **107**, 458–64.

31. Widimsky, P., Gregor, P., Cervenka *et al.* (1988) Severe diffuse hypokinesis of the remote myocardium – the main cause of cardiogenic shock? An echocardiographic study of 75 patients with extremely large myocardial infarctions. *Cor Vasa*, **30**(1), 27–34.

32. Rogers, W.J., Segall, P.H., McDaniel, H.G. *et al.* (1979) Prospective randomized trial of glucose–insulin–potassium in acute myocardial infarction. Effects on myocardial hemodynamics, substrates and rhythm. *Am. J. Cardiol*, **43**, 801–9.

33. Kloner, R.A. (1993) Does reperfusion injury exist in humans? *J. Am. Coll. Cardiol.*, **21**, 537–45.

34. Gutovitz, A.L., Sobel, B.E. and Roberts, R. (1978) Progressive nature of myocardial injury in selected patients with cardiogenic shock. *J. Am. Coll. Cardiol.*, **41**(3), 469–75.

35. Fuchs, R.M., Heuser, R.R., Yin, F.C. and Brinker, J.A. (1982) Limitations of pulmonary wedge V waves in diagnosing mitral regurgitation. *Am. J. Cardiol.*, **49**, 849–54.

36. Lorell, B., Leinbach, R.C., Pohost, G.M. *et al.* (1979) Right ventricular infarction. Clinical diagnosis and differentiation from cardiac tamponade and pericardial constriction. *Am. J. Cardiol.*, **43**, 465–71.

37. Eisenberg, P.R., Barzilai, B. and Perex, J.E. (1984) Noninvasive detection by Doppler echocardiography of combined ventricular septal rupture and mitral regurgitation in acute myocardial infarction. *J. Am. Coll. Cardiol.*, **4**, 617–20.

38. Mueller, H., Ayres, S.M., Giannelli, S. *et al.* (1971) Effect of isoproterenol, *l*-norepinephrine, and intraaortic counterpulsation on hemodynamics and myocardial metabolism in shock following acute myocardial infarction. *Circulation*, **XLV**, 335–51.

39. Chatterjee, K., Parmley, W.W., Ganz, W. *et al.* (1973) Hemodynamic and metabolic responses to vasodilator therapy in acute myocardial infarction. *Circulation*, **XLVIII**, 1183–93.

40. Fuchs, R.M., Brin, K.D., Brinker, J.A. *et al.* (1983) Augmentation of regional coronary blood flow by intra-aortic balloon counterpulsation in patients with unstable angina. *Circulation*, **68**, 117–23.

41. Weber, K.T. and Janick, J.S. (1974) Intraaortic balloon counterpulsation. *Ann. Thorac. Surg.*, **17**, 602.

42. Buckley, M.J., Leinbach, R.C., Kastor, J.A. *et al.* (1970) Hemodynamic evaluation of intra-aortic balloon pumping in man. *Circulation*, **XLI & XLII** (suppl. II), 130–4.

43. Willerson, J.T., Curry, G.C., Watson, J.T. *et al.* (1975) Intraaortic balloon counterpulsation in patients in cardiogenic shock, medically refractory left ventricular failure and/or recurrent ventricular tachycardia. *Am. J. Med.*, **58**, 183–91.

44. Kantrowitz, A., Krakauer, J.S., Rosenbaum, A. *et al.* (1969) Phase-shift balloon pumping in medically refractory cardiogenic shock. *Arch. Surg.*, **99**, 739–43.

45. O'Rourke, M.F., Sammel, N. and Chang, V.P. (1979) Arterial counterpulsation in severe refractory heart failure complicating acute myocardial infarction. *Br. Heart J.*, **41**, 308–16.

46. Scheidt, S., Wilner, G., Mueller, H. *et al.* (1973) Intra-aortic balloon counterpulsation in cardiogenic shock: Report of a cooperative clinical trial. *N. Engl. J. Med.*, **288**, 979–84.

47. O'Rourke, M.F., Norris, R.M., Campbell, T.J. *et al.* (1981) Randomized controlled trial of intraaortic balloon counterpulsation in early myocardial infarction with acute heart failure. *Am. J. Cardiol.*, **47**, 815–20.

48. Pennington, D.G., Kanter, K.R., McBride, L.R. *et al.* (1988) Seven year's experience with the Pierce–Donachy ventricular assist device. *J. Thorac. Cardiovasc. Surg.*, **96**, 901–11.

49. Portner, P.M., Oyer, P.E., Pennington, D.G. *et al.* (1989) Implantable electrical left ventricular assist system: Bridge to transplantation and future. *Ann. Thorac. Surg.*, **47**, 142–50.

50. Joyce, L.D., Johnson, K.E., Toninato, C.J. *et al.* (1989) Results of the first 100 patients who received symbion total artificial hearts as a bridge to cardiac transplantation. *Circulation*, **80** (suppl. III), 192–201.

51. Gacioch, G.M., Ellis, S.G., Lee, L. *et al.* (1992) Cardiogenic shock complicating acute myocardial infarction: The use of coronary angioplasty and the integration of the new support devices into patient management. *J. Am. Coll. Cardiol.*, **19**, 647–53.

52. Shawl, F.A., Domanski, M.J., Hernandez, T.J. and Punja, S. (1989) Emergency percutaneous cardiopulmonary bypass support in cardiogenic shock from acute myocardial infarction. *Am. J. Cardiol.*, **64**, 967–70.

53. Pennington, D.G., Merjavy, J.P., Cood, J.E. *et al.* (1984) Extracorporeal membrane oxygenation for patients with cardiogenic shock. *Circulation*, **70** (suppl. I), 130–7.

54. Lincoff, A.M., Popma, J.J., Bates E.R. *et al.* (1990) Successful coronary angioplasty in two patients with cardiogenic shock using the Nimbus Hemopump support device. *Am. Heart J.*, **120**, 970–2.

55. Baldwin, R.T., Radovancevic, B., Conger, J.L. *et al.* (1993) Peripheral organ perfusion augmentation during left ventricular failure. *Texas Heart Inst. J.*, **20**, 275–80.

56. Reimer, K.A. and Jennings R.B. (1979) The wavefront phenomenon of myocardial ischemic cell death. II. Transmural progression of necrosis within the framework of ischemic bed size (myocardium at risk) and collateral flow. *Lab. Invest.*, **40**, 633.

57. Hochman, J.S. and Choo, H. (1987) Limitation of myocardial infarct expansion by reperfusion independent of myocardial salvage. *Circulation*, **75**, 299–306.

58. Hale, S.L. and Kloner, R.A. (1988) Left ventricular topographic alterations in the completely healed rat infarct caused by early and late coronary artery reperfusion. *Am. Heart J.*, **116**, 1508–13.

59. Hahn, R., Brown, R., Mogtader, A. *et al.* (1993) Early benefits of late coronary reperfusion on reducing myocardial infarct expansion; echo findings and ultrastructural basis. *J. Am. Coll. Cardiol.*, **21**, 301A.

60. Kemper, F.T., Leavitt, M. and Parisi, A.F. (1988) Acute reduction in functional infarct expansion with late coronary reperfusion: Assessment with quantitative two-dimensional echocardiography. *J. Am. Coll. Cardiol.*, **11**, 192–200.

61. Brown, E.J., Swinford, R.D., Gadde, P. and Lillis, O. (1991) Acute effects of delayed reperfusion on myocardial infarct shape and left ventricular volume: A potential mechanism of additional benefits from thrombolysis therapy. *J. Am. Coll. Cardiol.*, **17**, 1641–50.
62. Schuster, E. and Bulkley, H.B. (1980) Ischemia at a distance after acute myocardial infarction: A cause of early post-infarction angina. *Circulation*, **62**, 3.
63. Steinberg, J.S., Hochman, J.S., Morgan, C.D. *et al.* (1993) The effects of thrombolytic therapy administered 6–24 hours after myocardial infarction on the signal-averaged ECG: Results of a multicenter randomized trial (abstract). *J. Am. Coll. Cardiol.*, **21**, 225A.
64. Kim, C.B. and Braunwald, E. (1993) Potential benefits of late reperfusion of infarcted myocardium: The open artery hypothesis. *Circulation*, **88**, 2426–36.
65. ISIS-2 (Second International Study of Infarct Survival) Collaborative Group (1988) Randomized trial of intravenous streptokinase, oral aspirin, both or neither among 17,187 cases of suspected acute myocardial infarction. *Lancet*, **ii**, 349–60.
66. Hsia, J., Hamilton, W.P., Kleinman, N. *et al.* (1990) The heparin–aspirin reperfusion trial (HART): A randomized trial of heparin versus aspirin adjunctive to tissue plasminogen activator-induced thrombolysis in acute myocardial infarction. *N. Engl. J. Med.*, **323**, 1433.
67. Bleich, S.D., Nichols, T., Schumacher, R. *et al.* (1989) The role of heparin following coronary thrombolysis with tissue plasminogen activator (t-PA). *Circulation*, **80** (suppl. II), 113.
68. The GUSTO Investigators (1993) An international randomized trial comparing four thrombolytic strategies for acute myocardial infarction. *N. Engl. J. Med.*, **329**, 673–82.
69. Kennedy, J.W., Gensini, G.C., Timmis, C.G. and Maynard C. (1985) Acute myocardial infarction treated with intracoronary streptokinase: A report of the society for cardiac angiography. *Am. J. Cardiol.*, **55**, 871–7.
70. Prewitt, R.M., Gu, S., Garber, P.J. and Ducas, J. (1992) Marked systemic hypotension depresses coronary thrombolysis induced by intracoronary administration of recombinant tissue-type plasminogen activator. *J. Am. Coll. Cardiol.*, **20**, 1626–33.
71. Prewitt, R.M., Gu Shian, Schick, U. and Ducas, J. (1994) Intraaortic balloon counterpulsation enhances coronary thrombolysis induced by intravenous administration of a thrombolytic agent. *J. Am. Coll. Cardiol.*, **23**, 791–8.
72. Gurbel, P.A., Anderson, R.D., MacCord, C.S. *et al.* (1994) Arterial diastolic pressure augmentation by intra-aortic balloon counterpulsation enhances the onset of coronary artery reperfusion by thrombolytic therapy. *Circulation*, **89**, 361–5.
73. Lew, A.S., Weiss, A.T., Shah, P.K. *et al.* (1984) Extensive myocardial salvage and reversal of cardiogenic shock after reperfusion of the left main coronary artery by intravenous streptokinase. *Am. J. Cardiol.*, **54**, 450–2.
74. Alosilla, C.E., Bell, W.W., Ferree, J. and Torre A.D.L. (1985) Thrombolytic therapy during acute myocardial infarction due to sudden occlusion of the left main coronary artery. *J. Am. Coll. Cardiol.*, **5**, 1253–6.
75. Gruppo Italiano per lo studio della streptokinasi nell'Infarto Micardico (GISSI) (1986) Effectiveness of intravenous thrombolytic treatment in acute myocardial infarction. *Lancet*, **i**, 397–401.
76. Fibrinolytic Therapy Trialists (FTT) Collaborative Group (1994) Indications for fibrinolytic therapy in suspected acute myocardial infarction: Collaborative overview of early mortality and major morbidity results from all randomized trials of more than 1000 patients. *Lancet*, **343**, 315–22.
77. Mundth, E.D., Buckley, M.J., Leinbach, R.C. *et al.* (1973) Surgical intervention for the complications of acute myocardial ischemia. *Ann. Surg.*, **178**, 379–88.
78. Miller, M.G., Weintraub, R.M., Hedley-Whyte, J. *et al.* (1974) Surgery for cardiogenic shock. *Lancet*, **i**, 1342–5.
79. Johnson, S.A., Scanlon, P.J., Loeb, H.S. *et al.* (1977) Treatment of cardiogenic shock in myocardial infarction by intra-aortic balloon counterpulsation and surgery. *Am. J. Med.*, **62**, 687–92.
80. Ehrich, D.A., Biddle, T.L., Kronenberg, M.W. and Yu, P.N. (1977) The hemodynamic reponse to intra-aortic balloon counterpulsation in patients with cardiogenic shock complicating acute myocardial infarction. *Am. Heart J.*, **93**, 274–9.
81. Bardet, J., Masquet, C., Kahn, J.C. *et al.* (1977) Clinical and hemodynamic results of intra-aortic balloon counterpul-sation and surgery for cardiogenic shock. *Am. Heart J.*, **93**, 280–8.
82. Subramanian, V.A., Roberts, A.J., Zema, M.J. *et al.* (1980) Cardiogenic shock following acute myocardial infarction: Late functional results after emergency cardiac surgery. *NY State J. Med.*, **80**, 947–52.
83. DeWood, M.A., Notske, R.N., Hensley, G.R. *et al.* (1980) Intra-aortic balloon counterpulsation with and without reperfusion for myocardial infarction shock. *Circulation*, **61**, 1105–12.
84. Kirklin, J.K., Blackstone, E.H., Zorn, G.L. Jr *et al.* (1985) Intermediate-term results of coronary artery bypass grafting for acute myocardial infarction. *Circulation*, **71** (suppl.II), 175–8.
85. Phillips, S.J., Zeff, R.H., Skinner, J.R. *et al.* (1986) Reperfusion protocol and results in 738 patients with evolving myocardial infarction. *Ann. Thorac. Surg.*, **41**, 119–25.
86. Laks, H., Rosenkranz, E. and Buckberg, G.D. (1986) Surgical treatment of cardiogenic shock after myocardial infarction. *Circulation*, **74** (suppl. III), 11–16.
87. Guyton, R.A., Archidi, J.M. Jr, Langford, D.A. *et al.* (1987) Emergency coronary bypass for cardiogenic shock. *Circulation*, **76** (suppl. V), 22–7.
88. Bolooki, H. (1989) Emergency cardiac procedures in patients in cardiogenic shock due to complications of coronary artery disease. *Circulation*, **79** (suppl. I), 137–48.
89. Beyersdorf, F., Sarai, K., Wendt, T. *et al.* (1990) Prolonged abnormalities of LV regional wall motion after normal reperfusion of patients with preoperative cardiogenic shock. *J. Thorac. Cardiovasc. Surg.*, **38**, 165–74.

90. Allen, B.S., Buckberg, G.D., Fontan, F.M. *et al.* (1993) Superiority of controlled surgical reperfusion versus percutaneous transluminal coronary angioplasty in acute coronary occlusion. *J. Thorac. Cardiovasc. Surg.*, **105**, 864–83.

91. Quigley, R.L., Milano, C.A., Smith, L.R. *et al.* (1993) Prognosis and management of anterolateral myocardial infarction in patients with severe left main disease and cardiogenic shock. The left main shock syndrome. *Circulation*, **88**, II-65–II-70.

92. O'Neill, W.W., Erbel, R., Laufer, N. *et al.* (1985) Coronary angioplasty therapy of cardiogenic shock complicating acute myocardial infarction (abstract). *Circulation*, **72** (suppl. III), 309.

93. Shani, J., Rivera, M., Greengart, A. *et al.* (1986) Percutaneous transluminal coronary angioplasty in cardiogenic shock (abstract). *J. Am. Coll. Cardiol.*, **7** (suppl. A), 219A.

94. Heuser, R.R., Maddoux G.L., Goss, J.E. *et al.* (1986) Coronary angioplasty in the treatment of cardiogenic shock: The therapy of choice (abstract). *J. Am. Coll. Cardiol.*, **7** (suppl. A), 219A.

95. Brown, T.M., Jannone, L.A., Gordon, D.F. *et al.* (1985) Percutaneous myocardial reperfusion reduces mortality in acute myocardial infarction complicated by cardiogenic shock (abstract). *Circulation*, **72** (suppl. III), 309.

96. Laramee, L.A., Rutherford, B.D., Ligon, R.W. *et al.* (1988) Coronary angioplasty for cardiogenic shock following myocardial infarction (abstract). *Circulation*, **78** (suppl. II), 634.

97. Lee, L., Erbel, R., Brown, T.M. *et al.* (1991) Multicenter registry of angioplasty therapy of cardiogenic shock: Initial and long-term survival. *J. Am. Coll. Cardiol.*, **17**, 599–603.

98. Disler, L., Haitas, B., Benjamin, J. *et al.* (1987) Cardiogenic shock evolving myocardial infarction: Treatment by angioplasty and streptokinase. *Heart Lung*, **16**, 649–52.

99. Verna, E., Repetto, S., Boscarini, M. *et al.* (1989) Emergency coronary angioplasty in patients with severe left ventricular dysfunction or cardiogenic shock after acute myocardial infarction. *Eur. Heart J.*, **20**, 958–66.

100. Meyer, P., Blanc, P., Baudouy, M. and Morand, P. (1990) Treatment de choc cardiogenique primaire par angioplastie transluminale coconarienne a la phase aigue de l'infartus. *Arch. Mal. Coeur*, **83**, 329–4.

101. Eltchaninoff, H., Simpfendorfer, C. and Whitlow, P.L. (1991) Coronary angioplasty improves both early and 1 year survival in acute myocardial infarction complicated by cardiogenic shock (abstract). *J. Am. Coll. Cardiol.*, **17**, 167A.

102. Yamamoto, H., Hayashi, Y., Oka, Y. *et al.* (1992) Efficacy of percutaneous transluminal coronary angioplasty in patients with acute myocardial infarction complicated by cardiogenic shock. *Jpn. Circ. J.*, **56**, 815–21.

103. Seydoux, C., Goy, J.J., Beuret, P. *et al.* (1992) Effectiveness of percutaneous transluminal coronary angioplasty in cardiogenic shock during acute myocardial infarction. *Am. J. Cardiol.*, **69**, 968–9.

104. Dunkman, W.B., Leinbach, R.C., Buckley, M.J. *et al.* (1972) Clinical and hemodynamic results of intraaortic balloon pumping and surgery for cardiogenic shock. *Circulation*, **46**, 465–77.

105. Beyerdorf, F., Kirsh, M., Buckberg, G.D. and Allen, B.S. (1992) Warm glutamate/asparate-enriched blood cardioplegic solution for perioperative sudden death. *J. Thorac. Cardiovasc. Surg.*, **104**, 1141–7.

106. O'Neill, W.W. (1992) Angioplasty therapy of cardiogenic shock: Are randomized trials necessary? *J. Am. Coll. Cardiol.*, **19**, 915–17.

107. Raneses, R., Grines, C., Almany, S. *et al.* (1992) Hemodynamic parameters 12-hours after onset of cardiogenic shock can predict survival (abstract). *J. Am. Coll. Cardiol.*, **19**, 363A.

108. Grines, C.L., Growne, K.F., Marco, J. *et al.* (1993) For the primary angioplasty in myocardial infarction study group: A comparison of immediate angioplasty with thrombolytic therapy for acute myocardial infarction. *N. Engl. J. Med.*, **328**, 673–9.

109. Zijlstra, F., Jan De Boer, M., Hoorntje, J.C.A. *et al.* (1993) A comparison of immediate coronary angioplasty with intravenous streptokinase in acute myocardial infarction. *N. Engl. J. Med.*, **328**, 680–4.

110. Gibbons, R.J., Holmes, D.R., Reeder, G.S. *et al.* for the Mayo Coronary Care Unit and Catheterization Laboratory Groups (1993) Immediate angioplasty compared with the administration of a thrombolytic agent followed by conservative treatment for myocardial infarction. *N. Engl. J. Med.*, **328**, 685–91.

111. Ohman, E.M., George, B.S., White, C.J. *et al.* (1993) The use of aortic counterpulsation to improve sustained coronary artery patency during acute myocardial infarction: Results of a randomized trial (abstract). *J. Am. Coll. Cardiol.*, **21**, 397A.

12

Mechanical Complications

M. T. Camacho, D. D. Muehrcke and F. D. Loop

In the USA, annual hospital admissions for suspected acute myocardial infarction total approximately 1.7 million; the diagnosis is confirmed in about one-third of these patients.[1] Prior to the beginning of thrombolytic therapy in 1980, hospital mortality rates averaged 10%.[2] Since the introduction of fibrinolytic therapy, early mortality may be reduced to ≤5%.[3] In the past, arrhythmias were the leading cause of death during the acute phase of myocardial infarction. Currently, myocardial failure is the most common cause of death. A subset of these deaths secondary to myocardial failure are the result of mechanical complications, which in the past could not be effectively treated by surgical intervention. Today there is good evidence that aggressive surgical management in selected cases may improve survival rates significantly in patients with mechanical complications.[4–7] This review highlights the key points in the diagnosis and treatment of patients with mechanical complications of acute myocardial infarction, which include ventricular septal defect, papillary muscle rupture, and left ventricular rupture.

Ventricular Septal Defect

Ventricular septal defect (VSD) is an infrequent but serious complication of myocardial infarction. Latham[8] is credited with first describing this entity in his lectures on the heart published in 1845. The first antemortem diagnosis of an acquired ventricular septal defect was not made until 1923 by Brunn.[9] Sager,[10] in 1932, established the clinical association between myocardial infarction and septal rupture. Subsequent reports noted the incidence[11–13] and palliative medical management of these patients until 1956, when Cooley[14] performed the first successful surgical repair of an acquired defect in a patient 9 weeks after the diagnosis of septal rupture.

The principal treatment of postinfarction VSD during the early 1960s was aggressive medical management, even though it was well recognized that survivors were rare following medical therapy alone. Surgical treatment was generally reserved for patients who survived at least 6 weeks. This delay allowed for scarring at the edges of the defect. It was thought that a secure and long-lasting closure of the septal defect was dependent on this process.[15–17] By the late 1960s, however, early repair was proposed for patients whose condition was deteriorating despite medical therapy.[17,18] More recently, improved surgical techniques,[19–21] enhanced myocardial protection,[22] and improved perioperative mechanical[23–25] and pharmacologic support have led to increasingly favorable results in the surgical management of patients with postinfarction VSD.

Incidence and Pathogenesis

Rupture of the interventricular septum is a rare complication of myocardial infarction. Although autopsy studies reveal an 11% incidence of myocardial free-wall rupture following myocardial infarction,[26] septal perforation is much less frequent with an incidence of 1–2%.[27–29] Septal rupture occurs through a zone of necrotic myocardial tissue, and is most likely to occur within the first week of myocardial infarction. Selzer[30] reported an average time of 2.6 days (range, 1–6 days) from infarction to septal rupture. Ten years later, Hutchin[29] reported an average time from infarction to rupture of 4 days (range 0.5–7 days). More recent data have suggested that the initial treatment of myocardial infarction by way of thrombolysis may shorten the time interval between infarction and septal rupture[31] as well as affect the outcome of surgical therapy (see below).

The average age of patients suffering a postinfarction VSD is 62.5 years.[30] There is evidence to suggest that the average age is increasing.[29,32–34] Men are affected more commonly than women. In most instances, septal rupture occurs as a complication of an individual's first myocardial infarction.[29,32,33,35] Coronary anatomy studied at autopsy or by angiography usually demonstrates coronary artery occlusion with poor or no collateral flow.[36] The lack of collateral flow noted acutely may be secondary to associated arterial disease, anatomic configuration, or myocardial edema. Associated coronary artery disease is frequent: Hill and associates,[37] in reviewing the cases of 19 patients with postinfarction VSD, found one-vessel disease in 64%, two-vessel disease in 7%, and three-vessel disease in 29% of their patients.

Not infrequently, there are multiple septal defects. Swithinbank[38] reported five instances of multiple VSDs from his own group of 46 patients (incidence, 10.9%), and the first of three patients reviewed by Kitamura and associates[28] had two VSDs. A successful clinical outcome is related to the adequacy of closure of the septal defects; therefore, multiple defects must be sought preoperatively if possible and certainly at the time of the operative repair.

Because postinfarction VSD is invariably associated with transmural infarction, ventricular aneurysms are commonly associated with postinfarction VSD and often contribute dramatically to the hemodynamic decline of patients. The reported incidence ranges from 35%[28] to 68%,[37] whereas the incidence of ventricular aneurysm following myocardial infarction without septal rupture is considerably less at 12.4%.[39]

Associated conditions that may increase likelihood of postinfarction VSD include hypertension,[26,35,40,41] anticoagulation therapy,[26,42] advanced age,[26] and possibly thrombolytic therapy.[31]

The uninterrupted natural course of patients suffering postinfarction VSD has been well documented and is abysmal. Sanders[40] reported that 54% of patients die within the first week and 92% in the first year after rupture. Oyamada[43] found that 24% of 157 patients with myocardial infarction and septal rupture died within the first 24 hours, 65% in 2 weeks, and 81% within 8 weeks. Oyamada and Sanders reported that approximately 7% of these patients live longer than 1 year. This poor prognosis results from a sudden volume load imposed on both ventricles in the heart already compromised by a large myocardial infarction and often by additional coronary artery disease in areas other than that already infarcted, a ventricular aneurysm, ischemic mitral valve dysfunction, or a combination of these. Significant impairment of cardiac output routinely leads to peripheral organ failure and death in the majority of patients.

Recently, Westaby *et al.*[31] reported an earlier presentation of ventricular septal rupture in patients treated with thrombolysis after acute myocardial infarction. The mean interval between symptomatic onset of myocardial infarction and the development of septal rupture was 24 hours for those patients treated with early thrombolytic therapy and 6 days for those who were not. Microscopic observation of the infarcted myocardium revealed that muscle bundles were dissected by blood rendered incoagulable by thrombolytic therapy together with the histologic features of reperfusion injury. Patients treated with thrombolytic therapy had a higher operative mortality rate when their septal defects were repaired. The implication of early rupture after thrombolysis is that repair must be undertaken at a time when the infarcted muscle is extremely friable. This requires more extensive excision and repair, and is reflected in a higher mortality rate.[31] Thus, thrombolytic therapy may affect the presentation and outcome of postinfarction VSDs.

Diagnosis

The development of a loud systolic murmur, usually within the first week following an acute myocardial infarction, is the most consistent finding of postinfarction VSD. Coincident with the onset of the murmur, there is usually an abrupt decline in the patient's clinical course with congestive failure and often cardiogenic shock; 50% of patients have recurrent chest pain.[29] The differential diagnosis includes rupture of the interventricular septum vs mitral regurgitation secondary to papillary muscle rupture, dysfunction, or left ventricular dilatation. The characteristic harsh systolic murmur is heard over a wide area, including the middle of the left sternal border and the apical area, depending on the location of the septal defect. Not infrequently the murmur radiates to the left axilla, thereby mimicking mitral regurgitation.[30] There is an associated thrill in 48–62% of patients.[38,44]

Septal rupture may be differentiated from mitral valve dysfunction by right heart catheterization using the Swan–Ganz catheter. This technique is quick, relatively safe,[45,46] and can often be performed at the bedside. With septal rupture, there is an oxygen saturation 'step-up' between the right atrium and the pulmonary artery. From the oxygen saturation samples, the pulmonary-to-systemic flow ratio can be calculated. There is a rough linear correlation between shunt size and septal defect size.[47] Left-sided and right-sided pressure measurements assess the degree of biventricular failure and are helpful in monitoring the response to perioperative therapy. Right ventricular pressure, although elevated, is usually less than systemic pressure. Although biventricular failure is frequently present, right-sided failure is more prominent in patients with postinfarction VSD, whereas left-sided failure and refractory pulmonary edema are more prominent in patients with ruptured papillary muscle. The morphology of the pulmonary capillary wedge pressure tracing is often helpful in differentiating acute mitral regurgitation from septal rupture. However, Miller and coworkers[36] reported that one-third of patients with postinfarction VSD also have some mitral regurgitation secondary to left ventricular dysfunction; only rarely is septal rupture also associated with ruptured papillary muscle.[48]

Recently Jones *et al.*[49] demonstrated the prognostic significance of right and left ventriculograms in a multivariant retrospective study of 60 patients. They showed that right ventricular shortening fraction, which is a single ventriculogram view measurement that approximates to the ejection fraction, correlated with short-term survival. Moreover, left ventricular shortening fraction correlated with long-term survival. More recently, we have concluded that left ventriculography is unnecessary at the time of coronary arteriography and the extra iodinated contrast may cause renal failure.

Chandraranta and associates[50] reported the use of echocardiography (M-mode) to examine three patients with postinfarction VSD. The only consistent finding was right ventricular dilatation. Normally directed septal motion was present in all patients. Other authors[51,52] have obtained more specific information, including VSD location and its approximate size, using two-dimensional echocardiography. Not all septal defects can be visualized on echocardiography, however, as they may consist of multiple small defects or serpiginous tunnels through the septal wall, most notably in the trabeculated portion of the septum, and appear as turbulence on echo. Nevertheless, the use of color flow Doppler echocardiography to accomplish early diagnosis of ventricular septal rupture has contributed greatly to speeding the referral of these critically ill patients to tertiary centers for definitive surgical repair.[53]

Preoperative Management

In view of the dismal natural course of patients who are not surgically treated, the diagnosis of postinfarction septal rupture can be regarded as its own indication for operation. Much of the current controversy concerning septal rupture centers around the timing of surgical intervention. As noted in the introduction, the first attempts at surgical repair were undertaken in patients who had survived for one or more months after septal rupture. The success of these operations, plus the data showing that myocardial fibrotic healing is not complete for 6–8 weeks, led to the erroneous early belief that operation should be performed only in these survivors. With the earlier recognition of this complication and the same successful late operative results, some surgeons attempted to further alter the natural course of these patients, attempting surgical repair during the acute period, particularly in patients with hemodynamic deterioration soon after infarction and septal rupture. Surgical repairs in patients presenting less than 1 month after infarction with intractable failure were performed with increasing success. This led Honey and coworkers [54] to correctly conclude in their 1967 case report that 'it is probable that the lower mortality of late operations is not due so much to the progress of reparative fibrosis of the infarcted muscle surrounding the defect, as the fact that the worst risk cases have already died'.

The safety of early operation was substantiated in 1971 by a report by Buckley and associates, who described five patients who had undergone operation for anterior or apical septal rupture.[55] Gaudiani and his colleagues at Stanford reviewed their experience in 43 patients up to 1980.[56] They observed that operative mortality depended substantially on the presence or absence of preoperative cardiogenic shock. They concluded that 'the inverse relationship between early operation and chance of survival was primarily a measure of the severity of the illness in the patients who required early operation'.

Pharmacologic management should be instituted initially in an attempt to stabilize patients hemodynamically. The purpose of this therapy is to reduce systemic vascular resistance in patients with an adequately maintained systemic blood pressure. Vasodilators may be used in an attempt to decrease the left-to-right shunting associated with the mechanical defect and thus increase cardiac output. Infusion of nitroprusside, in doses not sufficient to cause systemic hypotension, may also be effective in increasing cardiac output. The capacity of nitroprusside to decrease left-to-right shunting and pulmonary hypertension is not consistent.[57] Intravenous nitroglycerin can be used as a vasodilator and may provide improved myocardial blood flow in these patients with significant ischemic cardiac disease.[58] Inotropic agents, used alone, may increase cardiac output but, without changes in the pulmonary–systemic flow ratio (Q_p/Q_s), will markedly increase left ventricular work and myocardial oxygen consumption. Vasopressor agents that increase systemic afterload further increase the pulmonary–systemic flow ratio, lowering cardiac output and greatly augmenting myocardial oxygen consumption. Nevertheless, the profound level of cardiogenic shock in some of these patients precludes vasodilator treatment, often necessitating vasopressor support as the patient is prepared for transfer to the operating room. Pharmacologic therapy is neither a substitute for, nor reason to delay, definitive surgical repair of the defect.

Intra-aortic balloon counterpulsation (IABC) offers the most important available means of temporary hemodynamic support.[59] The IABC reduces left ventricular afterload, thus increasing systemic cardiac output and decreasing the Q_p/Q_s ratio.[24] This beneficial effect of the IABC may be expected to decrease myocardial oxygen consumption, while also providing an increase in perfusion pressure to the coronary arteries and other peripheral organs during diastole. Efforts to close these defects in the catheterization laboratory with a 'clam-shell' device have not, to date, met with success, but may in the future as this technology evolves.[60,61]

Operative Technique

The first operations for repair of postinfarction VSD employed an approach through the right ventricle with incision of the right ventricular outflow tract, as has been used in approaching some congenital VSDs.[14] This approach proved inadequate because of limited exposure (particularly when the defect was located toward the apex of the heart), injury to normal right ventricular muscle, interruption of coronary collaterals, and failure to eliminate the paradoxically expanding segment of infarcted left ventricular wall. Subsequently, a left-sided transinfarct approach (left ventriculotomy) was described, which led to more successful technical results.[19,21,62–64]

Techniques for closure of postinfarction VSD have evolved based on the following six principles: (1) a clear understanding of the anatomy and location of the VSD as well as any associated coronary artery disease; (2) expeditious establishment of hypothermic total cardiopulmonary bypass and meticulous attention to myocardial protection; (3) transinfarct approach to the VSD with the site of left ventriculotomy determined by the location of transmural infarction; (4) inspection of the papillary muscles and concomitant replacement of the mitral valve only if there is frank papillary muscle rupture; (5) closure of the VSD without tension; and (6) buttressing of suture lines with pledgets or strips of Teflon felt or similar material to prevent sutures from cutting through friable muscle.

Adherence to these principles facilitates individualized approaches to anterior, apical, and inferoposterior septal defects. Small defects beneath anterior infarcts may sometimes be simply closed by approximation of the septal margin of the defect to the right ventricular free wall. Larger anterior septal defects require patch closure to avoid tension on friable myocardium.

A different technique is used to close apical defects[21] (Figure 12.1). The initial incision is made through the infarcted apex of the left ventricle. Debridement of necrotic myocardium results in amputation of the apex of the left ventricle and septum. The resulting defect is closed by approximating the remaining apical portion of the left and right ventricular free wall to the apical septum. A row of interrupted mattress sutures is placed through a buttressing felt strip, the left ventricular wall, an additional strip of felt, the septum, a third strip of felt, the right ventricular wall, and a final strip of felt. The sutures are tied after all have been placed, and the closure is reinforced with an additional over-and-over suture. Large defects may require septal replacement with a prosthetic patch, which is then incorporated in the ventriculotomy closure.

The greatest technical challenge has been the successful management of inferoposterior septal defects, which are associated with transmural infarction in the distribution of the posterior descending and/or circumflex coronary arteries.[65] Early attempts at primary closure of these lesions were usually followed by reopening of the defect either intraoperatively or early postoperatively because the sutures tore out from the soft myocardium that was necessarily closed under tension. The principles already outlined have evolved in part from the analysis of such early experiences.

For inferoposterior septal defects (Figures 12.2–12.6) the heart is retracted as for bypass grafting to the posterior descending artery. The margins of the infarct are best identified prior to aortic cross-clamping, and may involve the diaphragmatic aspects of both ventricles or of the left ventricle only. The incision is made into the infarct of the left ventricle (Figure 12.2) and necrotic muscle debrided both to provide exposure of the VSD

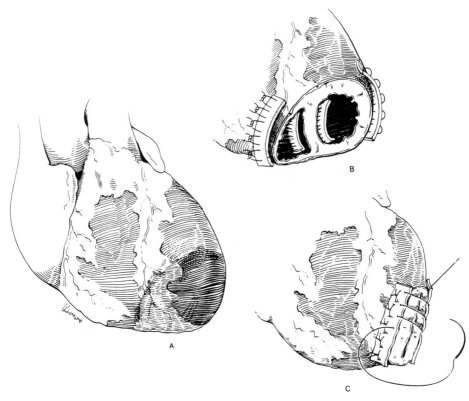

Figure 12.1   Repair of an apical ventricular septal defect. (A) Large apical aneurysm with underlying ventricular septal defect. (B) Interrupted suture repair is performed by excising the apex of the right and left ventricles including the ventricular septal defect with reapproximation of the left and right ventricular free walls along with the septum using Teflon felt strips for hemostasis. (C) Over-and-over suture reinforcement of the repair for further hemostasis.

and to avoid subsequent tearing out of sutures. The VSD may often be seen best from the patient's left side. The papillary muscles to the mitral valve are inspected, and mitral valve replacement or repair is undertaken only if there is frank papillary muscle rupture. When indicated, replacement of the mitral valve is accomplished through a separate conventional left atrial approach to avoid unnecessary tearing of friable ventricular muscle while exposing the mitral valve.

A small inferior septal defect may be closed by approximating the edge of the septum to the diaphragmatic right ventricular free wall using mattress sutures and buttressing strips of Teflon felt as shown in Figures 12.2–12.6. The same principles apply as in closure of a large anterior defect; however a patch is used to close the septum. Pledgeted mattress sutures are placed from the right side of the septum to the exterior (Figure 12.3). Small septal defects may be closed directly to the posterior ventricular wall. Circumferential sutures are then placed around the margins of the free left ventricular wall defect, which remains after the infarctectomy and after the VSD is closed (Figure 12.4). These sutures are then placed through a separate epicardial patch of low-porosity woven Dacron and then through additional felt pledgets (Figure 12.5). The Dacron patch may be baked in albumin to make it impervious to blood, or collagen-impregnated woven Dacron grafts may be used[66] (Figure 12.6).

The basic principles outlined above apply to all septal defects, irrespective of location. Each technique results in elimination of both the left-to-right shunt and the paradoxically

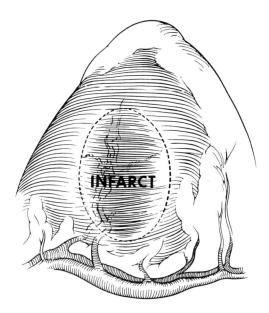

Figure 12.2 Diaphragmatic myocardial infarction of the left ventricle with an inferiorly based ventricular septal defect seen from the surgeon's view after dislocating the heart.

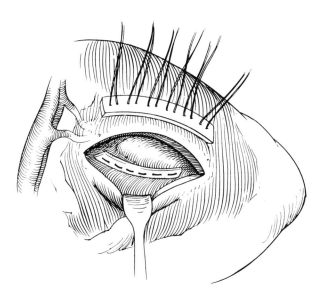

Figure 12.3 Placement of Teflon sutures circumferentially around the ventricular septal defect and subsequently through the free left ventricular wall inferiorly and reinforced with further Teflon sutures.

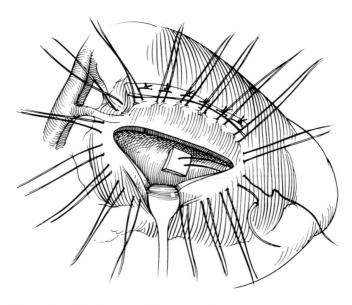

Figure 12.4 Circumferential placement of interrupted sutures and preparation for closing the left ventricular aneurysmectomy.

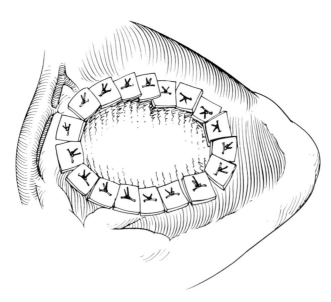

Figure 12.5 Closure of infarctectomy site with a Dacron patch to ensure the appropriate geometric shape of the inferior wall of the heart, which leads to left hemostatic bleeding problems as there is less tension on the repair.

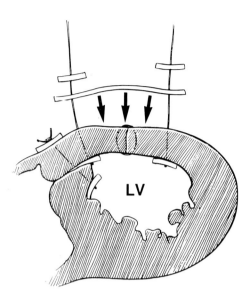

Figure 12.6 Schematic drawing of repair where the ventricular septal defect is closed directly to the ventricular free wall and the infarctectomy site is closed with a Dacron patch to ensure the geometric shape of the ventricle.

expanding segment of infarcted myocardium. Our policy at the time of VSD repair is to routinely perform aortocoronary grafts[67] to major epicardial coronary arteries that have severe proximal stenosis.

The concomitant bypassing of associated coronary artery disease along with acute VSD repair has been a controversial point in the past.[68] One of the authors[67] reviewed an experience in 75 patients who had undergone coronary angiography and repair of a postinfarction VSD. The incidence of two- or three-vessel coronary artery disease was 70% of patients and bypass grafts were performed in 64% of the patients, a level that was similar to the average rate of bypass grafting reported by eight recent large series of patients suffering postinfarction VSD.[68,69] Coronary atherosclerosis outside the distribution of the infarct is commonly associated with postinfarction VSDs and represents a frequently encountered clinical problem in this group of patients. After separating out patients with one-vessel disease, a difference in hospital survival between patients having bypass for two- or three-vessel disease and those not being bypassed, yet with a similar degree of coronary artery disease, could not be demonstrated. Patients undergoing revascularization, however, demonstrated significantly improved long-term survival when compared with patients who were not bypassed, despite each group having a similar extent of coronary artery disease (Figure 12.7). In patients with postinfarction ventricular septal rupture, coronary artery disease is related etiologically to the septal defect. Therefore, it is not surprising that survival is improved when the underlying problem is addressed. Miller and colleagues have previously reported a generalized lack of collateral flow between the coronary arteries in patients suffering postinfarction VSD.[36] This observation may help explain the benefit of concomitant bypass grafting for patients undergoing VSD repair. The lack of collateral blood flow effectively separates regions of the myocardium, and the additional blood supply provided by bypassing proximal lesions may overcome the lack of collaterals. The poor long-term outcome of patients with unbypassed two- and three-vessel coronary artery disease supports performance of coronary angiography in all patients being considered for VSD repair.

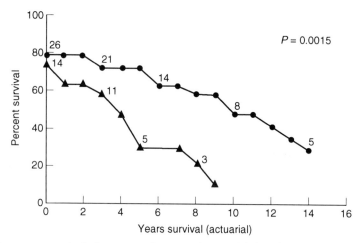

Figure 12.7   Long-term survival of patients with ventricular septal defect after myocardial infarction with two- or three-vessel coronary artery disease, comparing the long-term survival between those patients who underwent coronary artery bypass (●——●) and those not bypassed (▲——▲).

Another recent trend that has been recognized is the increasing age of patients presenting for VSD repair.[34] Daggett's group recently reviewed the number of patients operated on for each 5-year period between 1965 and 1990 at the Massachusetts General Hospital (Figure 12.8). The proportion of patients over the age of 70 years had significantly increased since 1975. Moreover, they were unable to demonstrate a difference in the operative mortality and long-term survival between the younger (<70 years) and older patients (>70 years) (Figure 12.9). The hospital mortality was 27.6% in patients over

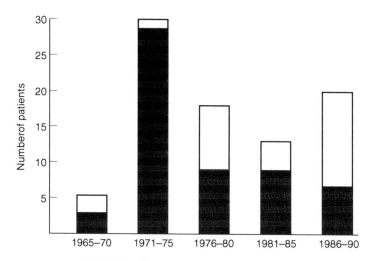

Figure 12.8   Increasing age of patients presenting with ventricular septal defects after myocardial infarction. The incidence of patients presenting for surgical repair over the age of 70 years has increased since 1975 and currently the majority of people presenting for repair are over the age of 70 years. ▨, age <70 years; □, ≥70 years.

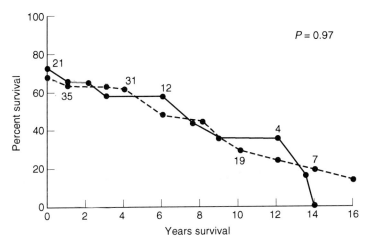

Figure 12.9 The long-term survival of patients younger and older than 70 years of age. No difference was found in the long-term survival of these two age groups in patients undergoing ventricular septal defect repair after myocardial infarction. ●——●, >70 years; ●- - -●, ≤70 years.

the age of 70 years, which was similar to the 25% mortality rate reported by Skillington in patients over the age of 65 years.[68] These mortality rates are an improvement over the 47% mortality rate reported by Weintraub in a series of 12 patients over the age of 65 years who underwent VSD repair prior to 1980.[32] Interestingly, Weintraub et al.[32] were able to show that there was no difference in hospital costs incurred by the older patients compared to the younger patients operated upon during the same time period.

Postoperative Management

Patients requiring IABC preoperatively appear to benefit from postoperative support with the device over a 24–72 hour period. More recently, Nasu et al.[70] compared the postoperative use of the left ventricular assist device (LVAD) with IABC in 18 patients with postinfarction septal rupture or free-wall rupture. Of 15 patients managed with IABC, nine survived and six died of organ dysfunction and sepsis; no deaths were due to low cardiac output. Of three patients in whom an LVAD was inserted, all were weaned from support. One patient died 6 days later due to cardiac arrhythmia, and a second patient died of massive air embolism due to IABC balloon rupture 2 days after LVAD removal. Both renal function and cardiac index improved to a significantly greater extent in the LVAD group. All six nonsurvivors in the IABC group suffered renal deterioration requiring renal assist procedures. In comparison, creatinine clearance in the three LVAD patients returned to greater than 20 ml min^{-1} within 1 week. Cardiac index rose from 2.0 to 2.5 l min^{-1} m^{-2} in the IABC group, and from 2.1–2.7 l min^{-1} m^{-2} to 4.1–4.8 l min^{-1} m^{-2} in the LVAD group. Only small doses of catecholamines were used. It appeared that use of the LVAD resulted in a more physiologic circulation without the need for high-dose inotropic support and hence with less organ deterioration. Previous studies in dogs[71,72] support this premise. Mickleborough[72] found significantly more myocardial necrosis and decreased compliance and systolic function in dogs treated with IABC after ischemic arrest, compared to dogs treated with LVAD and low-dose inotropic support. These studies suggest that early aggressive use of left ventricular support combined with low-dose inotropes may result in improved organ recovery in patients with cardiogenic shock.

A number of these patients demonstrate a small persistent left-to-right shunt after surgery. Alvarez[72] reported a 44% incidence of persistent postoperative shunts, with the Q_p/Q_s ratio ranging from 1.1:1 to 1.8:1 (mean 1.3:1). After a 14-month mean follow-up, no new shunts were detected and no change in shunt size occurred.

Because of the large amount of prosthetic material used in the repair, these patients should be anticoagulated for 6–8 weeks. Thereafter, warfarin is discontinued (when the patient has not had a mechanical valve placed) based on Daggett's experience of five long-term survivors suffering cerebral hemorrhage 2 or more months postoperatively.[74] Presumably, once the prosthetic material becomes endothelialized, anticoagulation is not needed.

Survival

Using an early operative approach, current overall hospital mortality rates of 25% can be expected in most patients.[69] Mortality tends to be lower for anteriorly located VSDs and lowest for patients with apical VSDs. Five-year and ten-year survival rates of 73% and 48% in patients bypassed with two- and three-vessel coronary artery disease have been reported in centers in the USA experienced in this problem.[69] At follow-up, 90% of patients are in New York Heart Association Function Class I or II postoperatively.[68,69]

The recent advance in the management of patients with postinfarction VSD have helped to decrease the operative mortality rate to 10% in one series.[73] The addition of CABG seems to improve long-term survival; however, it has little effect on hospital mortality. Recent technical improvements[66,69,75,76] have helped to decrease postoperative bleeding and may preserve ventricular function.

Patients presenting for repair today tend to be older and more likely to have received thrombolytic agents, which may complicate their repair. Survival and quality of life after successful repair is excellent even in patients over 70 years of age.

Papillary Muscle Rupture

Mitral regurgitation resulting from acute myocardial infarction can be the result of several different pathologic processes. The distinction between transient ischemic dysfunction, partial rupture, and complete rupture carries therapeutic significance. While the first two forms of mitral regurgitation may not require surgical intervention, the latter may be rapidly fatal without operation. Mitral incompetence from papillary muscle rupture has been recognized for a long time as a rare and frequently catastrophic complication of acute myocardial infarction. Merat is credited with first describing papillary muscle rupture at autopsy.[77] An antemortem diagnosis was not made until 1948 by Davison.[78] Mitral incompetence without papillary muscle rupture, occurring as an acute or chronic complication of ischemic heart disease, was described by Burch[79] in 1963. The first successful surgical correction of papillary muscle rupture was performed by Austen[80] in 1965.

Incidence and Pathology

The incidence of papillary muscle rupture as a complication of acute myocardial infarction has been reported to be between 0.5 and 5%.[81–85] Only about one-half of the patients developing acute mitral regurgitation soon after myocardial infarction will have suffered an actual rupture of the papillary muscle. One-third of these patients will have a complete disruption of the papillary muscle, resulting in flailing of both the anterior and posterior mitral leaflets. Two-thirds will have ruptured one or more heads of the papillary muscle.

The natural history of acute mitral incompetence complicating myocardial infarction depends on the extent of papillary muscle rupture.[86] With total rupture of a papillary muscle, only 25% of patients survive more than 24 hours. However, survival after partial papillary rupture is over 70%[87] in the first 24 hours, and 50% at 1 month. Patients surviving longer than 1 month have, by definition, chronic ischemic mitral insufficiency.

The anterolateral papillary muscle is ruptured in about 25% of patients, and the posteromedial papillary muscle in about 75% of patients with complete rupture. Moreover, the majority of patients suffering acute mitral incompetence due to acute infarction have suffered an inferior left wall infarction, and many suffer a coexisting right ventricular infarction. Most papillary muscle ruptures are the result of the patient's first myocardial infarction and tend to occur more frequently in patients with less severe coronary artery disease compared with those patients without muscle rupture.[88] Presumably, as in patients suffering postinfarction ventricular septal rupture, there is a lack of collateral flow between the coronary arteries. This lack of collateral flow noted acutely may be secondary to associated arterial disease, anatomic configuration or myocardial edema. The most likely explanation for the development of lethal mitral insufficiency following inferior wall myocardial infarctions has to do with the coronary anatomy. The anterolateral papillary muscle has a dual blood supply from the left anterior descending artery and circumflex coronary arteries. The posteromedial papillary muscle is usually supplied by a single vessel, most often the right coronary artery or alternatively the circumflex artery in a left dominant coronary system. Because of the dual blood supply to the anterolateral papillary muscle, an anterior wall infarction is unlikely to injure the anterolateral papillary muscle. In contrast, a posterior wall infarction is more likely to result in ischemic damage to the posteromedial papillary muscle due to its singular blood supply. Clinical evidence of rupture of the posteromedial papillary muscle is observed 2.5–12 times more frequently than the anterolateral papillary muscle.[7,59,88–91]

In addition to the location of the infarct and subsequent extent of papillary muscle dysfunction, the degree of left ventricular dysfunction influences survival. Preoperative left ventricular ejection fraction is the main determinant of hospital survival after mitral replacement and coronary bypass grafting in patients with ischemic mitral regurgitation.[92] Hospital mortality was 28% when the preoperative ejection fraction was greater than 35% and 40% when ejection fraction was less than 35%. The length of the interval between infarction and operation did not affect the hospital survival. The concomitant grafting of associated coronary artery disease is presumed to benefit patients over the long term. None-the-less, the addition of coronary artery revascularization to the mitral valve repair or replacement due to an acute myocardial infarction has not been shown to increase hospital mortality and because of the etiologic relationship between the two, bypass grafting should be performed at the time of surgery.[93]

Diagnosis

Acute papillary muscle rupture usually presents as profound congestive hart failure 3–10 days following infarction. Unlike VSDs, which occur with large myocardial infarctions, papillary muscle rupture may often complicate small infarctions.[83,94] The rapid clinical deterioration occurs because neither the left atrium, nor the left ventricle, have had time to adapt to the sudden development of regurgitation. Left atrial pressures are markedly increased leading to acute pulmonary edema despite excellent left ventricular function. Systemic vascular resistance rises as a compensatory mechanism to increase the blood pressure in response to a decrease in cardiac output. This creates a positive feedback loop increasing afterload further, increasing the regurgitant left ventricular ejection fraction and not only potentiating the congestive failure but decreasing further the forward cardiac output. The combination of increasing workload and a dilated volume-over-loaded ventricle with stretched hypoxic myocardial cells leads to cardiogenic shock and subsequent multiorgan system failure if not treated appropriately.

The diagnosis of acute mitral regurgitation can usually be easily diagnosed in the postinfarction period. Acute mitral regurgitation must be differentiated from a post-infarction ventricular septal rupture, which may share both a similar clinical presentation as well as a similar holosystolic murmur that radiates to the axilla. Typically a patient suffering acute postinfarction mitral regurgitation will show tall U-waves in the pulmon-ary capillary wedge pressure tracings, pulmonary edema, and confirmation of mitral pathology on the echocardiogram. These diagnostic signs are not, however, consistently present. Silent, severe mitral regurgitation can be present without a murmur or notice-able U-wave.[95] Patients suffering from silent, severe mitral regurgitation may appear to have massive pump failure rather than papillary muscle dysfunction. Moreover, large U-waves may be seen in patients with postinfarction ventricular septal rupture.[89] The ECG may show only minor changes, particularly since the extent of myocardial infarction is usually limited and most patients have not sustained previous infarctions.[86]

Horskotte found bedside hemodynamic studies to be unreliable for assessing the degree of mitral regurgitation: right ventricular filling pressures were normal in 82% of patients and significant U-waves were present in only 32% of patients.[96] Bedside echocardiography therefore is the best test to confirm mitral regurgitation and also to determine its etiology. Echocardiograpohy may delineate complete rupture by demon-strating a mobile mass appearing in the left atrium during systole and the left ventricle during diastole.[97] Although the most reliable examination, echocardiography cannot always accurately distinguish between severe papillary muscle dysfunction, partial, or complete papillary muscle rupture (Figures 12.10a–e). The clinical signs of complete rupture are usually so significant that Swan–Ganz catheterization reveals characteristic U-waves, and the therapeutic use of IABC will allow stabilization before coronary angiography.

Preoperative Management

In general, complete rupture of a papillary muscle is incompatible with life; rupture of a limited number of papillary heads or chordae attachments do not usually lead to such rapid hemodynamic compromise, and most patients survive without immediate sur-gery.[6] The early treatment of a patient suffering acute mitral regurgitation following myocardial infarction should include afterload reduction with pharmacologic agents, and usually IABC, diuretic therapy, coronary vasodilators, and pressor support for hypotension. In unstable patients, cardiac catheterization may not be possible, and surgery may need to be performed as a life-saving procedure.[89,98,99]

In patients suffering limited papillary muscle rupture with only moderate mitral regurgitation, the use of IABC, combined with afterload reduction employing nitroprus-side, may be effective in establishing hemodynamic stability. Sodium nitroprusside directly affects both arterial and venous smooth muscles and reduces afterload and left ventricular end-diastolic volume; mitral annual dilatation and consequent mitral regurgi-tation are reduced.[100] It is further suggested that sodium nitroprusside may have a beneficial effect on left ventricular and left atrial compliance.[101]

Afterload reduction using IABC is extremely useful in these patients. In a review of six patients with postinfarction papillary rupture, IABC decreased pulmonary capillary wedge pressure from 25 mmHg to 20 mmHg with a significant decrease in U-wave amplitude. Cardiac output rose from 3.1 to 3.7 l min^{-1}. IABC has a physiologic advantage

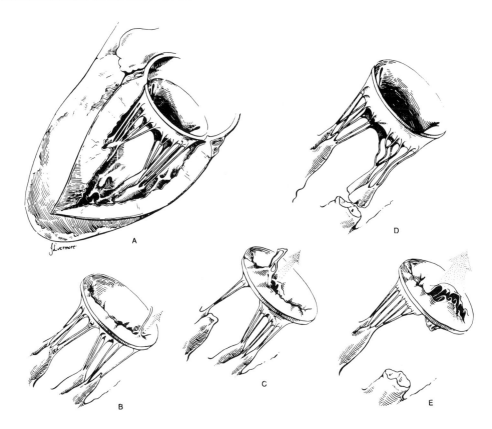

Figure 12.10 Mitral regurgitation after myocardial infarction due to papillary head rupture. (A) Normal annulus, chordae leaflets, and papillary structures. (B) Ruptured posterolateral chordae with mild posterolateral regurgitant jet at the commissure. (C) Partial papillary head rupture of the anterolateral papillary muscle with moderate mitral regurgitation of the anterolateral commissure. (D) Complete rupture of the posteromedial papillary muscle. (E) Severe regurgitation with anterior and posterior mitral leaflet flail segments due to the loss of the posterolateral papillary muscle.

over pressors and inotropic agents, in that the latter can increase systemic output, but can adversely affect myocardial ischemia.[102] IABC helps to decrease ischemia by increasing coronary perfusion, decreasing myocardial oxygen demand, and reducing afterload without lowering systemic blood pressure significantly.

Surgery is essential when left-sided heart failure persists despite maximal medical therapy. The definition of left-sided heart failure includes the manifestations of low cardiac output with elevated left-sided filling pressures, a pulmonary capillary wedge pressure greater than 20 mmHg, mean arterial pressure less than 60 mmHg for over 1 hour in a previously normotensive patient, a cardiac index less than $2.0\,l\,min^{-1}\,m^{-2}$, and urine output less than 20 ml hour^{-1} for 4 hours associated with progressive acidosis. These patients are particularly vulnerable to cardiac arrest and demand expeditious evaluation followed promptly by surgery. Mitral valve replacement is necessary in most patients following complete papillary muscle rupture. In a select few patients, mitral valve reconstruction may be considered. As mentioned above, coronary bypass grafting should be included for significantly narrowed coronary arteries of adequate caliber to ensure viable myocardium.

Surgical Results

Early surgical reports indicate that perioperative survival could be improved by delayed operation to allow healing of acute infarction.[4] However, several reports have shown a high early mortality rate without surgery. In one series, 9 out of 17 patients died before surgery was performed; moreover, the interval from papillary muscle rupture to death was less than 3 days in seven cases.[94] Currently, excellent results have been obtained with early operation in an effort to preserve myocardial function in patients with acute mitral regurgitation. Nishimura reported seven patients with postinfarction papillary muscle rupture who were operated on within 4 days of diagnosis with a 100% perioperative survival; six of these seven patients were alive at an average of 9.7 months postoperatively.[103] Killen demonstrated an actuarial 5-year survival of 75% in nine patients who underwent operation within 3 days of postinfarction papillary muscle rupture.[104] In 1985, Tepe studied 11 patients who underwent surgical correction within 1 month of acute myocardial infarction and found that the interval from onset of shock to operative treatment averaged 1.7 days for survivors and 9.3 days for nonsurvivors.[105]

Mitral valve replacement is currently the most common operation performed for postinfarction papillary rupture. Combined mitral valve replacement and coronary revascularization in patients with ischemic mitral regurgitation is associated with an operative mortality rate of 20% and an actuarial survival rate of 85%. Recently, techniques of mitral valve repair have evolved such that up to 77% of patients with ischemic mitral valve regurgitation (either partial or complete chordal or papillary muscle rupture) can be repaired.[106] There is increasing evidence to suggest that if the mitral valve can be repaired, these patients have a lower operative mortality rate and better left ventricular function and improved long-term survival.

Two of the most commonly used techniques of mitral valve repair are the resection of a flail segment of the posterior leaflet (Figure 12.11) and the reattachment of a completely ruptured papillary muscle head to an adjacent papillary muscle (Figure 12.12). Spence has conducted experiments suggesting that repair of ruptured papillary muscle preserves left ventricular function better than mitral valve replacements.[107] Kay reported on 101 mitral valve repair operations for ischemic mitral regurgitation with a perioperative mortality rate of only 2%.[108] Rankin and coworkers noted that mitral valve repair was associated with better hospital survival than mitral valve replacements in patients with postinfarction papillary muscle rupture requiring acute operations. Survival was independent of type of repair used. Improved results in the repair group may be due to technical simplification, preservation of mitral apparatus, and decreased need for anticoagulation.[109] The long-term results of mitral valve repair have also been excellent. Deloche reports that at 15 years after operation there was freedom from thromboembolism in 94% of patients, from endocarditis in 97% of patients, from anticoagulation-induced hemorrhage in 96%, and from reoperation in 87%. Along with lower operative mortality these figures are superior to the overall results of valve replacement.[110]

Improved survival after mitral valve repair is partially attributed to preservation of papillary chordal support. Several reports suggest that preserving the continuity of the mitral leaflets and the ventricular free wall improves long-term ventricular function and survival.[107,111–113] The Cleveland Clinic experience over a 5-year period with mitral valve repair for ischemic mitral regurgitation was similar.[106] During this period ischemia was identified as a cause of mitral regurgitation in 84 patients. Of these, 65 patients (77.4%) underwent mitral valve repair; 11 patients (17%) had acute and 54 (83%) had chronic mitral regurgitation. Valve prolapse was present in 26 patients (40%) and resulted from papillary muscle rupture in eight and papillary muscle infarction with elongation in 18. All patients had associated myocardial revascularization followed by transatrial valvuloplasty. Multiple techniques were employed to achieve valve competence: leaflet resection in three, chordal shortening in 15, papillary muscle reimplantation in 10,

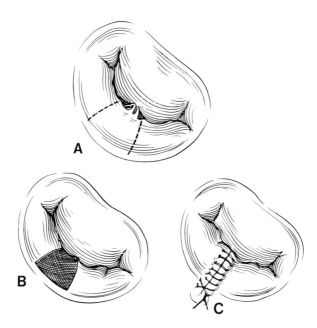

Figure 12.11 Quadrangular resection of the posterior leaflet of the mitral valve. (A) Ruptured chordae to the middle scallop of the posterior leaflet of the mitral valve. (B) Quadrangular excision of flail section including ruptured chordae. (C) Annular plication and interrupted suture repair of medial and lateral segments of the posterior mitral leaflet allowing for a competent mitral valve.

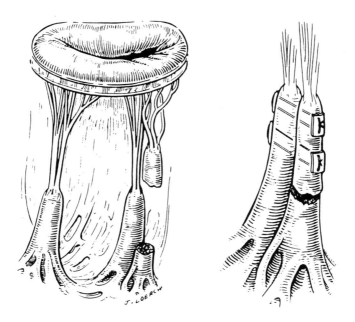

Figure 12.12 Repair of a totally ruptured papillary muscle head. On the left is the findings at surgery of a ruptured papillary head. On the right is a repair technique where the ruptured papillary head is sutured to an adjacent papillary head for competence of the posterior medial papillary support structure.

papillary muscle shortening in three, and annuloplasty in 63. There were six (9.2%) hospital deaths. In comparison with acute mitral regurgitation, those with chronic mitral regurgitation had worse ventricular function. Preoperative variables associated with increased risk of hospital death were poor functional classification and need for preoperative IABC. We identified incomplete revascularization, restricted leaflet motion, and perioperative morbidity such as stroke, myocardial infarction, renal failure, prolonged respiratory distress, and use of IABC as predictors of late mortality. Interestingly, at a mean follow-up of 3.1 ± 1.6 years, patients with valve prolapse had a 96% survival and those with restricted motion had a 48% survival.

Recent advances in the management of patients with postinfarction mitral regurgitation have helped to decrease the operative mortality, especially when the valve can be repaired. The addition of coronary artery bypass grafting to this patient population seems appropriate in an effort to improve long-term survival. Recent technical improvements have helped to preserve left ventricular function and may extend survival further. Current repair techniques are well documented and long lasting.

Left Ventricular Rupture

Rupture of the left ventricular free wall is a catastrophic complication that is fatal in the vast majority of patients. Few patients remain stable enough to have rupture confirmed by diagnostic testing.[114–116] The first recorded description of myocardial rupture after myocardial infarction was in 1649 by William Harvey, who reported on the post-mortem finding of a rent in the wall of the left ventricle.[117] It was not until 1815 that the coexistence of myocardial damage and coronary artery atherosclerosis was reported by Hodgson.[118] Left ventricular rupture is the third most common cause of death after acute myocardial infarction, following cardiogenic shock and dysrhythmia.[119] Some investigators report that up to 20% of fatal acute myocardial infarctions are the result of rupture,[114] and it is believed that this disorder is associated with an approximate mortality of 98%. Although ventricular wall rupture is 5–10 times more common than either VSD or papillary muscle rupture as a complication of myocardial infarction, most of what is known about rupture comes from autopsy studies, mainly because the diagnosis is rarely made before death. However, there are rare case reports of life-saving cardiac surgery after this event.[120–122] Unfortunately, this dismal record persists despite advances in many other areas of cardiac surgery.

Cardiac rupture usually occurs in an area of fresh infarction, often within 3–6 days of the onset of symptoms. The perforation may be a direct pathway from the endocardium to epicardium, or may be an irregular, circuitous pathway partially occluded by thrombus.[123] The myocardial rupture does not usually occur as a ventricular 'blow out'. Most pathologists believe it begins as a small endocardial rent similar to aortic dissection.[124,125] The formation of a pseudo or false aneurysm is probably the subacute form of this disease. A false aneurysm is distinguished from a true aneurysm in that the wall of the false aneurysm is made of parietal pericardium rather than myocardium.[126] Generally, these differences can be distinguished at cardiac catheterization by the appearance of the mouth of the aneurysm, which is characteristically narrow in a false aneurysm and quite broad in a true aneurysm. The diagnosis of an early pseudoaneurysm of the left ventricle should prompt urgent surgical intervention as these are inherently unstable lesions with a poor prognosis if untreated.

Clinically, cardiac rupture tends to occur in older patients without a significant past history of cardiac disease.[116] Women are affected more than men. Whether hypertension adds a significant risk is controversial. Cardiac rupture is characterized by sudden chest pain, sinus bradycardia, and signs of tamponade including electromechanical dissociation, which occurs most frequently during the first week after infarction. Typically, an otherwise stable postinfarction patient becomes hemodynamically unstable. Right-sided heart catheterization will often show tamponade physiology with equalization of diastolic pressure in all chambers. Left and right ventricular pressure tracings will reveal early diastolic pressure elevation known as the 'square root sign'. Inability to produce a palpable pulse by cardiopulmonary resuscitation is a frequent finding. London[127] reported an autopsy series of 1001 consecutive cases of acute myocardial infarction that included 47 cases of cardiac rupture. Anticoagulation administration, hypertension, diabetes, and time to ambulation were not correlated with risk of rupture. In approximately half of the cases, cardiac rupture was located in the anterior wall near the septum or the apex. Most patients had sustained transmural infarctions and had poor collateral flow to the infarcted area. Thrombosis superimposed on an atherosclerotic lesion was the primary lesion, although more recent data suggest that thrombosis may be found in up to 90% of patients with acute myocardial infarctions.

Echocardiography is helpful in diagnosing the presence of a new or increasing pericardial effusion secondary to cardiac rupture. However, diagnosis of the defect itself by this means is uncommon. Those surviving patients in whom false aneurysm develops often demonstrate an unusual bulge in the ventricle on the lateral chest X-ray. The diagnosis can be confirmed by ventriculography. Conventional contrast ventriculography is preferable to radionuclide ventriculography because of its clearer definition of the ventricle and it is often useful to define the coronary anatomy before surgery. Obviously, a high index of suspicion and optimal preoperative support are required to establish the diagnosis and proceed with emergency surgery.

Once a diagnosis of postinfarction free wall rupture is considered, pericardiocentesis is performed on unstable patients as both a diagnostic maneuver and a therapeutic intervention. Stable patients can undergo echocardiography followed by cardiac catheterization to assess the need for coronary revascularization. Patients who are too unstable to undergo cardiac catheterization should undergo surgery as soon as a diagnosis is made; coronary revascularization may be done empirically for coronary lesions palpated at surgery.[89]

Some authors have advocated the use of IABC for initial stabilization.[128] This seems unlikely to be of benefit because the pathophysiology of this lesion mimics pericardial tamponade. Treatment should include volume expansion and pressure support, pericardiocentesis, and immediate organization for surgery. Patients with subacute rupture who are unstable should similarly have volume and pressure support, echocardiography and possible pericardiocentesis, and surgery. Patients with subacute rupture and stable hemodynamics may undergo cardiac catheterization. In the presence of hemorrhagic fluid from pericardiocentesis, a decision about cardiac catheterization should be made and an operating room readied.[117]

Most authors recommend infarctectomy and closure with reinforced sutures such as those used with strips of felt Teflon (Figure 12.13). Large defects may require a Dacron patch to prevent distortion of ventricular geometry. Few acute cases survive to operation, and of those that do, friable, newly infarcted myocardial tissue may make repair a difficult technical challenge.[122] Nunez and coworkers described a technique of covering the perforation with a patch sewn on with continuous polypropylene sutures; they reported 57% survival.[129] In 1988, Padro and associates[130] described a sutureless repair using a Teflon patch fixed with cyanoacrylate surgical glue. Thirteen patients with subacute free-wall postinfarction rupture, all of whom showed sudden cardiac deterioration with signs of tamponade and two of whom had sustained cardiac arrest, underwent operation. They achieved a 100% hospital survival, and 100% survival at follow-up extending to 5 years (mean, 26 months).

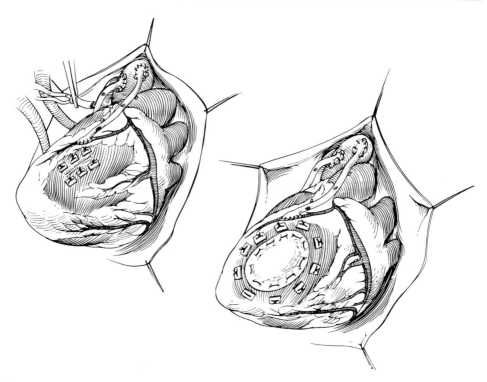

Figure 12.13   Free-wall perforation of the left ventricle. On the left is a direct suture repair of a small rupture. On the right is a Dacron patch closure of a larger rupture. Note the coronary artery bypass grafting which was also done at the time of surgery.

Summary

VSD, free wall rupture, and papillary muscle dysfunction or rupture present the most serious mechanical complications of acute myocardial infarction. Whereas a majority of patients presenting with cardiogenic shock after myocardial infarction will have an etiology of massive left ventricular necrosis alone, a small but consistent percentage will include those patients with these potentially treatable complications. The increased familiarity of interventionalists as well as cardiologists with the use of vasodilator and inotropic agents to treat pulmonary edema and shock in the acute phase of myocardial infarction now allows stabilization of a large number of these patients. However, in order to make a major impact on survival, definitive diagnosis and treatment must follow. Surgery now offers improved survival, especially with VSD and mitral valve dysfunction. All patients who experience acute deterioration after myocardial infarction, and those who develop a new murmur, should be investigated promptly. Early coronary angiography and ventriculography are important in identifying these patients with operable anatomy. IABC is frequently helpful in stabilizing these patients. Their survival is dependent upon rapid, early diagnosis and treatment by an experienced and skilled team of cardiologists and cardiac surgeons.

References

1. National Center for Health Statistics (1987) Utilization of short stay hospitals, United States, 1987. *Vital Health Stat.,* **31**, 197.
2. Braunwald, E. (1992) *Heart Disease,* 4th edn, p. 1200. Philadelphia: W.B. Saunders.
3. Sobel, B.E. (1989) Coronary thrombolysis and the new biology. *J. Am. Coll. Cardiol.,* **14**, 858.
4. Cohn, L.H. (1981) Surgical management of acute and chronic cardiac complications due to myocardial infarction. *Am. Heart J.,* **102**, 1049–60.
5. Fox, A.C., Glassman, E. and Isom, O.W. (1979) Surgically remediable complications of myocardial infarction. *Prog. Cardiovasc. Dis.,* **21**, 461–83.
6. Miller, D.C. and Stinson, E.B. (1981) Surgical management of acute mechanical defects secondary to myocardial infarction. *Am. J. Surg.,* **141**, 677–83.
7. Vlodaver, Z. and Edwards, J.E. (1977) Rupture of ventricular septum or papillary muscle complicating myocardial infarction. *Circulation,* **55**, 815–22.
8. Latham P.M. (1975) Lecture XXIV: Case of rupture of the heart. *Lectures on the subjects connected with Clinical Medicine comprising diseases of the heart.* London: Longmans, Brown, Green and Longmans 2, 168,1845.
9. Brunn, F. (1923) Rupture of interventricular septum. *Weim. Arch. F. Inn. Med.,* **6**, 533–44.
10. Sager, R.V. (1932) Coronary thrombosis: perforation of the infarcted ventricular septum. *Arch. Intern. Med.* **53**, 140.
11. Edmondson, H.A. and Hoxie, H.T. (1942) Hypertension and cardiac rupture: a clinical and pathological study of seventy-two cases, in thirteen of which rupture of the interventricular septum occurred. *Am. Heart J.,* **24**, 719.
12. Diaz-Rivera, R.S. and Mildler, A.J. (1948) Rupture of the heart following acute myocardial infarction. Incidence in a public hospital with five illustrated cases including one of perforation of the interventricular septum diagnosed antemortem. *Am. Heart J.,* **35**, 126.
13. Malloy, G.K., White, P.D. and Salcedo-Salger, J. (1939) The speed of healing of myocardial infarction: a study of the pathologic anatomy in seventy cases. *Am. Heart J.,* **18**, 647.
14. Cooley, D.A., Belmonte, B.A., Zeis, L.B. and Schur, S. (1957) Surgical repair of ruptured interventricular septum following acute myocardial infarction. *Surgery,* **41**, 930.
15. Diacoff, G.P. and Rhodes, M.L. (1968) Surgical repair of ventricular septal rupture and ventricular aneurysms. *JAMA,* **203**, 457.
16. Dobell, A.R., Scott, H.J., Cronin, R.F. and Reid, E.A. (1962) Surgical closure of interventricular septal perforation compounding myocardial infarction. *J. Thorac. Cardiovasc. Surg.,* **43**, 802.
17. Grismere, J.T., Raab, D.E., Berman, D.A. *et al.* (1966) Successful repair of a ruptured ventricular septum complicating a recent myocardial infarction. *Am. J. Cardiol.,* **18**, 120.
18. Stinson, E.B., Becker, J. and Shumway, N.E. (1969) Successful repair of a postinfarction VSD and biventricular aneurysm. *J. Thorac. Cardiovasc. Surg.,* **58**, 20.
19. Heimbecker, R.D., Lemire, G. and Chen, C. (1968) Surgery for massive myocardial infarction. *Circulation,* **37** (suppl. 2), II-3.
20. Lajos, T.Z., Green, D.G., Bunnell, I.L. *et al.* (1969) Surgery for acute myocardial infarction. *Ann. Thorac. Surg.,* **8**, 452.
21. Daggett, W.M., Burwell, L.R., Lawson, D.W. and Austen, W.G. (1970) Resection of acute ventricular aneurysm and ruptured interventricular septum after myocardial infarction. *N. Engl. J. Med.,* **283**, 1507.
22. Daggett, W.M., Randolph, J.D., Jacobs, M. *et al.* (1987) The superiority of cold oxygenated dilute blood cardioplegia. *Ann. Thorac. Surg.,* **43**, 397–402.
23. Freeny, P.C., Shattenberg, T.T., Danielson, G.K. *et al.* (1971) Ventricular septa defect and ventricular aneurysm secondary to acute myocardial infarction. *Circulation,* **43**, 360.
24. Gold, H.K., Leinbach, R.C., Sanders, C.A. *et al.* (1973) Intra-aortic balloon pumping for ventricular septal defect or mitral regurgitation complicating myocardial infarction. *Circulation,* **47**, 1191.
25. Daggett, W.M., Guyton, R.A., Mundth, E.D. *et al.* (1977) Surgery for postmyocardial infarct ventricular septal defect. *Ann. Surg.,* **186**, 260.
26. Lundberg, S. and Soderstrom, J. (1962) Perforation of the interventricular septum in myocardial infarction. *Acta Med. Scand.,* **172**, 413.
27. Lee, W., Cardon, L. and Slodki, S. (1962) Perforation of the interventricular septum. *Arch. Intern. Med.,* **109**, 135.
28. Kitamura, S., Mendez, A. and Kay, J. (1971) Ventricular septal defect following myocardial infarction. *J. Thorac. Cardiovasc. Surg.,* **61**, 186.
29. Hutchins, G. (1979) Rupture of the interventricular septum complicating myocardial infarction: pathologic analysis of ten patients with clinically diagnosed perforations. *Am. Heart J.,* **97**, 165.
30. Selzer, A., Gerbode, F. and Kerth, W.J. (1969) Clinical, hemodynamic and surgical consideration of rupture of the interventricular septum after myocardial infarction. *Am. Heart J.,* **78**, 598.
31. Westaby, S., Parry, A., Ornerod, O. *et al.* (1992) Thrombolysis and post-infarction ventricular septal rupture. *J. Thorac. Cardiovasc. Surg.,* **104**, 1506–9.
32. Weintraub, R.M., Thurer, R.L., Wei, J. and Aroesty, J.M. (1983) Repair of postinfarction ventricular septal defect in the elderly. *J. Thorac. Cardiovasc. Surg.,* **85**, 191.
33. Daggett, W.M., Buckley, M.J., Akins, C.W. *et al.* (1982) Improved results of surgical management of postinfarction ventricular septal rupture. *Ann. Surg.,* **196**, 269.

34. Muehrcke, D.D., Blank, S. and Daggett, W.M. (1992) Survival after repair of postinfarction ventricular septal defect in patients over the age of 70. *J. Cardiovasc. Surg.*, **7**, 290.
35. Roberts, W.C., Ronan, J.A. Jr and Harvey, W.P. (1975) Rupture of the left ventricular free wall (LVFW) or ventricular septum (VS) secondary to acute myocardial infarction (AMI): an occurrence virtually limited to the first transmural AMI in a hypertensive individual. *Am. J. Cardiol.*, **35**, 166.
36. Miller, S., Dinsmore, R.E., Greene, R. and Daggett, W.M. (1978) Coronary ventricular and pulmonary abnormalities associated with rupture of the intraventricular septum complicating myocardial infarction. *AJR*, **131**, 571.
37. Hill, D., Lary, D., Derth, W. and Gerbode, F. (1975) Acquired ventricular septal defects. *J. Thorac. Cardiovasc. Surg.*, **70**, 444.
38. Swithinbank, J.M. (1959) Perforation of the interventricular septum in myocardial infarction. *Br. Heart J.*, **21**, 562.
39. Abrams, D., Edilist, A., Luria, M. and Miller, A. (1963) Ventricular aneurysms. *Circulation*, **27**, 164.
40. Sanders, R.J., Kern, W.H. and Blount, S.G. (1956) Perforation of the interventricular septum complicating myocardial infarction. *Am. Heart J.*, **51**, 736.
41. Edmondson, H.A. and Hoxie, H.J. (1942) Hypertension and cardiac rupture. *Am. Heart J.*, **24**, 719.
42. Lang, H.F. and Aarseth, S. (1950) The influence of anticoagulation therapy on the occurrence of cardiac rupture and hemopericardium following heart infarction: a controlled study of a selected treated group based on 1,044 autopsies. *Am. Heart J.*, **56**, 257.
43. Oyamada, A. and Queen, F.B. (1961) Spontaneous rupture of the interventricular septum following acute myocardial infarction with some clinico-pathologic observations on survival in five cases. Presented at the Pan Pacific Pathology Congress, Tripler US Army Hospital, 12 October.
44. Radford, M.J., Johnson, R.A. and Daggett, W.M. (1981) Ventricular septal rupture: a review of clinical and physiologic features and an analysis of survival. *Circulation*, **64**, 545.
45. Meister, S.G. and Helfant, R.H. (1972) Rapid bedside differentiation of ruptured interventricular septum from acute mitral insufficiency. *N. Engl. J. Med.*, **16**, 1024.
46. Amsterdam, E.A., DeMaria, A.N, Lee, G. *et al.* (1978) Hemodynamic evaluation in acute myocardial infarction. *Adv. Cardiol.*, **23**, 132.
47. Heikkila, J., Karesoja, M. and Luomanmaki, K. (1974) Ruptured interventricular septum complicating acute myocardial infarction. *Chest*, **66**, 675.
48. Daggett, W.M., Mundth, E.D., Gold, H.K. *et al.* (1974) Early repair of ventricular septal defect complicating inferior myocardial infarction. Presented at 28th Annual Meeting of the American Heart Association, Dallas, Texas, November 1974. *Circulation*, **50** (suppl. III), 112.
49. Jones, M.T., Schofield, P.M., Drake, S.F. *et al.* (1981) Surgical repair of acquired ventricular septal defects: determinants of early and late outcome. *J. Thorac. Cardiovasc. Surg.*, **93**, 680–6.
50. Chandraratna P.A.N., Balachandran, P.K., Shah, P.M. and Hodges, M. (1975) Echocardiographic observations on ventricular septal rupture complicating acute myocardial infarction. *Circulation*, **51**, 506.
51. Farcot, J., Boisante, L., Rigaud, M. *et al.* (1980) Two-dimensional echocardiographic visualization of ventricular septal rupture after acute anterior myocardial infarction. *Am. J. Cardiol.*, **45**, 370.
52. Mintz, G.S., Victor, M.F., Kotler, M.N. *et al.* (1981) Two-dimensional echocardiographic identification of surgically correctable complications of acute myocardial infarction. *Circulation*, **64**, 91.
53. Harrison, M.R., MacPhail, B., Gurley, J.C. *et al.* (1989) Usefulness of color Doppler flow imaging to distinguish ventricular septal defect from mitral regurgitation complicating acute myocardial infarction. *Am. J. Cardiol.*, **64**, 697–70.
54. Honey, M., Belcher, J.R., Hansan, M. and Gibbons, J.R.P. (1967) Case reports: successful early repair of acquired ventricular septal defect after myocardial infarction. *Br. Heart J.*, **29**, 453.
55. Buckley, M.J., Mundth, E.D., Daggett, W.M. *et al.* (1971) Surgical therapy for early complications of myocardial infarction. *Surgery*, **70**, 814.
56. Gaudiani, V.A., Miller, D.C. and Stinson, E.B. (1981) Postinfarction ventricular septal defect: an argument for early operation. *Surgery*, **89**, 48.
57. Tecklenberg, P.L., Fitzgerald, J., Allaire, B.L. *et al.* (1976) Afterload reduction in the management of postinfarction ventricular septal defect. *Am. J. Cardiol.*, **38**, 956.
58. Chiarello, M., Gold, H.K., Leinbach, R.D. *et al.* (1976) Comparison between the effects of nitroprusside and nitroglycerine on ischemic injury during acute myocardial infarction. *Circulation*, **54**, 766.
59. Buckley, M.J., Mundth, E.D., Daggett, W.M. *et al.* (1973) Surgical management of ventricular septal defect and mitral regurgitation complicating acute myocardial infarction. *Ann. Thorac. Surg.*, **16**, 598.
60. Benton, J.P. and Barker, R.S. (1992) Transcatheter closure of ventricular septal defect: a new surgical approach to the care of the patient with acute ventricular septal rupture. *Heart Lung*, **21**, 356–64.
61. Landymere, R.W., Marble, A.E. and Cameron, C. (1988) Transvenous closure of acquired ventricular septal defects. *Am. J. Cardiol.*, **4**, 277–80.
62. Daggett, W.M. and Buckley, M.J. (1980) The surgical treatment of postinfarction ventricular septal defect: indications, techniques and results. In Moran, J. and Michaelis, L.L. (eds) *Surgery for the Complications of Myocardial Infarction*. Grune & Stratton.
63. Javid, H., Hunter, J.A., Najafi, H. *et al.* (1972) Left ventricular approach for the repair of ventricular septal perforation and infarctectomy. *J. Thorac. Cardiovasc. Surg.*, **63**, 14.
64. Brandt, B. III, Wright, C.B. and Ehrenhaft, J.L. (1979) Ventricular septal defect following myocardial infarction. *Ann. Thorac. Surg.*, **27**, 580.

65. Daggett, W.M. (1984) Surgical technique for early repair of posterior ventricular septal rupture. *J. Thorac. Cardiovasc. Surg.*, **84**, 306.
66. Westaby, M.S., Parry, A., Giannopoulos, N. *et al.* (1993) Replacement of the thoracic aorta with collagen-impregnated woven Dacron grafts. *J. Thorac. Cardiovasc. Surg.*, **106**, 427–33.
67. Muehrcke, D.D., Daggett, W.M., Buckley, M.J. *et al.* (1992) Survival following post-infarction ventricular septal defect repair: effect of coronary grafting. *Ann. Thorac. Surg.*, **57**, 876–83.
68. Skillington, P.D., David, R.H., Luff, A.D. *et al.* (1990) Surgical treatment for infarct-related ventricular septal defects: Improved early results combined with analysis of late functional status. *J. Thorac. Cardiovasc. Surg.*, **99**, 798–808.
69. Smyllie, J., Southerland, G.R., Vaissen, C. *et al.* (1989) Range of coronary artery lesions and the requirement for coronary angiography in post-infarct ventricular defects (abstract). *Br. Heart J.*, **61**, 114.
70. Nasu, M., Masahiko, S., Fujiwara, H. *et al.* (1991) Recovery of end-state organ dysfunction by circulatory assist. *ASAIO Trans.*, **37**, M345–M347.
71. Sukehiro, S. and Flameng, W. (1990) Effects of left ventricular assist for cardiogenic shock on cardiac function and organ blood flow distribution. *Ann. Thorac. Surg.*, **50**, 374–83.
72. Mickleborough, L.L., Rebeyka, K., Wilson, G.J. *et al.* (1987) Comparison of left ventricular assist and intra-aortic balloon counterpulsation during early reperfusion after ischemic arrest of the heart. *J. Thorac. Cardiovasc. Surg.*, **93**, 597–608.
73. Alvarez, J.M., Brady, P.W. and Ross, D.E. (1992) Technical improvements in the repair of acute postinfarction ventricular septal rupture. *J. Cardiovasc. Surg.*, **3**, 198.
74. Daggett, W.M. (1978) Surgical management of ventricular septal defect complicating myocardial infarction. *W. J. Surg.*, **2**, 753.
75. Komeda, M., Freuess and David, T.E. (1990) Surgical repair of postinfarcted ventricular septal defect. *Circulation*, **82** (suppl. 4), 243.
76. Jatene, A.D. (1985) Left ventricular aneurysmectomy, resection or reconstruction. *J. Thorac. Cardiovasc. Surg.*, **89**, 321–31.
77. Merat, F.B. (1803) Observations sur une lesions organique du coeur par ruptures des collonnes charneus du ventricle gauche. *J. Med. Chir. Pharmacol. (Paris)*, **6**, 587.
78. Davison, S. (1948) Spontaneous rupture of a papillary muscle of the heart. *J. Mt Sinai Hosp.*, **14**, 941–53.
79. Burch, G.E., DePasquale, N.P. and Phillips, J.H. (1963) Clinical manifestations of papillary muscle dysfunction. *Arch. Intern. Med.*, **112**, 158.
80. Austen, W.G., Sanders, C.A., Averill, J.H. and Friedlich, A.L. (1965) Ruptured papillary muscle; report of a case with successful mitral valve replacement. *Circulation*, **32**, 597–601.
81. Sanders, R.J., Neubuerger, K.T. and Ravin, A. (1957) Rupture of papillary muscles: occurrence of rupture of the posterior muscle in posterior myocardial infarction. *Dis. Chest*, **31**, 316–23.
82. Cederquiest, L. and Soderstrom, J. (1964) Papillary muscle rupture in myocardial infarction; a study based upon an autopsy material. *Acta Med. Scand.*, **176**, 287–92.
83. Wei, J.Y., Hutchins, G.M. and Bulkley, G.H. (1979) Papillary muscle rupture in fatal acute myocardial infarction: a potentially treatable form of cardiogenic shock. *Ann. Intern. Med.*, **90**, 149–53.
84. Agozzino, L., Falco, A., de Viro, F. *et al.* (1992) Surgical pathology of the mitral valve: gross and histological study of 1288 surgically excised valves. *Int. J. Cardiol.*, **37**, 79–89.
85. Chwa, E., Gonzalez, A., Bahr, R.D. *et al.* (1992) Papillary muscle rupture: a reversible cause of cardiogenic shock. *Md Med. J.*, **41**, 893–7.
86. Clements, S.D., Story, W.E., Hurst, J.W. *et al.* (1985) Ruptured papillary muscle, a complication of myocardial infarction, clinical presentation, diagnosis, and treatment. *Clin. Cardiol.*, **8**, 93–103.
87. Kirklin, J.W. and Barratt-Boyes, B. (1986) Postinfarction ventricular septal defect. In: Kirklin, J.W. and Barratt-Boyes, B.G. (eds) *Cardiac Surgery*, pp. 301–10. New York: John Wiley.
88. Barbour, D.J. and Roberts, W.C. (1986) Rupture of a left ventricular papillary muscle during acute myocardial infarction: analysis of 22 necropsy patients. *J. Am. Coll. Cardiol.*, **8**, 558–65.
89. Dresdale, A.R. and Paone, G. (1991) Surgical treatment of acute myocardial infarction. *Henry Ford Hosp. Med. J.*, **39**, 245–50.
90. Nunley, D.L. and Starr, A. (1983) Papillary muscle rupture complicating acute myocardial infarction: treatment with mitral valve replacement and coronary bypass surgery. *Am. J. Surg.*, **145**, 574–7.
91. Morrow, A.G., Cohen, L.S., Roberts, W.C. *et al.* (1968) Severe mitral regurgitation following acute myocardial infarction and ruptured papillary muscle: hemodynamic findings and results of operative treatment in four patients. *Circulation*, **37** (suppl. 2), 124–32.
92. Radford, M.J., Johson, J.A., Buckley, M.J. *et al.* (1979) Survival following mitral valve replacement for mitral regurgitation due to coronary artery disease. *Circulation*, **60** (suppl. I), 39–47.
93. Kouchoukos, N.T. (1981) Surgical treatment of acute complications of myocardial infarction. *Cardiovasc. Clin.*, **11**, 141–9.
94. Nishimura, R.A., Schaff, H.V., Shub, C. *et al.* (1983) Papillary muscle rupture complicating acute myocardial infarction: analysis of 17 patients. *Am. J. Cardiol.*, **51**, 373–7.
95. Goldman, A.P., Glover, M.U., Mick, W. *et al.* (1991) Role of echocardiography/Doppler in cardiogenic shock: silent mitral regurgitation. *Ann. Thorac. Surg.*, **52**, 296–9.

96. Horstkotte, D., Schulte, H.D., Niehues, R. *et al.* (1993) Diagnostic and therapeutic considerations in acute, severe mitral regurgitation experience in 42 consecutive patients entering the intensive care unit with pulmonary edema. *J. Heart Valve Dis.*, **2**, 512–22.
97. Roelandt, J.R., Smyllie, J.H. and Sutherland, G.R. (1989) The surgical complications of acute myocardial infarction: color Doppler evaluation. *Int. J. Card. Imaging*, **4**, 45–7.
98. Bolooki, H. (1989) Emergency cardiac procedures in patients in cardiogenic shock due to complications of coronary artery disease. *Circulation*, **80** (suppl. I), 137–48.
99. Replogle, R.L. and Campbell, C.D. (1989) Surgery for mitral regurgitation associated with ischemic heart disease: results and strategies. *Circulation*, **79** (suppl. I), 122–5.
100. Chatterjee, K. and Parmley, W.W. (1977) The role of vasodilatation therapy in heart failure. *Prog. Cardiovasc. Dis.*, **19**, 301–7.
101. Yoran, C., Yellen, E.L. and Becker, R.M. (1979) Mechanism or reduction of mitral regurgitation with vasodilatation therapy. *Am. J. Cardiol.*, **43**, 773–9.
102. Maroko, P.R., Kjekshus, J.K., Sobel, B.E. *et al.* (1971) Factors influencing infarct size following experimental coronary artery occlusions. *Circulation*, **43**, 67–82.
103. Nishimura, R.A., Schaff, H.V., Gersh, B.J. *et al.* (1986) Early repair of mechanical complications after acute myocardial infarction. *JAMA*, **256**, 47–50.
104. Killen, D.A., Reed, W.A., Wathanacharoen, S. *et al.* (1983) Surgical treatment of papillary muscle rupture. *Ann. Thorac. Surg.*, **35**, 243–8.
105. Tepe, N.A. and Edmunds, L.H. (1985) Operation for acute postinfarction mitral insufficiency and cardiogenic shock. *J. Thorac. Cardiovasc. Surg.*, **89**, 525.
106. Hendren, W.G., Nemec, J.J., Lytle, B.W. *et al.* (1991) Mitral valve repair for ischemic mitral insufficiency. *Ann. Thorac. Surg.*, **52**, 1246–52.
107. Spence, P.A., Peniston, C.M., Mihic, N. *et al.* (1986) A physiological approach to surgery for acute rupture of the papillary muscle. *Ann. Thorac. Surg.*, **42**, 27–30.
108. Kay, G.L., Kay, J.H., Zubiate, P. *et al.* (1986) Mitral valve repair for mitral regurgitation secondary to coronary artery disease. *Circulation*, **74**, 188.
109. Rankin, J.S., Feneley, M.P., Hickey, M.S.J. *et al.* (1988) A clinical comparison of mitral valve repair vs. valve replacement in ischemic mitral regurgitation. *J. Thorac. Cardiovasc. Surg.*, **95**, 165–77.
110. Deloche, A., Jebara, V.A., Relland, J.Y.M. *et al.* (1990) Valve repair with Carpentier techniques. The second decade. *J. Thorac. Cardiovasc. Surg.*, **99**, 990–1002.
111. Hansen, D.E., Cahill, P.D., Derby, G.C. and Miller, D.C. (1987) Relative contributions of the anterior and posterior mitral chordae tendinae to canine global left ventricular systolic function. *J. Thorac. Cardiovasc. Surg.*, **93**, 45.
112. David, T.E., Strauss, H.D., Mesher, E. *et al.* (1981) Is it important to preserve the chordae tendinae and the papillary muscles during mitral valve replacement? *Can. J. Surg.*, **24**, 236.
113. David, T.E., Uden, D.E. and Strauss, H.D. (1983) The importance of the mitral apparatus in left ventricular function after correction of mitral regurgitation. *Circulation*, **68** (suppl. II), 76.
114. Spiekerman, R.C., Brandenburg, J.T., Achor, R.P. *et al.* (1962) The spectrum of coronary heart disease in a community of 30 000. A clinicopathologic study. *Circulation*, **25**, 57–65.
115. van Tassel, R.A. and Edwards, J.E. (1972) Rupture of the heart complicating myocardial infarction: analysis of 40 cases including nine examples of left ventricular false aneurysm. *Chest*, **61**, 104.
116. Bates, R.J., Beutler, S., Resnekov, L. *et al.* (1977) Cardiac rupture: challenge in diagnosis and management. *Am. J. Cardiol.*, **40**, 429–37.
117. Stout, B., Ferrell, L., Wray, T. and Mayes, C. (1991) Myocardial rupture. *Postgrad. Med.*, **90**, 115–22.
118. Duke, M. (1993) A historical review of rupture of the heart. *Conn. Med.*, **57**, 91.
119. Friedberg, C.K. (1969) General treatment of acute myocardial infarction. *Circulation*, **40**, 252–60.
120. Aravot, D.J., Dhalla, N., Banner, N.R. *et al.* (1989) Combined septal perforation and cardiac rupture after myocardial infarction. *J. Thorac. Cardiovasc. Surg.*, **97**, 815–20.
121. Held, P., Dellborg, M., Larsson, S. *et al.* (1985) Successful repair of extensive inferior myocardial infarction with septal and free wall rupture. *Chest*, **87**, 540–1.
122. Pugsley, W. and Treasure, T. (1986) Surgery for acute myocardial infarction: ventricular septal rupture and mitral regurgitation. *Curr. Opin. Cardiol.*, **1**, 859–63.
123. Dhatta, B.N., Bowes, V.F. and Silver, M.D. (1975) Incomplete rupture of the heart with diverticulum formation. *Pathology*, **7**, 179–85.
124. Freeman, W.J. (1958) The histologic patterns of ruptured myocardial infarcts. *Arch. Pathol. Lab. Med.*, **65**, 646–53.
125. Schechter, D.C. (1974) Cardiac structural and functional changes after myocardial infarction. III. Parietal rupture and pseudoaneurysm. *NY State J. Med.*, **74**, 1011–17.
126. Roberts, W.G. and Morrow, A.G. (1967) Pseudoaneurysm of the left ventricle. *Am. J. Med.*, **43**, 639–44.
127. London, R.E. and London, S.B. (1965) Rupture of the heart. *Circulation*, **31**, 202–7.
128. Steigel, M., Zimmern, S.H. and Robicsek, F. (1987) Left ventricular rupture following coronary occlusion treated by streptokinase infusion: successful surgical repair. *Ann. Thorac. Surg.*, **44**, 413–15.
129. Nunez, L., de la Llana, R. Lopez-Sendon, J. *et al.* (1983) Diagnosis and treatment of subacute free wall ventricular rupture after infarction. *Ann. Thorac. Surg.*, **35**, 525–9.
130. Padro, J.M., Mesa, J.M., Silvestre, J. *et al.* Subacute cardiac rupture: repair with a sutureless technique. *Ann. Thorac. Surg.*, **55**, 20–4.

13

Non-Q-Wave, Incomplete Infarction

L. A. Piérard

Introduction

The most appropriate management after an acute myocardial infarction relies on the identification of patients at high and low risk and the anticipation of the nature of increased risk that are essential components of daily clinical practice.

There are two separate periods of risk after an acute infarction: an early vulnerable period of several weeks and a longer period of lower risk during the subsequent months and years. Early mortality is mainly determined by a large-size infarction and left ventricular remodeling and failure. These two deleterious characteristics are usually related to the occurrence of complete, transmural necrosis of a large area at risk. Patients with a nontransmural, incomplete infarction most frequently have a different natural history. The degree of myocardial damage is less and generally limited to the subendocardium. The early mortality is lower and the in-hospital complications are less frequent. However, because of epicardial salvage and greater instability, it is an unstable state and the long-term prognosis of these patients is not better, as they are at higher risk of recurrent cardiac events.

There are two different types of incomplete infarction. It may occur 'naturally' after spontaneous reperfusion, resolution of coronary spasm or recruitment of available collaterals. Incomplete infarction is also increasingly observed as a result of thrombolytic therapy or immediate angioplasty: myocardial salvage improves left ventricular function but increases the incidence of residual ischemia.

The distinction between transmural and nontransmural infarction is thus clinically important. It is not accurately obtained by observation of the ECG. No definite relation exists between the presence or absence of Q wave and the extension of necrosis into the thickness of the ventricular wall. However, a number of reports have indicated that non-Q-wave infarctions differ from Q-wave infarctions on pathophysiologic, prognostic and therapeutic aspects.

Concepts

Transmural vs Subendocardial Myocardial Infarction

Acute myocardial infarction occurs most frequently as a result of total coronary artery occlusion by a fresh thrombus.[1] In the absence of collateral circulation, persistence of this occlusion leads to transmural progression of necrosis, as a wavefront phenomenon,[2] resulting in a transmural infarct. Infarct size is determined not only by transmural extent but also by the site of coronary artery occlusion. A large transmural infarction with extensive myocardial damage is associated with left ventricular dysfunction and early mortality.[3] Transmural infarction and persistence of coronary occlusion, especially of the left anterior descending artery, increase the risk of infarct expansion, characterized by acute dilatation and thinning of the necrotic wall with alteration of geometric morphology of the left ventricle.[4,5] A transmural infarct, especially if expanded, may be associated with several severe complications: myocardial aneurysm formation,[6] cardiac rupture,[7] global left ventricular remodeling[8,9] and early mortality.[10] Acute pericarditis[11] and pericardial effusion[12] are also determined by transmural lesions.

Persistence or rapid restoration of coronary blood flow in the area at risk limits necrosis to the subendocardium, with significant preservation of myocardium, resulting in a nontransmural, incomplete or even abortive infarction. Transient hypoperfusion or nonperfusion followed by reperfusion leads to histologically observable contraction-band necrosis in the myocardium.[13] Several different mechanisms may account for nontransmural or incomplete infarction. The infarct-related artery may never be completely occluded and the infarct may be the consequence of severe imbalance between oxygen supply and demand in the presence of severe atherosclerotic obstruction and increased myocardial oxygen consumption. Another possibility is that coronary thrombosis may be followed by rapid spontaneous reperfusion; this occurs in 15–20% of cases.[1,14] Adequate collateral circulation may also be already developed at the time of coronary thrombosis, which maintains retrograde perfusion of the affected region. In the thrombolytic and interventional era, nontransmural infarction is frequently the result of the infusion of a thrombolytic agent leading to coronary artery reperfusion or of immediate coronary angioplasty.

Preservation of subepicardial viability explains why nontransmural infarction is rarely complicated by infarct expansion, rupture, pericarditis or pericardial effusion. This viable myocardium is usually stunned[15] for several days or even longer. Functional recovery occurs frequently but progressively. The extent and timing of recovery depend on several factors, such as the duration of coronary occlusion, rapidity of lysis of the thrombus, severity of residual atherosclerotic narrowing, changes in vasomotor tone or myocardial oxygen needs. Viable myocardium may, however, be at jeopardy because of the severity or instability of the infarct-related arterial plaque. Thus, nontransmural, incomplete infarction has two prognostically different characteristics: progressive functional recovery, thus better regional and global left ventricular function – the good point – and increased risk of residual ischemia and recurrent cardiac events – the bad point.

Nonspecificity of Electrocardiography to Distinguish between Transmural and Nontransmural Infarction

Despite experimental evidence and a mass of clinical–pathologic correlations, the ECG has been used for several decades, not only to diagnose acute myocardial infarction, but also to classify two types of lesions – transmural and nontransmural – from the presence or absence of Q waves.

However, an abnormal Q wave on the standard 12-lead ECG is not an accurate predictor of the presence of transmural necrosis. The subendocardial region is not electrically silent; thus, a number of subendocardial or nontransmural infarcts are accompanied by pathologic Q waves, as demonstrated by clinical[16] and experimental[17] studies. Q waves reflect abnormal myocardial electrical activity[18] but do not imply irreversibility of the underlying process. Persistence of viable tissue in a high proportion of Q-wave regions has been demonstrated by positron emission tomographic studies.[19]

On the other hand, the absence of Q waves may be related to the inability to detect infarct-related Q waves on the standard 12-lead ECG; this is frequent in patients with true posterior transmural infarction.

Thus, abundant evidence indicates that there is no relation between the presence or absence of Q waves and the extent of necrosis into the thickness of the ventricular wall.[21–23] Therefore, the terms 'transmural' and 'subendocardial' cannot be used from analysis of the ECG. After discussions in the literature,[24,25] the use of the terms 'Q-wave' or 'non-Q-wave' infarct has progressively emerged and is now well accepted.

Non-Q-Wave Infarction: a Heterogeneous Group of Abnormalities

The replacement of the old terminology of transmural vs subendocardial infarction by Q-wave vs non-Q-wave infarction does not resolve all problems. There are a number of electrocardiographic difficulties in distinguishing the two infarct types, because of several limitations: the lead system, the lack of uniformity in electrocardiographic criteria, the use of the initial ECG vs serial ECG changes, the type of ST segment shifts, the presence or absence of previous myocardial infarction.

The dominant electrocardiographic feature of non-Q-wave infarction is ST segment depression with or without T-wave inversion. However, this is not a specific pattern: independent confirmation of myocardial necrosis is required from a significant rise and fall in MB creatine kinase activity. As very sensitive methods are now available for myocardial enzyme detection, many episodes of acute ischemic syndromes that would have previously been categorized as unstable angina are now considered as non-Q-wave infarction, with significant release of enzymes into the blood.

The standard 12-lead ECG provides only a fraction of the total available surface potential information. Thus, it cannot distinguish between absence of abnormal Q waves anywhere on the thoracic surface, called by Montague *et al.*[26] 'true' non-Q-wave infarctions, and abnormal Q waves outside the conventional electrode sites, called 'missed' Q-wave infarction.

The electrocardiographic criteria of diagnostic Q waves are not uniform. In the Minnesota code, a codable Q wave is 1 mm or more in depth and 0.02 s or more in duration.[27] Some authors consider as significant a Q-wave duration of longer than 0.03 s or a Q-wave amplitude that is greater than 25% of the following R wave.[28] An abnormal Q wave is more usually defined as one that has a duration of 0.04 s or longer.[29] A significant reduction of R-wave amplitude is considered as a Q-wave infarction by some authors[30] and not by others.[31] However, the amount of R-wave reduction is not standardized. The criteria of true posterior myocardial infarction may also vary. Usually, 'Q-wave' posterior infarction is diagnosed in the presence of initial R waves in lead V1 and V2 that have a duration of 0.04 s or longer, with an R/S ratio equal to or greater than 1.[32] This classification is not included in the Minnesota coding system.

In most acute studies, acute ST segment elevation during prolonged chest pain is considered as a marker of transmural ischemia and a forerunner of transmural necrosis. Early use of thrombolytic therapy is recommended in patients who present with this pattern. A significant proportion of such patients who receive early thrombolytic therapy evolve non-Q wave infarction.[33] Even in the absence of thrombolytic therapy, ST-segment elevation during the early hours is not an invariable harbinger of subsequent Q-wave development.[34] On the other hand, some patients with initial non-Q-wave infarction will develop Q waves during hospitalization even in the absence of reinfarction; this temporal delay between the initial event and the electrocardiographic development of Q waves has been called temporal lag in the ECG.[35] Thus, the distinction between Q wave and non-Q wave requires the analysis of serial ECGs obtained during the first days and cannot be determined from only one recording, especially not the admission ECG.

Finally, several abnormalities of the baseline ECG preclude the classification of acute myocardial infarction: left bundle branch block, ventricular preexcitation, cardiomyopathies and ventricular pacing. A history of previous Q-wave infarction also reduces the accuracy of ECG diagnosis because myocardial scars can produce distortion in the electrical field.[36]

Thus, the ECG terminology is imprecise; however, clinical data support the concept of non-Q-wave acute myocardial infarction as a distinct, if heterogeneous, clinical entity.

Differences in Patients with Q-Wave and Non-Q-Wave Infarction

Despite the above-mentioned limitations, Q-wave vs non-Q-wave infarction has been used as a categorical variable in many published studies. A number of clinical characteristics of patients with non-Q-wave infarction have been compared to those with Q-wave infarction. Despite variations from study to study, substantial differences have emerged during the last decade (Table 13.1).

Prevalence of Non-Q-Wave Infarction

The prevalence of the non-Q-wave subtype has been estimated to be 30–40%. It is higher in subgroups of patients, such as those with previous coronary artery bypass surgery.[37] It is widely accepted that the frequency of non-Q-wave infarction is increasing. This can be explained in part by a greater sensitivity of enzymatic methods, the use of multiparametric approaches to diagnosis,[38] and especially by a more widespread use of aggressive management of acute infarction with thrombolytic therapy and coronary angioplasty. It can be estimated that the incidence of non-Q-wave infarction has grown from 25% in the 1970s to nearly 50% in the 1990s.

Table 13.1 Differences between non-Q-wave and Q-wave infarcts

Variable	Non-Q-wave infarct	Q-wave infarct
Prevalence	Increasing	Decreasing
Peak of onset	Evening hours	Morning hours
Occlusion of the IRV	Rare (±30%)	Frequent (90%)
Collateral circulation	Frequent	Rare
Incidence of prior infarction	Higher	Lower
Prodromal symptoms	Frequent	Rare
Peak CK level	Lower	Higher
Time to peak CK level	Shorter	Longer
Left ventricular ejection fraction	Higher	Lower
High Killip class	Rare	Frequent
Functional recovery	Frequent	Rare
Incidence of spontaneous ischemia	Higher	Lower
Recurrent infarction	More frequent	Less frequent
Early mortality	Lower	Higher
Late mortality	Higher	Lower
Total mortality	Similar	Similar

CK, creatine kinase; IRV, infarct-related vessel.

Pathophysiologic Features

A circadian variation in the frequency of onset of acute myocardial infarction has been observed in numerous studies, with a peak of onset occurring in the morning.[39] Increased platelet aggregability and lower fibrinolytic activity have also been reported during the early morning hours.[40] In contrast, an increased incidence of onset during the evening hours was found in patients with non-Q-wave infarction.[41]

De Wood *et al.* have demonstrated a high incidence of complete thrombotic occlusion of the infarct-related coronary artery in patients with Q-wave myocardial infarction.[1] The same investigators observed a much lower incidence (32%) of complete occlusion of the relevant vessel after non-Q-wave infarction.[31] The rate of complete occlusion increased between the first and the seventh day and collateral circulation was usually present when the infarct-related artery was completely occluded. Thus, non-Q-wave infarction frequently results from partial thrombotic occlusion of a coronary vessel or total occlusion of an artery with available collaterals. These anatomic characteristics imply that non-Q-wave infarction is often an incomplete infarction with persistence of some degree of perfusion and of tissue viability.

Clinical Characteristics

Patients with non-Q-wave infarction more frequently have a prior history of myocardial infarction, previous angina pectoris and prodromal symptoms.[42,43] Some authors have reported a higher mean age and a greater proportion of women and of nonsmokers in the absence of Q-waves, but these differences were not found in other studies.

Numerous findings indicate that the size of non-Q-wave myocardial infarction is usually smaller than that of Q-wave infarction. Peak creatine kinase level is lower;[44] time to peak creatine kinase level is shorter,[45] suggesting spontaneous thrombolysis.

Because of this limited infarct size, regional and global ventricular function is significantly better in patients with non-Q-wave infarction: left ventricular ejection fraction, as measured by radionuclide angiography[42] or contrast ventriculography[46] is higher. Regional wall motion abnormalities more frequently improve in the affected area in patients with non-Q-wave infarction.[47]

The hospital course of patients with non-Q-wave infarction is less frequently complicated when compared to patients with Q-wave infarctions: Killip class >I and congestive heart failure are less frequent; there are fewer atrial tachyarrhythmias and fewer intraventricular conduction defects.[48] In concordance with these findings, most studies have reported a significantly lower in-hospital mortality in patients with a non-Q-wave infarction.[49,50]

Natural History and Long-Term Prognosis

Q-wave infarction is generally associated with occluded coronary arteries, a large infarct size and no residual ischemia. Patent but severely stenotic coronary arteries leading to smaller infarcts and more residual ischemia are frequently observed in non-Q-wave infarction.

Left ventricular remodeling and function during healing differ substantially after Q-wave vs non-Q-wave infarction. In an experimental study, Jugdutt *et al.* demonstrated that the Q-wave group had greater infarct size, greater transmural extent, more infarct expansion, more thinning, greater cavity dilatation and regional asynergy, and higher incidence of aneurysm, left ventricular thrombus and ventricular arrhythmias.[51] The prognosis is worse during healing after a Q-wave event and the highest risk period is observed during the first 3 months.[52]

Global left ventricular size decreases and regional wall motion improves in non-Q-wave infarction during the year after the acute event. This recovery begins within the first 3 months and may be related to recovery of reversible ischemic myocardium or scar contraction.[53] Similar improvement may also be observed after Q-wave infarction in the 1-year survivors.

Despite the favorable short-term prognosis of patients with a non-Q-wave infarction, long-term prognosis is not improved: the early advantage is lost during follow-up, late mortality is much greater and total mortality equalizes over 3–5 years in the two groups. The vulnerable period is much longer after a non-Q-wave event and begins early in the clinical course. Most studies have demonstrated a higher rate of residual myocardial ischemia at predischarge exercise testing,[42] of early spontaneous postinfarction ischemia[54,55] and of early recurrent infarction.[56] After hospital discharge, residual angina and late infarction rate are more frequent when the original infarct is of the non-Q-wave type.[42,46] Reinfarction occurs most often in the same territory.

Risk Stratification of Patients with Non-Q-Wave Infarction

Prognosis after acute myocardial infarction depends essentially on left ventricular dysfunction, residual jeopardized myocardium and complex ventricular arrhythmias. A large infarct and poor residual left ventricular function are the major determinants of early mortality. High-risk patients may be identified during hospitalization by clinical characteristics, such as pulmonary congestion[57] and occurrence of specific complications, such as bundle branch block or atrioventricular block.[52] Different mechanisms explain late mortality and late nonsurvivors are less reliably identified by in-hospital characteristics. The type of infarction may have significant prognostic implication.

Because of the higher incidence of infarct extension and reinfarction, it has been proposed that early aggressive intervention with coronary arteriography and revascularization be performed in patients with a non-Q-wave infarction. Such a systematic approach is not warranted in each patient. Stratification into high-risk and low-risk subgroups is thus essential in the management of the individual patient (Table 13.2) (see also Chapter 16).

Clinical and Electrocardiographic Factors

Age is an important risk factor, In a large population of more than 2 000 patients, it was shown that in patients ≤70 years of age with or without previous infarction, a non-Q-

Table 13.2 Factors associated with high- and low-risk in patients with non-Q-wave infarction

Higher risk	Lower risk
Greater age	No in-hospital ST segment depression
History of congestive heart failure	Absence of definable ST-T abnormalities
Pulmonary congestion	Nonlocalizable infarction
Postinfarction ischemia	Killip class I
Infarct extension	Normal symptom-limited stress test
ST segment depression at admission	
Persistent ST segment depression	
ST segment elevation at discharge	
Ischemia during low-level stress test	
ST changes during Holter monitoring	

wave event did not carry an increased risk of death within 1 year. In contrast, older patients with non-Q-wave infarction had a higher mortality during the year after hospital discharge than those with Q-wave infarction, particularly in the absence of prior infarction.[58] In the Diltiazem Reinfarction Study Research Group, older age and a history of congestive heart failure were independently predictive of mortality after acute non-Q-wave infarction.[59] Prognosis after non-Q-wave infarction also deteriorates if infarct extension[60] or postinfarction ischemia – angina with transient ST–T changes – occurs during hospitalization.[54]

Several electrocardiographic characteristics also permit stratification of patients with non-Q-wave infarction into high-risk subgroups. Some are recorded at baseline: ST segment depression[61] or ST segment changes in two or more leads during pain;[62] other factors have significance at hospital discharge, such as ST elevation.[59] Persistent ST depression at baseline and discharge is a highly significant and independent predictor of poor prognosis;[59] it is associated with early mortality at 3 months, but not with mortality between 3 and 12 months.[63] On the other hand, patients with non-Q-wave infarction and no in-hospital ST depression are at extremely low risk.[63]

The significance of infarct location is more controversial. Some authors have presented data that suggest that anterior non-Q-wave infarction is associated with greater mortality.[64,65] Others have not found such differences in localizable infarcts, but excluded patients with cardiogenic shock.[66] Nonlocalizable infarcts are at lower risk but represent a heterogeneous group.[66] Absence of definable ST–T wave abnormalities is associated with a favourable short-term and long-term outcome.[67]

Exercise Testing and Electrocardiographic Monitoring

The residual ischemic burden may be determined by use of low-level or symptom-limited exercise testing and/or by ambulatory electrocardiographic ST segment monitoring before or after hospital discharge. Early low-level exercise testing has only a limited role after an uncomplicated non-Q-wave infarction, but is useful in patients with clinical markers of higher risk, such as the presence of pulmonary congestion: patients who develop ischemia in this cohort have an increased incidence of cardiac events in the year after the infarction (odds ratio >3).[68] A symptom-limited exercise test performed before hospital discharge provides a significantly greater cardiovascular stress than does a low-level test and an ischemic response is observed twice as frequently.[69] The exercise ECG aims to identify severe coronary artery disease in survivors of non-Q-wave and Q-wave infarction. Long-term infarct-free survival is indeed more related to the presence of severe coronary disease rather than to the occurrence of a non-Q-wave or Q-wave infarction.[70,71] Compared to patients with Q-wave infarction, more patients with non-Q-wave infarction develop transient episodes of ST segment depression, their ischemic threshold is significantly lower and ischemic episodes are significantly longer.[72] ST changes during Holter monitoring are associated with a poor prognosis. This technique is useful in the stratification of patients who are unable to perform an exercise stress test.[73]

Thus the risk of a second myocardial infarction and cardiac death is largely related to the extent of residual myocardium at jeopardy. Early coronary arteriography is warranted in patients who develop pulmonary congestion or other clinical signs of left ventricular dysfunction during hospital stay and in patients in whom early postinfarction angina occurs, particularly if angina is accompanied by ECG signs of ischemia.[74] In the asymptomatic patients, early exercise testing is the most rational method to stratify patients at high and low risk. It must be emphasized that this management is equally applicable to patients with Q-wave and non-Q-wave infarctions.[75]

Identification of Incomplete Infarction

Besides conventional electrocardiographic analysis, other methods are available to identify patients with an incomplete acute myocardial infarction (Table 13.3). Body surface potential maps can improve substantially the accuracy of the diagnosis of Q-wave vs non-Q-wave infarction.[76]

Recognition of Reperfusion

Nonangiographic manifestations, such as rapid resolution of chest pain, rapid decrease in ST segment elevation and abrupt rise in serum MB creatine kinase activities, are helpful in recognizing that coronary artery reperfusion has occurred, but myocardial reperfusion may sometimes be followed by reperfusion injury and absence of myocardial viability.

Significance of a Small Enzyme Rise

A small enzyme increase may be related to complete necrosis of a small area at risk, but it may often represent an incomplete infarction, especially in the presence of extensive acute ST segment changes, or transient heart failure, indicating a clinical–enzyme mismatch. In a series of 723 consecutive patients with acute myocardial infarction not treated by a thrombolytic agent, we have shown that patients with a low peak creatine kinase level ($\leqslant 650$ iu l^{-1}) had a poorer long-term outcome (3-year posthospital mortality rate, 26% vs 17% $P < 0.01$), especially in the presence of a Q-wave infarction (mortality 31% vs 16%; $P < 0.001$). Mortality was not significantly different in subgroups of patients with a non-Q-wave event: 17% in patients with low peak creatine kinase vs 29% in those with peak creatine kinase > 650 iu l^{-1} (NS). The prognostic implications of a small enzyme rise was thus independent of the type of infarction.[44] In this study population, previous infarction, angina before infarction, anterior location of a Q-wave infarction and pulmonary congestion were more frequently observed in nonsurvivors. The peak creatine kinase level was the most significant parameter for distinguishing between early and late nonsurvivors.[52] A majority of late nonsurvivors who had a low peak MB creatine kinase level probably had an incomplete infarction with myocardium at jeopardy.

Detection of Myocardial Viability

After an ischemic insult followed by restoration of myocardial blood flow, there may be a mismatch between perfusion which has been normalized and contractility, which may remain reduced.[15] This stunned myocardium usually recovers its function spontaneously, but slowly. Noncontractile segments observed by echocardiography or ventriculography early after the acute event may correspond to stunning or necrosis,

Table 13.3   Identification of incomplete infarction

Body surface potential maps
Small enzyme rise
Low-dose dobutamine responsive wall motion
Normal perfusion of the risk area with positron emission tomography
Contrast enhancement within the risk area with myocardial contrast echocardiography
Homozonal ischemia during stress echocardiography

---

which are important features and need to be distinguished. Stunned myocardium exhibits contractile reserve and responds to inotropic stimulation with a significant increase in myocardial thickening.[77] We have shown that this state can be identified by a low-dose dobutamine infusion coupled with echocardiographic monitoring.[78] Stunned myocardium has also been identified as exhibiting regional asynergy in segments exhibiting normal perfusion with positron emission tomography. In all patients with stunned myocardium, an increase in systolic wall thickening was observed during dobutamine infusion in the affected area and functional recovery was demonstrated in all patients on the follow-up echocardiographic study. In contrast, patients who did not respond to dobutamine had no subsequent functional improvement.

In another study, low-dose dobutamine-responsive wall motion and non-Q-wave myocardial infarction independently identified reversible dysfunction.[79] Dobutamine-responsive wall motion was sensitive in all infarct locations, but non-Q-wave event was sensitive only in anterior infarction.

Hibernating myocardium is another possible outcome of non-Q-wave infarction. In this situation, asynergy is accompanied by perfusion metabolic mismatch, i.e. decreased perfusion and high glucose uptake.[78] Some inotropic reserve is usually present, but functional recovery may be modest if a revascularization procedure is not performed.

Detection of Jeopardized Myocardium

In addition to conventional exercise stress testing, several imaging modalities may help to identify myocardium at jeopardy in the same territory of the infarct-related vessel. Pharmacologic stress echocardiography is one of the available methods; high-dose dobutamine or dipyridamole may be used. Residual ischemia in the infarct zone will be identified by the development of asynergy in a normal adjacent zone,[80] or by improvement of contractility at low dose followed by a deterioration at high dose in affected segments.[81] Such identification has prognostic significance as it is associated with an increased risk of cardiac events.[82]

Therapeutic Management of Non-Q-Wave Infarction

Thrombolytic Therapy

The selection of patients for thrombolytic therapy represents one of the first clinical decisions when the diagnosis of acute myocardial infarction is established. The admission ECG is used in the decision-making process. Patients are considered for thrombolysis when ST segment elevation is present, which suggests transmural ischemia. An accurate diagnosis of non-Q-wave infarction can only be obtained by analysis of serial ECG recordings. When fibrinolytic treatment has been given, the subsequent ECGs are of course influenced by the result of the therapy. The widespread use of thrombolysis is thus a major determinant of the evolution to a non-Q-wave event by aborting transmural necrosis.

On the other hand, ST segment depression frequently represents the electrocardiographic pattern of the 'naturally occurring' non-Q-wave or incomplete infarction. Thrombolytic therapy in this situation is not beneficial and may be detrimental.[83] However, it is important to distinguish between true subendocardial anterior infarction and true posterior transmural infarction. In this regard, the T wave is more important than the ST segment. A negative T wave in the precordial leads is an accurate indicator of the involvement of the anterior wall. Positive T waves with upsloping ST-segment depression are usually associated with posterior wall infarction related to left circumflex occlusion; thrombolysis may be warranted in this condition.

Anticoagulants and Platelet-Active Drugs

Whether or not thrombolytic therapy has been used, the patients with a non-Q-wave infarction are more likely to have a patent infarct-related artery and an increased risk of reocclusion. Prevention of reocclusion of the infarct-related artery after thrombolytic therapy or prevention of complete occlusion in patients with a 'naturally occurring' non-Q-wave event are essential components of therapeutic management. In unstable coronary disease, both platelets and thrombin play a primary role. Since the ISIS-2 study,[84] oral aspirin is definitely an established agent. Although there is not yet a consensus regarding the ideal dose of aspirin, the current recommendation is 160 mg chewed immediately on admission, if patients are not already taking aspirin, and 160 mg daily thereafter.

Anticoagulation is useful in conjunction with a thrombolytic agent and aspirin. Heparin is at present the most frequently used agent, but its efficacy remains limited, with the problem of rebound coagulation after cessation of its infusion.[85] Specific thrombin inhibitors are more potent than heparin for the prevention of platelet-mediated arterial thrombosis. They act not only on surface thrombin, but also on clot-bound thrombin. However, rebound thrombin generation associated with recurrent ischemic events was observed after cessation of argatroban therapy in patients with unstable angina.[86] Such a rebound phenomenon was not seen in a recent pilot trial of hirudin (recombinant desulfatohirudin) as adjunctive therapy to thrombolysis in acute myocardial infarction.[87] Hirudin was found to be a promising agent compared with heparin and will be evaluated in larger trials.

Platelet-active drugs are beneficial, not only as adjunctive therapy to thrombolysis, but also for secondary prevention effects. In the Persantine–aspirin reinfarction study, combined mortality and reinfarction was reduced by only 7% in the Q-wave group, but 48% among patients in the non-Q-wave group who received active treatment.[88]

Cardiovascular Drugs

After initial therapy, the clinician usually initiates a treatment aimed at secondary prevention after acute myocardial infarction. Several important issues to be considered in this choice are still unresolved. Does the use of thrombolytic therapy influence the choice of the agent? Do all risk strata receive similar benefit from treatment? How should one apply the results of clinical trials to specific subgroups of patients? In particular, should the selection of medication be made according to the electrocardiographic type of infarction? This is a difficult question, because the effects of few drugs have been specifically assessed in prospective studies recruiting patients with non-Q-wave infarctions; in contrast, the effects of other drugs have only been analyzed by *post-hoc* analysis of the non-Q-wave subgroup within a trial, which may raise biases.[89]

Calcium channel blockers

Many large multicenter trials have assessed the effects of calcium channel blockers in patients with myocardial infarction. In most studies, no distinction was made between Q-wave and non-Q-wave infarctions. The results of these studies are disappointing. Six trials compared nifedipine to placebo or to other cardiovascular drugs: none showed a favorable effect of nifedipine on mortality or reinfarction.[90] In two studies, patients assigned to nifedipine experienced reinfarction more frequently[91] or death.[92]

The effects of verapamil were studied in the Danish Verapamil Infarction Trials (DAVIT I and II). DAVIT I showed no beneficial effect on outcome, but used intravenous bolus at admission followed by early oral administration of verapamil 120 mg three times daily.[93] In DAVIT II, treatment started in the second week after admission.[94] There was no significant difference in 18-month mortality rates between verapamil and placebo, but a significant reduction in major cardiac events was found in the verapamil group. The positive effect was found in patients without heart failure.

In contrast with the above-mentioned studies, most clinical trials with diltiazem have prospectively considered the electrocardiographic type of infarction. In particular, the Diltiazem Reinfarction Study has only recruited patients with non-Q-wave infarction: 287 received diltiazem (90 mg every 6 hours) and 189 received placebo.[30] Treatment was initiated 24–72 hours after the onset of infarction and continued for up to 14 days. Diltiazem significantly reduced early reinfarction by 51.2% (90% confidence interval, 7–67%) [diltiazem = 6.3% (18/287) vs placebo = 12.9% (27/289)] and refractory postinfarction angina by 49.7% (90% confidence interval, 6–73%) [diltiazem = 3.5% (10/287) vs placebo = 6.9% (20/289)]. The drug was well tolerated, despite concurrent treatment with β-blockers in 61% of patients. Mortality was similar in the two groups.

The Multicenter Diltiazem Postinfarction Trial was a large, prospective study of 2466 patients with Q-wave or non-Q-wave infarction who were randomized 3–15 days after the acute event to placebo or diltiazem 240 mg daily and followed for 25 ± 8 months.[95] Diltiazem had no overall effect on mortality or cardiac events in the study population as a whole. There was a significant interaction between diltiazem and radiographic pulmonary congestion, a covariate specified prior to unblinding: diltiazem was associated with a reduced number of cardiac events in patients without pulmonary congestion but with an excess number of cardiac events in patients with pulmonary congestion. Among the 634 patients with non-Q-wave infarction there was a 34% reduction in the cumulative incidence of 1-year cardiac death and nonfatal reinfarction (diltiazem = 8% (25/296) vs placebo = 15% (50/338); $P = 0.0296$). Thus, those patients with non-Q-wave infarction and/or normal left ventricular function appear to benefit from diltiazem.[96] However, the reduced incidence of reinfarction observed with diltiazem in patients with non-Q-wave infarction is limited to the first 6 months after the acute event; the late rate of reinfarction is not influenced by the drug.[97] The stabilization by diltiazem of the coronary lesion that caused the acute infarction may be related to the decrease in heart rate and blood pressure, but also possibly to the antiplatelet effect of the drug or to its ability to reduce coronary arterial vasoconstriction or spasm. The role of diltiazem as an adjunctive therapy to thrombolysis is currently under investigation.

β-Blockers

Many large randomized trials have evaluated the utility of β-blockers after acute myocardial infarction. Pooled data indicate an approximately 25% reduction in both recurrent infarction and mortality.[98] None of these studies has specifically tried to demonstrate the effects of β-blockers in patients with non-Q-wave infarction. Retrospective, *post-hoc* analysis of the Beta-Blocker Heart Attack Trial[99] did not detect benefit for treatment with propranolol in the non-Q-wave subgroup. Similarly, in the MIAMI trial, metoprolol administration to this sub-group was associated with an increased risk of cardiac events, compared with the placebo group.[100] In contrast, a significant decrease in mortality was found among patients with non-Q-wave infarction in the timolol-treated group in the Norwegian β-blocker trial.[101] The hypothesis that β-blockers are ineffective or potentially harmful in patients with an incomplete infarction has not been confirmed.

Immediate administration of metoprolol reduced the incidence of recurrent ischemia and nonfatal reinfarction in the TIMI phase II trial.[102] β-Blockers appeared to be particularly beneficial as an adjunctive therapy in patients in the low-risk group.

Antiarrhythmic drugs

Frequent ventricular premature complexes in the period after myocardial infarction are associated with an increased risk of sudden death. The Cardiac Arrhythmia Suppression Trial (CAST) was designed to test the hypothesis that reduction of asymptomatic frequent ventricular premature complexes would reduce mortality. Patients assigned to flecainide or encainide had a significantly higher cardiac mortality than those assigned to placebo.[103] A *post-hoc* subgroup analysis showed that patients with non-Q-wave infarction treated with antiarrhythmics experienced a much greater excess of mortality compared with patients with Q-wave infarction, with relative risks differing by a factor of five.[104] The much greater increase in cardiac arrest rate in patients with non-Q-wave infarction was observed during the late follow-up period. These antiarrhythmic drugs could exert their deleterious effect on ischemic myocardium, a situation more likely to occur after an incomplete infarction.

Revascularization Procedures

Coronary angioplasty may be performed immediately after hospital admission to restore patency of the infarct-related coronary artery.[105] This strategy has recently been shown to result in better left ventricular function and lower risk of death and recurrent myocardial infarction than treatment with intravenous streptokinase (Chapter 4).[106] Myocardial salvage obtained by immediate angioplasty leads to a high incidence of incomplete infarction.

The procedure can also be considered after thrombolytic therapy in selected patients who develop spontaneous angina or ischemia postinfarction and in those who have an abnormal predischarge exercise or stress test. In contrast, prophylactic angioplasty is not superior to conservative treatment in patients with no evidence of recurrent ischemia.[102] Angioplasty is also safe in patients with naturally occurring non-Q-wave infarction.[107] Angiographic restenosis rate is similar to that in the general angioplasty population. Successful coronary angioplasty early after a non-Q-wave myocardial infarction may result in recovery of regional myocardial dysfunction.[108]

If the coronary anatomy is not suitable for angioplasty or if disease in the left main coronary artery is present, coronary artery bypass surgery is recommended to control residual ischemia after a non-Q-wave event.

Conclusions

An incomplete infarction has several characteristics: infarct size is smaller, the infarct-related artery is more frequently patent and there is a higher risk of residual ischemia or recurrent cardiac event in the follow-up period. Non-Q-wave infarction is frequently, but far from always, an incomplete infarction. Many patients in the thrombolytic era have an incomplete infarction, despite the development of abnormal Q waves during hospitalization. Several other methods are available to demonstrate the incompleteness of the infarction. Identification of a high-risk subset of patients is essential for appropriate management. The risk is related to the quantity of jeopardized myocardium. Different stress modalities may be used to stratify risk and select patients who require coronary angiography and a revascularization procedure.

References

1. De Wood, M.A., Spores, J., Notske, R. *et al.* (1980) Prevalence of total coronary occlusion during the early hours of transmural myocardial infarction. *N. Engl. J. Med.*, **303**, 897–902.
2. Reimer, K.A., and Jennings, R.B. (1979) The 'wavefront phenomenon' of myocardial ischemic cell death: transmural progression of necrosis within the framework of ischemic bed size (myocardium at risk) and collateral flow. *Lab. Invest.*, **40**, 633–44.
3. Galvani, M., Ottani, F., Ferrini, D. *et al.* (1993) Patency of the infarct-related artery and left ventricular function as the major determinants of survival after Q-wave acute myocardial infarction. *Am. J. Cardiol.*, **71**, 1–7.
4. Hutchins, G.M. and Bulkley, B.H. (1978) Infarct expansion versus extension: two different complications of acute myocardial infarction. *Am. J. Cardiol.* **41**, 1127–32.
5. Pirolo, J.S., Hutchins, G.M. and Moore, G.W. (1986) Infarct expansion: pathologic analysis of 204 patients with a single myocardial infarct. *J. Am. Coll. Cardiol.*, **7**, 349–54.
6. Hochman, J.S. and Bulkley, B.H. (1982) Pathogenesis of left ventricular aneurysms: an experimental study in the rat model. *Am. J. Cardiol.*, **50**, 83–8.
7. Schuster, F.H. and Bulkley, B.H. (1979) Expansion of transmural myocardial infarction: a pathophysiologic factor in cardiac rupture. *Circulation*, **60**, 1532–8.
8. Weisman, H.G., Bush, D.E., Mannisi, J.A. and Bulkley, B.H. (1985) Global cardiac remodeling after acute myocardial infarction: a study in the rat model. *J. Am. Coll. Cardiol.*, **5**, 1355–62.
9. Jeremy, R.W., Hackworthy, R.A., Bautovich, G. *et al.* (1987) Infarct artery perfusion and changes in left ventricular volume in the month after acute myocardial infarction. *J. Am. Coll. Cardiol.*, **9**, 989–95.
10. Eaton, L.W., Weiss, J.L., Bulkley, B.H. *et al.* (1979) Regional cardiac dilatation after acute myocardial infarction: recognition by two-dimensional echocardiography. *N. Engl. J. Med.*, **300**, 57–62.
11. Erhardt, L.R. (1974) Clinical and pathological observations in different types of acute myocardial infarction. A study of 84 patients decreased after treatment in coronary care unit. *Acta Med. Scand.*, Suppl. 560, 1–78.
12. Piérard, L.A., Albert, A., Henrard, L. *et al.* (1986) Incidence and significance of pericardial effusion in acute myocardial infarction as determined by two-dimensional echocardiography. *J. Am. Coll. Cardiol.*, **8**, 517–20.
13. Freifeld, A.G., Schuster, E.H. and Bulkley, B.H. (1983) Nontransmural versus transmural myocardial infarction: a morphologic study. *Am. J. Med.*, **75**, 423–32.
14. Schwartz, H., Leiboff, R.L., Katz, R.J. *et al.* (1985) Arteriographic predictors of spontaneous improvement in left ventricular function after myocardial infarction. *Circulation*, **71**, 466–72.
15. Braunwald, E. and Kloner, R.A. (1982) The stunned myocardium: prolonged post-ischemic ventricular dysfunction. *Circulation*, **66**, 1146–9.
16. Savage, R.M., Wagner, G.S., Ideker, R.E. *et al.* (1977) Correlation of postmortem anatomic findings with electrocardiographic changes in patients with myocardial infarction. *Circulation*, **55**, 279–85.
17. Abildskov, J.A., Wilkinson, R.S., Vincent, W.A. and Cohen, W. (1961) An experimental study of the electrocardiographic effects of localized myocardial lesions. *Am. J. Cardiol.*, **8**, 485–92.
18. De Pasquale, N.P., Burch, G.E. and Phillips, J.H. (1964) Electrocardiographic alterations associated with electrically 'silent' areas of myocardium. *Am. Heart J.*, **68**, 697–705.
19. Brunken, R., Tillisch, J., Schwaiger, M. *et al.* (1986) Regional perfusion, glucose metabolism, and wall motion in patients with chronic electrocardiographic Q wave infarctions: evidence for persistence of viable tissue in some infarct regions by positron emission tomography. *Circulation*, **73**, 951–63.
20. Montague, T.J., Johnstone, D.E., Spencer, C.A. *et al.* (1986) Non-Q wave acute myocardial infarction: body surface potential map and ventriculographic patterns. *Am. J. Cardiol.*, **58**, 1173–80.
21. Cook R.W., Edwards, J.E. and Pruit, R.D. (1958) Electrocardiographic changes in acute subendocardial infarction. I. Large subendocardial and large nontransmural infarcts. *Circulation*, **18**, 603–10.
22. Cook, R.W., Edwards, J.E. and Pruit, R.D. (1958) Electrocardiographic changes in acute subendocardial infarction. II. Small subendocardial infarcts. *Circulation*, **18**, 613–18.
23. Raunio, H., Rissanen, V., Romppanen, T. *et al.* (1979) Changes in the QRS complex and ST segment in transmural and subendocardial myocardial infarctions. A clinicopathologic study. *Am. Heart J.*, **98**, 176–84.
24. Spodick, D.H. (1983) Q-wave infarction versus S-T infarction. Nonspecificity of electrocardiographic criteria for differentiating transmural and nontransmural lesions. *Am. J. Cardiol.*, **51**, 913–15.
25. Phibbs, B. (1983) 'Transmural' versus 'subendocardial' myocardial infarction: electrocardiographic myth. *J. Am. Coll. Cardiol.*, **1**, 561–4.
26. Montague, T.J., MacKenzie, B.R., Henderson, M.A. *et al.* (1988) Acute non-Q wave myocardial infarction. A distinct clinical entity of increasing importance. *Can. Med. Assoc. J.*, **139**, 487–93.
27. Edlavitch, S.A., Crow, R., Burke, G.L. and Baxter, J. (1991) Secular trends in Q wave and non-Q wave acute myocardial infarction – The Minnesota Heart Survey. *Circulation*, **83**, 492–503.
28. Horan, L.G., Flowers, N.C. and Johnson, J.C. (1971) Significance of the diagnostic Q wave of myocardial infarction. *Circulation*, **43**, 428–37.

29. Myers, G.B., Klein, H.A. and Hiratza, T. (1949) Correlation of electrocardiographic and pathologic findings in posterolateral infarction. *Am. Heart J.*, **38**, 837–62.
30. Gibson, R.S., Boden, W.E., Théroux, P. *et al.* and the Diltiazem Reinfarction Study Group (1986) Diltiazem and reinfarction in patients with non-Q wave myocardial infarction. *N. Engl. J. Med.*, **315**, 423–9.
31. De Wood, M.A., Stifter, W.F., Simpson, C.S. *et al.* (1986) Coronary arteriographic findings soon after non-Q wave myocardial infarction. *N. Engl. J. Med.* **315**, 417–23.
32. Chou, T.C. (1991) Myocardial infarction, myocardial injury and myocardial ischemia. In: *Electrocardiography in Clinical Practice*, 3rd. edn, pp. 119–94. Philadelphia: W.B. Saunders.
33. Chouhan, L., Hajar, H.A., George, T. and Pomposiello, J.C. (1991) Non-Q and Q wave infarction after thrombolytic therapy with intravenous streptokinase for chest pain and anterior ST segment elevation. *Am. J. Cardiol.*, **68**, 446–50.
34. Boden, W.E., Gibson, R.S., Schechtman, K.B. *et al.* and the Diltiazem Reinfarction Study Research Group (1989) ST segment shifts are poor predictors of subsequent Q wave evolution in acute myocardial infarction. *Circulation*, **79**, 537–48.
35. Kleiger, R.E., Boden, W.E., Schechtman, K.B. *et al.* and the Diltiazem Reinfarction Study Group (1990) Frequency and significance of late evolution of Q waves in patients with initial non-Q wave acute myocardial infarction. *Am. J. Cardiol.*, **65**, 23–7.
36. Abbott, J.A. and Scheinman, M.M. (1973) Nondiagnostic electrocardiogram in patients with acute myocardial infarction. Clinical and anatomic correlations. *Am. J. Med.*, **55**, 608–15.
37. Waters, D.D., Pelletier, G.B. and Haché, M. (1984) Myocardial infarction in patients with previous coronary artery bypass surgery. *J. Am. Coll. Cardiol.*, **3**, 909–15.
38. Carpeggiani, C., L'Abbate, A., Marzullo, P. *et al.* (1989) Multiparametric approach to diagnosis of non-Q wave acute myocardial infarction. *Am. J. Cardiol.*, **63**, 404–8.
39. Muller, J.E., Stone, P.E., Turi, Z.G. *et al.* and the MILIS Study Group (1985) Circadian variation in the frequency of onset of acute myocardial infarction. *N. Engl. J. Med.*, **313**, 1315–22.
40. Rosing, D.R., Brakman, P., Redwood, D.R. *et al.* (1970) Blood fibrinolytic activity in man: diurnal variation and the response to varying intensities of exercise. *Circ. Res.*, **27**, 171–84.
41. Hjalmarson, A., Gilpin, E.A., Nicod, P. *et al.* (1989) Differing circadian patterns of symptom onset in subgroups of patients with acute myocardial infarction. *Circulation*, **80**, 267–75.
42. Gibson, R.S., Beller, G.A., Gheorghiade, M. *et al.* (1986) The prevalence and clinical significance of residual myocardial ischemia 2 weeks after uncomplicated non-Q wave infarction: a prospective natural history study. *Circulation*, **73**, 1186–98.
43. Ogawa, H., Hiramori, K., Haze, K. *et al.* (1986) Comparison of clinical features of non-Q wave and Q wave myocardial infarction. *Am. Heart J.*, **111**, 513–18.
44. Piérard, L.A., Dubois, C., Albert, A. *et al.* (1989) Prognostic significance of a low peak serum kinase level in acute myocardial infarction. *Am. J. Cardiol.*, **63**, 792–6.
45. Huey, B.L., Gheorghiade, M., Crampton, R.S. *et al.* (1987) Acute non-Q wave myocardial infarction associated with early ST segment elevation: evidence for spontaneous coronary reperfusion and implications for thrombolytic trials. *J. Am. Coll. Cardiol.*, **9**, 18–25.
46. Coll, S., Castaner, A., Sanz, G. *et al.* (1983) Prevalence and prognosis after a first nontransmural myocardial infarction. *Am. J. Cardiol.*, **51**, 1585–8.
47. Mahias-Navarte, H., Adams, K.F. and Willis, P.W. (1987) Evolution of regional left ventricular wall motion abnormalities in acute Q wave and non-Q wave myocardial infarction. *Am. Heart J.*, **113**, 1369–75.
48. Hutter, A.M. Jr., De Sanctis, R.W., Flynn, T. and Yeatman, L.A. (1981) Nontransmural myocardial infarction: a comparison of hospital and late clinical course of patients with that of matched patients with transmural anterior and transmural inferior myocardial infarction. *Am. J. Cardiol.*, **48**, 595–602.
49. Geltman, E.M., Ehsani, A.A., Campbell, M.K. *et al.* (1979) The influence of location and extent of myocardial infarction on long-term ventricular dysrrhythmia and mortality. *Circulation*, **50**, 805–14.
50. Thanavaro, S., Krone, R.J., Kleiger, F.E. *et al.* (1980) In-hospital prognosis of patients with nontransmural and transmural infarctions. *Circulation*, **61**, 29–33.
51. Jugdutt, B.I., Tang, S.B., Khan, M.I. and Basualdo, C.A. (1992) Functional impact of remodeling during healing after non Q wave versus Q wave anterior myocardial infarction in the dog. *J. Am. Coll. Cardiol.*, **20**, 722–31.
52. Piérard, L.A., Chapelle, J.P., Albert, A. *et al.* (1989) Characteristics associated with early (≤3 months) versus late (>3 months to ≤3 years) mortality after acute myocardial infarction. *Am. J. Cardiol.*, **64**, 315–18.
53. Picard, M.H., Wilkins, G.T., Ray, P.A. and Weyman, A.E. (1992) Progressive changes in ventricular structure and function during the year after acute myocardial infarction. *Am. Heart J.*, **124**, 24–31.
54. Bosch, X., Theroux, P., Waters, D.D. *et al.* (1987) Early postinfarction ischemia: clinical, angiographic, and prognostic significance. *Circulation*, **75**, 988–95.
55. Piérard, L.A., Albert, A. and Kulbertus, H.E. (1992) Predictors of spontaneous predischarge ischemia following acute myocardial infarction. *Clin. Cardiol.*, **15**, 260–4.
56. Marmor, A., Sobel, B.E. and Roberts, R. (1981) Factors presaging early recurrent myocardial infarction ('extension'). *Am. J. Cardiol.*, **48**, 603–10.
57. Dwyer, E.M., Greenberg, H., Case, R.B. and the Multicenter Postinfarction Research Group (1986) Association between transient pulmonary congestion during acute myocardial infarction and high incidence of death in six months. *Am. J. Cardiol.*, **58**, 900–5.

58. Nicod, P., Gilpin, E., Dittrich, H. *et al.* (1989) Short- and long-term clinical outcome after Q wave and non-Q wave myocardial infarction in a large patient population. *Circulation*, **79**, 528–36.

59. Schechtman, K.B., Capone, R.J., Kleiger, R.E. *et al.* and the Diltiazem Reinfarction Study Research Group (1989) Risk stratification of patients with non-Q wave myocardial infarction. The critical role of ST segment depression. *Circulation*, **80**, 1148–58.

60. Maisel, A.S., Ahnve, S., Gilpin, E. *et al.* (1985) Prognosis after extension of myocardial infarct: the role of Q wave or non-Q wave infarction. *Circulation*, **71**, 211–17.

61. Krone, R.J., Greenberg, H., Dwyer, E.M. *et al.* and the Multicenter Diltiazem Postinfarction Trial Research Group (1993) Long-term prognostic significance of ST segment depression during acute myocardial infarction. *J. Am. Coll. Cardiol.*, **22**, 361–7.

62. Cohen, M., Hawkins, L., Greenberg, S. and Fuster, V. (1991) Usefulness of ST segment changes in ≥2 leads on the emergency room electrocardiogram in either unstable angina pectoris or non-Q wave myocardial infarction in predicting outcome. *Am. J. Cardiol.*, **67**, 1368–73.

63. Schechtman, K.B., Capone, R.J., Kleiger, R.E. *et al.* and the Diltiazem Reinfarction Study Group (1990) Differential risk patterns associated with 3 month as compared with 3 to 12 month mortality and reinfarction after non-Q wave myocardial infarction. *J. Am. Coll. Cardiol.*, **15**, 940–7.

64. Stone, P.H., Raabe, D.S., Jaffe, A.S. *et al.* for the Milis Group (1988) Prognostic significance of location and type of myocardial infarction: independent adverse outcome associated with anterior location. *J. Am. Coll. Cardiol.*, **11**, 453–63.

65. Kao, W., Khaja, F., Foldstein, S. and Gheorghiade, M. (1989) Cardiac event rate after non-Q wave acute myocardial infarction and the significance of its anterior location. *Am. J. Cardiol.*, **64**, 1236–42.

66. Schechtman, K.B., Kleiger, R.E., Boden W.E. *et al.* (1991) The relationship between 1-year mortality and infarct location in patients with non-Q wave myocardial infarction. *Am. Heart. J.*, **123**, 1175–81.

67. Boden, W.E., Kleiger, R.E., Gibson, R.S. *et al.* and the Diltiazem Reinfarction Study Research Group (1989) Favourable long term prognosis in patients with non-Q wave acute myocardial infarction not associated with specific electrocardiographic changes. *Br. Heart. J.*, **61**, 396–402.

68. Krone, R.J., Dwyer, E.M., Greenberg, H. *et al.* and the Multicenter Post-Infarction Research Group (1989) Risk stratification in patients with first non-Q wave infarction: limited value of the early low level exercise test after uncomplicated infarcts. *J. Am. Coll. Cardiol.*, **14**, 31–7.

69. Juneau, M., Colles, P., Théroux, P. *et al.* (1992) Symptom-limited versus low level exercise testing before hospital discharge after myocardial infarction. *J. Am. Coll. Cardiol.*, **20**, 927–33.

70. Miranda, C.P., Herbert, W.G., Dubach, P. *et al.* (1991) Post-myocardial infarction exercise testing. Non-Q wave versus Q wave correlation with coronary angiography and long-term prognosis. *Circulation*, **84**, 2357–65.

71. Fox, J.P., Beattie, J.M., Salih, M.S. *et al.* (1990) Non-Q wave infraction: exercise test characteristics, coronary anatomy and prognosis. *Br. Heart J.*, **63**, 151–3.

72. Mickley, H., Pless, P., Nielsen, J.R. and Moller, M. (1993) Residual myocardial ischaemia in first non-Q versus Q wave infarction: maximal exercise testing and ambulatory ST segment monitoring. *Eur. Heart J.*, **14**, 18–25.

73. Petretta, M., Bonaduce, D., Bianchi, V. *et al.* (1992) Characterization and prognostic significance of silent myocardial ischemia on predischarge electrocardiographic monitoring in unselected patients with myocardial infarction. *Am. J. Cardiol.*, **69**, 579–83.

74 Bosch, X., Théroux, P., Pelletier, G.B. *et al.* (1991) Clinical and angiographic features and prognostic significance of early postinfarction angina with and without electrocardiographic signs of transient ischemia. *Am. J. Med.*, **91**, 493–501.

75. Moss, A.J. and Benhorin, J. (1990) Prognosis and management after a first myocardial infarction. *N. Engl. J. Med.*, **322**, 743–53.

76. Kornreich, F., Montague, T.J. and Rautaharju, P.M. (1991) Identification of first acute Q wave and non-Q wave myocardial infarction by multivariate analysis of body surface potential maps. *Circulation*, **84**, 2442–53.

77. Ellis, S.G., Wynne, J., Braunwald, E. *et al.* (1984) Response of reperfusion-salvaged stunned myocardium to inotropic stimulation. *Am. Heart J.*, **107**, 13–19.

78. Piérard, L.A., De Landsheere, C.M., Berthe, C. *et al.* (1990) Identification of viable myocardium by echocardiography during dobutamine infusion in patients with myocardial infarction after thrombolytic therapy: comparison with positron emission tomography. *J. Am. Coll. Cardiol.*, **15**, 1021–31.

79. Smart, S.C., Sawada, S., Ryan, T. *et al.* (1993) Low-dose dobutamine echocardiography detects reversible dysfunction after thrombolytic therapy of acute myocardial infarction. *Circulation*, **88**, 405–15.

80. Bolognese, L., Sarasso, S., Bongo, A.S. *et al.* (1991) Dipyridamole echocardiography test: a new tool for detecting jeopardized myocardium after thrombolytic therapy. *Circulation*, **84**, 1100–7.

81. Piérard, L.A., De Landsheere, C., Berthe, C. *et al.* (1992) Identification of viable myocardium: dobutamine echocardiography versus positron emission tomography. In: Hanrath, P. (ed.) *Cardiovascular Imaging by Ultrasound*, pp. 143–57. Kluwer Academic Publishers.

82. Bolognese, L., Rossi, L., Sarasso, G. *et al.* (1992) Silent versus symptomatic dipyridamole-induced ischemia after myocardial infarction: clinical and prognostic significance. *J. Am. Coll. Cardiol.*, **19**, 953–9.

83. The TIMI III B Investigators (1994) Effects of tissue plasminogen activator and a comparison of early invasive and conservative strategies in unstable angina and non-Q wave myocardial infarction. Results of the TIMI III B trial. *Circulation*, **89**, 1545–56.

84. ISIS 2 (Second International Study of Infarct Survival) Collaborative Group (1988) Randomized trial of intravenous streptokinase, oral aspirin, both or neither among 17 187 cases of suspected acute myocardial infarction: ISIS 2. *Lancet*, **ii**, 349–60.
85. Théroux, P., Waters, D., Lam, J. *et al.* (1992) Reactivation of unstable angina after the discontinuation of heparin. *N. Engl. J. Med.*, **327**, 141–5.
86. Gold, H.K., Torres, F.W., Garabedian, H.D. *et al.* (1993) Evidence for a rebound coagulation phenomenon after cessation of a 4-hour infusion of a specific thrombin inhibitor in patients with unstable angina pectoris. *J. Am. Coll. Cardiol.*, **21**, 1039–47.
87. Cannon, C.P., McCabe, C.H., Henry, T.D. *et al.* for the TIMI 5 investigators (1994) A pilot trial of recombinant desulfatohirudin compared with heparin in conjunction with tissue-type plasminogen activator and aspirin for acute myocardial infarction: results of the thrombolysis in myocardial infarction (TIMI) 5 trial. *J. Am. Coll. Cardiol.*, **23**, 993–1003.
88. Klimt, C.R., Knatterud, G.I., Stamler, J. and Meier, P. (1986) Persantine–aspirin reinfarction study: II. Secondary coronary prevention with Persantine and aspirin. *J. Am. Coll. Cardiol.*, **7**, 251–69.
89. Yusuf, S., Wittes, J. and Probstfield, J. (1990) Evaluating effects of treatment in subgroups of patients within a clinical trial: the case of non-Q wave myocardial infarction and beta blockers. *Am. J. Cardiol.*, **66**, 220–2.
90. Gibson, R.S. (1989) Current status of calcium channel-blocking drugs after Q wave and non-Q wave myocardial infarction. *Circulation*, **80** (suppl. IV), 107–19.
91. Report of the Holland Interuniversity Nifedipine/Metoprolol Trial (HINT) Research Group (1986) Early treatment of unstable angina in the coronary care unit: a randomized, double blind, placebo controlled comparison of recurrent ischaemia in patients treated with nifedipine or metoprolol or both. *Br. Heart J.*, **56**, 400–13.
92. Muller, J.E., Morrison, J., Stone, P.H. *et al.* (1984) Nifedipine therapy for patients with threatened or acute myocardial infarction: a randomized double-blind, placebo-controlled comparison. *Circulation*, **69**, 740–7.
93. The Danish Study Group on Verapamil in Myocardial Infarction (1984) Verapamil in acute myocardial infarction. *Eur. Heart J.*, **5**, 516–28.
94. The Danish Study Group on Verapamil in Myocardial Infarction (1990) Effect of verapamil on mortality and major events after acute myocardial infarction (The Danish Verapamil Infarction Trial II – DAVIT II). *Am. J. Cardiol.*, **66**, 779–85.
95. The Multicenter Diltiazem Postinfarction Trial Research Group (1988) The effect of diltiazem on mortality and reinfarction after myocardial infarction. *N. Engl. J. Med.*, **319**, 385–92.
96. Boden, W.E., Krone, R.J., Kleiger, R.E. *et al.* and the Multicenter Diltiazem Postinfarction Trial Research Group (1991) Electrocardiographic subset analysis of diltiazem administration on long-term outcome after acute myocardial infarction. *Am. J. Cardiol.*, **67**, 335–42.
97. Wong, S.C., Greenberg, H, Hager, W.D. and Dwyer, E.M. (1992) Effects of diltiazem on recurrent myocardial infarction in patients with non-Q wave myocardial infarction. *J. Am. Coll. Cardiol.*, **19**, 1421–5.
98. Furberg, C.D. (1987) Secondary prevention trials after acute myocardial infarction. *Am. J. Cardiol.*, **60**, 28A–32A.
99. Gheorghiade, M., Schultz, L., Tilley, B. *et al.* (1990) Effects of propranolol in non-Q wave acute myocardial infarction in the beta blocker heart attack trial. *Am. J. Cardiol.*, **66**, 129–33.
100. The MIAMI Trial Research Group (1985) Mortality. *Am. J. Cardiol.*, **56**, 15G–22G.
101. Pedersen, T.R. (1983) The Norwegian multicenter study of timolol after myocardial infarction. *Circulation*, **67** (suppl. I), 49–53.
102. TIMI Study Group (1989) Comparison of invasive and conservative strategies after treatment with intravenous tissue plasminogen activator in acute myocardial infarction. Results of the thrombolysis in myocardial infarction (TIMI). Phase II trial. *N. Engl. J. Med.*, **320**, 618–27.
103. The Cardiac Arrhythmia Suppression Trial (CAST) Investigators (1989) Special Report. Preliminary report: effect of encainide and flecainide on mortality in a randomized trial of arrhythmia suppression after myocardial infarction. *N. Engl. J. Med.*, **321**, 406–12.
104. Akiyama, T., Pawitan, Y., Greenberg, H. *et al.* and the CAST investigators (1991) Increased risk of death and cardiac arrest from encainide and flecainide in patients after non-Q wave acute myocardial infarction in the cardiac arrhythmia suppression trial. *Am. J. Cardiol.*, **68**, 1551–5.
105. Lange, R.A. and Hillis, L.D. (1993) Immediate angioplasty for acute myocardial infarction. *N. Engl. J. Med.*, **328**, 726–8.
106. De Boer, J., Hoorntje, J.C.A., Ottervanger, J.P. *et al.* (1994) Immediate coronary angioplasty versus intravenous streptokinase in acute myocardial infarction: left ventricular ejection fraction, hospital mortality and reinfarction. *J. Am. Coll. Cardiol.*, **23**, 1004–8.
107. Alfonso, F., Macaya, C., Iniguez, A. *et al.* (1990) Percutaneous transluminal coronary angioplasty after non-Q wave acute myocardial infarction. *Am. J. Cardiol.*, **65**, 835–9.
108. Suryapranata, J.J., Serruys, P.W., Beatt, K. *et al.* (1990) Recovery of regional myocardial dysfunction after successful coronary angioplasty early after a non-Q wave myocardial infarction. *Am. Heart J.*, **120**, 261–9.

14

Right Ventricular Infarction

H. E. Kulbertus

The right ventricle seems to be naturally protected against ischemia. Its wall is rather thin and its muscle mass small; it functions at low pressure and therefore its oxygen demands are considerably lower than those of the left ventricle. In addition, because the systolic pressure it generates is low, coronary perfusion takes place throughout systole and diastole.

The right ventricular free wall is perfused by the right coronary artery via acute marginal branches. However, its anterior aspects are supplied by the left anterior descending artery and by conus branches.[1] Finally, although this is not unanimously accepted,[2,3] the right ventricle seems to receive some blood directly from the right ventricular cavity through a system of Thebesian veins.[4] Collateral flow to the right ventricular myocardium through the moderator band artery, which originates from the left anterior descending artery, may also help protect against massive infarction in the presence of a proximal right coronary artery occlusion.[5] An extensive network of collaterals from the left anterior descending and conus arteries also exists.

In spite of this, a proximal right coronary artery occlusion before the origin of the acute marginal vessels generally causes a significant right ventricular infarction with necrosis of the posterior wall of the right ventricle. When the occlusion is distal to the origin of some marginal branches, but proximal to the origin of others, the extent of the right ventricular necrosis is more limited. With distal occlusion, no infarction occurs.[1]

The frequency of right ventricular infarction in autopsy series varies widely, probably because of differences in the populations studied, as well as in the definition of right ventricular infarction and in the techniques used for its pathologic diagnosis. Thus, the autopsy incidence varies from 1 to 85% and the amount of involvement ranges from 2 to 92% of the right ventricle.[6] Erhardt et al.[7] found right ventricular infarction in 43% of patients dying from an inferior infarction. Isner and Roberts,[8] in their autopsy series, described a 24% incidence of right ventricular infarction, the figure reaching 50% in the presence of a transmural posterior septal infarction. Isolated right ventricular infarction is extremely rare and has been reported in no more than 5% of autopsied cases with myocardial infarction.[1,9] Theoretically, it can be found only in patients with a left dominant coronary artery system in whom the territory of the small right coronary artery comprises only the right ventricle, but not the left ventricular inferior free wall. Early papers reported right ventricular involvement in cases of anterior infarction; later reports however failed to confirm these findings.[1]

Whether right ventricular hypertrophy predisposes to right ventricular infarction remains uncertain. Most authors believe that coronary perfusion remains well preserved in states of right ventricular hypertrophy provided the coronary arteries are normal.[10] Wade noted, however, that right ventricular hypertrophy was 1.5 times more frequent in autopsy specimens with right ventricular vs left ventricular infarction.[11] Similarly, Ratliff and associates[12] demonstrated in a swine model that when right ventricular hypertrophy had been induced before occlusion of the right coronary artery, right ventricular infarction was frequently observed in association with septal and left ventricular posterior wall necrosis. In spite of these observations, the consensus seems to be that right ventricular hypertrophy is not mandatory or even frequent in cases of right ventricular infarction.[1,5,7,13]

Pathophysiology

We have previously reviewed the hemodynamic consequences of right ventricular infarction.[14] Right ventricular infarction leads to loss of contraction of the right ventricular wall. Animal experiments, in which the right ventricle was thoroughly cauterized, showed that the force generated by the left ventricle can be transmitted to the inactive right ventricle.[15] The muscular spirals forming the ventricular myocardium encircle both ventricles. Thus tension developed during left ventricular contraction can be transferred to the thinner right ventricle and blood contained in the latter can be propelled through the pulmonary circulation. If the left ventricle is intact, normal cardiac output and pressures may be maintained. It was therefore widely accepted for a long time that the right ventricle was not really indispensable to sustain the overall cardiac function.

In the clinical setting of right ventricular infarction, the situation is somewhat different.[15] First of all, after cauterization, the ventricle forms a stiff conduit that renders coupling to left ventricular contraction very efficient.[15] In right ventricular infarction, the right ventricular wall is considerably less rigid. Secondly, right ventricular infarction is generally associated with left ventricular infarction and, therefore, occurs in the presence of impaired left ventricular contractility and compliance. This explains why right ventricular infarction is often attended by signs of right ventricular failure and systemic circulatory collapse.

Goldstein et al.[16,17] were the first to demonstrate the role of the intact pericardium in the presence of a right ventricular infarction. They occluded the right coronary artery in open-chest dogs without opening the pericardium. They observed an elevation and equalization in right- and left-sided cardiac filling pressures, associated with a decrease of cardiac output. When they incised the pericardium, the mean arterial pressure and cardiac output rose. After coronary occlusion but before the pericardium was opened, volume loading resulted in a significant increase in left ventricular end-diastolic pressure associated with a small increase of cardiac output and left ventricular volume. After pericardial incision, left ventricular end-diastolic pressure slightly decreased but left ventricular volume and cardiac output significantly increased to values higher than those observed after volume loading performed before pericardiotomy. These results underlined the restrictive role of the pericardium on cardiac output and demonstrated that the intact, restraining pericardium limits the cardiac output and systemic perfusion in the presence of a significant right ventricular infarction. It appears therefore that the hemodynamic derangements seen in the presence of right ventricular infarction are primarily mediated by the restraining influence of the pericardium. One should add that when the left ventricular wall is involved in the infarction, the required left ventricular filling pressures are higher than normal and further increase the right ventricular afterload, which leads to depression of right ventricular systolic function.[18] This, in association with the pericardial restraint, creates a low-output state.[1]

Diagnosis of Right Ventricular Infarction

The diagnosis of right ventricular infarction is based on clinical findings, the ECG, biochemical measurements, echocardiographic, radionuclide and hemodynamic

Table 14.1 Sensitivity, specificity, predictive value and diagnostic efficiency of electrocardiographic alterations

Criteria	Sensitivity	Specificity	Predictive value, test positive	Predictive value, test negative	Efficiency
ST increase in lead V4R	100%	68.2%	66.7%	100%	80.6%
	(76.8–100)	(45.1–86.1)	(43.0–85.4)	(78.2–100)	(64.0–91.8)
ST increase in lead V4R higher than in leads V1–V3	78.6%	100%	100%	88%	91.7%
	(49.2–95.3)	(77.2–99.8)	(61.5–99.8)	(67.4–97.3)	(73.9–96.9)

From Ref. 23 with permission.
The 95% confidence limits are indicated in parentheses.

studies. It should be stressed that extensive right ventricular necrosis is not absolutely necessary for serious hemodynamic alterations to develop if there is stunning of adjacent noninfarcted areas within the right ventricular territory.

The diagnosis of a right ventricular infarction should be suspected in patients suffering an acute transmural inferior infarction who present with hypotension, sometimes severe enough to induce shock and oliguria, elevated jugular venous pressure and clear lung fields.[19] In the presence of a right ventricular infarction, a Kussmaul's sign is often detected.[20,21] The jugular venous pressure is high and shows a characteristic pattern with a rapid Y descent greater than the X descent.[22] Tricuspid incompetence may be observed together with a right-sided third sound.[9] A paradoxical pulse may occur but it is extremely infrequent.

Electrocardiographic Findings

There are no entirely reliable electrocardiographic criteria for anterior right ventricular necrosis. Conversely, posterior right ventricular necrosis may be identified by the presence of a Q wave or ST-segment elevation in the right precordial leads (V4R, V3R, V1, V2, V3). The highest sensitivity and specificity are reached in lead V4R. The criterion of ST-segment elevation in lead V4R being higher than that in leads V1–V3 offers the highest specificity and efficiency in the diagnosis (Table 14.1, Figure 14.1).[23]

Cardiac Isoenzyme Measurements

In the presence of a right ventricular infarction, the enzyme release is higher than that which would be expected for the extent of concomitant left ventricular necrosis. In a series of 39 consecutive patients with inferior infarction, Isner and colleagues demonstrated that hemodynamically documented right ventricular infarction was present in nearly all patients whose peak creatine kinase value exceeded 2000 iu l^{-1}.[24]

Echocardiography

By combining several views, in particular the subcostal approach, cross-sectional echocardiography allows a detailed investigation of right ventricular volumes and global

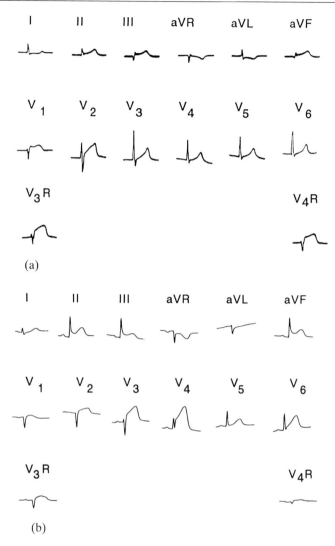

Figure 14.1 Examples of the electrocardiographic tracings recorded in two patients with a documented right ventricular infarction. (a), ST segment elevation in V3R–V4R is higher than in V1–V3. (b), ST segment elevation is present in V3R–V4R but less than in conventional right precordial leads.

contractility and, even more interestingly, a semiquantitative analysis of local contractility. In the presence of major ischemia or infarction,[1,9] echocardiography demonstrates right ventricular dilatation (Figure 14.2), which is particularly obvious during the first hours of the event, and, in almost all cases, some disorders of segmental contractility (akinesia, dyskinesia) at the level of the inferior wall of the right ventricle. Paradoxical septal motion may also be seen.[1,9] Early opening of the pulmonic valve may be seen in cases when the pressure generated by right atrial contraction approximates the pulmonary artery pressure.[25,26] Bellamy and colleagues[20] found that cross-sectional echocardiography had a sensitivity of 82% and a specificity of 93% for the diagnosis of right ventricular myocardial infarction detected by equilibrium-gated blood pool scintigraphy. Echocardiography is also quite useful for differential diagnosis, for example to rule out a

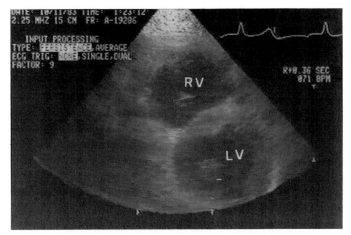

Figure 14.2 End-systolic stop-frame image of a cross-sectional echocardiogram obtained in parasternal short-axis view in a patient with right ventricular infarction. The inferior segment of the left ventricular free wall is akinetic. The right ventricle is enlarged and its free wall is akinetic. RV, right ventricle; LV, left ventricle.

pericardial effusion.[9] Finally, it is of great value for the detection of some of the complications associated with right ventricular infarction, which will be discussed later.[9]

Radioisotopic Investigations

Two radionuclide techniques are of value in the diagnosis of right ventricular myocardial infarction but both have their limitations.

Myocardial Scintigraphy with Technetium-99^m Pyrophosphate

This technique has been widely used especially in the early 1980s.[14,27] We have demonstrated uptake of the radionuclide in the right ventricle in 27.5% of 178 consecutive patients with acute inferior wall myocardial infarction. Right ventricular infarction was diagnosed when an area of pyrophosphate uptake was noted in the left anterior oblique view just behind the sternum and forward of the interventricular septum. Areas of right ventricular pyrophosphate uptake were graded 0 to 2 as indicated in Figure 14.3 (grade 0: no right ventricular uptake; grade 1: right ventricular uptake limited to the inferior wall of the right ventricle; grade 2: massive right ventricular uptake involving both the inferior and anterolateral wall of the right ventricle). Patients with grade 2 were those who, in the acute stage, presented more often with clinical signs of right failure and those in whom the right ventricular dysfunction persisted.[27] Using the same technique, Wackers *et al.*[28] described the prevalence of right ventricular involvement in inferior wall infarction to be nearly 40%. The limitations of this technique are obvious. Positivity of the study is manifest only 48–72 hours after the acute infarction. In addition, the presence of radioactivity in bone, cartilage and chest wall may render the evaluation difficult. In some cases, generally with extensive right ventricular infarction, the thallium-201 myocardial scintiscan may show abnormal right ventricular fixation confined to the

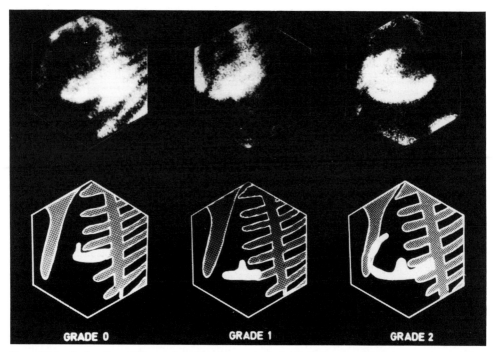

Figure 14.3   Technetium-99^m pyrophosphate images in the LAO (40°) view with diagrams corresponding to the classification into three grades: grade 0, no right ventricular uptake; grade 1, inferior right ventricular uptake; grade 2, inferior and anterolateral right ventricular uptake. (From Ref. 27 with permission).

infundibular region. This may reflect the increased perfusion and hemodynamic overload of the remaining viable territory.[27]

Multigated Blood Pool Scintigraphy Using Technetium-99^m Albumin

This technique, also called radionuclide angiography, overcomes the geometric problems inherent in most methods of right ventricular volume calculation. It is therefore probably the best method for the study of global right ventricular function and for the measurement of right ventricular ejection fraction.[27,29] Right ventricular akinesis can also be assessed by Fourier phase and amplitude analysis[27]. It is generally agreed that, in the presence of a right ventricular infarction, multigated blood pool scintigraphy usually demonstrates a clearcut lowering of right ventricular ejection fraction and dilatation of the right ventricle. It must be pointed out, however, that such disorders of global right ventricular function are of limited diagnostic and prognostic interest: they are indeed variable and reversible and can disappear quickly during the evolution of the disease.[9] The diagnosis therefore should rely on the demonstration of segmental akinesis. However, the superimposition of left ventricular activity does not always permit a satisfactory assessment of the contractile properties of the inferior wall of the right ventricle with this technique.

Right ventricular dysfunction or dilatation has been observed consistently in approximately 40% of patients with acute inferior infarcts.[1] Using criteria of right ventricular ejection fraction below 40% combined with segmental akinesis or dyskinesis, Sterling and associates[30] found that the sensitivity of radionuclide angiography was 92% and its specificity 82% for the diagnosis of hemodynamically significant right ventricular infarction.

Hemodynamic Findings

Bedside right-sided heart catheterization was the first technique to be used for the diagnosis and assessment of right ventricular infarction.[19] Two signs are useful for the diagnosis of right ventricular infarction: (1) a disproportionate elevation of right ventricular filling pressures (mean right atrial pressure or telediastolic right ventricular pressure) as compared to the filling pressures of the left side (pulmonary capillary wedge pressure); and (2) abnormalities in the right atrial and right ventricular pressure waveform.

A right atrial pressure of 10 mmHg or greater and a right atrial to pulmonary artery wedge pressure ratio of 0.8 or greater may represent a reasonable lower limit to identify hemodynamically significant right ventricular damage.[31]

As to the pressure curves, a right atrial tracing with an initial Y descent deeper than the X descent indicates severe right ventricular dysfunction.[22] A diastolic dip–plateau pattern in the right ventricular pressure tracing may be observed due to reduced right ventricular compliance. Right atrial and pulmonary artery pressure curves may look very similar due to a lack of elevation of the right ventricular pressure during systole.[14] Lopez-Sendon et al.[32] reported on the hemodynamic findings in 22 patients who had right ventricular infarction documented at necropsy. They concluded that: (1) equalization of right and left atrial pressures was highly specific but its sensitivity for the diagnosis of right ventricular infarction was only 45%; (2) a Y descent greater than the X descent was also highly specific, but insensitive; (3) a right atrial pressure of 10 mmHg or above, with the right atrial pressure no less than 5 mmHg below the pulmonary capillary wedge pressure was a rather sensitive (73%) and highly specific (100%) sign; and (4) the highest sensitivity (82%) was observed by the combination of the last two criteria. Volume loading significantly increases the identification of right ventricular infarction by hemodynamic criteria in patients with inferior transmural infarction.[31] However, volume loading should be performed with great care. Ideally, it should be limited to patients in whom the initial pulmonary artery wedge pressure is below 15 mmHg. Normal saline solution is infused in increments of 200 ml until the pulmonary artery wedge pressure reaches 15 mmHg, but does not exceed 20 mmHg.

Complications of Right Ventricular Infarction

The acute stage of right ventricular infarction is often characterized by the occurrence of one or several of the following complications. As in any other form of myocardial infarction, ventricular tachycardia or fibrillation may be observed.[27] Transient atrial fibrillation, right atrial paralysis, sinus node dysfunction or high-grade atrioventricular block are not infrequent in this clinical setting; they may add to the hemodynamic embarrassment because of the important role that the atrial contribution makes to cardiac output in the presence of an acute myocardial infarction complicated by left ventricular failure or by the involvement of the right ventricle.[1,9,27,33] Right ventricular free wall rupture, septal rupture and right ventricular papillary muscle rupture have all been observed after right ventricular infarction.[1,9]

Significant tricuspid regurgitation is observed in up to 35% of cases.[34] It is generally secondary to papillary muscle dysfunction but may occasionally be due to a papillary

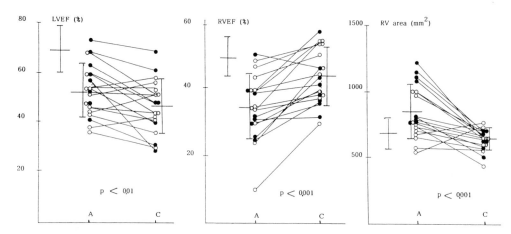

Figure 14.4 Comparison between the left ventricular ejection fraction (LVEF), right ventricular ejection fraction (RVEF) and right ventricular area (RV area) calculated from gated blood pool scintigraphy during hospitalization (acute phase, A) and in the chronic phase (C) 3–4 months after the infarction among 19 patients with right ventricular infarction. On the left of each diagram, mean ± SD of the value among normal subjects. Open circles, grade 1 by technetium-99^m pyrophosphate myocardial scintigraphy; filled circles, grade 2. (From Ref. 27 with permission).

muscle rupture or to right ventricular chamber enlargement. The presence of acute tricuspid incompetence is an ominous sign associated with an increased in-hospital mortality.[34] If the patient survives the acute phase, tricuspid regurgitation generally disappears with time and the need for surgical replacement of the tricuspid valve in the long term is extremely rare.[35]

Right-to-left shunts at the atrial level may develop following the increase of right atrial pressure in the presence of a preexisting atrial septal defect or patent foramen ovale. The shunts may result in profound hypoxia. Such shunts are best demonstrated by contrast echocardiography or by color Doppler echocardiography.[9,36–38]

Cardiogenic shock is one of the most prominent complications in the acute stage of right ventricular infarction.[1,9,14] It often develops early in the course of the disease and is usually rapidly reversible. However, in some cases it may be extremely severe, persist and be the cause of death. The prognosis of cardiogenic shock appears primarily determined by the extent of the associated lesion of the left ventricle but the impaired right ventricular contractility resulting in left ventricular underfilling undoubtedly plays a significant role.

Management of Right Ventricular Infarction

It is difficult to assess the exact benefit that patients with right ventricular infarction may derive from thrombolytic therapy. The difficulty arises from the fact that in the natural course of the disease, right ventricular ejection fraction recovers within days or weeks following the acute infarction (Figure 14.4). It may, in some instances, remain depressed but improvement is the rule. This goes along with the resolution of the right-sided congestive heart failure.

However, there exist some indications that myocardial reperfusion may be helpful. Schuler and associates observed a significant improvement in right ventricular ejection fraction after 1 month in their patients in whom successful intracoronary thrombolysis (with optional coronary angioplasty) has been achieved (improvement from 30% to 43%)

compared with those in whom therapy had failed (33% to 32%).[39] In patients with proximal right coronary artery occlusion treated with intracoronary streptokinase, Braat *et al.*[33] found a higher right ventricular ejection fraction than in patients not submitted to thrombolytic therapy. In the TIMI 2 trial, patients with patent infarct-related arteries had a significantly lower incidence of right ventricular infarction than those with occluded arteries, whereas patients with evidence of right ventricular infarction had a significantly greater incidence of occluded arteries at angiography.[40] One may therefore conclude that it is appropriate to use thrombolytic therapy in patients with right ventricular infarction although the long-term benefit, as compared to nonthrombolytic treatment, is probably less than in left ventricular infarcts. In the presence of severe hemodynamic embarrassment, however, rapid revascularization by thrombolysis[41], percutaneous transluminal coronary angioplasty or coronary artery bypass grafting[43] may be successful.

The primary goal of medical therapy in right ventricular infarction is to maintain an adequate left ventricular preload. Therefore, diuretics, morphine sulfate and nitrates should be avoided or used with great caution. Intravenous volume loading constitutes an interesting strategy.[44] Indeed volume administration elevates right-sided pressures, thereby increasing passive flow through the low-resistance pulmonary circulation and thus improves the left ventricular preload and increases the systemic output. This may require as much as 1–2 l of fluid within the first hours after the infarct and a maintained perfusion of up to 200 ml hour^{-1} later on.[1,9,14,19,46] Careful hemodynamic monitoring is mandatory during intravenous volume loading. The latter may indeed be remarkably efficacious in some cases. In others, it may aggravate right ventricular dilatation and failure. In some cases it may even unmask a latent left ventricular dysfunction and precipitate pulmonary edema.[9,45] If cardiac output does not improve under volume loading, dobutamine may be tried; its administration has been reported to induce a significant increase in cardiac index, right ventricular stroke volume and right ventricular ejection fraction.[9,13,45] Of course, if the left ventricular necrosis is severe, afterload reduction therapy is justified. Finally, if volume expansion and inotropic therapy fail to improve the low-output state in patients with evidence of left ventricular dysfunction, intraaortic balloon counterpulsation has been advocated.[14,27,46,47] It can reduce the right ventricular afterload by lowering left atrial pressure. Simultaneous use of dobutamine and counterpulsation has been reported.[48]

In cases of right ventricular infarction with shock and no response to all forms of therapy, one may be tempted, on the basis of the results of Goldstein,[16,17] to resort to a pericardectomy. To the best of our knowledge this has been performed in only one patient who experienced a dramatic transient hemodynamic improvement but eventually died from multiorgan failure.[1]

Bradyarrhythmias should be adequately treated. Sinus bradycardia may respond to atropine. If atrial fibrillation supervenes, the patient should be cardioverted. Indeed, it is important in this condition to maintain an adequate atrial contraction because the atrial contribution to cardiac output is of paramount importance in the presence of decreased right ventricular compliance. If right ventricular systolic function is depressed, the atrial contraction wave can be transmitted directly to the pulmonary artery.[14] Therefore, if high-grade heart block develops in the course of a right ventricular infarction, dual chamber pacing should be preferred. It has consistently been shown to induce a dramatic increase in cardiac output as compared to ventricular pacing.[49–51] However, the insertion of a temporary pacemaker is not without danger. Cases of right ventricular perforation, particularly following thrombolysis or anticoagulation, have been reported.[1] In addition, the catheter contact with a particularly irritable right ventricular myocardium may induce ventricular tachycardia or fibrillation.[52]

Finally, if the infarction is complicated by profound hypoxia, surgical[53] or balloon catheter[54] closure of a right-to-left shunt through a patent foramen ovale has produced favorable results.

Prognosis

Right ventricular involvement during acute inferior wall myocardial infarction is a strong independent predictor of major complications in the acute stage of the disease.[55] The prognosis, however, seems mainly determined by the extent of left ventricular lesions.[14] In spite of the severe and frequent complications of the acute stage, the long-term prognosis is usually favorable. Complete clinical recovery is common and right-sided congestive heart failure classically disappears.

References

1. Setaro, J.F. and Cabin, H.S. (1992) Right ventricular infarction. *Cardiol. Clin.*, **10**, 69–90.
2. Laurie, W. and Woods, J.D. (1963) Infarction (ischaemic fibrosis) in the right ventricle of the heart. *Acta Cardiol.*, **78**, 399.
3. Rackley, C.E. and Russell, R.O. (1974) Right ventricular function in acute myocardial infarction. *Am. J. Cardiol.*, **33**, 927–9.
4. Farrer-Brown, G. (1968) Vascular pattern of myocardium or right ventricle of human heart. *Br. Heart J.*, **30**, 679–86.
5. Haupt, H.M., Hutchins, G.M. and Moore, G.W. (1983) Right ventricular infarction: role of the moderator band artery in determining infarct size. *Circulation*, **67**, 1268–72.
6. Andersen, H.R., Falk, E. and Nielsen, D. (1987) Right ventricular infarction: frequency, size and topography in coronary heart disease: a prospective study comprising 107 consecutive autopsies from a coronary care unit. *J. Am. Coll. Cardiol.*, **10**, 1233–32.
7. Erhardt, L.R., Sjogren, A. and Wahlberg, I. (1976) Single right-sided precordial lead in the diagnosis of right ventricular involvement in inferior myocardial infarction. *Am. Heart J.*, **91**, 571–6.
8. Isner, J.M. and Roberts, W.C. (1978) Right ventricular infarction complicating left ventricular infarction secondary to coronary disease: frequency, location, associated findings and significance from analysis of 236 necropsy patients with acute or healed myocardial infarction. *Am. J. Cardiol.*, **42**, 885–94.
9. Daubert, J.C., de Place, C., Descaves, C. *et al.* (1988) L'infarctus du ventricule droit: acquisitions récentes et perspectives d'avenir. *La revue du Praticien, Cardiologie*, **19**, 1254–61.
10. Ferlinz, J. (1982) Right ventricular function in adult cardiovascular disease. *Prog. Cardiovasc. Dis.*, **25**, 225–67.
11. Wade, W.G. (1959) The pathogenesis of infarction of the right ventricle. *Br. Heart J.*, **21**, 545.
12. Ratliff, N.B., Peter, R.H., Ramo, B.W. *et al.* (1970) A model for the production of right ventricular infarction. *Am. J. Pathol.*, **58**, 471–9.
13. Ratliff, N.B. and Hackel, D.B. (1980) Combined right and left ventricular infarction: pathogenesis and clinicopathologic correlations. *Am. J. Cardiol.*, **45**, 217–21.
14. Kulbertus, H.E., Rigo, P. and Legrand, V. (1985) Right ventricular infarction: pathophysiology, diagnosis, clinical course and treatment. *Mod. Concepts Cardiovasc. Dis.*, **54**, 1–5.
15. Furey, S.A., Zieske, H.A. and Levy, M.N. (1984) The essential function of the right ventricle. *Am. Heart J.*, **107**, 404–10.
16. Goldstein, J.A., Vlahakes, G.J., Verrier, E.D. *et al.* (1982) The role of right ventricular systolic dysfunction and elevated intrapericardial pressure in the genesis of low output in experimental right ventricular infarction. *Circulation*, **65**, 513–22.
17. Goldstein, J.A., Vlahakes, G.J., Verrier, E.D. *et al.* (1983) Volume loading improves low cardiac output in experimental right ventricular infarction. *J. Am. Coll. Cardiol.*, **2**, 270–8.
18. Cabin, H.S. (1986) The pathophysiology of right ventricular myocardial infarction. *J. Intensive Care Med.*, **1**, 241.
19. Cohn, J.N., Guiha, N.H., Broder, M.I. and Limas, C.J. (1974) Right ventricular infarction: clinical and hemodynamic features. *Am. J. Cardiol.*, **33**, 209–14.
20. Bellamy, G.R., Rasmussen, H.H., Nasser, F.N. *et al.* (1986) Value of two-dimensional echocardiography, electrocardiography, and clinical signs in detecting right ventricular infarction. *Am. Heart J.*, **112**, 304–9.
21. Dell'Italia, L.J., Starling, M.R. and O'Rourke, R.A. (1983) Physical examination for exclusion of hemodynamically important right ventricular infarction. *Ann. Intern. Med.*, **99**, 608–11.
22. Coma-Canella, I. and Lopez-Sendon, J. (1980) Ventricular compliance in ischemic right ventricular dysfunction. *Am. J. Cardiol.*, **45**, 555–61.
23. Lopez-Sendon, J., Coma-Canella, I., Alcasena, S. *et al.* (1985) Electrocardiographic findings in acute right ventricular infarction: sensitivity and specificity of electrocardiographic alterations in right precordial leads V4R, V3R, V1, V2 and V3. *J. Am. Coll. Cardiol.*, **6**, 1273–9.
24. Isner, J.M. (1988) Right ventricular myocardial infarction. In: Konstam, M.A. and Isner, J.M. (eds) *The Right Ventricle*, p. 87. Boston: Kluwer Academic Publishers.
25. Lopez-Sendon, J., Garcia-Fernandez, M.A., Coma-Canella, I. *et al.* (1983) Segmental right ventricular function after acute myocardial infarction: two-dimensional echocardiographic study in 63 patients. *Am. J. Cardiol.*, **51**, 390–6.
26. Legrand, V. and Rigo, P. (1982) Premature opening of the pulmonary valve in right ventricular infarction. *Acta Cardiol.*, **37**, 227–31.

27. Legrand, V., Rigo, P., Smeets, J.P. *et al.* (1983) Right ventricular myocardial infarction diagnosed by 99m technetium pyrophosphate scintigraphy: clinical course and follow-up. *Eur. Heart J.*, **4**, 9–19.
28. Wackers, F.J.T., Lie, K.I., Sokole, E.B. *et al.* (1978) Prevalence of right ventricular involvement in inferior wall infarction assessed with myocardial imaging with thallium-201 and technetium-99m pyrophosphate. *Am. J. Cardiol.*, **42**, 358–62.
29. Rodrigues, E.A., Dewhurst, N.G., Smart, L.M. *et al.* (1986) Diagnosis and prognosis of right ventricular infarction. *Br. Heart J.*, **56**, 19–26.
30. Starling, M.R., Dell'Italia, L.J., Chaudhuri, T.K. *et al.* (1984) First transit and equilibrium radionuclide angiography in patients with inferior transmural myocardial infarction: criteria for the diagnosis of associated hemodynamically significant right ventricular infarction. *J. Am. Coll. Cardiol.*, **4**, 923–30.
31. Dell'Italia, L.J., Starling, M.R., Crawford, M.H. *et al.* (1984) Right ventricular infarction: identification by hemodynamic measurements before and after volume loading and correlation with non invasive techniques. *J. Am. Coll. Cardiol.*, **4**, 931–9.
32. Lopez-Sendon, J., Coma-Canella, I. and Gamallo, C. (1981) Sensitivity and specificity of hemodynamic criteria in the diagnosis of acute right ventricular infarction. *Circulation*, **64**, 515–25.
33. Braat, S.H., de Zwaan, C., Brugada, P. *et al.* (1984) Right ventricular involvement with acute inferior wall myocardial infarction identifies high risk of developing atrioventricular nodal conduction disturbances. *Am. Heart J.*, **107**, 1183–7.
34. Daubert, J.C., Langella, B., Besson, C. *et al.* (1983) Etude prospective des critères diagnostiques et pronostiques de l'atteinte ventriculaire droite à la phase aiguë des infarctus inféro-postérieurs. *Arch. Mal. Coeur*, **76**, 991–1003.
35. Descaves, C., Daubert, J.C., Langella, B. *et al.* (1985) L'insuffisance tricuspidienne des infarctus du myocarde biventriculaire. *Arch. Mal. Coeur*, **78**, 1287–98.
36. Krueger, S.K. and Lappe, D.L. (1988) Right-to-left shunt through patent foramen ovale complicating right ventricular infarction: successful percutaneous catheter closure. *Chest*, **94**, 1100–1.
37. Manno, B.V., Bemis, C.E. and Carver, J. (1983) Right ventricular infarction complicated by right to left shunt. *J. Am. Coll. Cardiol.*, **1**, 554.
38. Rietveld, A.P., Merrman, L., Essed, C.E. *et al.* (1983) Right to left shunt, with severe hypoxemia, at the atrial level in a patient with hemodynamically important right ventricular infarction. *J. Am. Coll. Cardiol.*, **2**, 776–9.
39. Schuler, G., Hofmann, M., Schwarz, F. *et al.* (1984) Effect of successful thrombolytic therapy on right ventricular function in acute inferior wall myocardial infarction. *Am. J. Cardiol.*, **54**, 951–7.
40. Berger, P.B., Ruocco, N.A. and Timm, T.C. (1989) The impact of thrombolytic therapy on right ventricular infarction complicating inferior myocardial infarction: results from thrombolysis in myocardial infarction II. *Circulation*, **80**, II-313.
41. Fujita, M., Sasayama, S. and Sakwai, T. (1987) Intracoronary thrombolysis in evolving isolated right ventricular infarction. *Cathet. Cardiovasc. Diagn.*, **13**, 54.
42. Moreyra, A.E., Suh, C., Porway, M.N. and Kostis, J.B. (1988) Rapid hemodynamic improvement in right ventricular infarction after coronary angioplasty. *Chest*, **94**, 197–200.
43. Goldstein, J.A., Barzilai, B., Rosamond, T.L. *et al.* (1990) Determinants of hemodynamic compromise with severe right ventricular infarction. *Circulation*, **82**, 359–68.
44. Guiha, N.H., Limas, C.J. and Cohn, J.N. (1974) Predominant right ventricular dysfunction after right ventricular destruction in the dog. *Am. J. Cardiol.*, **33**, 254–8.
45. Dell'Italia, L.J., Starling, M.R., Blumhardt, R. *et al.* (1985) Comparative effects of volume loading, dobutamine, and nitroprusside in patients with predominant right ventricular infarction. *Circulation*, **72**, 1327–35.
46. Miller, D.C., Moreno-Cabral, R.J., Stinson, E.B. *et al.* (1980) Pulmonary artery balloon counterpulsation for acute right ventricular failure. *J. Thorac. Cardiovasc. Surg.*, **80**, 760–3.
47. Moran, J.M., Opravil, M. and Gorman, A.J. (1984) Pulmonary artery balloon counterpulsation for right ventricular failure: II. Clinical experience. *Ann. Thorac. Surg.*, **38**, 254.
48. Iqbal, M.Z. and Liebson, P.R. (1981) Counterpulsation and dobutamine: their use in treatment of cardiogenic shock due to right ventricular infarct. *Arch. Intern. Med.*, **141**, 247–9.
49. Topol, E.J., Goldschlager, N., Ports, T.A. *et al.* (1982) Hemodynamic benefit of atrial pacing in right ventricular myocardial infarction. *Ann. Intern. Med.*, **96**, 594–7.
50. Love, J.C., Haffajee, C.I., Gore, J.M. and Alpert, J.S. (1984) Reversibility of hypotension and shock by atrial or atrioventricular sequential pacing in patients with right ventricular infarction. *Am. Heart J.*, **108**, 5–13.
51. Matangi, M.F. (1987) Temporary physiologic pacing in inferior wall acute myocardial infarction with right ventricular damage. *Am. J. Cardiol.*, **59**, 1207–8.
52. Lopez-Sendon, J., Lopez de Sa E., Gonzalez-Maqueda, I. *et al.* (1990) Right ventricular infarction as a risk factor for ventricular fibrillation during pulmonary artery catheterization using Swan–Ganz catheters. *Am. Heart J.*, **119**, 207–9.
53. Bansal, R.C., Marsa, R.J., Holland, D. *et al.* (1985) Severe hypoxemia due to shunting through patent foramen ovale: a correctable complication of right ventricular infarction. *J. Am. Coll. Cardiol.*, **5**, 188–92.
54. Uppstrom, E.L., Kern, M.J., Mezei, L. *et al.* (1988) Balloon catheter closure of patent foramen ovale complicating right ventricular infarction: improvement of hypoxia and intracardiac venous shunting. *Am. Heart J.*, **116**, 1092–7.
55. Zehender, M., Kasper, W., Kauder, E. *et al.* (1993) Right ventricular infarction as an independent predictor of prognosis after acute inferior myocardial infarction. *N. Engl. J. Med.*, **328**, 981–8.

15

Late Use of Angiotensin-converting Enzyme Inhibitors

R. Gorlin

Introduction

Secondary prevention has become an increasingly prominent motivation in our strategy to control the consequences resulting from the primary damage of an acute myocardial infarction. I shall consider the sequelae of an infarct, which lead to change in heart size, shape, and function, and how these affect clinical complications and prognosis, and finally how angiotensin-converting enzyme (ACE) inhibitors may modify the overall outcome.

Background

Myocardial infarction is a complex end result of deprivation of segmental coronary blood supply. Tissue asphyxia leads to myocyte swelling with distortion of organelles such as mitochondria, nuclei, and sarcolemmal membranes. Not only do the myocytes sustain damage, but there is disruption of intracellular fibrous scaffolding, thus unbinding the myocyte. Edema develops, neutrophils infiltrate (if there is any flow at all), and myocytes begin to slip away from each other. The process of thinning and expansion of the infarct zone has begun, all within the first 48 hours.[1] The entire sequence of events is shown in Figure 15.1. Many factors influence this initial process. Figure 15.2 shows the biophysical forces that lead to increased local infarct size, thinning, expansion, and permanent bulging with frank dyskinesis or akinesis.[2] This is affected by the following.

1. Loss of integrity of the wall related to completeness and suddenness of blood flow deprivation. This in turn affects not just the topographic, but the transmural, extent of the infarct. The more of the wall thickness that is damaged, the less resisting force to deformation.
2. Loss of scaffolding functions of the intercellular fibrous network and turgid vasculature to contain the damaged segment.
3. Size and location of the infarct: anterior infarcts tend to be larger, and the anterior apex is thinner than elsewhere in the left ventricle and with a correspondingly sharp angle of curvature.
4. Left ventricular systolic contractile forces both pull on the perimeter of the infarct segment and, via intracavitary pressure, exert force against its surface, both during systole and diastole.

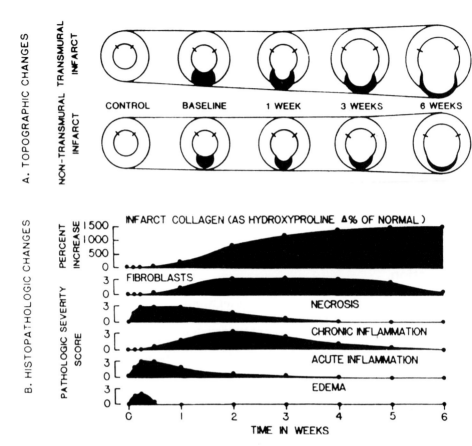

Figure 15.1 Histopathologic and topographic changes during infarct healing. Lower panel: The dynamic nature of histopathologic changes in the infarct substrate from 194 canine hearts studied at 10 time intervals between time zero and 6 weeks after permanent coronary artery ligation. (Data from Ref. 1; Jugdutt, B.I. and Amy, R.W. (1986). Healing after myocardial infarction in the dog: Changes in infarct hydroxyproline and topography. *J. Am. Coll. Cardiol.*, **7**, 81–102 and Pfeffer, J.M., Pfeffer, M.A., Fletcher, P.J. and Braunwald, E. (1991) Progressive ventricular remodeling in rat with myocardial infarction. *Am. J. Physiol.*, **260**, H1406–H1414). Upper panel: A schematic of topographic changes from maps of the transmural and nontransmural infarcts among those hearts for five selected time intervals. (From Ref. 2.)

These theoretic considerations are borne out by studies showing that infarct expansion occurs most frequently in the anterior left ventricular segment,[3] most often in association with hypertension, and is most prominent when the related coronary artery remains occluded and with little evidence of collateral flow.[4,5] Mortality after myocardial infarction appears to correlate both with expansion and with poor segmental perfusion.

The Effects of Infarct Expansion on Uninfarcted Ventricular Size and Shape

While most of the immediate increase in cardiac volume can be attributed to increase in the length as well as decrease in the thickness of the infarcted segment, this early effect on cardiac volume is dominant primarily in the first 48–72 hours.[6] Over the next few weeks, while the length of the infarct expanded by 13%, the length of the uninfarcted

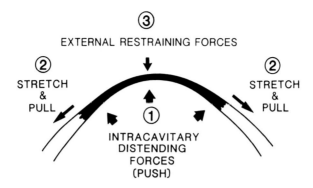

Figure 15.2 Major mechanical remodeling forces acting on the infarction segment during healing. (From Ref. 2.)

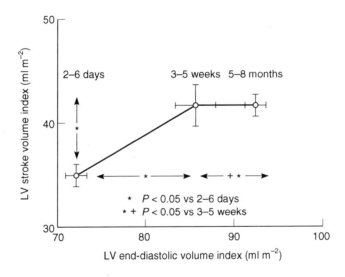

Figure 15.3 Left ventricular stroke volume index and end-diastolic volume index after myocardial infarction. Note progressive dilatation as a function of time without increase in stroke volume. (From Ref. 9.)

contracting segment increased by 19%.[7] This is undoubtedly attributable to early activation of myocardial hypertrophy, a feature demonstrated in the experimental animal.[8]

As time progresses there is little or no further 'give' to the infarct scar with maturation of fibrous tissue and diminution of chronic inflammation (Figure 15.1). Yet the heart gets larger. This is partly due to the Starling effect and to the impact of lost segmental contraction on the residual viable tissue[9] (Figure 15.3). The rest of the myocardium must either increase its fiber shortening distance per beat or increase its initial length to maintain stroke volume.[10] The latter Starling effect dominates in the early stages but, as

Table 15.1 Approaches to remodeling and dilatation following myocardial infarction

Favorable	Unfavorable
Thrombolysis (reperfusion)	Closed infarct-related artery
Angiotensin-converting enzyme inhibitors	Nonsteroidal anti-inflammatory drugs
Nitrates (?)	Steroids
	Exercise training

shown in the studies of Ertl, 'useless' dilatation ultimately appears by 6 months. The heart is now enlarged, altered in shape (remodeled to a spheroidal configuration), exhibits asymmetrical hypertrophy, and often shows diminished contractile performance.

Hypertrophy is a response to the altered stress–strain relationships brought about by the geometric distortions of a segmental ventricular scar. The process is mediated by expression of multiple growth-enhancing genes, dependent, at least in part, on activation of the sympathetic nervous system and the renin–angiotensin–aldosterone (RAA) system. Norepinephrine, for example, is released from nerve endings into the tissues after myocardial infarction. It has now been well established that there is a resident RAA system in the heart[11] that becomes activated during acute myocardial infarction and may be a crucial factor in the genesis of myocardial hypertrophy through the growth-enhancing actions of angiotensin II.

Consequences of Cardiac Enlargement after Myocardial Infarction

Diminished exercise tolerance,[4] the development of congestive failure,[5] and augmented mortality[12,13] all are associated with cardiac enlargement. This therefore gave rise to the hypothesis that limitation of dilatation (and perhaps preservation of contractile state as well) improves all three outcomes.

Approaches to the Problem

The major approaches have been to limit the size of the myocardial infarction through reperfusion therapy, to diminish geometric expansion of myocardial infarction through changes in ventricular pressure–volume dynamics, or to alter the biochemical response to injury both in repair of myocardial infarction and in the compensatory growth/ remodeling response of the residual uninfarcted cardiac muscle (Table 15.1).

The focus of this chapter will be the manifold actions of ACE inhibitors, which may inhibit the dilatation process and alter the natural history following myocardial infarction.

ACE Inhibitors

To understand these enzyme inhibitors, it is necessary to trace the history back to the discovery in the 1930s of a highly vasoactive peptide termed angiotonin by Page, hypertensin by Braun-Menendez, and finally called angiotensin. Skeggs[14] later determined that while renin converted angiotensinogen to angiotensin I, an enzyme was required to cleave off two amino acids and form the biologically active octapeptide,

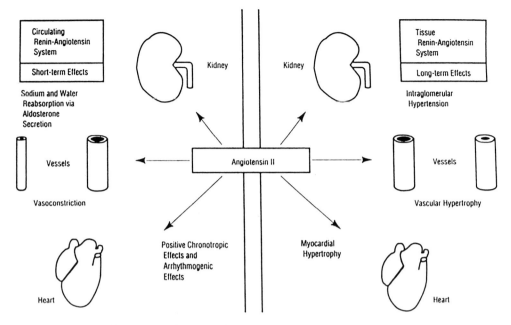

Figure 15.4 Relative roles of circulating and tissue renin–angiotensin systems. The circulating renin–angiotensin system exerts short-term regulation on cardiovascular homeostasis. The tissue renin–angiotensin system influences the cardiovascular system through long-term structural changes. To the left are effects attributable to circulating angiotensin II (endocrine-like), released primarily from the kidney (endocrine), and to the right the paracrine-like tissue-localized angiotensin system (renin, angiotensinogen, ACE and receptor sites for angiotensin II). (From Dzau, V.J. (1993) Tissue renin–angiotensin system in myocardial hypertrophy and failure. *Arch. Intern. Med.*, **153**, 937–42.

angiotensin II. ACE is the same as kininase II, which catalyzes bradykinin. ACE was shown to be blocked by a chemical constituent of pit viper venom.

As shown in Figure 15.4, angiotensin II has a wide array of actions, some mediated via the circulation and others at local tissue sites. Acute activation of this system leads to increased sympathetic activity, vasoconstriction, aldosterone and antidiuretic hormone (ADH) release, and amongst many other actions, chemotaxis of neutrophils.

The hemodynamic end results of an increase in angiotensin II concentration are venoconstriction, producing increased preload to the heart effecting diastolic dilatation, arteriolar and aortic constriction, producing increased afterload/impedance that inhibits cardiac contraction, probably decreased myocardial compliance (stiffness), and, finally, hypervolemia from salt and water retention.

At the tissue level, angiotensin II acts to stimulate growth through expression of a wide variety of growth genes. Consequently, angiotensin II can cause myocyte and connective tissue hypertrophy and vascular smooth muscle hypertrophy.

ACE inhibitors have been shown to inhibit virtually all the above mentioned acute effects of angiotensin II and apparently some of the less immediately responsive growth-enhancing factors as well. Their role in controlling hypertension and left ventricular hypertrophy and in modulating congestive failure has been well established. Thus it seems logical that ACE inhibitors might have a role in the care of the patient after myocardial infarction. The inhibitors reduce the activation of the RAA system that occurs with acute myocardial infarction;[11] modify the subtle physiological changes of heart failure that may be present following myocardial infarction; and, finally, they might alter the enlargement and remodeling process by diminishing loading and by inhibiting

Table 15.2   Efficacy of angiotensin-converting enzyme inhibition derives from pluralistic actions

Mechanical unloading
Systemic arteriolar dilatation
Systemic venous dilatation
Myocardial relaxation (compliance)

Improved organ perfusion
Release of selective vasoconstriction

Inhibition/excitation of multiple neurohormonal systems, both primary and secondary
Inhibition
   Angiotensin II
   Aldosterone
   Norepinephrine
   Arginine–vasopressin

Excitation
   Bradykinin
   Prostacyclin
   Prostaglandin E_2

Tissue-based renin–angiotensin–aldosterone systems and circulating humoral effects (paracrine and endocrine)

hypertrophy[15] (Table 15.2). In an elegant series of experiments in the rat graded infarction model, Pfeffer *et al.*[16] demonstrated that captopril, one of the first ACE inhibitors, could reduce ventricular volume, diminish remodeling and prolong survival in all but the largest infarcts. Thus these actions seemed to transcend purely hemodynamic unloading. This research set the stage for a number of subsequent human investigations.

Side-Effects and Major Adverse Reactions to ACE Inhibitors

Given the fact that there are both circulating and tissue components of the RAA system, it is surprising how few major side-effects there are.[17]

Hypotension is of major concern and is particularly prevalent when there is high renin activity. Hypotension, for example, was seen in the CONSENSUS II Trial[18] when enalapril was administered parenterally on the first day of an acute myocardial infarction. It is probably inadvisable to use ACE inhibitors at such a time of circulatory instability. Clearly 'first-dose' effects can be avoided through upward titration of the dose from a small to the full amount in days, and oral administration seems to be better tolerated than intravenous dosing, at least on the first day.

Hyperkalemia occurs and is directly attributable to inhibition of aldosterone. Creatinine often increases a small amount (up to 2.0 mg dl^{-1}) primarily related to reduced efferent constriction distal to the kidney glomerulus with a fall in filtration pressure and rate.

Unwanted side-effects include angioedema, dose-related agranulocytosis, cough (seen in about 5–10% of patients), rash, and dysgeusia. The cough is only occasionally so troubling to the patient as to warrant discontinuance, although the physician may interpret cough as a sign of worsening heart failure, which it is not.

Hepatic and renal function, blood count and electrolytes should be checked at 1 month after administration and every 3–4 months thereafter. One theoretic concern is whether inhibition of growth factor (angiotensin II) might limit tissue repair and regeneration, not unlike the effects of steroids and nonsteroidal antiinflammatory drugs, which inhibit scar formation following myocardial infarction.[19]

Uses of ACE Inhibitors in Myocardial Infarction

The thrust of this chapter is concerned primarily with therapy after acute myocardial infarction but one cannot overlook the fact that when ACE inhibitors were given for frank heart failure, the results were usually favorable and did not induce severe hypotension.[20–22] The clinician has several ACE inhibitors from which to choose (Table 15.3).

A number of long-term studies of ACE inhibitors have been performed in patients after myocardial infarction. The endpoints examined were heart size, response to exercise testing, development of heart failure, incidence of recurrent myocardial infarction or unstable angina, and mortality (Table 15.4). These endpoints will be discussed in the following sections.

Heart size or function

Among the first human studies were those of Pfeffer and colleagues.[23] They carried out a small trial in patients who had sustained a first anterior myocardial infarction who had no heart failure and an ejection fraction around 0.45. They were randomized to captopril (up to 50 mg) three times daily or placebo 2–4 weeks after myocardial infarction and followed for 1 year. The key findings of this trial were that left ventricular dilatation and distortion of shape (sphericity) correlated with a large myocardial infarction and persistently occluded infarct-related artery. These findings were significantly ameliorated by administration of captopril (Figure 15.5). Left ventricular filling pressures were less and heart failure scores were lower in the ACE inhibitor-treated group.

Sharpe and coworkers administered captopril to three different groups of patients recovering after myocardial infarction to address the question of timing as well as effectiveness of pharmacologic intervention. These researchers used echocardiographic methods to determine left ventricular size and function. In the first study they enrolled 60 patients with all types of Q-wave myocardial infarction, with depressed ejection fraction (<0.45) yet no clinical heart failure.[24] Patients were randomized 1 week after myocardial infarction to captopril 25 mg three times daily, furosemide 40 mg daily or placebo. The salient findings were an increase in end-diastolic volume at 1 year in the placebo and furosemide groups but no increase in the captopril group, while captopril administered induced a significant reduction in end-systolic volume and 10% increase in ejection fraction.

These same researchers studied yet another group of 90 patients, using the same agents and deriving similar findings.[25] Clinical heart failure developed in six patients receiving placebo and in one each in the captopril and furosemide groups.

The next set of observations were designed to test the value of even earlier administration of ACE inhibitors.[26] One hundred patients were administered 50 mg of captopril

Table 15.3 FDA approved angiotensin-converting enzyme inhibitors

Generic name	Manufacturer's brand name
Quinapril	Accupril
Ramipril	Altace
Captopril	Capoten
Benazepril	Lotensin
Fosinopril	Monopril
Lisinopril	Prinivil, Zestril
Enalapril	Vasotec
Cilazapril	Not marketed in USA

Table 15.4 Large clinical trials of angiotensin-converting enzyme inhibitors

Study	Age (years)	Gender	Entry criteria	Agent	Initiation	Duration (months)	Primary endpoint	Secondary endpoints
CONSENSUS II (n = 6090)	65.8	Male 74%	AMI	Enalapril 1 mg i.v. Titrate p.o. to 20 mg q.d.	First 24 hours	6	Death Enalapril 11.0% Placebo 10.2%	Worsening CHF (NS) Enalapril 27% Placebo 30% Re MI (NS)
AIRE (n = 2006)	65	Male 74%	AMI & CHF	Ramipril 2.5 mg b.i.d. 2 days then 5 mg b.i.d.	3–10 days	15	Death Ramipril 17.0% Placebo 22.0%	C-V events Ramipril 17% Placebo 34%
SAVE (n = 2231)	59.4	Male 82%	AMI EF ≤0.40	Captopril 50 mg t.i.d.	3–16 days	36	Death Captopril 20.0% Placebo 25%	Risk reduction C-V disease 37% CHF 22% Re MI 25%

AMI, acute myocardial infarction; CHF, congestive heart failure; C-V, cerebrovascular; EF, ejection fraction; NS, not significant; Re MI, reinfarction.

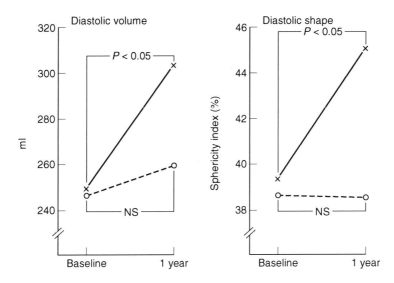

Figure 15.5 Effects of load-reducing therapy with captopril on left ventricular diastolic volume and shape in patients with a large infarct and an occluded infarct-related artery. ×, placebo; ○, captopril. (From Lamas, G.A. and Pfeffer, M.A. (1991) Left ventricular remodeling after acute myocardial infarction: Clinical course and beneficial effects of angiotensin-converting enzyme inhibition. *Am. Heart J.,* **121,** 1194–202.

or placebo twice daily 24–48 hours after the onset of acute myocardial infarction. The differences between the treated and control groups were essentially the same as in the earlier trials, although ventricular volumes generally increased less with treatment when it was initiated at 24–48 hours than at 1 week. Oldroyd[27] also reported that although dilatation had already begun by the first 3–7 days, the increase was less in the ACE inhibitor-treated group than among controls.

Sharpe *et al.*[28] examined the effect of therapy given *late* to those patients in the above-mentioned study[24] who had not been on captopril. Upon conclusion of the first trial at 1 year, 27 previously untreated patients were placed on open-label ACE inhibitors. This group exhibited an ejection fraction averaging 0.33. Even when begun 1 year after myocardial infarction, therapy led to partial reversal of dilatation along with improvement in ejection fraction (to have a control group not receiving ACE inhibitors was considered to be unethical under the circumstances) (Figure 15.6).

Ray *et al.*[29] also reported similar inhibitory effects on ventricular volumes with captopril, but most significantly this group showed that the favorable effects persisted 30 days after withdrawal from active agent. This suggests that remodeling forces rather than simply degree of dilatation may have been changed by the drug.

Exercise capacity following myocardial infarction

The effects of administration of ACE inhibitors on exercise capacity in patients recovering after myocardial infarction are mixed. Pfeffer *et al.*[23] reported a persistent increase in exercise capacity during 1 year of therapy with captopril treatment after myocardial infarction compared with placebo. Lamas *et al.*[4] reporting on the same patient population, stated that exercise capacity correlated inversely with the degree of chamber deformation or remodeling (sphericity), although ACE inhibitors still conferred an additional benefit even on those patients with the most deformed left ventricles. Similarly, Kleber *et al.*[30] described an inverse relationship between dilatation and exercise

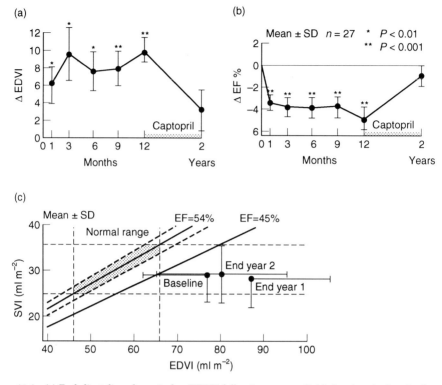

Figure 15.6 (a) End-diastolic volume index (EDVI) following myocardial infarction during the first year with placebo or frusemide and the second year with open captopril treatment. (b) Ejection fraction (EF) following myocardial infarction during the first year with placebo or frusemide treatment and the second year with open captopril treatment. (c) Ventricular function at baseline (approximately 1 week post-infarction) and at the end of the first and second years. The normal range is outlined. Note shift in values off captopril and then on captopril at 1 year. SVI, stroke volume index. (From Ref. 28.)

capacity. On the other hand, neither Oldroyd[27] nor Dickstein et al.[31] reported any change in exercise capacity with the use of captopril or enalapril respectively. This is similar to findings in the VHeFT II study.[32]

Clinical endpoints following acute myocardial infarction

This section will consider issues of morbidity, such as development of heart failure and recurrent myocardial infarction, and mortality (all-cause and cardiovascular) as affected by treatment with ACE inhibitors.

Heart failure has either been attenuated or its clinical emergence retarded by ACE inhibitors. This was suggested by some of the earlier relatively small trials[4,25] but data from two large trials, SAVE[33] and AIRE,[34] established a clearcut favorable effect on heart failure.

The details of trial size, agent dose, entry criteria, and time of administration, etc. are given in Table 15.4. In the SAVE trial the impact on emergence of heart failure in patients with decreased left ventricular dysfunction was judged by frequency of hospitalization or need for open-label ACE inhibitors. Figure 15.7 can be interpreted as showing either less heart failure at any time or a delay in achieving the same prevalence of failure in patients receiving captopril compared with placebo. Less heart failure was also associated with diminished mortality (see below).

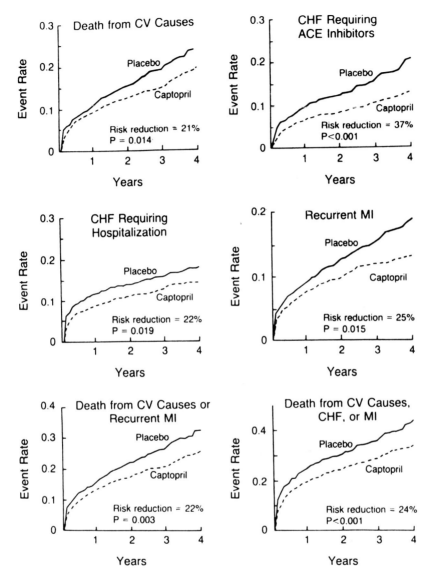

Figure 15.7 Life tables for cumulative fatal and nonfatal cardiovascular events. The bottom right panel shows the following events: death from cardiovascular causes, severe heart failure requiring ACE inhibitors or hospitalization, or recurrent myocardial infarction. For all the combined analyses, only the time to the first event was used. (CV, cardiovascular; CHF, congestive heart failure. (From Ref. 33.)

The AIRE trial[34] of patients who had heart failure during their index myocardial infarction reported a reduction of 19% in first validated secondary endpoints. The major morbid event attenuated other than death (see below) was severe refractory heart failure.

Recurrent myocardial infarction. An unexpected finding of the SOLVD Trial[35] was a reduction of myocardial infarction and unstable angina in both the treatment and prevention arms of the study, as well as diminution in cardiac death. Although almost

80% of the patients were believed to have ischemic heart disease as the basis for left ventricular dysfunction, the treatment effect was also seen in the putative nonischemic subgroup. The reduction in infarct frequency appeared to take place about 6 months after beginning treatment.

While a reduction of recurrent myocardial infarction was reported by the SAVE investigators,[33] the AIRE study[34] did not match these findings.

Whether these salutary effects can be attributed to favorable hemodynamics for myocardial perfusion, such as transmyocardial pressure gradient, subendocardial perfusion dynamics, to reduced afterload, or to inhibition of myocardial and vascular RAA systems *per se* in such a way as to prevent arterial occlusion is unknown.

The apparent, but unanticipated, reduction in the recurrence of myocardial infarction suggests that there may be other actions of ACE inhibitors on vascular biology. The existence of a tissue RAA system separate from circulating endocrine functions may provide important links for identifying and possibly reducing the risk for myocardial infarction. For example, ACE inhibition has favorable effects on diabetic–hypertensive renal vascular disease. Endothelial function may be restored to normal when dysfunctional[36] and inhibition of growth factors such as angiotensin II may retard atherogenesis,[37] although postangioplasty restenosis seems to be unaffected.[38] Conceivably inhibition of ACE, whatever its molecular form,[39] may alter coronary risk *per se*. As a minimum, the previously described reduction in recurrent myocardial infarction in some clinical trials is consistent with this hypothesis.

Mortality. Mortality was reported to be reduced in three of four studies. ISIS-4[40] was a study of 20 000 patients using a multifactorial design of various therapies following acute myocardial infarction. Results at 1 month demonstrated a modest but consistently favorable effect in those subgroups receiving captopril.

Consensus II[18] was a randomized trial of 6090 patients. This protocol called for enalapril to be given (up to 5 mg i.v.) on the first day of an acute myocardial infarction and 20 mg daily thereafter. At the end of 6 months the trial was discontinued owing to little or no difference between the treatment and placebo groups.

The SAVE trial[33] similarly showed no differences between control and ACE inhibitor-groups up to about 1 year, at which time the lines for all-cause mortality began to diverge, eventually resulting in 19% reduction in risk for the captopril-treated group (Figure 15.8). Death from cardiovascular causes was similarly reduced (Fig. 15.7). Sudden death and prevalence of ventricular tachycardia (by Holter monitor) were likewise diminished by ACE inhibitors.[41]

In a substudy of the SAVE Trial,[42] Sutton *et al.*[42] reported on the relationship between heart size and adverse events. In 512 patients, of whom 420 survived, both initial heart size and change in heart size with time predicted cardiovascular mortality and morbidity. Of those who had a major adverse event, all had an increase in heart size. Sixty-nine patients received placebo and 42 received captopril. This appeared to link not only dilatation and remodeling but also its modification to outcome. Kreulen *et al.*[4] and Douglas *et al.*[44] had previously reported that ventricular deformity as well as enlargement correlated with adverse outcome.

There was additional beneficial effect attributable to ACE inhibition beyond that attributable to β-blockers, aspirin and thrombolytics, respectively.[33–35]

The AIRE Trial of 2006 patients, in which ramipril or placebo were begun from the third to the tenth day after myocardial infarction, reported a significant 27% reduction in all-cause mortality. In contradistinction to both CONSENSUS II and SAVE, beneficial effects on mortality were achieved early, at 1 month (30%, $P <0.05$). Although no interaction was statistically significant, the authors reported that those not on diuretics (presumably with less heart failure) received less benefit; the same was true for those under 65 years of age.

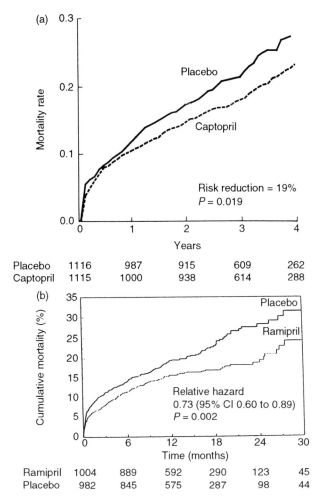

Placebo	1116	987	915	609	262
Captopril	1115	1000	938	614	288

Ramipril	1004	889	592	290	123	45
Placebo	982	845	575	287	98	44

Figure 15.8 (a) Cumulative all-cause postinfarction mortality in the SAVE Trial. The number of patients at risk at the beginning of each year are shown at the bottom. (From Ref. 33.) (b) All-cause mortality analyzed by intention-to-treat in the AIRE study. The numbers of patients at risk are shown at the bottom. (From Ref. 34.)

Discussion

As described at the beginning of this chapter, remodeling of the left ventricle and dilatation occur in a large number of patients with myocardial infarction, particularly those that are anterior or apically located and when they are large and approach full wall thickness in depth. A variety of interventions have been shown to limit this remodeling process. They include β-blockers during the first 48 hours to prevent 'remodeling', i.e. cardiac rupture,[46] reperfusion (especially thrombolysis) given either early or late,[47] and possibly parenteral nitrates during the first 48 hours of acute myocardial infarction.[48,49] Recent evidence indicates, however, that ACE inhibitors are probably the most important intervention after myocardial infarction that can be used to attenuate the remodeling process.[50]

Remodeling can be inhibited by reducing both systolic and diastolic tension through reduction in afterload, preload, and cardiac rate and through improved myocardial reperfusion. The latter not only provides nutrient flow but also serves as a scaffolding to support myocardial structural integrity. In virtually all studies a patent infarct-related artery is associated with improved outcome and less remodeling (see Chapter 5). Furthermore, a reduction in neurohormonal excess is beneficial both in the circulating and in the local tissue responses to acute myocardial infarction and to the often associated circulatory failure. Thus, the ACE inhibitors can play a role in inhibiting both mechanical and neurohormonal stimuli to remodeling. Remodeling depends in part on a hypertrophic process in cardiac muscle and noncontractile tissue. This is regulated, at least in part, by angiotensin II as well as norepinephrine. There are many unknowns in this equation, such as the release of atrial natriuretic peptide, particularly from the atria when they are distended and under high pressure. Relief of intracardiac tension may attenuate this compensatory response along with others.

It is important to discuss some of the differences amongst the various clinical trials of ACE inhibition, which bear on the premise that ACE inhibitors modify cardiac remodelling and in the process decrease both complications and overall mortality. The trials concerned are CONSENSUS II,[18] SAVE,[33] and AIRE.[34] Each had a different study design, timing of drug administration, and entry criteria. As shown in Table 15.4, the CONSENSUS II study called for the administration of intravenous enalaprilat on the very first day of the infarction, while SAVE and AIRE withheld ACE inhibitor administration for at least 3 days and often up to 16 days following myocardial infarction. Furthermore, three different ACE inhibitors were used, each with different properties, including a sulfhydryl group in captopril. Whether outcome depended on differences between the molecular entities in the same class is not known. Moreover, the entry criteria were often different. For example, all patients in CONSENSUS II who had met the criteria for an acute myocardial infarction were admitted irrespective of Q-wave status or circulatory complication. In SAVE, in addition to acute myocardial infarction, left ventricular systolic dysfunction as measured by ejection fraction was an entry criterion. All patients had either no major ischemia after myocardial infarction or such ischemia had been corrected by a revascularization or reperfusion procedure. Finally, the AIRE study stipulated that clinical heart failure be present at the time of the index myocardial infarction.

Adjunctive therapy was given during the trial with various interactions. For example, ACE inhibitors seem to have an effect separate from the known favorable results of thrombolytics, aspirin, and β-blockers. In AIRE, aspirin seemed to reduce the degree of benefit from ramipril, while β-blockers and ACE inhibitors seem to have additive effects in both AIRE and SAVE. In SAVE, ACE inhibitor effects likewise were additive to the favorable influence of a patent infarct-related artery. Finally, in the AIRE study, results were most favorable in patients receiving the most therapy for heart failure, suggesting that the severity of failure predicts the degree of response to ACE inhibition.[34]

Two of three clinical trials indicate that all-cause mortality and cardiovascular death were favorably affected. In the AIRE trial, which enrolled patients *with* heart failure post infarction, this beneficial effect was seen almost from the outset, while in SAVE, in which overt heart failure at the time of randomization was an exclusion criterion, it took fully 1 year before a benefit emerged. Benefit was progressive over the next 1.5–3 years, however, in both trials. The findings of CONSENSUS II are at variance but this may well have been related to the short duration of the study (6 months), the choice of ACE inhibitor, the decision to give the drug intravenously on the first day of myocardial infarction to patients with and without left ventricular dysfunction, and the high incidence of induced hypotension.

The other major issue was the emergence of heart failure. The results of all the studies, including CONSENSUS II, suggest either that the onset of heart failure was delayed or that its prevalence was reduced. There seems little doubt as well that ventricular size and shape can be favorably affected, although the magnitude of the effect related to how soon after the infarct medication was begun. Yet a favorable result could still be achieved even when the agent was administered as late as one year after the myocardial infarction. Change in heart size correlated well with the number of adverse events. Beneficial effects on volume and function of the left ventricle continued after termination of ACE inhibitor therapy, suggesting that true intervention in the remodeling process had occurred.

The data are less clear regarding recurrent myocardial infarction. Certainly, recurrent myocardial infarction occurred less frequently in the SOLVD trial, which reported on patients with heart failure, the majority of whom had had a previous myocardial infarction. The SAVE investigators, indeed, reported a reduction in this complication during follow-up but this was not seen in either the AIRE nor in the CONSENSUS II trials. Thus, this remains an area in which more data are required, including perhaps a separate clinical trial with recurrent myocardial infarction as primary endpoint and irrespective of the state of left ventricular function. There is evidence of a vascular RAA system that controls vascular growth, and there is experimental evidence suggesting that the atherosclerotic process may be attenuated by ACE inhibitors. It is sobering to realize that high levels of morbidity and mortality related to recurrent myocardial infarction and sudden cardiac death persist following a first acute myocardial infarction, despite all the above described successful interventions. These may call for innovative strategies targeted beyond attenuation of cardiac remodeling and enlargement.

Summary

A critical strategy in the care of the patient after myocardial infarction is reduction in late morbidity and mortality. Adverse consequences, such as death, heart failure, recurrent myocardial infarction and potentially fatal arrhythmias, seem to be associated with cardiac enlargement and a persistently occluded infarct-related artery. ACE inhibitors have been shown to attenuate remodeling after myocardial infarction in patients with cardiac dysfunction. For this and other reasons ACE inhibitors reduce the frequency of virtually all other anticipated morbid events. Therefore, they have a firm place in the management of patients recovering from myocardial infarction when there is associated left ventricular dysfunction, and are complementary to revascularization and to other established pharmaceutic agents, such as β-blockers, aspirin, and probably nitrates.

References

1. Erlebacher, J.A., Weiss, J.L., Weisfeldt, M.L. and Bulkley, B.H. (1984) Early dilation of the infarcted segment in acute transmural myocardial infarction: Role of infarct expansion in acute left ventricular enlargement. *J. Am. Coll. Cardiol.*, **4**, 201–8.
2. Jugdutt, B.I. (1993) Prevention of ventricular remodelling post myocardial infarction: Timing and duration of therapy. *Can. J. Cardiol.*, **9**, 103–14.
3. Piérard, L.A., Albert, A., Gilis, F. *et al.* (1987) Hemodynamic profile of patients with acute myocardial infarction at risk of infarct expansion. *Am. J. Cardiol.*, **60**, 5–9.
4. Lamas, G.A., Vaughan, D.E., Parisi, A.F. and Pfeffer, M.A. (1989) Effects of left ventricular shape and captopril therapy on exercise capacity after anterior wall acute myocardial infarction. *Am. J. Cardiol.*, **63**, 1167–73.
5. Jeremy, R.W., Hackworthy, R.A., Bautovich, G. *et al.* (1987) Infarct artery perfusion and changes in left ventricular volume in the month after acute myocardial infarction. *J. Am. Coll. Cardiol.*, **9**, 989–95.
6. Eaton, L.W., Weiss, J.L., Bulkley, B.H. *et al.* (1979) Regional cardiac dilatation after acute myocardial infarction. Recognition by two-dimensional echocardiography. *N. Engl. J. Med.*, **300**, 57–62.
7. McKay, R.G., Pfeffer, M.A., Pasternak, R.C. *et al.* (1986) Left ventricular remodeling after myocardial infarction: a corollary to infarct expansion. *Circulation*, **74**, 693–702.
8. Anversa, P., Loud, A.V., Levicky, V. and Guideri, G. (1985) Left ventricular failure induced by myocardial infarction. I. Myocyte hypertrophy. *Am. J. Physiol.*, **248**, H876–H882.

9. Ertl, G., Gaudron, P., Eilles, C. and Kochsiek, K. (1991) Serial changes in left ventricular size after acute myocardial infarction. *Am. J. Cardiol.*, **68**, 116D–120D.
10. Klein, M.D., Herman, M.V. and Gorlin, R. (1967) A hemodynamic study of left ventricular aneurysm. *Circulation*, **35**, 614–30.
11. Lindpaintner, K., Neidermaier, N., Drexler, H. and Ganten, D. (1992) Left ventricular remodeling after myocardial infarction: Does the cardiac renin–angiotensin system play a role? *J. Cardiovasc. Pharmacol.*, **20** (suppl. 1), S41–S47.
12. Hammermeister, K.E., Chikos, P.M., Fisher, I.L. and Dodge, H.T. (1979) Relationship of cardiothoracic ratio and plain film heart volume to late survival. *Circulation*, **59**, 89–95.
13. White, H.D., Norris, R.M., Brown, M.A. *et al.* (1987) Left ventricular end-systolic volume as the major determinant of survival after recovery myocardial infarction. *Circulation*, **76**, 44–51.
14. Skeggs, L.T., Kahn, J.R. and Shumway, N.P. (1956) Preparation and function of the angiotensin-converting enzyme. *J. Exp. Med.*, **103**, 295–9.
15. Michel, J.B., Lattion, A.L., Salzmann, J.L. *et al.* (1988) Hormonal and cardiac effects of converting enzyme inhibition in rat myocardial infarction. *Clin. Res.*, **62**, 641–50.
16. Pfeffer, J.M., Pfeffer, M.A. and Braunwald, E. (1985) Influence of chronic captopril therapy on the infarcted left ventricle of the rat. *Circ. Res.*, **57**, 84–95.
17. Lotvin, A. and Gorlin, R. (1993) Converting enzyme inhibitors: Current use. *ACC Current Journal Review*, **2**, 55–7.
18. Swedberg, K., Held, P., Kjekshus, J. *et al.* on behalf of the Consensus II Study Group (1992) Effects of the early administration of enalapril on mortality in patients with acute myocardial infarction. *N. Engl. J. Med.*, **327**, 678–84.
19. Jugdutt, B.I. and Basualdo, C.A. (1989) Myocardial infarct expansion during indomethacin or ibuprofen therapy for symptomatic post-infarction pericarditis. Influence of other pharmacologic agents during early remodeling. *Can. J. Cardiol.*, **5**, 211–21.
20. Brivet, F., Delfraissy, J.F., Giudicelli, J.F. *et al.* (1981) Immediate effects of captopril in acute left ventricular failure secondary to myocardial infarction. *Eur. J. Clin. Invest.* **11**, 369–73.
21. Mattioli, G., Ricci, S., Rigo, R. *et al.* (1986) Effects of captopril in heart failure complicating acute myocardial infarction and persistence of acute haemodynamic effects in heart failure after 3 years of treatment. *Postgrad. Med. J.*, **62** (suppl. 1), 164–6.
22. McAlpine, H.M., Morton, J.J., Leckie, B. and Dargie, H.J. (1987) Haemodynamic effects of captopril in acute left ventricular failure complicating myocardial infarction. *J. Cardiovasc. Pharmacol.*, **9** (suppl. 2), S25–S30.
23. Pfeffer, M.A., Lamas, G.A., Vaughan, D.E. *et al.* (1988) Effect of captopril on progressive ventricular dilatation after anterior myocardial infarction. *N. Engl. J. Med.*, **319**, 80–6.
24. Sharpe, N., Smith, H., Murphy, J. and Hannan, S. (1988) Treatment of patients with symptomless left ventricular dysfunction after myocardial infarction. *Lancet*, **i**, 256–9.
25. Sharpe, N., Murphy, J., Smith, H. and Hannan, S. (1990) Preventive treatment of asymptomatic left ventricular dysfunction following myocardial infarction. *Eur. Heart J.*, **11** (suppl. B), 147–56.
26. Sharpe, N., Smith, H., Murphy, J. *et al.* (1991) Early prevention of left ventricular dysfunction after myocardial infarction with angiotensin-converting-enzyme inhibition. *Lancet*, **337**, 872–6.
27. Oldroyd, K.G., Pe, M.P., Ray, S.G. *et al.* (1991) Effects of early captopril administration on infarct expansion, left ventricular remodeling and exercise capacity after acute myocardial infarction. *Am. J. Cardiol.*, **68**, 713–18.
28. Sharpe, N. (1991) Angiotensin-converting enzyme inhibitors in heart failure: A role after myocardial infarction. *J. Cardiovasc. Pharmacol.* **18** (suppl. 2), S99–S104.
29. Ray, S.G., Pye, M., Oldroyd, K.G. *et al.* (1993) Early treatment with captopril after acute myocardial infarction. *Br. Heart J.*, **69**, 215–22.
30. Kleber, F.X., Nussberger, J., Niemoller, L. and Doering, W. (1992) Mechanisms involved in cardiac enlargement and congestive heart failure development after acute myocardial infarction. *Cardiology*, **81**, 213–20.
31. Dickstein, K., Barvik, S. and Aarsland, T. (1991) Effect of long-term enalapril therapy on cardiopulmonary exercise performance in men with mild heart failure and previous myocardial infarction. *J. Am. Coll. Cardiol.*, **18**, 596–602.
32. Cohn, J.N., Johnson, G., Ziesche, S. *et al.* (1991) A comparison of enalapril with hydralazine–isosorbide dinitrate in the treatment of chronic congestive heart failure. *N. Engl. J. Med.*, **325**, 303–10.
33. Pfeffer, M.A., Braunwald, E., Moyé, L.A. *et al.* on behalf of the SAVE Investigators (1992) Effect of captopril on mortality and morbidity in patients with left ventricular dysfunction after myocardial infarction. Results of the Survival and Ventricular Enlargement Trial. *N. Engl. J. Med.*, **327**, 669–77.
34. The Acute Infarction Ramipril Efficacy (AIRE) Study Investigators (1993) Effect of ramipril on mortality and morbidity of survivors of acute myocardial infarction with clinical evidence of heart failure. *Lancet*, **342**, 821–8.
35. Yusuf, S., Pepine, C.J., Garces, C. *et al.* (1992) Effect of enalapril on myocardial infarction and unstable angina in patients with low ejection fractions. *Lancet*, **340**, 1173–8.
36. Becker, R.H.A., Wiemer, G. and Linz, W. (1991) Preservation of endothelial function by ramipril in rabbits on a long-term atherogenic diet. *J. Cardiovasc. Pharmacol.*, **18** (suppl. 2), S110–15.
37. Chobanian, A.V., Haudenschild, C.C., Nickerson, C. and Drago, R. (1990) Antiatherogenic effect of captopril in the Watanabe heritable hyperlipidemic rabbit. *Hypertension*, **15**, 327–31.
38. MERCATOR Study Group (1992) Does the new angiotensin converting enzyme inhibitor cilazapril prevent restenosis after percutaneous transluminal coronary angioplasty? *Circulation*, **86**, 100–10.
39. Tiret, L., Poirier, O., Lecerf, L. *et al.* Deletion polymorphism in the angiotensin-converting enzyme gene associated with parental history of myocardial infarction. *Lancet*, **341**, 991–2.

40. ISIS Collaborative Group (1993) ISIS-4: Randomised study of oral captopril in over 50,000 patients with suspected acute myocardial infarction (abstract). *Circulation*, **88**, I-394.
41. Packer, M., Rouleau, J.-L., Moyé, L.A. *et al.* (1993) Effect of captopril on ventricular arrhythmias and sudden death in patients with left ventricular dysfunction after myocardial infarction: SAVE Trial. *J. Am. Coll. Cardiol.*, **21**, 130A.
42. Sutton, MSt J., Pfeffer, M.A., Plappert, T. *et al.* for the SAVE Investigators (1994) Quantitative two dimensional echocardiographic measurements are major predictors of adverse cardiovascular events following acute myocardial infarction: The protective effects of captopril. *Circulation*, **89**, 68–75.
43. Kreulen, T., Gorlin, R. and Herman, M.V. (1973) Ventricular patterns and hemodynamics in primary myocardial disease. *Circulation*, **47**, 299–308.
44. Douglas, P.A., Morrow, R., Ioli, A. and Reichek, N. (1989) Left ventricular shape, afterload and survival in idiopathic dilated cardiomyopathy. *J. Am. Coll. Cardiol.*, **13**, 311–15.
45. Nabel, E.G., Topol, E.J., Galeana, A. *et al.* (1989) A randomized double-blind, placebo-controlled pilot trial of combined early intravenous captopril and tPA therapy in acute myocardial infarction (abstract). *Circulation*, **80** (suppl. II), II-112.
46. ISIS-1 (First International Study of Infarct Survival) Collaborative Group (1986) Randomised trial of intravenous atenolol among 16 027 cases of suspected acute myocardial infarction: ISIS-1. *Lancet*, **ii**, 57–66.
47. Bonaduce, D., Petretta, M., Villari, B. *et al.* (1990) Effects of late administration of tissue-type plasminogen activator on left ventricular remodeling and function after myocardial infarction. *J. Am. Coll. Cardiol.*, **16**, 1561–8.
48. Jugdutt, B.I. and Warnica, W. (1988) Intravenous nitroglycerin therapy to limit myocardial infarct size, expansion, and complications. Effect of timing, dosage, and infarct location. *Circulation*, **78**, 906–19.
49. Jugdutt, B.I., Tymchak, W., Humen, D. *et al.* (1990) Prolonged nitroglycerin versus captopril therapy on remodeling after transmural myocardial infarction (abstract). *Circulation*, **82**, III-442.
50. Gorlin, R. (1994) Prevention of remodeling of the heart after myocardial infarction. *Mt Sinai J. Med.*, (in press).

16

Risk Stratification

V. Figueredo and M. D. Cheitlin

Introduction

After myocardial infarction there is a loss of a variable amount of functional myocardium. If this loss is in the range of 40% during the infarction, most patients develop congestive heart failure and some progress to cardiogenic shock.[1] Those who survive an infarction of this size have markedly reduced ventricular function, and most demonstrate congestive heart failure. Between a small infarction, losing a minimum amount of functional myocardium, and the catastrophic loss of myocardium just described, are most myocardial infarctions. The remaining viable myocardium is the reserve left for heart function. A subsequent infarction, if survived, adds more nonfunctioning myocardium, further reducing this reserve.

Many studies have been done in patients after myocardial infarction to identify those factors that relate best to short- and long-term prognosis. In assessing prognosis the most important endpoints are those that, when they occur, irreversibly change the ultimate prognosis. These hard endpoints include death, reinfarction with further irreversible loss of myocardium, and life-threatening arrhythmias. Other endpoints used in studying the prognostic value of various risk stratification modalities in patients after myocardial infarction are the development of angina and the necessity for revascularization, either coronary artery bypass surgery or angioplasty. The latter group of endpoints are less useful in assessing prognosis, since they are 'soft' endpoints and do not change the patient's course irreversibly. Furthermore, the recommendation for revascularization is often a clinical decision, dependent on the beliefs and practice of the individual physician treating the patient, as well as the patient's wishes.

There is enormous experience with risk stratification in patients with chronic coronary artery disease, the lessons of which can be applied to risk stratification after acute myocardial infarction. However, the prognosis, even with the same findings on a risk stratification test, may be different and probably worse in patients after acute infarction than in patients with stable coronary artery disease, because of the short but finite period of lesion instability and left ventricular remodeling that occurs after an acute myocardial infarction. Still the principles are similar: that prognosis worsens with increasing left ventricular dysfunction and with the presence and amount of ischemic myocardium.

Beginning with the early landmark studies of Bruschke and colleagues[2] at the Cleveland Clinic, the long-term prognosis in patients with coronary artery disease was found to be related to the number of coronary arteries significantly obstructed as well as the resting systolic function of the left ventricle.[3] The more vessels involved, the worse the prognosis on follow-up. Additionally, for any degree of severity of coronary involvement, the lower the ejection fraction, the worse the prognosis.

Subsequent studies compared clinical findings and coronary arteriographic findings. Harris and colleagues[4] showed on univariate analysis a number of clinical findings and

Table 16.1 Medically treated patients with coronary artery disease: factors predicting survival

Clinical	Catheterization
NYHA Class IV heart failure	Number of significantly obstructed vessels
Progressive or unstable angina	Diffuse abnormal left ventricular contraction
Variant angina	Significant left branch coronary artery lesion
Peripheral vascular disease	Anterior left ventricular contraction abnormality
Resting ST–T wave changes	Arteriovenous oxygen difference
Nocturnal chest pain	Ejection fraction

Adapted from Ref. 4.
1214 patients; follow-up, 7 years; initial event 18% nonfatal myocardial infarction and 29% death; Cumulative event rate 49%.

other coronary arteriographic findings that were related to survival in patients with coronary artery disease. (Table 16.1). By examining these studies it is apparent that all the factors are related to: (1) left ventricular function, and (2) the amount of viable myocardium still in jeopardy because of obstructed coronary arteries.

A third prognostic indicator after myocardial infarction that has been found to be important is the presence of ventricular arrhythmias. Lown and colleagues[5] have classified ventricular ectopy into five grades, from unifocal, occasional premature ventricular contractions (PVCs) (frequent in the majority of patients with coronary disease) to the most serious, nonsustained ventricular tachycardia. The higher grades of ventricular ectopy, including early PVCs (R on T), multiform PVCs, and nonsustained ventricular tachycardia ('complex ventricular ectopy'), have been associated with a poor prognosis.[6] Furthermore, studies have shown that patients surviving infarction with significant ventricular ectopy in combination with abnormal left ventricular function have an even worse long-term prognosis.[7,8] Of note, ventricular ectopy at the time of the acute myocardial infarction is not predictive of late prognosis, whereas later ectopy, at the time of discharge from the hospital, has been shown to have adverse prognostic significance.

Therefore, the prognosis after myocardial infarction will depend on the amount of viable myocardium remaining, the amount of potentially ischemic myocardium subserved by obstructed coronary arteries, and the potential for the development of fatal arrhythmias. Given these facts, risk stratification must evaluate: (1) resting left ventricular function, (2) evidence for the presence and amount of potentially ischemic myocardium, and (3) the presence of serious ventricular arrhythmias.

The purpose of risk stratification after myocardial infarction is to identify those patients at highest risk for subsequent cardiac events and if possible to improve their prognosis by treating them with medication or revascularization. Exactly who will benefit from revascularization is still a matter of controversy and continuing investigation. One approach to this question is to look at the randomized studies that have been done (e.g.) the VA Cooperative Study,[9] the European Coronary Surgery Study,[10] and the CASS study[11] to examine the characteristics of patients who were benefited in terms of survival. From these studies and others, revascularization appears to decrease neither the incidence of arrhythmias nor reinfarction. As far as prolongation of life is concerned, the benefit is most evident in: (1) the symptomatic patient with left main coronary disease; (2) the patient with three-vessel disease and decreased ventricular function; and (3) possibly the patient with three-vessel disease including the left anterior descending coronary artery and with good ventricular function.

To the extent that the risk-stratification process identifies these patients, it is agreed that revascularization to prolong life is achievable. Whether patients with lesser degrees of obstructive disease, especially with good left ventricular function, benefit from revascularization is yet to be proved.

Risk Stratification by Clinical Findings

One of the most powerful clinical indicators of poor prognosis after myocardial infarction is age. Patients over 70–75 years of age have a relatively high in-hospital late mortality compared with younger patients; this is very evident in the placebo arms of the GISSI-I[12] and ISIS-2[13] trials and appears prominently in numerous other studies to be discussed.

The location and type of myocardial infarction is associated with the risk of in-hospital mortality. Anterior myocardial infarctions are known to have a higher in-hospital mortality than inferior-wall myocardial infarctions.[14] Patients with non-Q-wave myocardial infarctions have a better prognosis in the hospital but significant mortality after leaving the hospital, so that by the end of the first year the mortality of Q-wave and non-Q-wave myocardial infarctions are similar. It is also true that predischarge reinfarctions are more frequent after non-Q-wave than Q-wave infarctions.[15] These findings suggest that the non-Q-wave myocardial infarction is in essence a noncompleted infarct that therefore places these patients at higher risk for reinfarction and subsequent cardiac death.

During hospitalization for the acute myocardial infarction, subgoups have been identified as being at high risk (Table 16.2). One or more of these high-risk features is seen in 30–48% of patients with acute myocardial infarction.[16]

Spontaneous Ischemia

Those with spontaneous myocardial ischemia 24–48 hours after admission are at high risk of reinfarction and death. Myocardial ischemia can be manifested by spontaneous angina at rest or on minimal activity or by ST-segment depression of ECG even without angina, so-called 'silent ischemia'. Strictly speaking, 'silent ischemia' is a laboratory finding but probably has the same significance as spontaneous angina pectoris and so is mentioned here. Hamill and colleagues[17] showed that the mortality in patients with coronary artery disease on treadmill testing over a 7-year follow-up was identical whether the ischemia was manifested by angina alone, ST-segment depression alone, or both angina and ST-segment depression. Patients with silent ischemia by ST-segment shifts after myocardial infarction have a higher mortality than patients without silent ischemia. Tzivoni and colleagues[18] evaluated 224 low-risk patients after myocardial infarction with a treadmill test and an ambulatory ECG. Those with silent ischemia had four times the risk of cardiac events in a more than 2-year follow-up.

Clinical Congestive Heart Failure and/or Decreased Left Ventricular Ejection Fraction

Many attempts have been made to predict prognosis shortly after the onset of a myocardial infarction on the basis of clinical findings alone. Peel and colleagues[19]

Table 16.2 Subgroups during acute myocardial infarction at high risk for posthospital ischemic events

Spontaneous ischemia 24–48 hours after admission
Clinical congestive heart failure and/or left ventricular dysfunction
Complex and/or frequent ventricular ectopy at 5–7 days after acute event
History of previous myocardial infarction

developed a numeric score that correlated with the patient's prognosis 4 weeks after the myocardial infarction. The score was developed at the time of admission to the hospital using the patient's age, gender, history of ischemic heart disease, extent of the ECG changes, and the presence of shock, congestive heart failure, and rhythm and conduction disturbances.

Norris and colleagues,[20] studying 757 patients with acute myocardial infarction, devised a 'Coronary Prognostic Index' developed by assigning numeric weights to six variables selected by discriminate analysis: age, history of ischemic heart disease, ECG, location of infarction, systolic blood pressure, heart size on chest X-ray, and extent of pulmonary congestion.

Killip and Kimball[21] in their risk-stratification classification reported that the patient with acute myocardial infarction who had no signs of failure had an in-hospital mortality of 6%. In-hospital mortality was 17% in patients with an S_3 gallop and bibasilar rales, 38% in those with pulmonary edema, and 81% in those with cardiogenic shock.[21] They also showed that the incidence of life-threatening arrhythmias was related to the degree of left ventricular dysfunction.

The Multicenter Post-infarction Research Group[22] reported 866 patients who survived acute myocardial infarction (61% of those eligible) and followed them for 1–3 years (mean 22 months). They found four preselected factors which by multifactorial analysis contributed independently to the final survival model that they developed:

1. Ejection fraction <40%, the relative risk 2.4 (95% confidence intervals, 0.5–3.2).
2. PVCs ≥10 per hour, relative risk 1.6 (95% confidence intervals, 1–2.6).
3. Rales greater than bibasilar, relative risk 3.3 (95% confidence intervals, 2.1–5.2).
4. New York Heart Association class II–IV before the acute myocardial infarction, relative risk 1.9 (1.2–3.0).

When two or more risk factors coexist, the relative risk can be estimated by multiplying the relative risks of the individual factors. As an example, the relative risk for mortality of a patient with both a low ejection fraction and rales would be 7.9 (2.4 × 3.3); that is, the relative risk is 7.9 times the risk without these two factors present. Figure 16.1 shows on 2-year follow-up the estimated range of mortality according to the number of risk factors.

In the era of thrombolysis in acute myocardial infarction, it is not clear whether it is possible to use risk stratification to classify patients into high- and low-risk groups using clinical variables. Hillis and colleagues[23] evaluated the use of clinical risk factors in 3339 patients enrolled in the Phase II Thrombolysis in Myocardial Infarction (TIMI) trial. Patients known to be high risk, that is those with pulmonary edema and cardiogenic shock, were excluded. Before intravenous tissue plasminogen activator was given the presence of each of eight risk factors was noted: age ≥70 years, female gender, history of diabetes mellitus or previous myocardial infarction, ECG evidence of evolving anterior myocardial infarction or atrial fibrillation, evidence on physical examination of mild pulmonary congestion or systolic blood pressure <100 mmHg, and sinus tachycardia >100 beats min^{-1}. At 6 weeks 26% of the patients who had no risk factors had a mortality of 1.5%. Of the 74% of the population who had one or more risk factors, there was a 5.3% mortality ($P < 0.001$). Among those with one or more risk factors the mortality was related to the number of risk factors on admission and varied from 2.3% with one risk factor to 17.2% with four or more. In a follow-up study of many of these patients, the same clinical risk factors present on admission before thrombolysis predicted similar high- and low-risk prognostic groups 2 and 3 years later.[24]

McNamara and colleagues[25] found that an estimate of ventricular function in the patient after infarction can be made from knowledge of four clinically obtained findings: (1) anterior vs inferior myocardial infarction, (2) history of previous myocardial infarction, (3) pulmonary congestion on chest X-ray, and (4) creatine kinase over 1000 units. In a patient with none or one of these risk factors the chances were greater than 80% of

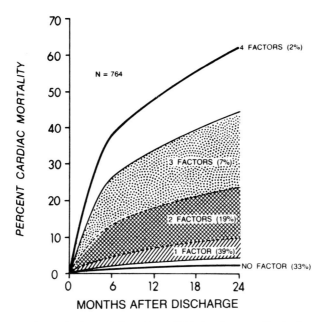

Figure 16.1 Range of mortality curves after myocardial infarction according to the number of risk factors. Risk factors were (1) NYHA Function Class II to IV before admission; (2) more than bibasilar rales; (3) 10 or more PVCs per hour; (4) radionuclide ejection fraction <0.40. The variation of risk within each zone reflects the relative risk for individual factors as well as the range of multiple active risks for combinations of two and three factors. The numbers in parentheses indicate the percentage of the population with the specified number of factors. (From Ref. 22 with permission.)

having an ejection fraction >40%. Two or more variables predicted a low ejection fraction with an accuracy of 60%. When three or more variables were present there was a predictive accuracy of a low ejection fraction of 84%.

Other researchers[26] have reported that the clinical findings of heart failure and an impaired ejection fraction after infarction are independent determinants of mortality.

Stratification of Risk by Enzyme Release

Ischemia to the point of myocardial necrosis releases intracellular cytoplasmic and mitochondrial structural elements, such as myosin and enzymes, into the interstitial space and then into the venous blood. Therefore, after an acute myocardial infarction enzymes such as creatine kinase (CK), serum aspartate transaminase (AST), and lactate dehydrogenase (LDH) are released in amounts related to the volume of infarcted myocardial muscle. Shell and associates[27] experimentally showed that the cumulative amount of CK released over time correlated closely with the grams of myocardium infarcted in animals.

The size of the myocardial infarction is a reflection of how much ventricular reserve is lost. Geltman and colleagues[28] showed that serial CK measurements allowed estimation of the volume of necrotic myocardium and that in-hospital mortality was related to the total release of CK. It was also shown that there were more arrhythmias in the patients with large infarcts, and multifactorial analysis substantiated the infarct size as an independent predictor of outcome. It is not clear whether the enhanced release of CK in patients with acute myocardial infarction who are revascularized by thrombolysis will accurately reflect the volume of ischemic myocardium.

Coronary Arteriography as a Means of Risk Stratification

Coronary arteriography for risk stratification after myocardial infarction has many advantages (Table 16.3).

1. Catheterization and coronary arteriography can be performed on an out-patient basis.
2. The location and severity of obstruction to coronary arteries and whether the myocardium which is served by that obstructed coronary artery is viable (jeopardized myocardium) are immediately known.
3. Coronary arteriography with left ventriculography provides an assessment of global and regional ventricular function.

There are, however, several limitations to this approach as a sole means of risk stratification.

Coronary arteriography soon after an acute myocardial infarction may show a greater degree of obstruction of the infarct-related coronary artery than would one done several weeks later. Acute Q-wave myocardial infarction is usually precipitated by rupture of a plaque with sudden, complete occlusion of a coronary artery. The sooner after onset of chest pain the angiogram is obtained, the more likely the vessel is to be totally occluded. This was shown by DeWood and colleagues,[29] where 87% of the patients had obstruction of the involved coronary artery with thrombus 0–24 hours after onset of chest pain, and only 65% had obstruction if angiography was performed 12–24 hours after onset of chest pain. DeFeyter and collegues[30] showed that within 6 hours of onset of chest pain angiography revealed an approximately 90% incidence of total occlusion in the infarct-related vessel. By 2 weeks, total occlusion was present in 53% and by 4 weeks in 45%. Acute myocardial infarction is precipitated by rupture of an atherosclerotic plaque, which may not be severely obstructed before rupture, and complete occlusion is caused by the thrombus. Subsequently, there is recanalization by fibrinolysis either spontaneously or with fibrinolytics and possibly remodeling of the arterial wall, leaving a lumen that is not critically obstructed. Coronary arteriography soon after an acute myocardial infarction might lead to inappropriate revascularization of a vessel that without intervention might later be patent with only a nonobstructive lesion.

There are a number of studies of patients who have had coronary arteriograms both before and after an acute myocardial infarction. There is no evidence to date that coronary arteriography can predict the plaque that is most likely to occlude. Little and colleagues[31] reported on 42 patients who had had a coronary angiogram before and up to 1 month after an acute myocardial infarction; 29 patients had an occluded coronary artery. Of these 29 patients 19 (66%) had a coronary artery that demonstrated less than 50% obstruction on the first coronary arteriogram. In 28 of these 29 patients (97%) the stenotic area was less than 70% before the acute infarct. Furthermore, there was no

Table 16.3 Risk stratification by cardiac catheterization and coronary arteriography in the patient following infarction. What can be learned?

Hemodynamics
Left ventricular funtion
Extent and severity of coronary artery disease
Estimation of amount of 'jeopardized' myocardium
Clues to the progress of stunned or hibernating myocardium

correlation between the time from the first coronary arteriogram to the infarct and the percent stenosis of the coronary artery causing the infarct. From these studies it is apparent that many myocardial infarcts occur due to rupture of a plaque that was only minimally obstructive before rupture and may explain why revascularization does not decrease the incidence of myocardial infarction compared to medical management.

Mark and colleagues[32] prospectively followed 283 patients who underwent two angiograms 4.5 years apart. They found that acute myocardial infarction was more likely to occur when occlusion occurred on a plaque that was less than 75% obstructive, whereas angina or no clinical change most often occurred when the occlusion involved a previously highly occlusive plaque. These data indicate that acute occlusion of a mildly stenotic coronary artery is more likely to cause acute myocardial infarction than occlusion of a highly stenotic artery. One possibility is that there is development of collateral circulation supplying jeopardized myocardium in the presence of a highly stenotic artery. The authors concluded that 85% of infarct-related lesions are not hemodynamically significant at the time of initial study. Although this does not negate the value of coronary arteriography as a prognostic indicator, it does limit the value of coronary arteriography in predicting future acute myocardial infarction and which vessel is likely to be the cause of future acute ischemic events.

Factors not related to the coronary pathology or amount of jeopardized myocardium may be important in the determination of the risk of developing a future coronary event. These factors could involve the composition of the plaque as well as the activation of the platelet–thrombin systems and is independent of the anatomic findings on coronary arteriography. Again, this does not negate coronary arteriography as a means of prognosticating risk but is a limitation of coronary arteriography as well as other methods of risk stratification in identifying all patients at risk of future ischemic events.

There is increasing evidence from lipid-lowering studies that lowering low-density lipoprotein (LDL) confers an advantage in terms of decreased ischemic events far beyond the amount of regression of plaque obstruction seen in repeated coronary arteriograms. [33,34] Whereas effective lipid lowering significantly decreases the rate of progression, there is evidence for only minimal regression in plaque obstruction. Despite this, in the Program on the Surgical Control of the Hyperlipidemias (POSCH)[33] and in the Familial Atherosclerosis Reduction Study (FATS)[34] the incidence of subsequent ischemic coronary events was reduced substantially, by 30% to 60%. One possible explanation for this is that there was a change in the lipid composition of the plaque, making it less vulnerable to rupture.

Another interesting finding is that of platelet hyperactivity, seen in some patients long after acute myocardial infarction. Trip and colleagues[35] studied platelet aggregability in 149 patients 3 months after an acute myocardial infarction. In 26 patients demonstrating abnormal platelet aggregability compared to 94 patients without such an abnormality, the mortality over a period of 5 years was 34.6% vs 6.4%, a relative risk ratio of 5.4 (95% confidence interval, 2.2–13.4), and the incidence of cardiac events was 46.2% vs 14.9%, a relative risk ratio of 3.1 (95% confidence interval, 1.6–5.8). Thus, here is another risk factor for ischemic events totally separate from the morphologic findings in the coronary arteries.

The major problem in routinely performing coronary arteriography as the sole method of risk stratification in patients with infarction is that the obstructive lesions in the coronary arteries are visualized without knowing their functional significance. The emotional pressure to revascularize myocardium served by an obstructed vessel is difficult to resist and, in fact, is resisted poorly, especially since angioplasty has become a primary means of revascularization. While surgery was the only revascularization procedure, restraint was exercised in sending patients to surgery with coronary disease where there was no evidence that surgery was superior to medical management. Since the advent of percutaneous transluminal coronary angioplasty (PTCA) such restraint is less evident, despite the fact that there still is no evidence that revascularization is superior to medical management in such patients.

Coronary arteriography is usually performed in the patient surviving myocardial infarction in order to identify those who would benefit from revascularization. Since anatomic arteriographic assessment alone is not sufficient to identify patients for revascularization and might lead to inappropriate revascularization in some patients, a more considered approach is to perform coronary arteriography only in those patients with evidence of persistent myocardial ischemia or depressed ventricular function. Coronary arteriography demonstrating a critical obstruction to vessels supplying large quantities of viable myocardium provides a good indication in these patients for revascularization. Such a scheme is proposed by Ross and colleagues[36] and is discussed later.

Studies of Left Ventricular Function and Perfusion

The predischarge assessment of left ventricular function after an acute myocardial infarction has been demonstrated to be one of the most accurate predictors of future cardiac events in the risk stratification work-up of these patients.[22,37–42] Several techniques for assessing left ventricular function of patients after infarction have been shown to have excellent prognostic value (Table 16.4). These include radionuclide ventriculography,[22,38,39,43] myocardial perfusion imaging with thallium-201 and technetium-99m sestamibi scintigraphy,[39,40] two-dimensional echocardiography,[41] and contrast ventriculography.[42]

The Multicenter Postinfarction Research Group[22] found a progressive increase in cardiac mortality during the first year after myocardial infarction as the predischarge left ventricular ejection fraction, determined by radionuclide ventriculography, fell below 0.40. A more recent study by Roig and colleagues,[37] found that resting radionuclide ventriculography was valuable in predicting future cardiac events in 93 patients following acute myocardial infarction over a 16 month follow-up period. Specifically, the presence of extensive (more than one area) regional wall motion abnormalities, or increased end-diastolic and end-systolic volume indices, were demonstrated by multivariate analysis to be independent predictors of future cardiac events. A recent study by Zaret and colleagues[38] found that a left ventricular ejection fraction of less than 0.30 as assessed by radionuclide ventriculography was still predictive of mortality in patients

Table 16.4 Resting left ventricular function: prognostic indicators after acute myocardial infarction

Technique	Parameter
Radionuclide ventriculography	Depressed left ventricular ejection fraction (e.g. <0.30 to 0.40)
	Increased end-diastolic volume index
	Increased end-diastolic volume index and greater than one area regional wall motion abnormality
Myocardial perfusion mapping Thallium-201 Technetium-99m sestamibi	Infarct size (e.g. reduction in activity involving >40% of the left ventricle)
Two-dimensional echocardiography	Abnormal wall motion score
	Depressed left ventricular ejection fraction
Contrast left ventriculography	Depressed left ventricular ejection fraction
	Increased end-systolic volume (e.g. >130 ml)

surviving infarction treated with thrombolytics, despite the significantly reduced mortality in these patients compared to those in the prethrombolytic era.

Assessment of infarct size using myocardial perfusion imaging techniques has also demonstrated prognostic value in risk stratification of patients after acute myocardial infarction.[39,40] Silverman and colleagues[44] demonstrated that a high thallium-210 defect score, corresponding to at least a moderated reduction of activity involving 40% of the left ventricle, within 15 hours of an acute myocardial infarction, was 93% predictive of mortality over a 9-month follow-up (sensitivity 86%, specificity 96%) in 42 patients.

In addition to the measurement of left ventricular ejection fraction and infarct size in patients following infarction, several studies have demonstrated alternative methods for assessing left ventricular function and predicting future cardiac events.[37,41,42] Bhatnagar and colleagues[41] described an abnormal wall motion score, derived by analyzing endocardial motion in 11 ventricular segments on two-dimensional echocardiography, which had high sensitivity (82%) and specificity (93%) for predicting future cardiac events in 47 patients surviving infarction over a 17-month follow-up period. White and colleagues[42] performed contrast left ventriculography in 605 patients 1–2 months after myocardial infarction. They found that postinfarction left ventricular dilatation, demonstrated by an increased end-systolic volume >130 ml, was an even better predictor of mortality after myocardial infarction than a left ventricular ejection fraction <0.4 or increased end-diastolic volume.

Thus, multiple methods that assess the degree of impairment of resting left ventricular function in patients after myocardial infarction have been shown to have prognostic value in risk stratification. Importantly, assessing resting left ventricular function in patients surviving infarction who have received thrombolytic therapy appears to have important prognostic value as well.

Exercise Electrocardiography

Increasing myocardial oxygen demand beyond the ability of an obstructed coronary artery to increase flow is the classic way of precipitating myocardial ischemia. The earliest technique used for increasing myocardial oxygen demand was exercise, and the first way in which myocardial ischemia was detected during exercise was by its effect on repolarization as detected by ST segment changes on the ECG. During exercise an ST-segment depression of ≥1 mm, flat or down-sloping, has been shown to be predictive of an increased incidence of coronary ischemic events, such as the development of angina pectoris, myocardial infarction, or sudden death.[45] Correlations of ST-segment depression with exercise and coronary arteriography defining the degree and location of the obstruction have been made.[46,47]

In 1979, Théroux and colleagues[48] performed heart-rate-limited, exercise treadmill tests in 210 patients 2 weeks after an acute myocardial infarction: 64 (30%) had ≥1-mm ST-segment depression, and 146 (70%) did not. The 1-year mortality was 27% in those with ≥1-mm ST-segment depression and 3% for those without ST-segment depression (Table 16.5). Subsequently, there were many reports of heart-rate-limited stress tests and later symptom-limited stress tests, done after myocardial infarction, which showed that the patients with ST-segment depression had a higher mortality and a higher incidence of reinfarction than those without ST-segment depression.[48–51] In these studies the patients were not necessarily consecutive and had mostly uncomplicated myocardial infarctions. The timing of the stress tests differed from 7 days to 3 weeks or later.

The degree of ST-segment depression and the level of exercise at which ST-segment depression occurred also indicated the severity and the extent of the ischemia. Although performed in patients with stable coronary artery disease, the following studies indicate

Table 16.5 Exercise test and coronary events within 1 year after acute myocardial infarction

Coronary event	No ischemia	Angina, ST depression, or both
None	70 (54%)	13 (16%)
Stable angina (coronary revascularization)	45 (35%)	43 (54%)
Unstable angina	4 (3%)	2 (3%)
Myocardial infarction	8 (6%)	5 (62%)
Death	3 (3%)	17 (21%)
Total	130	80

Adapted from Ref. 48.

the importance of the degree of ST-segment depression and the stage at which it occurs in predicting the severity of the coronary disease and prognosis. Ellestad and colleagues[52] showed that the workload at which significant ST-segment depression occurred is of prime importance in evaluating the severity of the disease and long-term prognosis. They performed Bruce protocol exercise treadmill tests on 266 patients with coronary artery disease and followed them for up to 6 years for the endpoints of death, myocardial infarction, or the progression of angina. The incidence of these combined endpoints increased the earlier during the exercise 2-mm ST-segment depression occurred. The incidence of ischemic events in a subject with 2.0-mm ST-segment depression occurring at 3 min on the Bruce protocol [1.7 m.p.h. (2.7 k.p.h.) at a 10% incline] was four times that of a subject requiring 7 min of exercise [4 m.p.h. (6.4 k.p.h.) at a 10% incline].

The patient with a previous myocardial infarction is at more risk than those without previous events. The incidence of a subsequent cardiac event in patients surviving infarction with ≥1-mm ST-segment depression without preceding myocardial infarction was 34% at 5 years; in patients with a prior infarction the incidence was 81% at 5 years.[53]

The magnitude of the ST-segment depression with exercise has been shown to be related to the extent and significance of the coronary obstruction. Cheitlin and colleagues[54] compared the results of submaximal Bruce protocol exercise treadmill testing with subsequent coronary arteriography in an attempt to predict the presence of significant lesions from the exercise ECG. Significant lesions considered to be 'high risk' were defined as: (1) left main coronary artery obstruction at 50% or greater diameter narrowing; (2) proximal left anterior descending and left circumflex coronary artery obstruction ≥75%; and (3) 90% left anterior descending coronary arterial obstruction prior to the first septal perforator. In those with ≥2-mm ST-segment depression, 24% had left main coronary arterial lesions, and 34 of 45 patients (75%) had one or more of these significant lesions. In patients with 1.0–1.9 mm of ST-segment depression, 10 of 31 (32%) had combined left anterior descending and left circumflex lesions or high-grade left anterior descending lesions. In patients with <1.0-mm ST-segment depression, 2 of 30 patients (7%) had a single 90% left anterior descending lesion. Therefore the risk of missing any of these 'significant' lesions would have been less than 5% if the patients with <1.0-mm ST-segment depressions had not been catheterized.

In 1983, DeBusk and colleagues[49] reported 702 consecutive men studied 21 days after an acute myocardial infarction. Risk stratification was performed on the patients segmentally as follows: Group I included patients with historic risk factors that significantly increased the risk of subsequent cardiac events (prior angina, myocardial infarction prior to the index infarction, and recurrent angina in the CCU). There were 62 patients in this group, 10% of the population, and they were not exercised. Group II included patients with clinical risk factors such as heart failure, unstable angina, and

Table 16.6 Exercise treadmill responses that predict multivessel disease and/or left main coronary artery disease

ECG variables	Downsloping ST-segment depression
	ST-segment depression ≥ 2 mm
	Early onset (≤ 3 min on the Bruce Protocol) ST-segment depression or elevation
	Prolonged duration (>8 min) of ST-segment depression
	Complex ventricular ectopy at low heart rate (<130 beats min^{-1})
Non-ECG variables	Low achieved heart rate (≤ 120 beats min^{-1})
	Hypotension during exercise (≥ 10 mmHg fall in systolic pressure from previous levels)
	Failure to increase systolic blood pressure over 10 mmHg
	Low achieved heart rate $\times$ blood pressure product ($\leq 15 \times 10^3$)
	Inability to exercise >3 min on the Bruce Protocol

other problems known to increase the risk of exercise testing or to make it difficult to do, such as peripheral vascular disease. There were 265 patients in this group, 40% of the population. Group III, the low-risk group, included patients who underwent symptom-limited Bruce protocol stress tests. There were 338 in this group, 50% of the population.

They followed the study population for 33.8 ± 23.2 months and at 6 months tabulated the rate of hard cardiac events; nonfatal reinfarction, fatal reinfarction, cardiac arrest, and sudden cardiac death. In Group I the rate was 17.7%, in Group II 6.4%, and Group III 4.4%. In Group III, 31 patients (9%) had a positive stress test (≥ 2-mm ST depression and a peak heart rate ≤ 135 beats min^{-1}), and 307 (91%) had a negative test. The rate of hard cardiac events within 6 months in the 31 patients with a positive stress test was 9.7% vs 3.9% in the 307 patients with a negative test. Therefore, of the 16 patients with hard events, 12 came from the group with a negative stress test.

Several facts are evident from this study:

1. The number of patients at 3 weeks after uncomplicated myocardial infarction with ST-segment depression with a symptom-limited stress test is low (less than 10%).
2. Most patients who suffer subsequent cardiac events are predicted clinically by having historic or clinical risk factors or for some other reason are not candidates for an exercise test. Therefore, the patients who can exercise will be a preselected group at low risk.
3. The patients with an uncomplicated infarction who can exercise can be divided into low-risk and high-risk groups; however, of all the patients after uncomplicated myocardial infarction who will suffer a cardiac event, most will not have been predicted by the development of ST-segment depression on a symptom-limited exercise test.

So far, the sign of ischemia in these exercise tests has been the development of ST-segment depression, but other exercise endpoints have been described that predict the presence of multivessel disease and/or left main coronary artery disease (Table 16.6) and for the uncomplicated infarction may be more predictive of future cardiac events than ST-segment depression.

Weld and colleagues[55] reported the 1-year follow-up after low-level exercise tests in 236 patients after myocardial infarction (Table 16.7). It is evident that the parameter most predictive of a 1-year cardiovascular mortality was the inability to exercise past stage 2 on the Bruce protocol (<6 min). The ability to exercise depends on myocardial function remaining the same or improving with exercise. With the development of ischemia, there is progressive diastolic and systolic left ventricular dysfunction and inability to maintain stroke volume.

Supportive of these studies is a report by de Feyter and colleagues,[56] who studied 179 consecutive patients 6–8 weeks after acute uncomplicated myocardial infarction.

Table 16.7 Exercise treadmill variables vs 1-year cardiovascular mortality in patients following myocardial infarction

Exercise variables	Death odds ratio at 1 year
ST depression $\geq$1 mm in V_5	1.92
ST depression $\geq$2 mm in V_5	2.17
Angina	2.11
PVC $\geq$3 hour^{-1}	4.32
PVC $\geq$10 hour^{-1}	6.30
PVC $\geq$100 hour^{-1}	7.76
PVC in pairs	9.20
Multiform PVCs	3.86
Nonsustained ventricular tachycardia	4.13
Duration of exercise $\leq$6 min	15.42

PVC, premature ventricular contractions.
Modified from Ref. 55.

Symptom-limited Bruce protocol treadmill tests were done as well as coronary arteriography on all patients, who were followed for a mean of 28 months. The patients were considered high risk by coronary arteriography if they had ejection fraction less than 30% or three-vessel disease, and by exercise treadmill if they could not exercise for $\geq$10 min (Table 16.8). The coronary arteriogram predicted all but one patient who died but less than half of the patients who had recurrent myocardial infarciton, whereas the exercise treadmill test predicted all 11 patients who died, and all but one (10/11) of those having recurrent myocardial infarction. Thus the patients who could walk for at least 10 min on the Bruce protocol represented a very low-risk group for subsequent cardiac events.

Mark and colleagues[57,58] devised a prognostic exercise treadmill score from data on a population of 2842 consecutive inpatients who had both cardiac catheterization and exercise treadmill testing using the Bruce protocol. Using a combination of duration of exercise, the presence or absence of angina during the test, and the maximal ST-segment deviation during or after exercise, they were able to develop a nomogram that provided an estimate of 5-year survival of 55–99%, and an average yearly mortality of 0.2–9% per year. Although these patients were not immediately post myocardial infarction, it is likely that similar results would be seen in these patients.[58] Similar approaches using clinical exercise test variables have been developed to predict three-vessel disease and left main coronary artery disease.[59]

Patients with acute myocardial infarction are increasingly being treated with thrombolytic agents with a high rate of reperfusion being achieved. It is not clear whether stress testing prior to discharge has the same prognostic value as it does in patients who have not had thrombolysis. Chaitman and colleagues[60] in the TIMI-II trial reported that

Table 16.8 Risk of cardiac death and recurrent myocardial infarction in patients following myocardial infarction (MI): risk stratification by coronary arteriography and exercise treadmill testing

	Catheterization			Exercise treadmill		
	N	Death	Recurrent MI	N	Death	Recurrent MI
High risk	46	10 (22%)	5 (11%)	121	11 (9%)	11 (9%)
Low risk	133	1 (1%)	7 (5%)	58	0	1 (2%)

Adapted from Ref. 56.

coronary revascularization in patients who develop ischemic chest discomfort or exercise-induced ST-segment depression results in a low 1-year mortality comparable to that found in patients who did not have these findings.

Exercise electrocardiography is a valuable test in assessing prognosis in patients with coronary artery disease. It is generally available with experienced personnel capable of performing it safely and is relatively inexpensive. After uncomplicated myocardial infarction patients can be divided into high- and low-risk groups for subsequent cardiac events using exercise electrocardiography, especially if all the information available on the treadmill test is utilized.

'Silent' Ischemia by Ambulatory ECG

With the onset of ischemia, ST-segment depression or elevation precedes the development of angina pectoris. With exercise testing, patients may develop ST-segment depression without experiencing any chest discomfort. With exercise testing, Weiner and colleagues[61] have shown that patients with coronary artery disease in the CASS Registry with ST-segment depression without angina had the same survival at 7 years as those with both ST-segment depression and angina. The survival of both of these groups was lower than that of patients without either ST-segment depression or angina on the exercise test. In patients with coronary artery disease having 24-hour ambulatory ECG during everyday activities, for every episode of ST-segment depression that occurs with angina, there are eight to ten episodes of silent ST-segment depression.[62]

After myocardial infarction, ambulatory ECG has been used to risk-stratify patients. Gottlieb and colleagues[63] studied 103 patients recovering from myocardial infarction with Lown Class III or greater ventricular arrhythmias and/or ejection fractions <40% with ambulatory ECG 8 days after admission. Thirty patients (29%) had episodes of ST-segment depression, more than 90% of which were silent. At 1 year of follow-up, mortality was 30% in those with silent ischemia compared with 11% of those without ($P < 0.05$). Silent ischemia was also a predictor of death or reinfarction.

Tzivoni and colleagues[18] reported on 224 low-risk patients with myocardial infarction who had an ambulatory ECG and Bruce protocol stress test before discharge. After 2 years of follow-up, those with silent ischemia had a fourfold increase in ischemic events compared to those without. In patients with both ischemia on exercise and on the ambulatory ECG, the event rate was 51% compared to a 20% event rate in those with a positive exercise test but without ischemia on the ambulatory ECG. Ambulatory 24-hour ECG can be used in patients surviving myocardial infarction who cannot exercise. However, it is not clear that finding silent ischemia on 24-hour ambulatory ECG adds any more prognostic information to the development of ST-segment depression on an exercise test. Hinderliter and colleagues[64] showed that patients with stable coronary artery disease who completed stage 3 of the Bruce protocol had little silent ischemia on 24-hour ambulatory ECG, suggesting that silent ischemia is a marker for more significant coronary artery disease just as ST-segment depression is at low exercise level on a stress test.

Exercise Myocardial Perfusion Imaging

The ACC/AHA Task Force,[65] in their 1990 report entitled 'Guidelines for the Early Management of Patients with Acute Myocardial Infarction', recommended exercise testing with electrocardiographic monitoring in the peridischarge period as the preferred procedure for risk stratification in patients after infarction with uncomplicated courses. However, this recommendation has recently been called into question given the improved diagnostic accuracy demonstrated with the addition of myocardial perfusion imaging to exercise treadmill testing.[66] As recomended by the ACC/AHA Task Force,[65] stress thallium-201 scintigraphy is certainly of benefit for risk stratification in patients surviving infarction with uninterpretable ECGs due to conduction abnormalities, marked ST–T wave abnormalities, or changes due to digoxin therapy. What is less clear is whether the improvement in diagnostic accuracy with the addition of myocardial perfusion imaging is worth the additional cost for routine risk stratification following myocardial infarction. To complicate the issue, recent studies have suggested that exercise thallium-201 scintigraphy may be less accurate for risk stratification of patients who have undergone a revascularization procedure following myocardial infarction (e.g. thrombolytic therapy or coronary angioplasty).[67–70]

Exercise thallium-201 scintigraphy has been shown in numerous studies to identify residual ischemic myocardium in patients following infarction with greater diagnostic accuracy than exercise testing with electrocardiographic monitoring.[44,67,68,71,72] With the advent of single photon emission computed tomographic (SPECT) thallium-201 scintigraphy the sensitivity for identifying ischemic myocardium has approached 96%. However, specificity (82–86%) has proven to be more of a problem with SPECT than planar imaging, primarily because of technical problems such as patient motion artifact during the longer acquisition time. Many laboratories now perform both planar and SPECT imaging techniques to corroborate findings. New technetium-99m perfusion agents, technetium-99m sestamibi, technetium-99m tetrofosmin, and technetium-99m teboroxime, are being evaluated as alternatives to thallium-201 scintigraphy given their greater ease of production, relatively short half-life, and favorable patient dosimetry. Initial reports have suggested that the sensitivity and specificity of these agents for the detection of coronary artery disease to be comparable to exercise thallium-201 scintigraphy.[73–76] An example of a technetium-99m sestamibi study in a patient following infarction is shown in Figure 16.2.

In addition to the demonstrated improvement in the detection of myocardium at risk, the prognostic value of exercise thallium-201 scintigraphy in identifying subsequent cardiac events following myocardial infarction has been shown to be superior to exercise electrocardiography alone.[44,71] Gibson and colleagues[71] compared submaximal exercise thallium-201 scintigraphy to submaximal exercise electrocardiography and coronary angiography in 140 patients within 2 weeks following myocardial infarction. With a mean follow-up of 16 months, they found that exercise thallium-201 scintigraphy was more sensitive (97%) than exercise electrocardiography (56%) or coronary angiography (74%) in predicting subsequent cardiac events (angina, reinfarction or death). In agreement with these findings, a study by Silverman and colleagues[44] found that the incidence of subsequent cardiac events in patients following infarction, classified as low risk by submaximal exercise thallium scintigraphy, submaximal exercise electrocardiography, or coronary angiography, was 6%, 27%, or 22%, respectively.

In contrast, Hung and colleagues[72] found that while submaximal exercise thallium-201 scintigraphy identified residual ischemic myocardium more frequently than exercise electrocardiography, no new prognostic information was provided with the addition of thallium-201 perfusion imaging to exercise electrocardiography regarding subsequent cardiac events. In a study by Moss and colleagues,[77] 936 patients were evaluated 1–6 months following myocardial infarction with exercise thallium-201 scintigraphy. Using exercise thallium-201 scintigraphy, only reversible thallium defects occurring in conjunction with increased lung uptake, a finding correlated with decreased left ventricular function, were predictive of future cardiac events. Because this represents such a small proportion of patients studied, they suggested that exercise thallium-201 scintigraphy was not useful in the risk stratification of patients following infarction. However, as pointed out in an editorial by Diamond,[78] this study demonstrated that risk stratification with exercise thallium-201 scintigraphy was not useful in patients surviving infarction

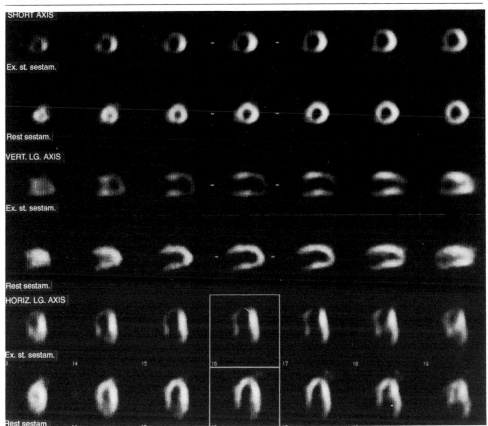

Figure 16.2 An example of a positive exercise study with supplemental technetium-99m sestamibi imaging in a 54-year-old male 7 days following an uncomplicated inferior myocardial infarction. Note, there are multiple perfusion defects present in the anterior, inferior, apical and septal areas. With rest, all areas reperfuse except for a small persistent infero-apical defect indicating the site of recent infarction. In each orientation, from left to right: short axis = apex to base; vertical long axis = septum to lateral wall; horizontal long axis = superior to inferior wall.

after hospital discharge. Current practice is to perform risk stratification on patients prior to discharge with consideration towards elective revascularization procedures.

Recent data have demonstrated the value of thallium-201 reinjection at rest in patients with apparent fixed defects on rest reperfusion imaging to better distinguish between scar and ischemic, but viable, myocardium.[79,80] Fixed thallium-201 defects on reperfusion imaging of less than 50% relative reduction in signal vs normally perfused myocardium have been found to represent viable, metabolically active myocardium that can improve with reperfusion.[66] While no studies have specifically addressed the effect of reinjection on long-term prognosis, the increased sensitivity for identifying potentially viable myocardium has resulted in revascularization of myocardium that was only identifiable as viable by reinjection. Dilsizian and colleagues[79] demonstrated that 49% of fixed defects became partially reversible following reinjection of thallium-201 at the time of reperfusion imaging. In this study, of 15 myocardial regions identified as viable by reinjection, 87% had normal thallium-201 scans and normal wall motion after coronary angioplasty. All eight defects that remained fixed following thallium-201 reinjection still had abnormal wall motion following revascularization.

Several recent studies have evaluated the prognostic value of exercise thallium-201 scintigraphy in patients surviving infarction who have undergone revascularization procedures.[67–70] These studies have suggested that extrapolation of findings from the prethrombolytic era may not be valid in revascularized patients. Similar to comparisons made in the prethrombolytic era, residual ischemia was significantly more prevalent as assessed by exercise thallium-201 testing than by electrocardiographic treadmill testing alone (55% vs 11%) in patients surviving infarction who had received thrombolytic therapy.[67] However, there are conflicting data regarding the prognostic value of exercise thallium-201 testing in patients surviving infarction who have undergone revascularization procedures. Dakik and colleagues[81] found that the size of a perfusion defect on exercise thallium-201 SPECT was predictive of future cardiac events during a 2-year follow-up of patients who received thrombolytic therapy following myocardial infarction. In contrast, Tilkemeier and colleagues[67] found that predischarge thallium-201 redistribution was much less sensitive for predicting future cardiac events in patients who received thrombolytics compared to those who did not receive thrombolytics (55% vs 81%).

To further complicate this issue, several recent studies have suggested that thallium-201 imaging early after a revascularization procedure may actually overestimate the extent of residual ischemic myocardium. Manyari and colleagues[69] found that thallium-201 perfusion imaging performed early after revascularization did not necessarily reflect residual coronary stenosis or reocclusion. Studies at 3.3 and 6.8 months demonstrated normal perfusion in the one-third of patients found to have thallium-201 defects with redistribution consistent with ischemia at 9 days. Although the mechanism of this false-positive result is unknown, the authors suggest several possibilities including persistent vasoconstriction distal to the angioplasty site, and hibernating or stunned myocardium. Sutton and Topol have arrived at similar conclusions.[70]

In summary, exercise thallium-201 scintigraphy has been demonstrated to have several advantages over exercise electrocardiography in risk stratification of patients following myocardial infarction. The error rate in falsely classifying patients at low risk for angina, reinfarction or cardiac death following myocardial infarction is significantly reduced with exercise thallium-201 scintigraphy.[66] Furthermore, thallium-201 perfusion imaging has the additional benefit of assessing the relative size and identifying the specific region of myocardium at risk. Myocardial perfusion imaging reveals the functional significance of angiographically documented lesions and probably correlates better with prognosis than the anatomic appearance of the lesion.

Because of this demonstrated improvement in the diagnostic accuracy of exercise thallium-201 scintigraphy over exercise electrocardiography, it has been suggested that exercise perfusion imaging be used for routine postinfarction risk stratification. One of the problems with exercise thallium-201 scintigraphy is the uneven availability of expertise and high-quality studies in all institutions. Given the substantial increased cost involved, cost–benefit analyses will need to be performed before this approach can be recommended. Furthermore, although exercise thallium scintigraphy has proven superior to exercise electrocardiography in risk stratification of patients who have not undergone revascularization procedures following infarction, its prognostic value in patients who received thrombolysis or coronary angioplasty is less clear. As more patients undergo revascularization procedures, an accurate method for risk stratification of these patients needs to be identified. Further studies using exercise testing with myocardial perfusion imaging will be necessary before this method can be recommended for routine risk stratification in these patients.

Myocardial Perfusion Imaging with Pharmacologic Agents

Pharmacologic myocardial perfusion imaging using dipyridamole or adenosine has proven invaluable for the evaluation of myocardium at risk in patients who are unable to exercise. These include patients with concomitant arthritis, claudication, orthopedic problems, neuromuscular diseases, or general disability. Pooled results from several studies of patients with stable coronary artery disease, who had undergone both exercise and dipyridamole thallium-201 planar scintigraphy, have demonstrated comparable sensitivity and specificity for identifying myocardium at risk.[82] With the advent of SPECT thallium-201 imaging with dipyridamole, a sensitivity of 92% and a specificity of 88% for identifying ischemic myocardium have been demonstrated.[83]

Large prospective randomized trials have not yet been performed to examine the efficacy of myocardial perfusion imaging with pharmacologic agents for risk stratification of patients following infarction. However, several smaller studies have suggested dipyridamole thallium-201 scintigraphy to be useful for postinfarction risk stratification.[84–88] For example, Brown and colleagues[88] performed dipyridamole thallium-201 scintigraphy and cardiac catheterization early (1–4 days) after acute myocardial infarction in 50 patients. Following multivariate logistic regression analysis, only thallium-201 redistribution in the infarct zone was predictive of in-hospital and late recurrent myocardial ischemic events. In their study, 45% of patients with a reversible thallium-201 defect in the infarct zone had a subsequent cardiac event compared to none of the patients with no evidence of redistribution. Importantly, there were no serious adverse effects using this dipyridamole thallium-201 scintigraphy protocol early after myocardial infarction.

Dobutamine has also been utilized as a pharmacologic stress agent with thallium-201 scintigraphy. Dobutamine increases myocardial metabolic demand through β and α-adrenergic receptor stimulation. Because of its lack of effect on adenosine receptors, dobutamine offers an alternative to dipyridamole and adenosine in patients with asthma or chronic obstructive pulmonary disease. The sensitivity and specificity for identifying myocardium at risk using dobutamine pharmacologic stress imaging has been shown to be comparable to exercise thallium-201 scintigraphy or myocardial perfusion imaging with dipyridamole or adenosine vasodilatory stress.[89] However, no studies have yet examined the predictive value of dobutamine stress with myocardial perfusion imaging techniques for risk stratification of patients following infarction.

Limited data exist regarding the diagnostic accuracy of dipyridamole thallium-201 scintigraphy in patients surviving infarction treated with thrombolytics. Jain and colleagues[90] found that thallium-201 SPECT scintigraphy with dipyridamole identified residual myocardial ischemia in 74% of patients approximately 5 days post infarction compared to 28% with symptom-limited exercise electrocardiography. However, Hendel and colleagues[91] found that dipyridamole thallium-201 scintigraphy was not predictive of reinfarction or death on a 2-year follow-up of 71 patients surviving infarction who received thrombolytic therapy (and frequently coronary angioplasty). Therefore, until further studies have been completed, caution should be exercised in extrapolating results from prethrombolytic studies to the use of pharmacologic stress myocardial perfusion imaging for risk stratification of patients who have received thrombolytic therapy following infarction.

In summary, pharmacologic myocardial perfusion imaging may have an important role for the evaluation of myocardium at risk in patients who are unable to exercise following infarction. At present pharmacologic myocardial perfusion imaging should not be considered as a replacement for exercise myocardial perfusion imaging in a patient able to exercise, as much useful clinical information is lost. This includes clinical parameters such as duration of exercise, heart rate and blood pressure responses, and reproduction of symptoms. In patients who have undergone revascularization procedures following infarction the role of pharmacologic myocardial perfusion imaging is not yet clear. Larger, prospectively defined and executed trials establishing the predictive value of pharmacologic myocardial perfusion imaging for risk stratification in patients surviving infarction will need to be performed.

Exercise Echocardiography

Exercise echocardiography has been demonstrated to be an acceptable alternative to exercise myocardial perfusion imaging for the evaluation of residual ischemic myocardium in patients surviving infarction.[92–96] Many institutions report equivalent accuracy for assessing myocardium at risk using echocardiographic and more established myocardial perfusion scintigraphy techniques.[92] Sensitivities of 86–97% and specificities of 64–88% for detecting coronary artery disease have been reported with exercise echocardiography.[92] Exercise echocardiography has several advantages over exercise with myocardial perfusion imaging. The technique is totally noninvasive and there is no radiation exposure. Echocardiography provides information regarding global and regional left ventricular size and function, as well as providing a comprehensive evaluation of all four cardiac chambers, valves and great vessels. The single greatest disadvantage of exercise echocardiography is the high degree of operator dependency. Although an early concern, exercise echocardiography is now becoming increasingly popular due to the recent introduction of digital image acquisition techniques. Digital acquisition provides high-quality single cardiac cycle images that can be displayed in a side-by-side, continuous loop format, which has improved the detection of more subtle ischemic-induced wall motion abnormalities.[93]

Several small prospective studies have demonstrated both the superiority of exercise echocardiography over exercise electrocardiography, as well as its equivalency to exercise myocardial perfusion imaging for identifying patients with coronary artery disease.[97–99] Quinones and colleagues[99] demonstrated an 88% concordance between exercise echocardiography and exercise thallium-201 SPECT for detecting coronary artery disease in 292 patients with suspected coronary artery disease. Overall sensitivities (74% vs 76%) and specificities (88% vs 81%) were comparable.

Although no large, prospective randomized trial has yet been undertaken, three small studies, comprising a total of 156 patients less than 3 weeks after an acute myocardial infarction, have demonstrated the predictive value of exercise echocardiography in risk stratification of patients following infarction.[94–96] During 3–11 month follow-up periods, the overall sensitivity and specificity for predicting future cardiac events were 63–80% and 78–95%, respectively. In patients with multivessel coronary artery disease, the sensitivity and specificity predicting future cardiac events were 77–82% and 88–95%, rspectively. Like other exercise imaging techniques, single-vessel disease, especially left circumflex arterial disease, remain the largest source of false-negative studies.[92]

Unfortunately, no data are presently available regarding the prognostic value of exercise echocardiography for predicting future cardiac events in patients who have undergone revascularization procedures following infarction.

Pharmacologic Stress Echocardiography

Preliminary work using pharmacologic stress echocardiography for risk stratification of patients after myocardial infarction has been encouraging.[100–105] Like pharmacologic myocardial perfusion imaging techniques, pharmacologic stress echocardiography has been shown to be a safe, accurate method for the diagnosis of coronary artery disease in patients unable to exercise.[106] In addition, pharmacologic stress echocardiography appears to be a promising technique for assessing the viability of myocardium that remains dysfunctional following revascularization after an acute myocardial infarction.[107,108]

Pharmacologic stress echocardiography was first tested as a technique for identifying coronary artery disease by Picano and colleagues[109] in 1985. Since then several small studies have demonstrated the prognostic value of pharmacologic stress echocardiography for identifying patients at risk for future cardiac events following infarction.[99–104] Dipyridamole echocardiography has been demonstrated to be superior to exercise electrocardiography in identifying residual myocardial ischemia and in predicting risk for future cardiac events in patients following infarction.[92,99,100] For example, Neskovic and colleagues[103] followed 93 patients surviving infarction for approximately 16 months following predischarge dipyridamole echocardiography. Dipyridamole echocardiography was found to have an accuracy of 82% (sensitivity 68%, specificity 92%) for predicting future cardiac events. They demonstrated that the prognosis during a 14-month follow-up period could be significantly improved in patients surviving infarction who underwent a revascularization procedure following a positive dipyridamole echocardiography study compared to those with negative studies who underwent revascularization.[102] Mortality was significantly reduced in patients with positive dipyridamole echocardiography studies who underwent revascularization after infarction compared to patients with positive dipyridamole echocardiography studies who did not (0.8% vs 7%, $P < 0.001$). In contrast, patients with negative dipyridamole echocardiography studies had no improvement in survival with revascularization after infarction when compared to patients with negative dipyridamole echocardiography studies who did not (6% vs 2%, P = NS). This study provides encouraging results. Further research examining the outcome of patients treated on the basis of risk stratification studies is needed.

Several studies examining the usefulness of dobutamine echocardiography in the patient after infarction are also encouraging;[102,105,110] they demonstrated a positive predictive accuracy of 76% and a negative predictive accuracy of 84% for dobutamine echocardiography in predicting future cardiac events.

Preliminary work using pharmacologic stress echocardiography for risk stratification of patients after myocardial infarction has been encouraging.[99–104] Additionally, preliminary work suggests that pharmacologic stress echocardiography is useful in predicting which patients will benefit from revascularization following myocardial infarction.[103]

Stress Radionuclide Ventricular Angiography

Several studies have reported the prognostic utility of exercise radionuclide ventriculography in patients following myocardial infarction.[36,42,71,110] Patients surviving infarction with normal resting left ventricular function (e.g. assessed by rest radionuclide ventriculography) who demonstrate abnormal function during exercise have been shown to be at an increased risk for subsequent cardiac events.[36] Similar to exercise echocardiography, exercise radionuclide ventriculography can provide information regarding alterations in global and regional left ventricular function in response to stress.

The normal left ventricle reponds to exercise stress with an increase in ejection fraction of at least 5% and more vigorous segmental contraction. During exercise the end-systolic volume index is decreased, while the systolic pressure–volume index is increased. Several studies have shown that patients surviving infarction who demonstrate a lack of increase, or a decrease, in left ventricular ejection fraction in response to exercise are more likely to suffer a subsequent cardiac event.[36,42,71,110] Similarly, an increase in end-systolic volume or a limited response of the systolic pressure–volume index to exercise have been shown to be prognostically valuable in patients following infarction.[36,110] For example, Corbett and colleagues[111] examined the clinical outcome over a 10-month period of 61 patients studied approximately 3 weeks following acute myocardial infarction using exercise radionuclide ventriculography. Failure of the left ventricular ejection fraction to increase by more than 5%, an increase in end-systolic volume of greater than 5%, or failure of the systolic pressure–volume index to increase by 35% or more, were highly predictive of subsequent cardiac events (sensitivity of 95–97%; specificity of 88–96%). In contrast, two studies have suggested that exercise radionuclide ventriculography has limited prognostic usefulness in patients following infarction.[112,113] However, these studies were carried out 1–4 months after myocardial infarction and excluded patients with interval cardiac complications.

A single study by Lim and colleagues[43] has evaluated the prognostic value of exercise radionuclide ventriculography following thrombolysis in patients who had suffered acute myocardial infarctions. Thirty-one revascularized patients underwent exercise radionuclide ventriculography, while remaining on their antiischemic medical regimens, within 3 months after myocardial infarction and thrombolysis. Twelve month follow-up demonstrated that a fall in left ventricular ejection fraction during exercise radionuclide ventriculography was strongly predictive of subsequent cardiac events.

Several studies have reported the prognostic utility of exercise radionuclide ventriculography in risk stratification of patients following myocardial infarction.[37,43,72,111] Unfortunately, there are few data comparing the predictive accuracy of exercise radionuclide ventriculography vs exercise myocardial perfusion imaging or echocardiography for risk stratification of patients following myocardial infarction.[72] Additionally, the limited information available is less encouraging regarding the use of pharmacologic agents with radionuclide ventriculography for assessing residual ischemia in patients following infarction.[114] Nevertheless, the development of new gated tomographic techniques and the introduction of newer technetium-labeled imaging agents that can provide both perfusion and function information will require further investigation, but appear to have the potential for providing improved prognostic assessment for patients post-infarction.

Positron Emission Tomography

Although limited data exist regarding the prognostic value of positron emission tomography (PET) for risk stratification of patients after an acute myocardial infarction, several small studies have suggested that PET imaging may prove valuable in these patients.[115–119] PET imaging has been shown to be more accurate than stress thallium-201 scintigraphy for identifying ischemic, but viable, myocardium in patients with coronary artery disease.[115,116] Brunken and colleagues[115] found that PET imaging (using[13]N-ammonia and[18]F-2-deoxyglucose to assess myocardial perfusion and glucose utilization, respectively) demonstrated persistent glucose metabolism in over half of myocardial segments with fixed (58%) or partially reversible (64%) stress thallium-201 defects in patients with coronary artery disease. This suggests that assessment of myocardial perfusion alone may underestimate the quantity of viable, but hypoperfused, myocardium in coronary artery disease patients. Tillisch and colleagues[117] found ^{13}N-ammonia and ^{18}F-2-deoxyglucose PET imaging to be an accurate method for predicting the improvement of regional myocardial contractile abnormalities after surgical revascularization. Of 41 abnormal wall motion segments diagnosed by radionuclide ventriculography, 35 were correctly predicted with PET imaging to be reversible with revascularization (85% positive predictive accuracy) and 24 of 26 wall motion abnormalities were correctly predicted to be irreversible (92% negative predictive accuracy).

A recent study by Tamaki and colleagues[118] compared the prognostic value of ^{18}F-2-deoxyglucose PET imaging, exercise thallium-201 scintigraphy, and coronary angiography for predicting postinfarction cardiac events. An increase in ^{18}F-2-deoxyglucose uptake was found to be the best predictor of future cardiac events among all clinical, angiographic, and radionuclide variables in this study. Yoshida and Gould[119] found that the demonstration of viable myocardium in the infarct area in 35 patients, as assessed by rubidium-82 PET imaging, was predictive of 3-year mortality. This was true regardless of left ventricular ejection fraction or infarct size. Interestingly, they found that for patients with low ejection fractions (<40%) or large scars (>23%), the degree of decrease in ejection fraction or infarct size was not predictive of mortality. Yet in these subgroups of patients the presence of viable myocardium was highly predictive of 3-year mortality. Importantly, this study demonstrated that patients who had demonstrated viable myocardium who underwent revascularization had improved survival compared to patients with viable myocardium who did not undergo revascularization. Patients without evidence for viable myocardium on PET imaging did no better with revascularization than patients who did not. This study not only provided data supporting the prognostic value of risk stratification studies, but also suggests that outcome can be altered by intervention based on the results of the studies.

Therefore, although the presently available data are limited, they do suggest PET imaging may have a role in the risk stratification of these patients. Additionally, patients surviving infarction with viable myocardium demonstrated by PET imaging may benefit from revascularization. Further studies are needed before PET imaging can be recommended for routine risk stratification in patients following infarction.

Detection of Ventricular Arrhythmias

The presence of ventricular ectopic activity in patients after myocardial infarction is associated with a greater risk of subsequent cardiac events, most notably sudden death.[120–122] Several electrocardiographic methods for risk stratification of patients surviving infarction have been evaluated. These include assessment of ventricular ectopic activity and intermittent ST-segment depression with ambulatory ECG (Holter) monitoring,[120–126] measurement of ventricular late potentials by signal-averaged electrocardiography,[125,127–129] induction of ventricular tachyarrhythmias by electrophysiologic testing,[130–133] and the measurement of heart rate variability index on ambulatory ECG monitoring.[131,134–137]

Ambulatory Electrocardiography

Numerous studies have demonstrated that frequent premature ventricular complexes (10 or more per hour) and complex premature ventricular complexes (multimorphic premature ventricular complexes, nonsustained ventricular tachycardia) represent variables predictive of subsequent cardiac mortality in patients surviving infarction independent of left ventricular function or evidence of residual myocardium at risk.[120–122] However, others have found ventricular ectopic activity to only be predictive of subsequent mortality and arrhythmic events in patients with significant left ventricular dysfunction.[123] Still others have suggested that ambulatory ECG monitoring is not prognostically valuable in risk stratification of patients after myocardial infarction.[124,125] These conflicting data, when taken together with the lack of demonstrated positive therapeutic effect of suppression of ventricular ectopic activity after myocardial infarction,[10] calls into question the routine use of ambulatory ECG monitoring after myocardial infarction. Studies, now underway, examining the benefit of other antiarrhythmic agents (e.g. amiodarone) in this patient population, may alter this recommendation.

In addition to the finding of ventricular ectopic activity on ambulatory ECG monitoring, the presence of intermittent ST-segment depression in the patient surviving infarction has been suggested as a predictor of subsequent cardiac events.[126] In the Beta Blocker Heart Attack Trial,[138] transient ST-segment depression of greater than 1-min duration during predischarge 24-hour ambulatory ECG monitoring had a prevalence of 21% in 3837 patients and a relative risk for mortality of 2.56 in patients not treated with propranolol. Patients surviving infarction with intermittent ST-segment depression who were treated with propranolol had a relative risk for mortality of 0.98, suggesting treated patients were less affected by the presence of intermittent ST-segment depression.

Signal-Averaged Electrocardigraphy

More recently, much attention has been given to the use of signal-averaged ECG monitoring for predicting subsequent sudden death and arrhythmic events in patients surviving infarction. The finding of low-amplitude late potentials together with an increased filtered QRS duration greater than 120 ms suggests diseased myocardium in which conduction is slowed and fragmented. This diseased myocardium serves as substrate for arrhythmogenesis. Although the frequency of late potentials has been reported to be reduced in the thrombolytic era,[125] several studies have demonstrated signal-averaged ECG to be independently predictive of future cardiac mortality and arrhythmic events in patients surviving infarction.[125,127,128]

A recent study by McClements and colleagues[125] assessed the predictive value of signal-averaged ECG, ambulatory ECG, and radionuclide ventriculography for identifying patients following infarction, of whom two-thirds received thrombolytic therapy, for sudden cardiac death and arrhythmic events over a 1-year follow-up period. Late potentials on signal-averaged ECG and depressed left ventricular ejection fraction were each found to be independently predictive of sudden death and sustained ventricular arrhythmias. In a recent meta-analysis[127] of three studies examining the predictive value of signal-averaged ECG and left ventricular ejection fraction for identifying future arrhythmic events in patients surviving infarction, an abnormal signal-average ECG was associated with a six-fold increase in risk for arrhythmic events independent of ejection fraction. The same authors[127] also performed a meta-analysis of four studies examining the predictive value of signal-averaged ECG vs ambulatory ECG for identifying future arrhythmic events in patients surviving infarction. Pooled results demonstrated that an abnormal signal-averaged ECG resulted in an eightfold increase in risk for subsequent arrhythmic events independent of the presence of frequent or complex ectopy on ambulatory ECG. In a summary of seven prospective studies assessing the prognostic value of signal-averaged ECG in patients surviving infarction, Gomes and colleagues[128] found the positive predictive value of the presence of late potentials to range from 8 to 27%, while the negative predictive value ranged from 96 to 99%. Thus, the practical application of signal-averaged ECG to postinfarction risk stratification is somewhat limited by a high false-positive rate. However, when the presence of late potentials was associated with postinfarction findings of depressed left ventricular ejection fraction and increased ventricular ectopy on ambulatory monitoring, arrhythmic event rates of greater than 50% have been demonstrated.[128] In contrast, the arrhythmic event rate in patients after infarction was less than 2% if all three tests were normal.

Whether all patients surviving infarction should undergo signal-averaged ECG for risk stratification remains unclear. Studies assessing the benefit of sending these patients with late potentials for electrophysiologic testing need to be performed. A recent report by Breithardt and colleagues[129] demonstrated a correlation between the absence of late potentials after myocardial infarction and successful thrombolytic therapy.

Electrophysiologic Testing

Programmed electrophysiologic ventricular stimulation has been recommended for routine use in risk stratification of patients with left ventricular impairment following infarction.[130] However, while some studies have shown a positive correlation between inducible ventricular tachycardia and subsequent arrhythmic events in patients after infarction (especially in the setting of reduced ejection fraction),[130,131] others have failed to demonstrate a prognostic value in risk stratification of these patients with electro-physiologic testing.[132] Furthermore, similar to signal-averaged ECG, the results of electrophysiologic testing in patients after uncomplicated myocardial infarction are hampered by the large number of false positives. Add to this the invasive nature of this technique and electrophysiologic testing does not appear well suited for routine risk stratification of the patient following infarction.

Pedretti and colleagues[133] recently demonstrated inducibility of sustained ventricular tachycardia to have a sensitivity of 81% and specificity of 97% for predicting future arrhythmic events in patients surviving infarction who were preselected by noninvasive techniques. These included patients who had two or more of the following: ejection fraction <0.4, ventricular late potentials, and high-grade ventricular ectopic activity. This group of patients demonstrated a high arrhythmic event rate of 65% over a 15-month follow-up. The authors suggest that given the high negative predictive value (99%) of electrophysiologic testing in these patients, no further treatment would be needed if they were noninducible. The authors further suggest that electrophysiologic testing for risk stratification of this subgroup of high-risk patients identified by noninvasive testing is warranted and that patients with inducible ventricular tachycardia should be considered for implantable cardioverter-defibrillators or therapy guided by electrophysiologic test-ing. However, prospective randomized examination will be required before electrophy-siologic testing or treatment based on its results can be recommended for risk stratification of all, or a subgroup of patients after myocardial infarction.

Heart Rate Variability

Heart rate variability on ambulatory ECG monitoring is an index of the sympathovagal interaction regulating heart rate. Reduced vagal tone decreases heart rate variability and predisposes to ventricular fibrillation. Several studies[134–137] have recently demonstrated the prognostic value of assessing heart rate variability for risk stratification of patients after myocardial infarction. Decreased heart rate variability has been demonstrated to be of equivalent or greater prognostic value for predicting subsequent cardiac mortality and arrhythmic events than the presence of late potentials on signal-averaged ECG or a depressed ejection fraction.[134–137] A recent study by Bigger and colleagues[137] found that abnormalities of heart rate variability and their predictive value for arrhythmic events in patients surviving infarction could be assessed from short (2–15 min) ECG recordings with comparable accuracy to 24-hour ambulatory ECG recordings. This would imply that assessment of heart rate variability could be obtained from the same recordings acquired for signal-averaged ECG measurements. The advantage of this is apparent from the findings that the positive predictive accuracy for subsequent arrhythmic events in patients after infarction for the combination of signal-averaged ECG and heart rate variability was shown to be 33% vs signal-averaged ECG or heart rate variability alone (17% for each test).[135] The ability to obtain heart rate variability simultaneously with other risk stratification tests (e.g. ambulatory and signal-averaged ECG) makes it an attractive method for predicting subsequent cardiac events after myocardial infarction.

Another indicator of disordered autonomic function in patients following infarction that may have prognostic significance is baroreflex sensitivity. A recent study by Farrell and colleagues[139] found depressed arterial baroreflex sensitivity, assessed by the phenyl-ephrine method, to have a higher positive accuracy (63.6%) for predicting inducible sustained monomorphic ventricular tachycardia at electrophysiologic testing compared to heart rate variability (45.5%), late potentials on signal-averaged ECG (38.5%), frequent ventricular ectopic activity on ambulatory ECG monitoring (22.7%), or depressed left ventricular ejection fraction (31.3%). Additional studies will be needed to assess the prognostic value of this method for risk stratification of patients surviving infarction.

Summary

The late prognosis after acute myocardial infarction is dependent on three interrelated factors: (1) the residual left ventricular function, (2) the remaining viable myocardium subserved by coronary arteries significantly obstructed by atherosclerotic plaque, and (3) the substrate for development of malignant arrhythmias. Clinical factors such as age, previous history of myocardial infarction, clinical congestive heart failure, and spontaneous angina pectoris are all indicators of poor prognosis and high risk. A clinical decision can be made that patients at high risk should have coronary arteriography and revascularization if possible. Patients without these high-risk historic or clinical factors can undergo risk stratification to look for left ventricular dysfunction, the presence and amount of potentially ischemic myocardium, and malignant arrhythmias by a number of techniques. The exercise test is the oldest, the most studied, the most inexpensive, and the most useful test for risk stratification of patients after acute myocardial infarction. When all the information obtainable during an exercise treadmill test is used, the ability to divide patients who have suffered uncomplicated infarctions into high- and low-risk groups for future cardiac events is excellent. Myocardial perfusion studies and wall motion studies during stress can yield additional information as to location and extent of the myocardium at risk.

Ross and colleagues[36] have developed an approach to risk stratification in patients who have survived an acute myocardial infarction that selects patients at high risk for coronary arteriography and follows the low-risk patients medically. They evaluated 1848 patients who survived beyond day 5 after an acute myocardial infarction and followed them until death or for at least 1 year and identified the following subgroups who were at high risk. For patients under age 75 years with severe resting ischemia in the hospital at any time after the first 24 hours the 1-year mortality was 18%. For those with a history of previous myocardial infarction and clinical or radiographic signs of left ventricular failure in the hospital, 1-year mortality was 25%. Among the remaining patients, those with exercise tests showing 2-mm ST-segment depression, the 1-year mortality was 11%. In patients who could not exercise, a resting radionuclide angiogram was done, and those with an ejection fraction between 0.20 and 0.44 had 12% 1-year mortality. All 'high-risk' patients together had a 1-year mortality of 16% and made up 55% of the population under age 75 years. They all had coronary arteriography and underwent revascularization when possible. All of the rest had 1-year mortality of 3% or less and did not have coronary arteriography. This retrospectively developed schema was then tested in a second group of 780 patients with similar results. For patients over age 75 years the 1-year mortality was 31%, and it was recommended that their management be highly individualized. Only those with severe symptomatic ischemia should have coronary arteriography with the purpose of selecting those for revascularization (Figure 16.3).

In 1990 the American College of Cardiology together with the American Heart Association published the ACC/AHA Task Force Report and Guidelines for the Management of Patients with Acute Myocardial Infarction.[64] In this report they recommended an algorithm for three strategies for predischarge or early postdischarge risk stratification (Figure 16.4).

Our approach to risk stratification follows the general recommendations outlined in the ACC/AHA Task Force Report. Patients who have clinically declared themselves to be at high risk should have coronary arteriography to identify those who are candidates for

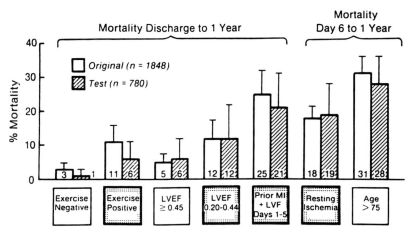

Figure 16.3 Mortality rates after acute myocardial infarction in two populations from day 6 to 1 year after hospital discharge. The groups are identified early in the admission for 'age >75 years' and 'resting ischemia' and 'from the time of hospital discharge' for the remaining groups. The vertical lines show 95% confidence limits for the percent mortalities. Coronary arteriography is recommended for the groups in stippled boxes. Not shown are the patients with ejection fractions of less than 0.20 and patients who had neither an exercise test not an ejection fraction measurement. LVEF, left ventricular ejection fraction; LVF, left ventricular failure; MI, myocardial infarction. (Adapted from Ref. 36 with permission.)

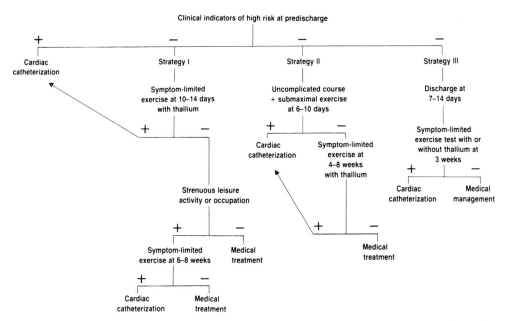

Figure 16.4 Strategies for predischarge or early postdischarge exercise evaluation. (From Ref. 65 with permission.)

revascularization. Patients who are clinically uncomplicated after infarction should have a heart-rate-limited stress test before discharge or alternatively a symptom-limited stress test 3 weeks after discharge. Those patients who can walk into the third stage of the Bruce protocol are treated medically. If there are signs of high risk, such as ST depression ≥2 mm in the first two stages, if the patient cannot walk more than 6 min on the Bruce protocol, if the blood pressure does not rise, or especially if it falls during the exercise, then the patients should go to coronary arteriography.

If the ECG is abnormal with ST-segment elevation or depression, radionuclide myocardial perfusion imaging with exercise or exercise wall motion study by echocardiography can be used depending on local experience. If the patient cannot exercise, pharmacologic stress agents can be used with radionuclide myocardial perfusion imaging techniques.

With the above approach, it is possible to detect and revascularize most of the high-risk patients surviving myocardial infarction. However, there is as yet no proof that revascularization is more effective than continued medical management except in the few subgroups where effectiveness is already established.

References

1. Wackers, F.J., Lie, K.I., Becker, A.E. *et al.* (1976) Coronary artery disease in patients dying from cardiogenic shock or congestive heart failure in the setting of acute myocardial infarction. *Br. Heart J.*, **38**, 906–10.
2. Bruschke, A.V.G., Proudfit, W.L. and Sones, F.M. Jr (1973) Progress study of 590 consecutive nonsurgical cases of coronary disease followed 5–9 years: I. Arteriographic correlations. *Circulation*, **47**, 1147–53.
3. Bruschke, A.V.G., Proudfit, W.L. and Sones, F.M. Jr (1973) Progress study of 590 consecutive nonsurgical cases of coronary artery disease followed 5–9 years: II. Ventriculographic and other correlations. *Circulation*, **47**, 1154–63.
4. Harris, P.J., Lee, K.L., Harrell, F.E. Jr *et al.* (1980) Outcome in medically treated coronary artery disease. Ischemic events: nonfatal infarction and death. *Circulation*, **62**, 718–26.
5. Lown, B. and Graboys, T.B. (1977) Sudden death: an ancient problem newly perceived. *Cardiovasc. Med.*, **2**, 219–26, 229, 231, 233.
6. Bigger, J.T. Jr and Weld, F.M. (1981) Analysis of prognostic significance of ventricular arrhythmias after myocardial infarction. Shortcomings of Lown grading system. *Br. Heart J.*, **45**, 717–24.
7. Schulze, R.A. Jr, Strauss, H.W. and Pitt, B. (1977) Sudden death in the year following myocardial infarction. Relation to ventricular premature contractions in the late hospital phase and left ventricular ejection fraction. *Am. J. Med.*, **62**, 192–9.
8. Rapaport, E. and Remedios, P. (1983) The highrisk patient after recovery from myocardial infarction: recognition and management. *J. Am. Coll. Cardiol.*, **1**, 391–400.
9. The VA Coronary Artery Bypass Surgery Cooperative Study Group (1992) Eighteen-year follow-up in the Veterans Affairs Cooperative Study of Coronary Bypass Surgery for stable angina. *Circulation*, **86**, 121–30.
10. European Coronary Surgery Study Group (1982) Long-term results of prospective randomised study of coronary artery bypass surgery in stable angina pectoris. European Coronary Surgery Study Group. *Lancet*, **ii**, 1173–80.
11. CASS Principal Investigators and their Associates (1983) Coronary Artery Surgery Study (CASS): a randomized trial of coronary artery bypass surgery. Survival data. *Circulation*, **68**, 939–50.
12. Gruppo Italiano per lo Studio della Streptochinasi nell'Infarto Miocardico Trial (1986) Effectiveness of intravenous thrombolytic treatment in acute myocardial infarction. *Lancet*, **i**, 349–60.
13. ISIS-2 (Second International Study of Infarct Survival) Collaborative Group (1992) Randomized trial of intravenous streptokinase, oral aspirin, both or neither among 17 187 cases of suspected acute myocardial infarction. *Lancet*, **339**, 753–70.
14. Hands, M.E., Lloyd, B.L., Robinson, J.S. *et al.* (1986) Prognostic significance of electrocardiographic site of infarction after correction for enzymatic size of infarction. *Circulation*, **73**, 885–91.
15. Nicod, P., Gilpin, E., Dittrich, H. *et al.* (1989) Short- and long-term clinical outcome after Q wave and non-Q wave myocardial infarction in a large patient population. *Circulation*, **79**, 528–36.
16. Kulick, D.L. and Rahimtoola, S.H. (1991) Risk stratification in survivors of acute myocardial infarction: routine cardiac catheterization and angiography is a reasonable approach in most patients (editorial). *Am. Heart J.*, **121**, 641–56.
17. Hamill, S.C. and Khandheria, B.K. (1990) Silent myocardial ischemia. *Mayo Clin. Proc.*, **65**, 374–83.
18. Tzivoni, D., Gavish, A., Zin, D. *et al.* (1988) Prognostic significance of ischemic episodes in patients with previous myocardial infarction. *Am. J. Cardiol.*, **62**, 661–4.
19. Peel, A.A.F., Semple, T., Wang, I. *et al.* (1962) A coronary prognostic index for grading the severity of infarction. *Br. Heart J.*, **24**, 745–60.

20. Norris, R.M., Brandt, P.W.T., Caughey, D.E. *et al.* (1969) A new coronary prognostic index. *Lancet*, **i**, 274–8.
21. Killip, T. 3rd and Kimball, J.T. (1967) Treatment of myocardial infarction in a coronary care unit. A two year experience with 250 patients. *Am. J. Cardiol.*, **20**, 457–64.
22. The Multicenter Postinfarction Research Group (1983) Risk stratification and survival after myocardial infarction. *N. Engl. J. Med.*, **309**, 331–6.
23. Hillis, L.D., Forman, S., Braunwald, E. and the TIMI Phase II Co-investigators (1990) Risk stratification before thrombolytic therapy in patients with acute myocardial infarction. *J. Am. Coll. Cardiol.*, **16**, 313–15.
24. Terrin, M.L., Williams, D.O., Kleiman, N.S. *et al.* (1993) Two- and three-year results of the Thrombolysis in Myocardial Infarction (TIMI) Phase II Clinical Trial. *J. Am. Coll. Cardiol.*, **22**, 1763–72
25. McNamara, R.F., Carleen, E. and Moss, A.J. (1988) Estimating left ventricular ejection fraction after myocardial infarction by various clinical parameters. *Am. J. Cardiol.*, **62**, 192–6.
26. Warnowicz, M.A., Parker, H. and Cheitlin, M.D. (1983) Prognosis of patients with acute pulmonary edema and normal ejection fraction after acute myocardial infarction. *Circulation*, **67**, 330–4.
27. Shell, W.E., Kjehshus, J.K. and Sobel, B.E. (1971) Quantitative assessment of the extent of myocardial infarction in the conscious dog by means of analysis of serial changes in serum creatine phosphokinase activity. *J. Clin. Invest.*, **50**, 2614.
28. Geltman, E.M., Ehsani, A.A., Campbell, M.K. *et al.* (1979) The influence of location and extent of myocardial infarction on long-term ventricular dysrhythmia and mortality. *Circulation*, **60**, 805–14.
29. DeWood, M.A., Spores, J., Notske, R. *et al.* (1980) Prevalence of total coronary occlusion during the early hours of transmural myocardial infarction. *N. Engl. J. Med.*, **303**, 897–902.
30. de Feyter, P.J., van den Brand, M., Serruys, P.W. and Wijns, W. (1985) Early angiography after myocardial infarction: what have we learned? *Am. Heart J.*, **109**, 194–9.
31. Little, W.C., Constantinescu, M., Applegate, R.J. *et al.* (1988) Can coronary angiography predict the site of a subsequent myocardial infarction in patients with mild-to-moderate coronary artery disease? *Circulation*, **78**, 1157–66.
32. Mark, W.I., Webster, M.B., Chesebro, J.H. *et al.* (1990) Myocardial infarction and coronary artery occlusion: a prospective 5-year angiographic study (abstract). *J. Am. Coll. Cardiol.*, **15**, 218A.
33. Buchwald, H., Varco, R.L., Matts, J.P. *et al.* (1990) Effect of partial ileal bypass surgery on mortality and morbidity from coronary heart disease in patients with hypercholesterolemia: Report of the Program on the Surgical Control of the Hyperlipidemias (POSCH). *N. Engl. J. Med.*, **323**, 946–55.
34. Brown, G., Albers, J.J., Fisher, L.D. *et al.* (1990) Regression of coronary artery disease as a result of intensive lipid-lowering therapy in men with high levels of apolipoprotein B. *N. Engl. J. Med.*, **323**, 1289–98.
35. Trip, M.D., Cats, V.M., van Capelle, F.J. and Vreeken, J. (1990) Platelet hyperactivity and prognosis in survivors of myocardial infarction. *N. Engl. J. Med.*, **322**, 1549–54.
36. Ross, J. Jr, Gilprin, E.A., Mason, E.B. *et al.* (1989) A decision scheme for coronary angiography after acute myocardial infarction. *Circulation*, **79**, 292–303.
37. Roig, E., Magrina, J., Garcia, A. *et al.* (1993) Prognostic value of exercise radionuclide angiography in low risk acute myocardial infarction survivors. *Eur. Heart J.*, **14**, 213–18.
38. Zaret, B.L., Wackers, F.J., Terrin, M. *et al.* and the TIMI investigators (1991) Does left ventricular ejection fraction following thrombolytic therapy have the same prognostic impact described in the prethrombolytic era? Results of the TIMI II Trial. *J. Am. Coll. Cardiol.*, **17**, 214A.
39. McClements, B.M. and Adgey, A.A. (1993) Value of signal-averaged electrocardiography, radionuclide ventriculo-graphy, holter monitoring and clinical variables for prediction of arrhythmic events in survivors of acute myocardial infarction in the thrombolytic era. *J. Am. Coll. Cardiol.*, **21**, 1419–27.
40. Miller, T.D., Christian, T.F., Hopfenspirger, M.R. *et al.* (1993) Infarct size measured by Tc99m Sestamibi scintigraphy identifies patients at increased risk of mortality. *Circulation*, **88**, I-487.
41. Bhatnagar, S.K., Moussa, M.A.A. and Al-Yusuf, A.R. (1985) The role of prehospital discharge two-dimensional echocardiography in determining the prognosis of survivors of first myocardial infarction. *Am. Heart J.*, **109**, 472–7.
42. White, H.D., Norris, R.M., Brown, M.A. *et al.* (1987) Left ventricular end-systolic volume as the major determinant of survival after recovery from myocardial infarction. *Circulation*, **76**, 44–51.
43. Lim, R., Dyke, L. and Dymond, D.S. (1991) Early prognosis after thrombolysis: value of exercise radionuclide ventriculography performed on anti-ischemic medication. *Int. J. Card. Imaging*, **7**, 125–31.
44. Silverman, K.J., Becker, L.C., Buckley, B.H. *et al.* (1980) Value of early thallium-201 scintigraphy for predicting mortality in patients with acute myocardial infarction. *Circulation*, **61**, 996–1003.
45. Ellestad, M.H. and Wan, M.K.C. (1975) Predictive implications of stress testing. Follow-up of 2700 subjects after maximum treadmill stress testing. *Circulation*, **51**, 363–9.
46. McConahay, D.R., McAllister, B.D. and Smith, R.E. (1971) Postexercise electrocardiography: correlations with coronary arteriography and left ventricular hemodynamics. *Am. J. Cardiol.*, **28**, 1–9.
47. Goldschlager, N., Selzer, A. and Cohn, K. (1976) Treadmill stress tests as indicators of presence and severity of coronary artery disease. *Ann. Intern. Med.*, **85**, 277–86.
48. Théroux, P., Waters, D.D., Halphen, C. *et al.* (1979) Prognostic value of exercise testing soon after myocardial infarction. *N. Engl. J. Med.*, **301**, 341–5.
49. DeBusk, R.F., Kraemer, H.C., Nash, E. *et al.* (1983) Stepwise risk stratification soon after acute myocardial infarction. *Am. J. Cardiol.*, **52**, 1161–6.

50. Krone, R.J., Gillespie, J.A., Weld, F.M. *et al.* (1985) Low-level exercise testing after myocardial infarction: usefulness in enhancing clinical risk stratification. *Circulation*, **71**, 80–9.
51. Madsen, E.B., Gilpin, E., Ahnve, S. *et al.* (1985) Prediction of functional capacity and use of exercise testing for predicting risk after acute myocardial infarction. *Am. J. Cardiol.*, **56**, 839–45.
52. Ellestad, M.H. (1975) *Stress Testing. Principles and Practice*, p.**167**, Philadelphia: F.A. Davis.
53. Ellestad, M.H. (1975) *Stress Testing. Principles and Practice*, p.**172**, Philadelphia: F.A. Davis.
54. Cheitlin, M.D., Davia, J.E., de Castro, C.M. *et al.* (1975) Correlation of 'critical' left coronary artery lesions with positive submaximal exercise tests in patients with chest pain. *Am. Heart J.*, **89**, 305–10.
55. Weld, F.M., Chu, K.L., Bigger, J.T. Jr and Rolnitzky, L.M. (1981) Risk stratification with low-level exercise testing 2 weeks after acute myocardial infarction. *Circulation*, **64**, 306–14.
56. de Feyter, P.J., van Eenige, M.J., Dighton, D.H. *et al.* (1982) Prognostic value of exercise testing, coronary angiography and left ventriculography 6–8 weeks after myocardial infarction. *Circulation*, **66**, 527–36.
57. Mark, D.B., Hlatky, M.A., Harrell, F.E. Jr *et al.* (1987) Exercise treadmill score for predicting prognosis in coronary artery disease. *Ann. Intern. Med.*, **106**, 793–800.
58. Mark, D.B., Shaw, L., Harrell, F.E. Jr *et al.* (1991) Prognostic value of a treadmill exercise score in outpatients with suspected coronary artery disease. *N. Engl. J. Med.*, **325**, 849–53.
59. Detrano, R., Janosi, A., Steinbrunn, W. *et al.* (1991) Algorithm to predict triple-vessel/left main coronary artery disease in patients without myocardial infarction. An interventional cross validation. *Circulation*, **83**, III-89–III-96.
60. Chaitman, B.R., McMahon, R.P., Terria, M. *et al.* for the TIMI Investigators (1993) Impact of treatment strategy on predischarge exercise test in the Thrombolysis in Myocardial Infarction (TIMI) II Trial. *Am. J. Cardiol.*, **71**, 131–8.
61. Weiner, D.A., Ryan, T.J., McCabe, C.H. *et al.* (1989) The role of exercise-induced silent myocardial ischemia in patients with abnormal left ventricular function. A report from the Coronary Artery Surgery Study (CASS) Registry. *Am. Heart J.*, **118**, 649–54.
62. Cohn, P.F. (1986) Silent myocardial ischemia: dimensions of the problem in patients with and without angina. *Am. J. Med.*, **80** (suppl. 4C), 3–8.
63. Gottlieb, S.O., Gottlieb, S.H., Achuff, S.C. *et al.* (1988) Silent ischemia on Holter monitoring predicts mortality in high-risk postinfarction patients. *JAMA*, **259**, 1030–5.
64. Hinderliter, A.L., Herbst, M.C., Graden, E.E. *et al.* (1990) Relationship of silent ischemia during daily activities to results of exercise testing. *Consultant* (*Philadelphia*), **30** (suppl.), 23–7.
65. ACC/AHA Task Force Report (1990) Guidelines for the early management of patients with acute myocardial infarction. *J. Am. Coll. Cardiol.*, **16**, 249–92.
66. Gibson, R.S. and Watson, D.D. (1991) Value of planar ^{201}TI imaging in risk stratification of patients recovering from acute myocardial infarction. *Circulation*, **84** (suppl. I), I148–62.
67. Tilkemeier, P.L., Guiney, T.E., LaRaia, P.J. and Boucher, C.A. (1990) Prognostic value of pre-discharge low-level exercise thallium testing after thrombolytic treatment of acute myocardial infarction. *Am. J. Cardiol.*, **66**, 1203–7.
68. Haber, H.L., Beller, G.A., Watson, D.D. and Gimple, L.W. (1993) Exercise thallium-201 scintigraphy after thrombolytic therapy with or without angioplasty for acute myocardial infarction. *Am. J. Cardiol.*, **71**, 1257–61.
69. Manyari, D.E., Knudtson, M., Kloiber, R. and Roth, D. (1988) Sequential thallium-201 myocardial perfusion studies after successful percutaneous transluminal coronary artery angioplasty: delayed resolution of exercise-induced scintigraphic abnormalities. *Circulation*, **77**, 86–95.
70. Sutton, J.M. and Topol, E.J. (1991) Significance of a negative exercise thallium test in the presence of a critical residual stenosis after thrombolysis for acute myocardial infarction. *Circulation*, **83**, 1278–86.
71. Gibson, R.S., Watson, D.D., Craddock, G.B. *et al.* (1983) Prediction of cardiac events after uncomplicated myocardial infarction: a prospective study comparing predischarge exercise thallium-201 scintigraphy and coronary angiography. *Circulation*, **68**, 321–36.
72. Hung, J., Goris, M.L., Nash, E. *et al.* (1984) Comparative value of maximal treadmill testing, exercise thallium myocardial perfusion scintigraphy and exercise radionuclide ventriculography for distinguishing high- and low-risk patients soon after acute myocardial infarction. *Am. J. Cardiol.*, **53**, 1221–7.
73. Kiat, H., Maddahi, J., Roy, L.T. *et al.* (1989) Comparison of technetium 99m methoxy isobutyl isonitrile and thallium 201 for evaluation of coronary artery disease by planar and tomographic methods. *Am. Heart J.*, **117**, 1–11.
74. Iskandrian, A.S., Heo, J., Kong, B. *et al.* (1989) Use of technetium-99m isonitrile (RP-30A) in assessing left ventricular perfusion and function at rest and during exercise in coronary artery disease, and comparison with coronary arteriography and exercise thallium-201 SPECT imaging. *Am. J. Cardiol.*, **64**, 270–5.
75. Hendel, R.C., McSherry, B., Karimeddini, M. and Leppo, J.A. (1990) Diagnostic value of a new myocardial perfusion agent, teboroxime (SQ-30.217), utilizing a rapid planar imaging protocol: preliminary results. *J. Am. Coll. Cardiol.*, **16**, 855–61.
76. Hendel, R.C., Parker, M., Wackers, F.J. *et al.* and the Tetrofosmin Study Group (1993) Is the interpretation of myocardial perfusion scans more consistent with Tc-99m tetrofosmin than thallium-201. *Circulation*, **88**, I-440.
77. Moss, A.J. and the Multicenter Myocardial Ischemia Research Group (1993) Detection and significance of myocardial ischemia in stable patients after recovery from an acute coronary event. *JAMA*, **269**, 2379–85.
78. Diamond, G.A. (1993) Postinfarction risk stratification. Is preventive war winnable? *JAMA*, **269**, 2418–19.
79. Dilsizian, V., Rocco, T.P., Freedman, N.M.T. *et al.* (1990) Enhanced detection of ischemic but viable myocardium by the reinjection of thallium after stress-redistribution imaging. *N. Engl. J. Med.*, **323**, 141–6.

80. Bisi, G., Sciagra, R., Santoro, G.M. *et al.* (1993) Evaluation of ^{99}Tc^m-teboroxime scintigraphy for the differentiation of reversible from fixed defects: comparison with ^{201}Tl redistribution and reinjection imaging. *Nuc. Med. Commun.*, **14** 520–8.
81. Dakik, H.A., Mahmarian, J.J. and Verani, M.S. (1993) Prognostic value of exercise thallium-201 tomography after acute myocardial infarction in the thrombolytic era. *Circulation*, **88**, I-487.
82. Okada, R.D., Glover, D.K. and Leppo, J.A. (1991) Dipyridamole ^{201}Tl scintigraphy in the evaluation of prognosis after myocardial infarction. *Circulation*, **84** (suppl. I), I132–9
83. Borges-Neto, S., Mahmarian, J.J., Jain, A. *et al.* (1988) Quantitative thallium-201 single photon emission computed tomography for assessing the presence, anatomic location and severity of coronary artery disease. *J. Am. Coll. Cardiol.*, **64**, 871–7.
84. Leppo, J.A., O'Brien, J., Rothendler, J.A. *et al.* (1984) Dipyridamole thallium-201 scintigraphy in the prediction of future cardiac events after acute myocardial infarction. *N. Engl. J. Med.*, **310** 1014–18.
85. Younis, L.T., Byers, S., Shaw, L. *et al.* (1989) Prognostic value of intravenous dipyridamole thallium scintigraphy after an acute myocardial ischemic event. *Am. J. Cardiol.*, **64**, 161–6.
86. Pirelli, S., Inglese, E., Suppa, M. *et al.* (1988) Dipyridamole–thallium-201 scintigraphy in the early post-infarction period: (safety and accuracy in predicting the extent of coronary disease and future recurrence of angina in patients suffering from their first myocardial infarction). *Eur. Heart J.*, **9**, 1324–31.
87. Nienaber, C.A., Spielmann, R.P., Salge, D. *et al.* (1990) Assessment of post-infarction jeopardized myocardium by vasodilation-thallium-201 tomography: impact on risk stratification. *Eur. Heart J.*, **11**, 1093–100.
88. Brown, K.A., O'Meara, J., Chambers, C.E. and Plante, D.A. (1990) Ability of dipyridamole–thallium-201 imaging one to four days after acute myocardial infarction to predict in-hospital and late recurrent myocardial ischemic events. *Am. J. Cardiol.*, **65**, 160–7.
89. Marwick, T., Willemart, B., D'Hondt, A.M. *et al.* (1993) Selection of the optimal nonexercise stress for the evaluation of ischemic regional myocardial dysfunction and malperfusion. *Circulation*, **87**, 345–54.
90. Jain, A., Hicks, R.R., Frantz, D.M. *et al.* (1990) Comparison of early exercise treadmill test and oral dipyridamole thallium-201 tomography for the identification of jeopardized myocardium in patients receiving thrombolytic therapy for acute Q-wave myocardial infarction. *Am. J. Cardiol.*, **66**, 551–5.
91. Hendel, R.C., Gore, J.M., Alpert, J.S. and Leppo, J.A. (1991) Prognosis following interventional therapy for acute myocardial infarction: utility of dipyridamole thallium scintigraphy. *Cardiology*, **79**, 73–80.
92. Armstrong, W.F. (1991) Stress echocardiography for detection of coronary artery disease. *Circulation*, **84** (suppl. I), I43–9.
93. Crawford , M.H. (1991) Risk stratification after myocardial infarction with exercise and doppler echocardiography. *Circulation*, **84** (suppl. I), 163–6.
94. Applegate, R.J., Dell'Italia, L.J. and Crawford, M.H. (1987) Usefulness of two-dimensonal echocardiography during low-level exercise testing early after uncomplicated acute myocardial infarction. *Am. J. Cardiol.*, **60**, 10–14.
95. Jaarsma, W., Visser, C.A., Funke Kupper, A.J. *et al.* (1986) Usefulness of two-dimensional exercise echocardiography shortly after myocardial infarction. *Am. J. Cardiol.*, **57**, 86–90.
96. Ryan, T., Armstrong, W.F., O'Donnell, J.A. and Feigenbaum, H. (1987) Risk stratification after acute myocardial infarction by means of exercise two-dimensional echocardiography. *Am. Heart J.*, **114**, 1305–16.
97. Marwick. T.H., Nemec, J.J., Pashkow, F.J. *et al.* (1992) Accuracy and limitations of exercise echocardiography in a routine clinical setting. *J. Am. Coll. Cardiol.*, **19**, 74–81.
98. Galanti, G., Sciagra, R., Comeglio, M. *et al.* (1991) Diagnostic accuracy of peak exercise echocardiography in coronary artery disease: comparison with thallium-201 myocardial scintigraphy. *Am. Heart J.*, **122**, 1609–16.
99. Quinones, M.A., Verani, M.S., Haichin, R.M. *et al.* (1992) Exercise echocardiography versus ^{201}Tl single-photon emission computed tomography in evaluation of coronary artery disease: analysis of 292 patients. *Circulation*, **85**, 1026–31.
100. Bolognese, L., Rossi, L., Sarasso, G. *et al.* (1992) Silent versus symptomatic dipyridamole-induced ischemia after myocardial infarction: clinical and prognostic significance. *J. Am. Coll. Cardiol.*, **19**, 953–9.
101. Landi, P., Orlandini, A., Sclavo, M.G. *et al.* and the EPIC Study Group (1991). The prognostic value of dipyridamole-echocardiography early after uncomplicated acute myocardial infarction: a large scale multicenter trial. *Circulation*, **84** (suppl. II), 208.
102. Sawada, S.G., Segar, D.S., Ryan, T. *et al.* (1990) Dobutamine stress echocardiography: assessment of prognosis after myocardial infarction. *Circulation*, **82** (suppl. III), 74.
103. Neskovic, A.N., Popovic, A.D., Babic, R. *et al.* (1993) Positive high-dose dipyridamole-echocardiography test after acute myocardial infarction is an excellent predictor of future cardiac events. *Circulation*, **88**, I-121.
104. Camerieri, A., Bianchi, F., Landi, P. *et al.* and the Echo Persantine International Cooperative Study Group (1993) Risk stratification with pharmacological stress echocardiography early after uncomplicated myocardial infarction: the impact of revascularization. *Circulation*, **88**, I-120.
105. Jaarsma, W., Cramer, J.M., Suttorp, M.J. *et al.* (1993) Risk stratification following thrombolysis in acute myocardial infarction with dobutamine stress echocardiography. *Circulation*, **88**, I-120.
106. Marcovitz, P.A. and Armstrong, W.F. (1992) Accuracy of dobutamine stress echocardiography in detecting coronary artery disease. *Am. J. Cardiol.*, **69**, 1269–73.
107. Bach, D.S. and Armstrong, W.F. (1992) Dobutamine stress echocardiography. *Am. J. Cardiol.*, **69**, 90H–96H.

108. Pirelli, S., Danzi, G.B., Massa, D. *et al.* (1993) Exercise thallium scintigraphy versus high-dose dipyridamole echocardiography testing for detection of asymptomatic restenosis in patients with positive exercise tests after coronary angioplasty. *Am. J. Cardiol*, **71**, 1052–6.

109. Picano, E., Distante, A., Masini, M. *et al.* (1985) Dipyridamole echocardiography test in effort angina pectoris. *Am. J. Cardiol.*, **56**, 452–6.

110. Berthe, C., Pierard, L.A., Hiernaux, M. *et al.* (1986) Predicting the extent and location of coronary artery disease in acute myocardial infarction by echocardiography during dobutamine infusion. *Am. J. Cardiol.*, **58**, 1167–72.

111. Corbett, J.R., Dehmer, G.J., Lewis, S.E. *et al.* (1981) The prognostic value of submaximal exercise testing with radionuclide ventriculography before hospital discharge in patients with recent myocardial infarction. *Circulation*, **64**, 535–40.

112. Fubini, A., Cecchi, E., Bobbio, M. *et al.* (1992) Value of exercise stress test, radionuclide angiography and coronary angiography in predicting new coronary events in asymptomatic patients after a first episode of myocardial infarction. *Int. J. Cardiol.*, **34**, 319–25.

113. Abraham, R.D., Harris, P.J., Roubin, G.S. *et al.* (1987) Usefulness of ejection fraction response to exercise one month after acute myocardial infarction in predicting coronary anatomy and prognosis. *Am. J. Cardiol.*, **60**, 225–30.

114. Coma-Canella, I., del Val Gomez Martinez, M., Rodrigo, F. and Castro Beiras, J. M. (1993) The dobutamine stress test with thallium-201 single-photon emission computed tomography and radionuclide angiography: postinfarction study. *J. Am. Coll. Cardiol.*, **22**, 399–406.

115. Brunken, R., Schwaiger, M., Grover-McKay, M. *et al.* (1987) Positron emission tomography detects tissue metabolic activity in myocardial segments with persistent thallium perfusion defects. *J. Am. Coll. Cardiol.*, **10**, 557–67.

116. Stewart, R.E., Schwaiger, M., Molina, E. *et al.* (1991) Comparison of rubidium-82 positron emission tomography and thallium-201 SPECT imaging for detection of coronary artery disease. *Am. J. Cardiol.*, **67**, 1303–10.

117. Tillisch, J., Brunken, R., Marshall, R. *et al.* (1986) Reversibility of cardiac wall-motion abnormalities predicted by positron tomography. *N. Engl. J. Med.*, **314**, 884–8.

118. Tamaki, N., Kawamoto, M., Takahashi, N. *et al.* (1993) Prognostic value of an increase in fluorine-18 deoxyglucose uptake in patients with myocardial infarction: comparison with stress thallium imaging. *J. Am. Coll. Cardiol.*, **22**, 1621–7.

119. Yoshida, K. and Gould, K.L. (1993) Quantitative relation of myocardial infarct size and myocardial viability by positron emission tomography to left ventricular ejection fraction and 3-year mortality with and without revascularization. *J. Am. Coll. Cardiol.*, **22**, 984–97.

120. Bigger, J.T. Jr, Fleiss, J.L., Kleiger, R. *et al.* (1984) The relationship among ventricular arrhythmias, left ventricular dysfunction, and mortality in the 2 years after myocardial infarction. *Circulation*, **69**, 250–8.

121. Moss, A.J., Davis, H.T., DeCamilla, J. and Bayer, L.W. (1979) Ventricular ectopic beats and their relation to sudden and nonsudden cardiac death after myocardial infarction. *Circulation*, **60**, 998–1003.

122. Ruberman, W., Weinblatt, E., Goldberg, J.D. *et al.* (1981) Ventricular premature complexes and sudden death after myocardial infarction. *Circulation*, **64**, 297–305.

123. Mukarji, J., Rude, R.E., Poole, W.K. and the MILIS Study Group (1984) Risk factors for sudden death after myocardial infarction: two year follow-up. *Am. J. Cardiol.*, **54**, 31–6.

124. Gomes, J.A., Winters, S.L., Stewart, D. *et al.* (1987) A noninvasive index to predict sustained ventricular tachycardia and sudden death in the first year after myocardial infarction: based on signal-averaged electrocardiogram, radionuclide ejection fraction and Holter monitoring. *J. Am. Coll. Cardiol.*, **10**, 349–57.

125. McClements, B.M. and Adgey, A.A.J. (1993) Value of signal-averaged electrocardiography, radionuclide ventriculography, Holter monitoring and clinical variables for prediction of arrhythmic events in survivors of acute myocardial infarction in the thrombolytic era. *J. Am. Coll. Cardiol.*, **21**, 1419–27.

126. Ruberman, W., Crow, R., Rosenberg, C.R. *et al.* (1992) Intermittent ST depression and mortality after myocardial infarction. *Circulation*, **85**, 1440–6.

127. Steinberg, J.S., Regan, A., Sciacca, R.R. *et al.* (1992) Predicting arrhythmic events after acute myocardial infarction using the signal-averaged electrocardiogram. *Am. J. Cardiol.*, **69**, 13–21.

128. Gomes, J.A., Winters, S.L. and Ip, J. (1993) Post myocardial infarction stratification and the signal-averaged electrocardiogram. *Prog. Cardiovasc. Dis.*, **35**, 263–70.

129. Breithardt, G., Borggrefe, M. and Karbenn, U. (1990) Late potentials as predictors of risk after thrombolytic therapy. *Br. Heart J.*, **64**, 174–6.

130. Bourke, J.P., Richards, D.A.B., Ross, D.L. *et al.* (1991) Routine programmed electrical stimulation in survivors of acute myocardial infarction for prediction of spontaneous ventricular tachyarrhythmias during follow-up: results, optimal stimulation protocol and cost-effective screening. *J. Am. Coll. Cardiol.*, **18**, 780–8.

131. Cripps, T., Bennett, E.D., Camm, A.J. and Ward, D.E. (1989) Inducibility of sustained monomorphic ventricular tachycardia as a prognostic indicator in survivors of recent myocardial infarction: a prospective evaluation in relation to other prognostic variables. *J. Am. Coll. Cardiol.*, **14**, 289–96.

132. Roy, D., Marchand, E., Théroux, P. *et al.* (1985) Programmed ventricular stimulation in survivors of acute myocardial infarction. *Circulation*, **72**, 487–94.

133. Pedretti, R., Etro, M.D., Laporta, A. *et al.* (1993) Prediction of late arrhythmic events after acute myocardial infarction from combined use of noninvasive prognostic variables and inducibility of sustained monomorphic ventricular tachycardia. *Am. J. Cardiol.*, **71**, 1131–41.

134. Cripps, T.R., Malik, M., Farrell, T.A. *et al.* (1991) Prognostic value of reduced heart rate variability after myocardial infarction: clinical evaluation of a new analysis method. *Br. Heart J.*, **65**, 14–19.

135. Farrell, T.G., Bashir, Y., Cripps, T. *et al.* (1991) Risk stratification for arrhythmic events in postinfarction patients based on heart rate variability, ambulatory ECG variables and the signal-averaged electrocardiogram. *J. Am. Coll. Cardiol.*, **18**, 687–97.
136. Odemuyiwa, O., Malik, M., Farrell, T. *et al.* (1991) Comparison of the predictive characteristics of heart rate variability index and left ventricular ejection fraction for all-cause mortality, arrhythmic events and sudden death after acute myocardial infarction. *Am. J. Cardiol.*, **68**, 434–9.
137. Bigger, J.T., Fleiss, J.L., Rolnitzky, L.M. and Steinman, R.C. (1993) The ability of several short-term measures of RR variability to predict mortality after myocardial infarction. *Circulation*, **88**, 927–34.
138. Wilson, A.C. and Kostis, J.B. for the BHAT Study Group (1992) The prognostic significance of very low frequency ventricular ectopic activity in survivors of acute myocardial infarction. *Chest*, **102**, 732–6.
139. Farrell, T.G., Paul, V., Cripps, T.R. *et al.* (1992) Baroreflex sensitivity and electrophysiological correlates in patients after acute myocardial infarction. *Circulation*, **83**, 945–52.

17

Meta-Analysis in the Evaluation of Therapies

M. D. Flather, M. E. Farkouh and S. Yusuf

Meta-analysis describes a systematic approach to quantitatively synthesizing information from a set of studies that address a related question. This approach has been extensively utilized to systematically pool information from clinical trials in cardiovascular medicine using methods that are now fairly well established. Meta-analysis is a tool which, if used properly, can allow the best possible appraisal of the *totality* of evidence concerning a particular therapy or management strategy. The purpose of this chapter is to review briefly the rationale and methodology of meta-analysis, describe its value in the evaluation of therapies for acute myocardial infarction (AMI), and to discuss its strengths and limitations utilizing specific examples.

Rationale for Meta-Analysis

It is believed that clinical practice could be improved by a systematic approach to appraising and synthesizing the available evidence on a particular therapeutic strategy. The use of the randomized controlled trial (RCT) is an important step towards the unbiased assessment of therapeutic strategies. The ability of RCTs to reliably detect moderate, plausible, and medically useful differences in treatment effects requires studies with several hundred to a few thousand endpoints. The development and implementation of large trials (or mega-trials) in myocardial infarction has been a key step towards this goal.[1] Meta-analysis provides a complementary approach whereby the information from all relevant randomized controlled trials is synthesized in a quantitative fashion.[2] If performed properly this technique can provide a relatively unbiased assessment of the benefits and risks of a particular treatment to help physicians in the clinical decision-making process.[3,4]

Principles and Practical Steps of Meta-Analysis

Fundamental Concepts

Most interventions in a common condition like AMI are likely to have at best only moderate effects (10%, 15% or 20% risk reductions) on major outcomes (e.g. death or major morbidity). Many treatments are only moderately effective, given the multiplicity of precipitating events, varying pathophysiologic processes and numerous complications in AMI[1]. Even if a therapy affected an important process in the pathogenesis of

AMI, it would be surprising if large benefits were achieved. This general judgment is supported by the experience with various interventions in AMI (Table 17.1) where the impact of treatments on mortality have only been moderate.

It is now recognized that the effects of a therapy on a specific outcome in different patients, and in related situations, are quite likely to differ in magnitude (i.e. 'quantitative interactions' are common and to be expected) but they are much less likely to differ in *direction* (i.e. 'qualitative interactions') or directional effects in which treatment is beneficial in one subgroup, but harmful in another, are much rarer especially if they were initially unanticipated.[2] Clearly, different trials with different patient populations are not exactly comparable, but it is reasonable to assume that if different trials address approximately the same question, then there will be a tendency for their results to point in the same direction. In individual trials, the play of chance may exaggerate, dilute or even reverse this tendency. However, on average, the collective direction (and estimate of treatment effect) will likely approximate the 'truth'[3,4] depending on the amount of information available from the trials.

Formulating the Question

The purpose of meta-analysis should be to provide a reliable answer to a specific question. It should not be regarded simply as a 'pooling process', of available trials that address a similar question in which the published data are reformatted and republished, thus providing very little extra information over and above a simple review of the individual trials. Specific questions (e.g. Do β-blockers, when started in the acute phase, reduce mortality after myocardial infarction?) are much more useful for patient care than broader ones (e.g. What are the pooled results of the available trials of β-blockers in ischemic heart disease?)[2,3] The questions to be addressed by meta-analysis are best framed in the context of the supposed mechanism of action of the intervention, and the known epidemiology of the disease of interest. It is recommended that every meta-analysis have a formal protocol that outlines the specific goals, the key steps, the statistical methods and any relevant definitions. This ensures consistency and rigor in approach.

Identification and Selection of Trials

The source material for a meta-analysis must be carefully identified and selected. The only reliable sources of data are individual unconfounded RCTs that address the question being studied. Key aspects of the quality of each trial must be critically appraised, in particular to ensure that true random allocation of treatment (without foreknowledge) was utilized for each trial.[4,5] Having formulated an appropriate question, all the relevant published or unpublished RCTs should be identified using all available useful methods: computer-aided searches (e.g. MEDLINE), scrutiny of reference lists of review articles, trial registries, consultation with colleagues, correspondence with pharmaceutical companies and manual searches where appropriate.[6] Publication bias, whereby smaller trials or those with 'negative' or unpromising results do not get published, is an important problem to consider when performing a meta-analysis.[4,7,8] In general, publication bias is likely to be more relevant in situations where only a few trials are available, or there are relatively few endpoints upon which to base a statistical inference. A careful log of trials that are excluded from the meta-analysis (with reasons for exclusion) is helpful in ascertaining whether subtle bias in selection of trials might have modified the results.

Table 17.1 A summary of the published results of meta-analyses of early interventions on mortality after acute myocardial infarction

Title	Year	Early intervention[a]	Follow-up duration	Total no. trials	Total no. patients	Total no. deaths	Death				
							Treatment	Control	P-value	Odds ratio[b] (95% CI)	NNT
β-Blocker[9]	1985	i.v. beta-blocker	7 days	27	11 309	399	194/5676 (3.4%)	205/5633 (3.6%)	NS	0.94 (0.76–1.14)	500
Fibrinolytic[16]	1985	i.v. streptokinase	6 weeks	24	5284	913	412/2672 (15.4%)	501/2612 (19.2%)	0.0003	0.76 (0.57–0.89)	26
Prophylactic lidocaine[17]	1988	i.m. or i.v. lidocaine	48 hours	14	9155	137	82/4616 (1.7%)	55/4539 (1.2%)	NS	1.38 (0.98–1.95)	−200
Nitrates[18]	1988	i.v. nitrates	7 days	10	2041	329	136/1021 (13.3%)	193/1020 (18.9%)	0.0006	0.65 (0.52–0.84)	12
Calcium channel blockers[19]	1990	Oral calcium channel blockers	Early	19	11 225	890	464/5604 (8.3%)	426/5621 (7.6%)	0.17	1.10 (0.96–1.26)	−143
Magnesium in suspected AMI[20]	1991	i.v. magnesium	1 month	7	1301	87	25/657 (3.8%)	53/644 (8.2%)	0.0008	0.45 (0.27–0.71)	23
Antiplatelet therapy[21]	1994	Antiplatelet therapy	1 month	9	18 773	1976	874/9388 (9.3%)	1102/9385 (11.7%)	<0.0001	0.77 (0.70–0.85)	42
Fibrinolytic therapy[22]	1994	Fibrinolytic therapy overall	35 days	9	58 600	6177	2820/29 315 (9.6%)	3357/29 285 (11.5%)	<0.0001	0.82 (0.78–0.87)	52
		0–6 hours from symptom onset with ST elevation or bundle branch block	35 days	9	28 824	3125	1 352/14 438 (9.4%)	1773/14 386 (12.3%)	<0.0001	0.74 (0.68–0.79)	35
		7–12 hours from symptom onset with ST elevation or bundle branch block	35 days	5	9308	1241	575/4683 (12.3%)	666/4625 (14.4%)	0.003	0.83 (0.74–0.94)	48
PTCA[23]	1994	Primary PTCA versus thrombolysis	6 weeks	5	955	43	15/473 (3.2%)	28/482 (5.8%)	–	0.54 (0.28–1.00)	38

[a] Within 72 hours of symptom onset.
[b] Odds ratio, proportion of events in treatment group compared with control.
AMI, acute myocardial infarction; 95% CI, 95% confidence intervals (%); i.m., intramuscular; i.v., intravenous; NNT, number needed to treat (estimated number of patients needed to be treated in order to prevent one adverse event; 1 (Absolute risk reduction); PTCA, percutaneous transluminal coronary angioplasty.
Note. The results in this table do not necessarily reflect the most recent estimates of treatment effects, but serve to illustrate the results of the relevant meta-analyses and allow broad comparisons to be made.

Table 17.2 Example of calculation of $O - E$ and its variance: hypothetical data[10]

	Allocated treatment	Allocated control	Both together
Dead	25	40	65
Alive	75	60	135
Total	100	100	200

O, 'observed' number of deaths in the treatment group = 25.
If a total of 65 die and treatment has no effect, then E, 'expected' no. of deaths in treatment group = 65/2 = 32.5.
Statistical calculation (treatment group only):
$O - E = 25 - 32.5 = -7.5$
NB Minus denotes benefit, and −7.5 suggests about 15 deaths avoided.
Finally, the 'variance' of $O - E = 32.5 \times (100/200) \times 135(200-1) = 11.0$.

Data Collection

Before embarking on the process of meta-analysis, it is essential to select the appropriate data points that will be used in the analysis. Descriptive, or demographic information will describe the baseline pre-randomization data (e.g. age, sex, location of ST elevation, etc.) and the postrandomization data will consist of the endpoints considered to be important (usually death plus major morbid events such as reinfarction and stroke) along with other relevant information, e.g. concomitant medication and length of follow-up.

The collection of the relevant data for a good meta-analysis is a time-consuming procedure because correspondence with the original trialists is essential to ensure completeness, and to discuss and resolve any issues or areas that are unclear.[9] A typical example may be an imbalance in the numbers of patients in the control and treatment groups in the published report because of some data-derived postrandomization exclusions. In the meta-analysis *all* randomized patients must be accounted for and included in the analysis on an intention-to-treat basis (as should also be the case in a good RCT).[2] Once the data have been collected they need to be computerized (if not already in a computer format) and then checked for inconsistencies and missing information. Most meta-analyses utilize the published data from the literature. However, the preferred method is to obtain individual data points from each patient in the trials, which allows much greater flexibility in checking of the data and subsequent analysis. The process of data collection and verification can take several years if there are a large number of trials, a large number of patients or both.

Analysis (Tables 17.2 and 17.3)

The statistical methods and assumptions involved in analyzing the data in a meta-analysis are now well accepted.[9–11] They do not implicitly assume that the real risk reductions in different trials (or different patient populations) are the same size, but that they will point in the same direction. The unjustified assumption that patients in one trial can be compared with patients in other trials (i.e. that 'apples' can be compared with 'oranges' is *not* made). The basic principle involved in the most commonly used statistical method (Peto and Yusuf modification of the Mantel–Haenszel approach) is to make

Table 17.3 Principle of unbiased combination of randomized trial results[10]

Trial 1	Result 1 (O − E)	Variance 1
Trial 2	Result 2 (O − E)	Variance 2
Trial 3	Result 3 (O − E)	Variance 3
	Overview result = grand total,	
Sum of separate[a] results	i.e. result 1 + result 2 + result 3	Sum of variances

[a]If treatment had no effect on outcome in any trial then each of the results, considered separately, would differ only randomly from zero, and so too would their grand total. (An overall test of whether the grand total differs from zero does not depend on the unjustified assumption that any real effects in different trials must be of similar size.)

comparisons of treatment with control only within one trial, and to avoid completely any direct comparisons of patients in another. This is achieved by calculating separately for each trial the standard quantity 'observed minus expected' (O−E) for the number of adverse outcome events (usually deaths) among treatment allocated patients. O−E will have a negative value if the treated group fared better than controls (and positive if it fared worse). The O−E values, one for each trial, are then added. The variance of the total of the individual O−E values is given by the sum of the individual variances of each O−E value. This method gives the results of each trial's appropriate 'weight' or emphasis in the overall assessment, which depends on the amount of statistical information provided by it (i.e. on the number of endpoints in a particular trial).[10] Other methods (e.g. the random effects model) have also been utilized for statistical inference in meta-analyses. These alterntive methods generally yield the same or similar results, although some might be more or less conservative than others. Additional techniques utilizing weighting by intervention effect (e.g. degree of cholesterol lowering) or by regression methods are also of value. A fuller discussion of these different statistical approaches can be found elsewhere.[12–15]

Interpretation of Results

The results of a meta-analysis should be intepreted in the light of knowledge of the biologic processes, known mechanisms of the treatment strategy under scrutiny, and the natural history of the condition under study. In many cases it is quite possible that even the combined results on the main endpoints of interest in a meta-analysis may not be enough to provide a clear interpretation of the data. In these cases it is important to review the data on other secondary and related endpoints.[3] For example, a reduction in fatal coronary heart disease (CHD) events of borderline significance is more plausible if it is accompanied by a reduction in nonfatal CHD events. In general, interpretation of the results of a meta-analysis should be conservative. Perhaps statistical significance for two-sided 'P' values should only be considered when differences between treatment and control are fairly extreme (i.e. $P < 0.001$), based on sufficiently large numbers of events (e.g. 500 or more) so that the results are generally robust. This would help to ensure that lack of data from a few small unpublished trials would not alter the conclusions. In addition, confidence intervals around the point estimate must always be considered. Confidence intervals which are wide (i.e. >30%) or overlap the point of equivalence suggest inherent unreliability of the point estimate. Currently, there is little evidence to suggest that the results of meta-analyses alone have a major influence on clinical practice, in contrast to the results of some large RCTs of treatment of AMI such as those evaluating thrombolytic therapy and aspirin. Meta-analyses that review the data from smaller trials tend to be used to generate or confirm hypotheses in preparation for a more definite RCT. These meta-analyses are not designed to provide definitive clinical recommendations. However, once large trials have been completed, meta-analyses of these studies enable more reliable *post-hoc* analyses of subgroup effects.

Summary of Principles Involved in Meta-Analysis

At its best, meta-analysis should provide a systematic, scientific, unbiased and comprehensive review of the available evidence from the relevant RCTs of a particular treatment strategy. This process involves all the care and rigor that can be applied to well-designed and implemented RCTs. If the source trials do not represent the complete information of the treatment strategy under scrutiny, then the results of the analysis may be flawed. The strength of the conclusions depend not only on the completeness of the available data, but also on the numbers of relevant endpoints. Conservative interpretation and use of the results of meta-analyses is advised, and should include critical appraisal of the meta-analysis itself, its robustness, a clear understanding of the plausibility of the results and its consistency across the individual RCTs and other relevant biologic or epidemiologic information.

Some Examples of Meta-Analyses of Treatment of AMI

There have been many comprehensive meta-analyses ('systematic overviews') reviewing treatments for AMI.[9,16–23] A summary of these is provided in Table 17.1, which includes a column for the number of patients that need to be treated to prevent one adverse event ('number needed to treat' or NNT). NNT is the reciprocal of the absolute risk reduction (or ARR, which is the difference between the event rate in the treatment and control groups expressed as a fraction) and may be a more useful way of expressing the clinical efficacy of a treatment than odds ratios or relative risk reductions.[24] Lower NNTs suggest more useful treatments (although the estimate of NNT is subject to the same statistical variability as the estimates of the odds ratio or relative risk reduction).

A meta-analysis of the 27 trials that compared early mortality after AMI between patients treated with early intravenous β-blockers (followed by oral β-blockers) vs control showed a nonsignificant trend towards mortality reduction with β-blockers.[9] These data were used to design the first of the International Studies of Infarct Survival, ISIS-1, a large trial of 16 000 patients.[25] The results of ISIS-1 showed a modest benefit of early intravenous β-blocker followed by oral therapy in AMI with a relative risk reduction of 15% ($P < 0.04$) in mortality, with similar reductions in nonfatal reinfarction and cardiac arrests. Similar experiences were found with a review of the small trials of long-term β-blockade after AMI.[26] Subsequent larger trials such as the Beta-Blocker Heart Attack Trial (BHAT) confirmed that long-term β-blockade reduced the risk of death and recurrent myocardial infarction by about one-quarter.[27]

In an effort to prevent early occurrence of ventricular fibrillation, after AMI, prophylactic lidocaine was utilized because of its effect in suppressing ventricular ectopy and ventricular tachycardia. However, the results of a meta-analysis of 14 RCTs showed no benefit of lidocaine in preventing early death.[17] The trials included in this meta-analysis were small, follow-up was short (48 hours) and only 137 endpoints were recorded upon which to base the comparison of lidocaine with control. No subsequent large trials have addressed this question but the results of the Cardiac Arrhythmia Suppression Trial (CAST), which showed that oral class I antiarrhythmic therapy (encainide, flecainide and moricizine) following AMI increased mortality,[28,29] were consistent with the results of the lidocaine meta-analysis.

Ten trials of early intravenous nitrate therapy in AMI in a total of 2000 patients showed a mortality reduction of about one-third.[18] Again, these trials were relatively small with only about 300 deaths. In the GISSI-3 trial, intravenous nitrates were compared with control in 19 000 patients with AMI.[30] Preliminary results show that there was a nonsignificant 6% reduction in mortality (odds ratio 0.94, 95% confidence interval 0.84–1.05). ISIS-4, which evaluated oral mononitrate in 50 000 patients with AMI, showed a similar result to GISSI-3.[31] These data suggest that results of the early meta-analysis may have been an overestimate of the treatment effect (due to the play of chance) or that routine nitrate treatment may be less relevant in the current era of management of AMI, which includes routine use of thrombolytic agents and aspirin for the treatment of patients with AMI.

The meta-analysis of calcium channel blockers demonstrated that there was no benefit for a class of agents that were once considered to be promising on theoretical grounds.[19] Although there was no significant difference observed between treatment and control groups ($P = 0.2$), the relatively large size of the meta-analysis (about 890 deaths) suggests that there is no rationale for the routine use of calcium channel blockers for the treatment of AMI patients. The meta-analysis of antiplatelet therapy in AMI[21] consisted mostly of the results of ISIS-2[32] with about a 20% risk reduction in mortality. Aspirin is now standard therapy for patients with AMI in most parts of the world.

More recently, percutaneous transluminal coronary angioplasty (PTCA) has been compared with thrombolytic therapy as primary treatment for AMI in a preliminary meta-analysis of five small trials.[23] With a total sample size of 955 patients and less than 50 deaths, any conclusions about the efficacy of primary PTCA must be drawn with considerable caution (although the data indicate a 46% risk reduction with wide confidence intervals). Larger trials will need to be performed to answer the question of primary PTCA in AMI more reliably.

An Example of How Meta-Analysis Has Helped to Evaluate Thrombolytic Therapy for AMI

Two important comprehensive meta-analyses (systematic overviews) have been influential in our understanding of the role of thrombolytic therapy in AMI.[16,22] An earlier meta-analysis of 24 small randomized trials involving a total of more than 5000 patients published in 1985 showed clearly that intravenous thrombolytic therapy (with most trials studying streptokinase) was associated with 22% relative risk reduction ($P < 0.001$; Table 17.1)[16] This in itself was a surprising result because although some of the trials were individually promising, there was a real fear that the hazardous side-effects (hemorrhagic stroke, major extracranial bleeding) would offset any potential benefit. Other important findings from this meta-analysis included: (1) generation of the hypothesis that thrombolytic therapy might be beneficial when given to patients presenting beyond 6 hours from symptom onset, (2) routine anticoagulation following intravenous thrombolysis may not be necessary, (3) the risk of excess strokes was minimal, and (4) a rigorously performed meta-analysis could show a clear treatment effect when the individual trials appeared less promising. These observations influenced the design of subsequent trials such as ISIS-2[32] and GISSI-I[33] and ensured a large enough sample size to detect a 20% reduction in mortality, inclusion of patients up to 24 hours after symptom onset, and simplification of the treatment regimen so that intravenous heparin was not mandatory. The results of ISIS-2 and GISSI-I trials confirmed the hypotheses generated by this meta-analysis. This is a good example of a meta-analysis with about 1000 endpoints (deaths) that yielded fairly robust statistical information, generated more definitive RCTs, and provided reliable information in its own right. However, there is little evidence to suggest that this meta-analysis had any immediate or direct influence on clinical practice. Certainly, the proportion of patients receiving thrombolytic therapy increased only after the publication of several definitive trials (ISIS-2,[32] GISSI,[33] AIMS,[34] and ASSET[35]).

Since the publication of the meta-analysis discussed above, nine large RCTs of more than 1000 patients have randomized patients to thrombolytic therapy or control.[32-40] The pooled results (death and major morbidity) from these trials have now been published.[22] Four of these trials independently showed clear evidence of benefit for thrombolytic therapy,[32-35] and it is therefore important to summarize the rationale for this further meta-analysis. Although it had been accepted that, overall, thrombolytic therapy was beneficial for patients with AMI presenting within 6 hours of the onset of symptoms, there was still uncertainty about: (1) the effects among patients presenting beyond 6 hours from symptom onset; (2) the benefit of thrombolytic therapy for patients with suspected MI presenting with ECGs not showing ST elevation (e.g. ST depression, bundle branch block, etc.); (3) the risk–benefit ratio of thrombolytic therapy in other important patient subgroups, e.g. the elderly, patients with prior MI or those at the extremes of blood pressure at entry. The major results of the Fibrinolytic Therapy Trialists' Collaboration report[22] (Table 17.1), which used individual patient data for each analysis, are summarized below.

1. Most of the benefit of thrombolytic therapy was observed in patients presenting with ST elevation or bundle branch block on the ECG within 12 hours from pain or symptom onset.
2. There was clear evidence of benefit for patients treated with thrombolytic therapy presenting 7–12 hours after symptom onset (Table 17.1).
3. The benefit of thrombolytic therapy with elapsed time from symptom onset was clearly delineated (Figure 5.7, p. 153) and amounted to a loss of about two lives for every 1000 patients treated for each 1-hour delay. Surprisingly, the relationship between benefit vs time was shown to be linear (except for the very early period of 0–2 hours where the benefits might be proportionately greater).
4. Early mortality (within 12–24 hours after randomization) for patients randomized to thrombolytic therapy was actually higher than controls (Table 17.4). This 'early hazard' associated with thrombolytic therapy was more than offset by the much larger later benefit. The causes of the early hazard are still uncertain, but cardiac rupture and reperfusion injury have been suggested as possible mechanisms since the majority of these early deaths are cardiac (as opposed to strokes or other vascular causes).
5. Within the categories of ST elevation or bundle branch block, presenting within 12 hours from symptom onset, the benefits of thrombolytic therapy were seen consistently across the major subgroups of the elderly, prior MI, diabetics, males and females, high and low blood pressure.

Limitations and Controversial Aspects of Meta-Analysis for Treatment of AMI

Magnesium in AMI

Before the presentation of the preliminary results of the Fourth International Study of Infarct Survival (ISIS-4) in 1993,[31] there was promising evidence from a small meta-analysis (less than 100 deaths: 3.8% deaths in the magnesium group vs 8.2% deaths in the control group; $P < 0.001$; Table 17.1) and a moderate-size RCT[41] (LIMIT-2 with about

Table 17.4 Proportional and absolute differences of fibrinolytic therapy on mortality during days 0–35

| Day of death | Deaths during days 0–35 | | Proportional reduction (95% CL) | Benefit per 1000 (95% CL) |
	Fibrinolytic (29 315)	Control (29 285)		
Day 0	695 (2.4%)	554 (1.9%)	−26% SD 6 (−38% to − 13%)	−5 SD 1** (−7 to −2)
Day 1	475 (1.7%)	549 (1.9%)	13% SD 6 (2% to 25%)	3 SD 1* (0–5)
Day 2–7	847 (3.0%)	1100 (3.9%)	23% SD 4 (16% to 31%)	9 SD 2*** (6–12)
Days 8–35	803 (2.9%)	1154 (4.3%)	32% SD 4 (24% to 39%)	13 SD 2*** (10–16)
All in days 0–35	2820 (9.6%)	3357 (11.5%)	18% SD 2 (13% to 23%)	18 SD 3*** (13–23)

*2P < 0.05; **2P < 0.001; ***2P < 0.00001.
Note This table illustrates the early hazard of thrombolytic therapy on the day of randomization (i.e. excess deaths in day 0) that is offset by the much larger later benefit, yielding a substantial overall benefit at 35 days.[22]
CL, Confidence Limits; SD, Standard Deviation.

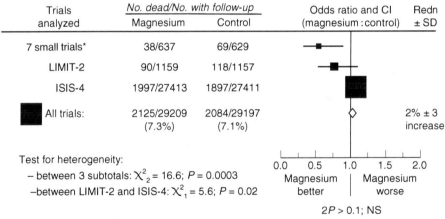

*Numbers updated from published report.[20]

Figure 17.1 Short-term mortality in trials of i.v. magnesium in acute myocardial infarction.[31]

200 deaths: 7.8% magnesium vs 10.3% placebo control; $P = 0.04$) that magnesium infusion reduced mortality after AMI. ISIS-4, which randomized 58 000 patients with about 4000 deaths, did not confirm these earlier observations. Mortality at 35 days was 7.3% in the magnesium group vs 6.9% in the control group ($P = $ NS).[31] The disagreement between these studies, which have addressed essentially the same question, has been the subject of controversy, fuelled by statistical evidence of heterogeneity between the meta-analysis, LIMIT-2 and ISIS-4 (Figure 17.1).

1. Were there any important differences between the patient populations in the earlier studies and ISIS-4? The broad baseline characteristics of these studies are summarized

Table 17.5 Comparison of patient populations between LIMIT-2[41] and ISIS-4[31]

	LIMIT-2	ISIS-4
Total number randomized	2316	57 820
Mean age (years)	62	62
Male	74%	74%
Prior MI	26%	17%
Confirmed MI	65%	92%
% treated within 6 hours of symptom onset	74%	40%
Infarct location		
Anterior	46%	39%
Inferior	46%	40%
Other	8%	21%
Concomitant Therapy		
Thrombolytic agent	36%	70%
Aspirin	66%	94%

MI, myocardial infarction.

in Table 17.5, which suggests some important differences in the proportions of patients receiving thrombolytic therapy and aspirin (many more patients received thrombolytic therapy and aspirin in ISIS-4 than LIMIT-2), and in the mean time from pain onset to randomization (patients were generally randomized earlier after pain onset in LIMIT-2 than ISIS-4).
2. Is it possible that delays in the administration of magnesium after thrombolytic therapy in ISIS-4 (compared to before, or at the initiation of, thrombolytic therapy in LIMIT-2) attenuated its benefit? Although not proven in humans, some animal studies suggest that elevated magnesium levels at the time of reperfusion may limit reperfusion injury. This hypothesis is not substantiated by the available data from:
   a. ISIS-4, in which patients randomized within 3 hours after symptom onset also did not show a reduction in mortality with magnesium (deaths/patients: magnesium = 342/4847 [7.1%]; control = 345/4865 [7.1%]).[31] Although the exact time of initiation of thrombolytic therapy and magnesium is not available, it is likely that by the time reperfusion was established (about 90–180 min after starting thrombolytic therapy) 'therapeutic' levels of magnesium would have been achieved in those patients allocated magnesium infusion.
   b. LIMIT-2 in which only about one-third of patients received thrombolytic therapy.[41] If magnesium only worked in patients who reperfused early, or in the presence of thrombolytic therapy, the effects in this group should have been very much larger than in those not receiving thrombolytic therapy. However, no such interaction was demonstrated in LIMIT-2, and the apparent benefit of magnesium in those receiving or not receiving thrombolytic therapy was similar.
   c. The meta-analysis of small trials in which very few patients would have received concomitant thrombolytic therapy.[20]
3. It is possible that the high rate of use of thrombolytic therapy (70%) and aspirin (94%) in ISIS-4 provided less of an opportunity for magnesium to be beneficial.
4. The paucity of events in the meta-analysis (<100 deaths) and LIMIT-2 (<200 events) made these results less robust. Even a small number of excess deaths from therapy in unpublished trials that the meta-analysts were unaware of may negate the apparently promising results of the meta-analysis and of LIMIT-2.

At present, there is no satisfactory explanation for the discrepancy between the results of the meta-analysis, LIMIT-2 and ISIS-4, but given the totality of the evidence, there is no convincing argument for the routine use of intravenous magnesium supplements for the treatment of AMI.

Limitations of Meta-Analysis

Although meta-analysis is a useful tool its limitations should be considered. First, there are several potential sources of bias. One form of bias is publication bias. This involves situations where whole studies are not available to be incorporated into a meta-analysis or partial data from identified trials are unavailable, and where the bias is introduced by the reporting of only promising parts of particular studies.[7,8] It is more likely that trials that report an interesting or a positive result are published than those that have a negative result. Therefore, a meta-analysis of published trials (or data) may well be more promising than the real effects of an intervention.

Another important form of bias that is not commonly recognized is that of the meta-analysts's bias. This is where the researcher conducting the meta-analysis identifies which area is 'worth' analyzing in detail. In general, only areas that are likely to be interesting or promising are chosen for in-depth analysis and publication. The biases of the meta-analyst are also introduced when the researcher determines which endpoints are to be evaluated. For example, secondary endpoints may only be reported if they were promising. By focusing only on the promising results, a statistically or extreme but spurious result may emerge.[4]

Secondly, the reliability of a meta-analysis is dependent upon the validity of the source evidence. If the individual randomized trials incorporated into a meta-analysis are of questionable validity, then this obviously will have a great impact on the validity of the entire meta-analysis. When interpreting the results of a meta-analysis it is important to consider that the *direction* of the overall treatment effect is generally more reliable than the quantitative estimate of the *magnitude* of the treatment effect.

Third, meta-analysis has generally been a retrospective exercise that has been undertaken after review of the easily accessible literature. One would have to identify retrospectively all of the relevant trials and it may be that if researchers are not rigorous enough that certain data will be overlooked.[5] This is best avoided by prospective registration of trials and development of protocols for meta-analysis while large trials are underway and prior to their results being available.

Fourth, meta-analyses are often carried out using data that are published as opposed to the original or raw data on each individual patient. When using published data there are a number of limitations that are immediately imposed on the scope of analyses and comparisons which may be carried out after the data have been obtained and checked. In addition, there are usually varying definitions of outcome of events and these definitions may have been chosen to maximize the apparent treatment effect. It is often not possible to define key subgroups utilizing similar definitions, thereby limiting the sensitivity of subgroup analysis. Without individual patient data, survival and multivariate analyses are difficult or may not be possible.

Cumulative Meta-Analysis: An Evaluation

Some investigators have recently proposed that RCTs addressing a similar question should be subject to a continuous pooling process that is updated as the results of each consecutive trial become available. This approach has been termed cumulative meta-analysis.[42,43] Proponents of this approach have suggested that performing a new meta-analysis whenever the results of a new trial of a particular therapy are published permits the study of trends in efficacy, and makes it possible to determine when a new treatment appears to be significantly effective or deleterious. It is also argued that cumulative meta-analysis provides up-to-date information on emerging and established therapies, and allows clinicians to keep abreast of the ever-expanding database on a particular question.

An example quoted to retrospectively support the concept of cumulative meta-analysis is that of thrombolytic therapy for AMI. It has been pointed out that although 33 RCTs of thrombolytic therapy were carried out between 1959 and 1988, a consistent and statistically significant reduction in total mortality (odds ratio 0.74; 95% confidence interval 0.59–0.92) was achieved in 1973 after only eight trials involving 2432 patients had been completed. The subsequent 25 trials, which enrolled an additional 35 542 patients, had little or no effect on this estimate of efficacy (although the precision of estimate improved substantially making it clinically more important). The implication here is that if the results of this cumulative meta-analysis had been used to determine clinical practice at $P < 0.01$ in favor of treatment, thrombolytic therapy would have been widely utilized about 15 years earlier than was actually the case. However, as discussed earlier, there was no change in clinical practice regarding the use of thrombolytic therapy even after the early formal meta-analysis published in 1985.

The factors influencing a widespread change in clinical practice for a common high-risk condition like AMI with potent agents like thrombolytics with potentially serious side-effects are multiple, complex and beyond the scope of this discussion. However, it is clear from these examples that physicians require very clear and extensive documentation of the efficacy and safety of such drugs before they are willing to use them widely. The available data on thrombolytic therapy in 1973 provided very little information on the risk–benefit ratio (i.e. the balance of strokes, major bleeds, and serious allergic reactions vs mortality reduction and other measures of improved outcome). In addition, the beneficial effects of these agents among important subgroups like the elderly and those presenting later after symptom onset would never have been described. Therefore, the argument that a technique such as cumulative meta-analysis would have facilitated the earlier use of thrombolytic therapy in AMI is not substantiated by historical facts; clinicians were not prepared to change practice on the strength of the evidence provided *before* the publication of the ISIS-2 study in 1988 (well after the first major meta-analysis and GISSI-1).[33] This conservatism is perhaps vindicated by the results of other interventions that have been shown to be beneficial in a meta-analysis, without corroborating evidence from subsequent mega-trials (e.g. magnesium and perhaps nitrates).

Currently, it has not been resolved when a meta-analysis, including cumulative meta-analysis, provides enough evidence about a particular therapy to cause widespread changes in clinical practice. There is uncertainty about the strength of the P value in this determination, as fairly extreme values (e.g. <0.001) can be achieved with meta-analysis involving less than 100 endpoints. Further, with multiple looks at the data there are increasing risks for a type I statistical error (where statistical differences are claimed between treatment and control when in truth none exists). Therefore, formal and perhaps extreme statistical rules for monitoring and interpreting cumulative meta-analysis (similar to monitoring an individual trial) should be employed.

Cumulative meta-analysis is likely to be a useful method for synthesizing and updating information from RCTs. It is an interesting concept that should be prospectively studied and validated as a research methodology. However, at the present time there is no evidence that it is a substitute for well-designed, well-powered large RCTs.

Conclusions

Meta-analysis has been shown to be a useful method of synthesizing evidence about therapeutic strategies in AMI from related RCTs. Meta-analyses of small trials, where the total number of endpoints are small to moderate (e.g. <500), should generally be regarded as useful for identifying promising therapies, generating hypotheses, and designing more definitive RCTs. Meta-analyses of large trials, which in themselves may have provided definitive answers to some of the main questions, help to provide more information on treatment effects in important subgroups, more detail on the balance of risk and benefits, and may also provide new insights on the treatment in question. Meta-analysis is currently the best way to view the totality of data from the RCTs designed to answer the same or related questions about a particular therapy. However, the impact of meta-analysis depends upon several factors, including consistency, biologic plausibility, robustness (number of endpoints) and degree of statistical significance.

References

1. Yusuf, S., Collins, R. and Peto, R. (1984) Why do we need some large, simple randomized trials? *Stat. Med.*, **3**, 409–20.
2. Peto, R. (1987) Why do we need systematic overviews of randomized trials? *Stat. Med.*, **6**, 233–40.
3. Yusuf, S. (1987) Obtaining medically meaningful answers from an overview of randomized clinical trials. *Stat. Med.*, **6**, 281–94.
4. Chalmers, T.C., Levin, H., Sacks, H.S. *et al.* Meta-analysis of clinical trials as a scientific discipline. I: Control of bias and comparison with large co-operative trials. *Stat. Med.*, **6**, 315–25.
5. Chalmers, T.C., Berrier, J., Sacks, H.S. *et al.* (1987) Meta-analysis of clinical trials as a scientific discipline. II: Replicate variability and comparisons of studies that agree and disagree. *Stat. Med.*, **6**, 733–44.
6. Collins, R., Gray, R., Godwin, J. and Peto, R. (1987) Avoidance of large biases and large random errors in the assessment of moderate treatment effects: The need for systematic overviews. *Stat. Med.*, **6**, 245–50.
7. Simes, R.J. (1987) Confronting publication bias: A cohort design for meta-analysis. *Stat. Med.*, **6**, 11–29.
8. Dickersin, K., Chan, S., Chalmers, T.C. *et al.* (1987) Publication bias and clinical trials. *Controlled Clin. Trials*, **8**, 343–53.
9. Yusuf, S., Peto, R., Lewis, J. *et al.* (1985) Beta blockade during and after myocardial infarction: An overview of the randomized trials. *Prog. Cardiovasc. Dis.*, **27**, 335–71.
10. Early Breast Cancer Trialists' Collaborative Group (1990) *Treatment of Early Breast Cancer*. Oxford: Oxford Medical Publications.
11. Pocock, S.J. and Hughes, M.D. (1990) Estimation issues in clinical trials and overviews. *Stat. Med.*, **9**, 657–71.
12. DerSimonian, R. and Laird, N. (1986) Meta-analysis in clinical trials. *Controlled Clin. Trials*, **7**, 177–88.
13. Buyse, M. and Ryan, L.M. (1987) Issues of efficiency in combining proportions of deaths from several clinical trials. *Stat. Med.*, **6**, 565–76.
14. Berlin, J., Laird, N.M., Sacks, H.S. and Chalmers, T.C. (1989) A comparison of statistical methods for combining event rates from clinical trials. *Stat. Med.*, **8**, 141–51.
15. Goodman, S.N. (1989) Meta-analysis and evidence. *Controlled Clin. Trials*, **10**, 188–204.
16. Yusuf, S., Collins, R., Peto, R. *et al.* (1985) Intravenous and intracoronary fibrinolytic therapy in acute myocardial infarction: Overview of results on mortality, reinfarction and side-effects from 33 randomized controlled trials. *Eur. Heart J.*, **6**, 556–85.
17. MacMahon, S., Collins, R., Peto, R. *et al.* (1988) Effects of prophylactic lidocaine in suspected acute myocardial infarction. *JAMA*, **260**, 1910–16.
18. Yusuf, S., Collins, R., MacMahon, S. and Peto, R. (1988) Effect of intravenous nitrates on mortality in acute myocardial infarction: An overview of the randomized trials. *Lancet*, **i**, 1088–92.
19. Held, P.H., Yusuf, S. and Furberg, C.D. (1989) Calcium channel blockers in acute myocardial infarction and unstable angina: An overview. *BMJ*, **299**, 1187–92.
20. Teo, K.K, Yusuf, S., Collins, R. *et al.* (1991) Effects of intravenous magnesium in suspected acute myocardial infarction: Overview of randomized trials. *BMJ*, **303**, 1499–503.
21. Antiplatelet Trialists' Collaboration (1994) Collaborative overview of randomized trials of antiplatelet therapy. I: Prevention of death, myocardial infarction, and stroke by prolonged antiplatelet therapy in various categories of patients. *BMJ*, **308**, 81–106.
22. Fibrinolytic Therapy Trialists' Collaboration (1994) Indications for fibrinolytic therapy in suspected acute myocardial infarction: Collaborative overview of early mortality and major morbidity results from all randomized trials of more than 1000 patients. *Lancet*, **343**, 311–22.
23. Michels, K.B. and Yusuf, S. (1994) The randomized controlled clinical trials of PTCA in acute myocardial infarction. A systematic overview (meta-analysis). *Circulation* (in press).
24. Laupacis, A., Sackett, D. and Roberts, R.S. (1988) An assessment of clinically useful measures of the consequences of treatment. *N. Engl. J. Med.*, **318**, 1728–33.
25. ISIS-1 (First International Study of Infarct Survival) Collaborative Group (1986) Randomized trial of intravenous atenolol among 16 027 cases of suspected acute myocardial infarction: ISIS 1. *Lancet*, **ii**, 57–66.
26. Yusuf, S. (1980) *Beta Adrenergic Blockade in Myocardial Infarction*. Oxford University: D Phil. Thesis.
27. Beta-blocker Heart Attack Trial Research Group (BHAT) (1983) A randomized trial of propranolol in patients with acute myocardial infarction. I: Mortality results. *JAMA*, **250**, 2814–19.
28. Echt, D.S., Liebson, P.R., Mitchell, L.B. *et al.* (1991) Mortality and morbidity in patients receiving encainaide, flecainide or placebo. The Cardiac Arrhythmia Suppression Trial. *N. Eng. J. Med.*, **324**, 781–8.

29. Greene, H.L., Roden, D.M., Katz, Rj *et al.* (1992) The Cardiac Arrhythmia Suppression Trial: First CAST . . . then CAST-II. *J. Am. Coll. Cardiol.*, **19**, 894–8.
30. Gruppo Italiano per lo studio della sopravvivenza nell' infarto miocardico. GISSI-3: effects of lisinopril and transdermal glyceryl trinitrate singly and together on 6-week mortality and ventricular function after acute myocardial infarction. *Lancet*, **334**, 1115–21.
31. ISIS-4 (1994) (Fourth International Study of Infarct Survival). Collaborative Group. ISIS-4: a randomized trial of oral captopril versus placebo, oral mononitrate versus placebo, and intravenous magnesium versus control among 58 043 patients with suspected acute myocardial infarction. *Lancet* (in press).
32. ISIS-2 (Second International Study of Infarct Survival) Collaborative Group. (1988) Randomized trial of intravenous streptokinase, oral aspirin, both, or neither among 17 187 cases of suspected acute myocardial infarction: ISIS-2. *Lancet*, **ii**, 349–60.
33. GISSI-1 (1986) Effectiveness of intravenous thrombolytic treatment in acute myocardial infarction. *Lancet*, **i**, 397–402.
34. AIMS Trial Study Group (1988) Effect of intravenous APSAC on mortality after acute myocardial infarction: Preliminary report of a placebo-controlled clinical trial. *Lancet*, **i**, 545–9.
35. Wilcox, R.G., Von der Lippe, G., Olsson, C.G. *et al.* (1988) Trial of tissue plasminogen activator for mortality reduction in acute myocardial infarction (Anglo-Scandinavian Study of Early Thrombolysis) (ASSET). *Lancet*, **ii**, 525–30.
36. ISIS-3 Collaborative Group (1992) ISIS-3: A randomized trial comparing SK vs tPA vs APSAC and comparing aspirin plus heparin vs aspirin alone in 41 298 suspected acute myocardial infarction. *Lancet*, **339**, 753–70.
37. EMERAS (Estudio Multicentrico Estreptoquinasa Republicas de America del Sur) Collaborative Group (1992) Randomized trial of late thrombolysis in patients with suspected acute myocardial infarction. *Lancet*, **342**, 767–72.
38. LATE Study Group (1986) Late assessment of Thrombolytic Efficacy (LATE) study with alteplase 6–24 hours after onset of acute myocardial infarction. *Lancet*, **342**, 759–66.
39. The ISAM Study Group A prospective trial of intravenous streptokinase in acute myocardial infarction (ISAM). *N. Engl. J. Med.*, **314**, 1465–71.
40. Rossi, P. and Bolognese, L. on behalf of Urochinasi per via Sistemica nell'infarto Miocardico (USIM) Collaborative Group (1991) Comparison of intravenous urokinase plus heparin vs heparin alone in acute myocardial infarction. *Am. J. Cardiol.*, **68**, 585–92.
41. Woods, K.L., Fletcher, S., Roffe, C. and Haider, Y. (1992) Intravenous magnesium sulphate in suspected acute myocardial infarction: Results of the second Leicester intravenous magnesium intervention trial (LIMIT-2) *Lancet*, **339**, 1553–8.
42. Lau, J., Antman, E.M., Jimenez-Silva, J. *et al.* (1992) Cumulative meta-analysis of therapeutic trials for myocardial infarction. *N. Engl. J. Med.*, **327**, 248–54.
43. Antman, E.M., Lau, J., Kupelnick, B. *et al.* (1992) A comparison of results of meta-analyses of randomized control trials and recommendations of clinical experts. *JAMA*, **268**, 240–8.

18

The Practical Implications Of Clinical Trials: Putting It All Together

D. Julian

The therapy of myocardial infarction is now based on sound scientific principles validated by large well-conducted randomized controlled trials. The results of these trials have certainly influenced practice,[1–3] yet effective agents, such as thrombolytic drugs, are underutilized while relatively ineffective therapy, such as calcium antagonists, is still frequently prescribed. Thus, Pashos *et al.*[3] report, from the 1992 US nationwide database of the SMS Corporation, that calcium antagonists were administered to 47% of acute myocardial infarction patients whereas only 19% received thrombolytic drugs. Why should physicians fail to apply the findings of clinical trials? Although ignorance plays a part, different interpretations of the data undoubtedly make a major contribution. Extrapolation from trials is not simple and among issues that need consideration in this regard are:

- Can the conditions that obtain in a clinical trial be replicated in routine care?
- Can the many drugs and interventions used in this context be safely and effectively combined?
- Can the overall results of trials be applied to all of the heterogeneous mix of patients with myocardial infarction studied?
- Can we extrapolate from those included in trials to the broad mass of patients in routine practice?

This chapter attempts to draw practical conclusions from the major trials of acute myocardial infarction in the light of these questions.

Reproducibility of Trial Conditions

Physicians may not be convinced that a trial has been carried out in conditions that are reproducible in everyday practice. It is true that many trials today involve a wide range of hospitals and one can assume that the findings of such trials are widely applicable. But even in such trials, the treatment under investigation is often monitored with a degree of care that may not obtain under nontrial conditions. This applies particularly to treatments that require close supervision, such as the complex schedule of administration of tissue-type plasminogen activator (t-PA) and heparin in the Global Utilization of Streptokinase and Tissue Plasminogen Activator for Occluded Coronary Arteries

(GUSTO) trial,[4] or that demand considerable technical expertise and facilities, as in the trials of percutaneous transluminal coronary angioplasty.[5,6] Physicians in some hospitals would need to be reassured that the necessary conditions are available for their implementation. Another more general issue is that of the reliability of drug administration. Errors in administration are not unusual, even in coronary care units, and the more complex the regimen the more likely they are to occur. Adherence by patients to the prescribed regimen is not a problem in the acute phase but becomes of importance in the long term. Considerable efforts are made during the conduct of trials to ensure compliance by patient education and such methods as pill-counting. One cannot assume that compliance to the same degree can be guaranteed in practice, particularly if several different drugs are prescribed. As Laurence and Bennett[7] have written 'It is unlikely that any patient will reliably take more than three medicines without special supervision'. This must apply to most patients following infarction today. This implies that we should, as far as possible, limit the number of drugs we prescribe and be particularly cautious about those whose value and safety has not been demonstrated in this context.

Multiple Drug Therapy and Drug Interactions

It is now usual for patients with acute myocardial infarction to be given several different pharmacologic agents simultaneously or in rapid succession. For instance, Casscells[8] in a recent editorial has recommended 'aspirin should be given first . . ., followed immediately by magnesium, then heparin. This regimen will help to prevent the procoagulant side-effects of tPA or streptokinase, which should be given next (in transmural infarction) followed by 6.5 mg captopril. Chest pain, ischaemic ST changes on the electrocardiogram, and hypertension should be treated with nitrates (although they had little effect on mortality in GISSI-3 or ISIS-4) and morphine, but watch out for hypotension and respiratory depression. . . . Residual tachycardia and hypertension should be carefully "blunted" with beta-blockers, except in patients with heart block or asthma. Lignocaine should be reserved for patients with ventricular tachycardia or increasingly frequent salvos of ventricular couplets, multifocal premature ventricular contractions, or R-on-T beats in the first 24 hours.'

Several of these drugs interact with each other or with other therapies used in myocardial infarction but clinical trials have not in most cases adequately addressed the question of whether any such interactions are beneficial or adverse. It is true that the factorial trials have done this with the two or three therapies under study. Thus, in ISIS-2[9], the beneficial effect of combining aspirin and streptokinase was demonstrated when it had been feared that the combination might be hazardous. Furthermore, it was possible to show that the addition of aspirin counteracted the increased risk of reinfarction due to the thrombolytic agent. In other non-factorial trials, agents may appear to enhance or diminish the effectiveness of this randomized treatment, but the relatively small size of the subgroups concerned makes it difficult to draw conclusions. For instance, in the AIRE trial[10] of ramipril after myocardial infarction, the drug was possibly more effective in those on diuretics and in those not on aspirin. If the relatively better effect in those on a diuretic was a true finding, was it due to a beneficial synergy between diuretics and the angiotensin-converting enzyme (ACE) inhibitor, or did those receiving a diuretic constitute a higher risk group in whom it was easier to demonstrate a benefit of an ACE inhibitor? Was the possible failure to show as much benefit in those on aspirin due to its known action in countering the effects of an ACE inhibitor[11] or was it due to the play of chance? If the former, did the almost universal use of aspirin contribute to the relatively minor benefit shown by ACE inhibitors in the ISIS-4[12] and GISSI-3[13] trials?

There are several potentially important pharmacologic interactions between drugs used in myocardial infarction. Thus, β-blockers depress hepatic blood flow and decrease the hepatic inactivation of lidocaine;[14] schedules for lidocaine should be modified accordingly. Intravenous nitroglycerin may induce heparin resistance by altering the activity of antithrombin III;[15,16] this necessitates closer monitoring of the activated partial thromboplastin time than is often undertaken. Many other relevant interactions have been recently extensively reviewed by Opie.[17]

Subgrouping and Extrapolation

Large trials are usually designed to answer with confidence only one or two major questions. But clinicians need to know whether the overall results of trials apply with sufficient force to specific subgroups of patients. While it is often realistic to suppose that if a treatment is effective overall, it exerts an effect in the same direction in most subgroups, this is not always the case and certainly the degree of benefit or harm may vary widely, particularly in the *absolute* risk reduction in patients of different prognosis. Furthermore, important categories of patient (for example elderly people or women) may be excluded or underrepresented in trials. Can we then extrapolate from the trial experience to such patients?

Subgroup Analysis

Yusuf and colleagues[18] have recently reviewed the analysis and interpretation of treatment effects in subgroups of patients in randomized clinical trials. They pointed out that interpreting the effects of subgroups is fraught with inferential problems, but recognize that subgroup analysis should help to identify either consistency of, or large differences in, the magnitude of treatment effects among different categories of patients. They defined what they termed *proper* and *improper* subgroups. A *proper* subgroup is characterized by a common set of 'baseline' parameters. These parameters include such unalterable characteristics as gender and age, and disease characteristics such as location of infarction. But they may also include other features at baseline such as concomitant drug therapy. An *improper* subgroup is defined as 'a group of patients characterized by a variable measured after randomization and potentially affected by treatment e.g. separate examination of patients with a patent coronary artery in a trial of a thrombolytic agent when patency is determined after initiating the randomized treatment'. They continue 'comparisons of responders to non-responders or compliers to non-compliers based on information collected after randomization are particularly egregious forms of improper subgroup analysis because response and adherence may be markers of a good prognosis, not necessarily measures of therapeutic efficacy'. In their article, Yusuf and colleagues dismissed 'improper' subgroups from further consideration.

The play of chance determines that, if many subgroups are analyzed, some will spuriously appear to differ in their response from the main body of patients. The more subgroups that are examined, the greater the potential for spurious findings. This problem can be limited if subgroups are defined in the original protocol. The issue can be addressed in a factorial trial in which patients can be randomized to one of four strategies as in ISIS-2,[9] in which patients received streptokinase, aspirin, both or neither. This allowed the interactions between the drugs to be studied. But there are many more subgroups of potential interest than can be dealt with in this way.

One approach to the problems of subgroups is to assume that all subgroups have a similar proportionate reduction in risk. By applying this proportionate reduction to the known risk in the placebo or comparison subgroup, one can estimate the absolute reduction in mortality that the treatment might achieve. One can then compare this with

Table 18.1 Electrical and mechanical complications in the acute phase and mortality[19]

| Risk group | Mortality (%) | | Relative risk |
	Propranolol	Placebo	
Electrical	5.2	10.9	0.48
Mechanical	10.4	16.8	0.62
Both	12.9	17.1	0.76
Neither	6.2	6.6	0.98

the findings in the study. Thus, in the Betablocker Heart Attack Trial[19] (Table 18.1), an overall 25% reduction in mortality was observed, but the mortality in the placebo group was very different depending upon whether there had been mechanical or electrical complications, or both, or neither. A proportionate risk reduction of the order of 25% in those with complications would have had a profound effect on mortality, whereas its effect in those without such complications would be small, and perhaps not justify the treatment. In fact, in the subgroup analysis it appeared that there was really no benefit in those without complications but there were large relative as well as absolute benefits in those with them.

Another example concerns the overview of all the major thrombolytic trials,[20] in which there was an overall 16% reduction in mortality due to thrombolytic therapy. If this were applied to those with a normal ECG, with a placebo mortality of 2.3% this would have represented a saving of life of seven lives per 1000 patients treated, a level at which one could question the wisdom of such treatment, particularly bearing in mind the rather similar risk of inducing hemorrhagic stroke. In fact, in the overview, there was no evidence of any benefit at all in this subgroup. On the other hand, the 24% reduction in mortality in those aged under 55 years (placebo mortality of 4.6%) saved only 11 lives per 1000 while a 16% reduction in those aged between 65 and 74 years (placebo mortality 16.1%) saved 27 per 1000. This illustrates the fact that the baseline risk of the individual patient is an important factor in decision-making and that the absolute reduction is, for practical purposes, of much greater relevance than the proportionate (relative) reduction.

Can any credulity be given to subgroup findings that are obtained by analysis of the data (data-derived observations) from clinical trials? It is accepted that such data form a valuable source for the generation of hypotheses, which may then be tested either by a new trial or in a meta-analysis of other trials. But such acquisition of additional data is not always feasible, so are there any guidelines for clinical decision-making when faced with apparent subgroup effects? The first issue is the statistical strength of that evidence. Has an appropriate statistical test of interaction been performed, was it significant and how many subgroups were investigated in order to detect this finding? The second issue is one of biologic plausibility. There must be at least an acceptable hypothesis to account for the finding. As the ISIS group have pointed out, it is not difficult to show that patients with a particular astrologic sign have a different outcome from those with other signs. This example is clearly ludicrous but it may have given subgroup analysis too bad a name. An example may illustrate this. It can be seen from Tables 18.2 and 18.3 that older patients and those with relative hypertension appeared to benefit particularly from intravenous β-blockade with atenolol in ISIS-1,[21] whereas those who were normotensive or younger did not. Is this likely to be a genuine finding? An examination of the causes of death in this study showed the chief benefit from the therapy was the prevention of cardiac rupture.[22] Rupture is known to occur particularly in the elderly and the relatively hypertensive, so a rational explanation is forthcoming for this unanticipated benefit seen

Table 18.2   Vascular mortality in ISIS-2[21]

Age (years)	Control	Atenolol
<55	1.2%	1.1%
55–64	4.0%	3.9%
>65	8.8%	6.8%

Table 18.3   Vascular mortality in ISIS-2[21]

Systolic blood pressure (mmHg)	Control	Atenolol
<120	6.8%	7.7%
120–159	4.3%	3.7%
>160	4.3%	2.9%

in these specific subgroups. It would then seem reasonable to select patients for treatment on this basis. There is, therefore, a case of utilizing the findings in relation to such subgroups when other evidence and biologic plausibility support their identification.

Extrapolation to Excluded Groups

Trials vary greatly from one another in the proportion of potentially eligible patients who are eventually recruited. When inclusion and exclusion criteria are precisely drawn, a high proportion of potential patients are apt to be excluded, whereas when these criteria are deliberately less stringent, it is likely that fewer will be excluded. In the former case, it is informative, by keeping a log of all patients included and excluded, to define the proportion of patients who have been excluded and the reasons for this. Patients are excluded from trials for a variety of different reasons.

1. Some are excluded because it is thought that there are coexisting disorders that place the patients at high risk from the therapy. Thus, in the case of thrombolytic drugs, those with previous stroke, recent surgery or bleeding diatheses have been excluded. One may question the need to exclude previous stroke (if known not to be hemorrhagic), but the other exclusion criteria seem appropriate and one would not wish to extrapolate from the trial to these groups. Similar considerations apply to the β-blocker trials, in which patients were excluded because of hypotension, bradycardia, or heart failure, and trials of ACE inhibitors in which hypotension and renal dysfunction were considered to be contraindications.
2. Some are excluded for quite arbitrary reasons, such as age or time after onset of symptoms. The exclusion of these categories of patient was a limitation in many of the earlier thrombolytic trials and may have had the effect of denying the benefits of this therapy to many of the elderly and those admitted late. If new data had not been forthcoming, it would have been reasonable to extrapolate the results of the trials to such patients, while bearing in mind the progressive increase in absolute benefit as age increases and the progressive reduction in benefit as time elapses after the onset of symptoms. Fortunately, further trials have now established the efficacy and safety of treatment in these groups.[20]

3. In some trials, patients are excluded because they or their physicians are committed to one or other of the therapies. This has particularly applied in the coronary surgery and angioplasty trials, resulting in a very small percentage (about 3%) of the potentially eligible patients being enrolled. As has been shown, however, in the Coronary Artery Surgery Study (CASS) registry,[23] deductions can be made from the information contained in a register of excluded cases. In this study, 780 patients were randomized to surgery or medical treatment, whereas a further 1315 were 'randomizable' but declined participation. Survival in the medically randomized and randomizable groups was similar, as was the case in the surgical groups. It is, therefore, reasonable to assume that the findings of trials such as CASS[24] and the Randomized Intervention Treatment of Angina (RITA) of angioplasty versus surgery[25] can be applied to a much higher proportion of patients with similar characteristics being considered for these procedures than were included in these trials.

Practical Application of the Results of Trials

The results of clinical trials are often not translated into action, for instance, the use of intravenous β-blockade in acute myocardial infarction. The ISIS-1 trial[21] of this therapy demonstrated a significant 14% reduction in mortality; evidence of this benefit was reinforced when the results were pooled with those of the marginally nonsignificant MIAMI study.[26] Should not these findings have been generally applied to patients with myocardial infarction? That they were not is shown by the small utilization of intravenous blockade in the succeeding ISIS trials; in ISIS-4 only 2% of UK and 26% of US patients were given intravenous β-blockade (L.P. Sleight, personal communication). The failure to apply these findings is in striking contrast to the rapid implementation of the findings of the thrombolytic and aspirin studies.[27]

One reason for the nonapplication of the findings of the intravenous β-blockade studies may have been due to the fact that in ISIS-1 the *absolute* reduction in mortality was relatively small – from 4.3% to 3.8%. These studies were carried out in relatively low-risk patients. Physicians may have been reluctant to extrapolate from such patients to those with more severe myocardial damage, in whom β-blockade might have adverse rather than beneficial effects. Of course, there are other cogent clinical indications for β-blockade, such as sinus tachycardia in the absence of heart failure and chest pain unresponsive to opiates. The figures quoted above suggest that β-blockade is underused, at least in the UK, for these purposes. The situation has, of course, changed since the introduction of thrombolysis but, in spite of TIMI II,[28] it remains unclear as to the added benefit of intravenous β-blockade in this context.

It will be interesting to observe the effect on practice of the findings in the ISIS-4[12] and GISSI-3[13] trials of ACE inhibitors. Both these trials have reported a marginal benefit from ACE inhibitors at 1 month when given routinely early in myocardial infarction. Neither showed a benefit from nitrates. ACE inhibitors are now recognized therapies for those with heart failure in acute myocardial infarction, and the SAVE[29] and AIRE[10] trials have established the role of ACE inhibitors in those who have experienced heart failure during the acute event or who have residual poor ventricular function. One suspects that no significant benefit would have been found in ISIS-4 and GISSI-3 had patients with heart failure been excluded. Indeed, a profound blood pressure fall was encountered in a sizeable proportion of patients treated with ACE inhibitors in these trials. In view of these observations, should ACE inhibitors be used routinely in myocardial infarction?

An additional but increasingly important factor influencing clinical decision-making is that of cost. Many clinicians, especially in Europe, choose streptokinase rather than tPA for this reason. Interestingly, it seems that angioplasty may not be a more expensive option than thrombolysis[30] and this will certainly, in part, determine the extent to which this technique is used in future.

Indications for Therapies Tested by Clinical Trials in Acute Myocardial Infarction

There are several standard therapies, such as opiates and oxygen, that have not been addressed by large clinical trials yet are essential in the management of myocardial infarction. There are other therapies in common use, such as the inotropic agents and diuretics, which have not, as yet, been adequately tested in this way. These have been discussed in previous chapters and will not be considered further here.

All Patients with Suspected Acute Myocardial Infarction

Aspirin is the only therapy tested by randomized controlled trials that is appropriate for all patients with suspected acute myocardial infarction for whom it is not contraindicated.

All Patients with the Clinical Features of Myocardial Infarction with ST Elevation (? and Bundle Branch Block)

All patients with these features seen within 6, and probably up to 12, hours of the onset of symptoms should be submitted either to thrombolytic therapy (as discussed in Chapters 2 and 3) or angioplasty (as discussed in Chapter 4). The choice between these therapies will depend largely on whether there are contraindications to thrombolysis and whether appropriate staff and facilities are available for prompt angioplasty.

Whether heparin is used as well as the thrombolytic depends upon the agent used. It should certainly be given with rtPA, but questionably so with streptokinase.

Opinions are divided upon whether the other therapies, namely β-blockade and ACE inhibitors, that have been shown to be beneficial in randomized clinical trials in the acute phase of infarction should be given to all patients for whom the agent is not contraindicated or only to those in whom there is a clear clinical indication (see Chapters 7 and 10). As discussed above, my personal preference is for the latter strategy.

Long-term Secondary Prevention after Infarction

All patients should be encouraged to give up smoking.[31] Effective programs for helping patients to quit have been devised[32] and should be implemented.

Serum lipids should be measured in every case and an attempt should be made to lower the total cholesterol level towards $5.2 \, \text{mmol} \, l^{-1}$ by diet or, if this fails, by lipid-lowering agents.[33]

A rehabilitation program with an exercise component should be available to all patients as a meta-analysis shows that this results in a significant reduction in subsequent mortality.[34]

There is sufficient evidence to warrant the use of aspirin in all patients after infarction unless either the patient is on an oral anticoagulant for a valid reason or there is a contraindication.[35]

ACE inhibitors should be prescribed for all patients without contraindications who have experienced heart failure during the acute event and also, probably, for those who have an ejection fraction less than 40% (Chapter 15).[10,28]

Opinions are divided as to whether β-blockers should be given to all patients for whom they are not contraindicated or whether it is acceptable to exclude those at low risk (Chapter 7).

There may be a case for prescribing diltiazem[36] or verapamil[37] for patients with a non-Q-wave infarction who do not have severely impaired left ventricular function to prevent reinfarction.

Nitrates, calcium antagonists, oral anticoagulants, angioplasty and coronary bypass surgery cannot now be regarded as routine and should be reserved for appropriate clinical indications.

References

1. Lamas, G.A., Pfeffer, M., Hamm, P. *et al.* (1992) Do the results of randomized trials of cardiovascular drugs influence medical practice? *N. Engl. J. Med.*, **327**, 241–7.
2. Thompson, P.L., Parsons, R.W., Jamrozik, K. *et al.* (1992) Changing patterns of medical treatment in acute myocardial infarction. *Med. J. Aust.*, **157**, 87–92.
3. Pashos, C.L., Normand, S.T., Garfinkle, J.B. *et al.* (1994) Trends in the use of drug therapies in patients with acute myocardial infarction, 1988–1992. *J. Am. Coll. Cardiol.*, **23**, 1023–30.
4. The GUSTO Investigators (1993) An international randomized trial comparing four thrombolytic strategies for acute myocardial infarction. *N. Engl. J. Med.*, **329**, 673–82.
5. Grines, C.L., Browne, K.F., Marco, J. *et al.* (1993) A comparison of immediate angioplasty with thrombolytic therapy for acute myocardial infarction. *N. Engl. J. Med.*, **328**, 673–9.
6. Zijlstra, F., de Boer, M.J., Hoorntje, J.C.A. *et al.* (1993) A comparison of immediate coronary angioplasty with intravenous streptokinase in acute myocardial infarction. *N. Engl. J. Med.*, **328**, 680–4.
7. Laurence, D.R. and Bennett, P.N. (1992) *Clinical Pharmacology*, p.24. Edinburgh: Churchill Livingstone.
8. Casscells, W. (1994) Magnesium and myocardial infarction. *Lancet*, **343**, 807–9.
9. ISIS-2 (Second International Study of Infarct Survival) Collaborative Group (1988) Randomized trial of intravenous streptokinase, oral aspirin, both, or neither among 17 187 cases of suspected acute myocardial infarction. ISIS-2. *Lancet*, **ii**, 349–60.
10. The AIRE Study Investigators, (1993) Effect of ramipril on mortality and morbidity of survivors of acute myocardial infarction with clinical evidence of cardiac failure. *Lancet*, **342**, 821–28.
11. Hall, D., Zeitler, H. and Rudolph, W. (1992) Counteraction of the vasodilator effects of enalapril by aspirin in severe heart failure. *J. Am. Coll. Cardiol.*, **20**, 1549–55.
12. ISIS-4. Awaiting publication.
13. GISSI-3 (1994) *Lancet* (in press).
14. Ochs, H.R., Carstens, G. and Greenblatt, D.J. (1980) Reduction in lidocaine clearance during continuous infusion and by coadministration of propranolol. *N. Engl. J. Med.*, **303**, 373–7.
15. Becker, R.C., Corras, J.M., Bovill, E.G. *et al.* (1990) Intravenous nitroglycerin–heparin resistance: a qualitative antithrombin III abnormality. *Am. Heart J.*, **119**, 1254–61.
16. Brack, M.J., More, R.S., Hubner, P.J.B. and Gerschlick, A.H. (1994) The effect of different nitrate preparations and the activated partial thromboplastin time. *Postgrad. Med. J.*, **70**, 100–3.
17. Opie, L.H. (1993) Interactions with cardiovascular drugs. *Curr. Probl. Cardiol.*, **18**, 529–84.
18. Yusuf, S., Wittes, J., Probstfield, J. and Tyroler, H.A. (1991) Analysis and interpretation of treatment effects in subgroups of patients in randomized clinical trials. *JAMA*, **266**, 93–8.
19. Furberg, C.D., Hawkins, C.M. and Lichstein, E. (1984) Effect of propranolol in postinfarction patients with mechanical or electrical complications. *Circulation*, **69**, 761–5.
20. Fibrinolytic Therapy Trialists' (FTT) Collaborative Group (1994) Indications for fibrinolytic therapy in suspected acute myocardial infarction: collaborative overview of early mortality and major major morbidity results from all randomized trials of more than 1000 patients. *Lancet*, **343**, 311–22.
21. ISIS-1 Collaborative Group (1986) Randomized trial of intravenous atenolol among 16 027 cases of acute myocardial infarction. ISIS-1. *Lancet*, **ii**, 57–66.
22. ISIS-1 (First International Study of Infarct Survival) Collaborative Group (1988) Mechanisms for the early mortality reduction produced by beta-blockade started early in acute myocardial infarction; ISIS-1. *Lancet*, **i**, 921–3.
23. CASS Principal Investigators and their Associates (1984) Coronary Artery Surgery Study (CASS): a randomized trial of coronary artery bypass surgery. Comparability of entry characteristics and survival in randomized patients and non-randomized patients meeting randomization criteria. *J. Am. Cardiol.*, **3**, 114–18.
24. CASS Principal Investigators and their Associates (1983) Coronary Artery Surgery Study (CASS): a randomized trial of coronary artery bypass surgery. Survival data. *Circulation*, **68**, 939–50.

25. RITA Trial Participants (1993) Coronary angioplasty versus coronary artery bypass surgery: Randomized Intervention Treatment of Angina (RITA) trial. *Lancet*, **341**, 573–80.
26. The MIAMI Trial Research Group (1985) Metoprolol in acute myocardial infarction (MIAMI). A randomized placebo-controlled international trial. *Eur. Heart J.*, **6**, 199–226.
27. Collins, R. and Julian, D.G. (1991) British Heart Foundation surveys (1987 and 1989) of United Kingdom treatment policies for acute myocardial infarction. *Br. Heart J.*, **66**, 250–5.
28. Roberts, R., Rogers, W.J., Mueller, H.S. *et al.* (1991) Immediate versus deferred beta-blockade following thrombolytic therapy in patients with acute myocardial infarction. Results of the Thrombolysis in Myocardial Infarction (TIMI) II-B study. *Circulation*, **83**, 422–37.
29. Pfeffer, M.A., Braunwald, E., Moyé, L.A. *et al.* (1992) Effect of captopril on mortality and morbidity in patients with left ventricular dysfunction after myocardial infarction. *N. Engl. J. Med.*, **327**, 669–77.
30. Reeder, G.S., Bailey, K.R., Gersh, B.J. *et al.* (1994) Cost comparison of immediate angioplasty versus thrombolysis followed by conservative therapy for acute myocardial infarction: a randomized prospective trial. *Mayo Clin. Proc.*, **69**, 5–12.
31. Åberg, A., Bergstrand, R., Johansson, S. *et al.* (1983) Cessation of smoking after myocardial infarction. Effects on mortality after 10 years. *Br. Heart J.* **49**, 416–22.
32. Taylor, C.B., Houston-Miller, N., Killen, J.D. and De Busk, R.F. (1990) Smoking cessation after acute myocardial infarction: effect of a nurse-managed intervention. *Ann. Intern. Med.*, **113**, 118–32.
33. Roussouw, J.E., Lewis, B. and Rifkind, B.M. (1990) The value of lowering cholesterol after myocardial infarction. *N. Engl. J. Med.*, **323**, 1112–19.
34. O'Connors, G.T., Buring, J.E., Yusuf, S. *et al.*(1989) An overview of randomized trials of rehabilitation with exercise after myocardial infarction. *Circulation*, **80**, 234–44.
35. Antiplatelet trialists' Collaboration (1994) Collaborative overview of randomized trials of antiplatelet therapy–1. Prevention of death, myocardial infarction, and stroke by prolonged antiplatelet therapy in various categories of patients. *BMJ*, **308**, 81–106.
36. The Multicenter Diltiazem Post-infarction Trial Research Group (1988) The effect of diltiazem on mortality and reinfarction after myocardial infarction. *N. Engl. J. Med.*, **319**, 385–92.
37. The Danish Study Group on Verapamil in Myocardial Infarction (1990) Effect of verapamil on mortality and major events after myocardial infarction (the Danish Verapamil Infarction Trial II-DAVIT II). *Am. J. Cardiol.*, **66**, 779–85.

Index

(*Italic* page numbers refer to figures and tables)